D1556517

Sinus Surgery
Endoscopic and Microscopic Approaches

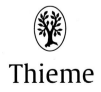

Thieme

Sinus Surgery
Endoscopic and Microscopic Approaches

Howard L. Levine, M.D.
Co-Director
Cleveland Nasal-Sinus and Sleep Center
Marymount Outpatient Care Center
Cleveland, Ohio
and
Adjunct Staff
Department of Otolaryngology–Head and Neck Surgery
Cleveland Clinic
Cleveland, Ohio

M. Pais Clemente, M.D., Ph.D.
Professor and Chairman
Department of Otorhinolaryngology
Porto University School of Medicine
Hospital de S. João
Porto, Portugal
Chairman Center for Optical Technologies (CETO)
Porto, Portugal
Chairman National Council for Smoking Prevention
Lisbon, Portugal

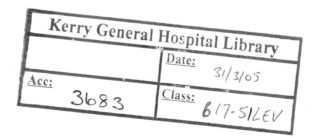
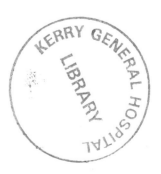
Thieme

New York • Stuttgart

Thieme Medical Publishers, Inc.
333 Seventh Ave.
New York, NY 10001

Editorial Assistant: Birgitta Brandenburg
Consulting Editor: Esther Gumpert
Director, Production and Manufacturing: Anne Vinnicombe
Production Editor: Becky Dille
Marketing Director: Phyllis Gold
Sales Director: Ross Lumpkin
Chief Financial Officer: Peter van Woerden
President: Brian D. Scanlan
Compositor: Compset Inc.
Printer: Everbest Printing Co.

Medical Illustrations by Haderer & Muller, Biomedical Art. E-mail address: biomedart@haderermuller.com.

Library of Congress Cataloging-in-Publication Data

Sinus surgery : endoscopic and microscopic approaches / [edited by] Howard L. Levine,
Manuel António Caldeira Pais Clemente.
        p. ; cm.
    Includes bibliographical references and index.
    ISBN 0-86577-972-4 (TMP : alk. paper)--ISBN 3-13-124791-6 (GTV : alk. paper) 1.
Paranasal sinuses--Surgery.
    [DNLM: 1. Paranasal Sinuses--surgery. 2. Endoscopy--methods. 3. Microsurgery--
methods. 4. Paranasal Sinus Diseases--surgery. WV 340 S6185 2005] I. Levine, Howard,
1944– II. Clemente, M. Pais
    RF421.S555 2005
    617.5'23059--dc22

                                                    2004016604

Important note: Medical knowledge is ever-changing. As new research and clinical experience broaden our knowledge,
changes in treatment and drug therapy may be required. The authors and editors of the material herein have consulted
sources believed to be reliable in their efforts to provide information that is complete and in accord with the standards accepted at the time of publication. However, in the view of the possibility of human error by the authors, editors, or publisher,
of the work herein, or changes in medical knowledge, neither the authors, editors, or publisher, nor any other party who has
been involved in the preparation of this work, warrants that the information contained herein is in every respect accurate or
complete, and they are not responsible for any errors or omissions or for the results obtained from use of such information.
Readers are encouraged to confirm the information contained herein with other sources. For example, readers are advised to
check the product information sheet included in the package of each drug they plan to administer to be certain that the information contained in this publication is accurate and that changes have not been made in the recommended dose or in the
contraindications for administration. This recommendation is of particular importance in connection with new or infrequently used drugs.

Some of the product names, patents, and registered designs referred to in this book are in fact registered trademarks or proprietary names even though specific reference to this fact is not always made in the text. Therefore, the appearance of a name
without designation as proprietary is not to be construed as a representation by the publisher that it is in the public domain.

Printed in China
5 4 3 2 1
TMP ISBN 0-86577-972-4
GTV ISBN 3 13 124791 6

Dedication

Dedicated to my mother, Edith, and in memory of my father, Sam, whose hard work and encouragement permitted me to become a physician.

Howard L. Levine

In memory of my mother, Amália, and in honor of my father, José, and former teachers of my residency training at Boston University School of Medicine, M. Stuart Strong, M.D., and Charles Vaughn, M.D., whose examples of dedication, encouragement, teaching, and passion for medicine and otorhinolaryngology have guided me throughout my medical and academic careers.

To my wife and colleague, Laudelina, for her inspiration, continuous help, and constant support with special appreciation and deep gratitude.

M. Pais Clemente

Table of Contents

Dedication v

Foreword xi

Preface xi

1. Surgical Anatomy of the Paranasal Sinus 1
   M. Pais Clemente
2. Physiology of the Paranasal Sinuses 57
   Desiderio Passàli, Giulio Cesare Passàli,
   Francesco Maria Passàli, and L. Bellussi
3. Imaging of the Paranasal Sinuses 64
   Todd W. Stultz and Michael T. Modic
4 Diagnosis and Management of Rhinosinusitis 90
   Howard L. Levine
5. The Relationships of Allergy and Asthma to Rhinosinusitis:
   Epidemiological, Mechanistic, and Clinical 100
   Michael Schatz and Raymond G. Slavin
6. Rhinosinusitis in Immunocompromised Hosts 113
   Desiderio Passàli, Maria Lauriello, Giulio Cesare Passàli,
   Francesco Maria Passàli, and L. Bellussi
7. Pediatric Rhinosinusitis 121
   Ken Kazahaya and Lawrence W. C. Tom
8. Headache and Rhinosinusitis.. 132
   Howard L. Levine
9. The Medical and Surgical Management of Allergic Fungal Rhinosinusitis 141
   Berrylin J. Ferguson
10. Surgical Approaches: Endonasal Endoscopic 148
    Howard L. Levine
11. Combined Microscopic and Endoscopic Technique (COMET Surgery)........ 162
    M. Pais Clemente
12. Minimally Invasive Endoscopic Sinus Surgery with
    Powered Instrumentation 207
    Peter Doble

13. Stereotactic Surgery 219
    Jack B. Anon and Ludger Klimek

14. The Frontal Sinus: The Endoscopic Approach 231
    Barry Schaitkin

15a. Lasers and Nasal and Sinus Surgery: KTP/532 Laser and
     Nasal and Sinus Surgery.. 241
     Howard L. Levine

15b. Nd:YAG Laser and the Treatment of Nasal and Sinus Pathology 245
     Michel Jakobowicz

16. Outcome and Results in the Surgical Management of Rhinosinusitis 256
    Howard L. Levine

17. Revision Endoscopic Sinus Surgery 260
    James A. Stankiewicz, HanJo Na, and James M. Chow

18. Complications, Management, and Avoidance 269
    Heinrich Rudert

19. Ophthalmologic Complications of Endoscopic Sinus Surgery 285
    Mark Levine

20. The Diagnosis of Allergic Fungal Sinusitis 290
    Berrylin J. Ferguson

21. Meningoencephaloceles and Cerebrospinal Fluid Leak............................ 300
    Howard L. Levine

22. Endoscopic Orbital Decompression.. 306
    Ralph B. Metson and Mathew Cosenza

23. Dacryocystorhinostomy... 312
    Ralph B. Metson

24. Anesthesia for Sinus Surgery 316
    Douglas Mayers and Margaret M. Hildebrandt

25. Postoperative Care of the Patient Undergoing Endoscopic Sinus Surgery..... 322
    Howard L. Levine

26. Nursing Care for Outpatient Endoscopic Sinus Surgery 325
    Barbara R. Bilski, Cindi L. Davis, and Howard L. Levine

Index 331

Foreword

The practical aspect of management of sinusitis is a challenging effort for the clinician or the surgeon who is actively involved in the management of this disease. The various options in the medical and surgical management of sinusitis could be confusing and pose a challenge in the choice of treatment. The causes of sinusitis and the effective management have changed recently with the current fungal hypothesis which is still not clearly understood.

This textbook makes some important contributions in the field of sinusitis. The authors who have written the informative chapters have addressed the questions that one is faced with in the clinical management of sinusitis. The contributing authors in this book are all well known in the field of rhinology and have had substantial experience in the clinical management of sinusitis. The basics of anatomy and the physiology of sinusitis with endoscopic diagnostic illustrations have been well presented. The controversial question of an allergic fungal etiology and the role of immunology has been described in an easily readable manner and answers most of the questions pertaining to it.

The combined endoscopic and microscopic technique in sinus surgery has been presented in an interesting format.

The ease of reading and the ability to understand the concepts in the management of sinusitis has been dealt with in an ideal manner. I would congratulate Dr. Howard Levine and his colleagues in the compiling of this book and would recommend this book to all practicing physicians as an ideal addition to their library.

Vijay Anand, M.D.

Foreword

Preface

When I began performing endoscopic sinus surgery in the early 1980's, there was little educational material for the neophyte surgeon. There were a handful of video tapes illustrating removal of concha bullosa and partial ethmoidectomy mainly emphasizing the area of the uncinate, hiatus semilunaris, and ethmoid bulla. There was a 35 mm slide series of sinus pathology from Dr. Wolgang Draf, Fulda, Germany showing various pathologies of the nose. Because traditional sinus surgery was done with a headlight and as an "open" procedure (Caldwell-Luc, intranasal ethmoidectomy) it was difficult to transfer those surgical techniques to endoscopic sinus surgery. I clearly remember studying each video tape attempting to learn the techniques of using instruments in the sinuses. The cadaver laboratory and examining office patients endoscopically provided an excellent method to gain the technical skills needed to manage the endoscopes and instruments in the nose.

As the early years went by, several sinus surgeons wrote textbooks and gave courses to help the new and young sinus surgeons. Some of these early writers included Drs. Wolfgang Draf, David Kennedy, Walter Messerklinger, Dale Rice, Steven Schaeffer, Heinz Stammberger, James Stankiwiecz, and Malke Wigand. From these early teachers so many of us learned so much and to them we owe thanks.

In 1993, Dr. Mark May and I decided to publish a "how-to" text of endoscopic sinus surgery for the "in-the-trenches" practitioner (*Endoscopic Sinus Surgery*, Thieme, New York). With so much having been written for the academic, this seemed appropriate. This new text of *Sinus Surgery: Endoscopic and Microscopic Approaches* follows and updates that early volume. It is an outgrowth from a sinus course taught by one of the authors (M. Pais Clemente) in Porto, Portugal for surgeons wanting an introduction to sinus surgery. This text may not provide all of the most sophisticated techniques and the erudite scientific theory, but is meant to provide information can that be easily used and assimilated by the young and less experienced physician. Use it as both a reference text and practical manual of sinus surgery. Use it to accompany other writings.

And most importantly, use it to enjoy the wonderful and challenging aspect of otolaryngology that I have learned to love over these many years.

Howard L. Levine

Acknowledgments

I have for many years enjoyed a great friendship and professional respect for Howard L. Levine, M.D. for his recognized contribution in the field of rhinology and dedication to medical care. This book reflects the spirit of such cooperation, support, and understanding. I acknowledge the valuable contributions of the other authors who have covered their assigned topics based on their expertise and related publications.

I wish to express my gratitude to the medical staff of my Department, with a special appreciation to Horácio F. Silva, M.D., Ph.D., an exceptional colleague, friend and co-worker, and also to Margarida Santos, M.D. and Fernando Vales, M.D. for their support and dedicated collaboration.

I would like to thank Daniel Muller, the medical artist responsible for the illustrations for Chapters 1 and 11, for his excellent artwork.

I'm also grateful to the staff at Thieme Medical Publishers, particularly Mrs. Esther Gumpert, for their editorial assistance.

M. Pais Clemente

List of Contributors

Jack B. Anon
Assistant Clinical Professor
Department of Otolaryngology
University of Pittsburgh
Pittsburgh, Pennsylvania

L. Bellussi
Associate Professor
ENT Department
University of Siena Medical School
Siena, Italy

Barbara R. Bilski, L.P.N.
Cleveland Nasal Sinus & Sleep Center
Cleveland, Ohio

James M. Chow
Professor
Department of Otolaryngology–Head and Neck Surgery
Loyola University Medical Center
Maywood, Illinois

M. Pais Clemente, M.D., Ph.D.
Professor and Chairman
Department of Otorhinolaryngology
Porto University School of Medicine
Hospital S. João
Porto, Portugal
Chairman Center for Optical Technologies (CETO)
Porto, Portugal
Chairman National Council for Smoking Prevention
Lisbon Portugal

Mathew J. Cosenza, D.O.
Department of Otolaryngology

Massachusetts Eye and Ear Infirmary
Boston, Massachusetts

Cindi L. Davis, R.N., B.S.N.
Peter Doble, M.D.
Berrylin Ferguson, M.D.
Associate Professor
Department of Otolaryngology
University of Pittsburgh School of Medicine
Pittsburgh, Pennsylvania

Margaret M. Hildebrandt, C.R.N.A.
Cleveland Anesthesia Group
and
Cleveland Clinic Foundation

Michael Jakobowicz, M.D.
Hopital La Pitie Salpetriere/
    Attache des Hopital de Paris
Attache d'Enseignement Clinique a la
    Faculte de Medicine Paris Quest
Membre de L'Academie l'ORL et CCF de Russie

Ken Kazahaya, M.D.
Director
Pediatric Skull Base Surgery
Division of Pediatric Otoloryngology
Children's Hospital of Philadelphia
and
Assistant Professor
Department of Otorhinolaryngology–Head and
    Neck Surgery
University of Pennsylvania School of Medicine
Philadelphia, Pennsylvania

Ludger Klimek, M.D., Ph.D.
Leiter des Zentrums fuer Rhinologie und Allergologie

Maria Lauriello, M.D.
Associate Professor
ENT Department
University of Siena
Policlinico Le Scotte

Howard L. Levine, M.D.
Co-Director
Cleveland Nasal-Sinus and Sleep Center
Marymount Outpatient Care Center
Cleveland, Ohio

Mark R. Levine, M.D.
Head Section of Oculoplastic Surgery
Case Western Reserve Surgery
School of Medicine
Cleveland, Ohio

Douglas Mayers, M.D., Ph.D.
Director
Ambulatary Surgery Center
Division of Anesthesiology
The Cleveland Clinic Foundation–Beachwood
Cleveland, Ohio

Ralph B. Metson, M.D., F.A.C.S
Professor
Department. of Otolaryngology
Massachusetts Eye and Ear Infirmary
Boston, Massachusetts

Michael Modic, M.D.
Chairman
Division of Radiology
Cleveland Clinic Foundation
and
Professor of Radiology
The Ohio State University
Cleveland, Ohio

HanJo Na, M.D.
Associate Professor
Department of Otolaryngology
Chosun University Hospital
KwangJu, South Korea

Desiderio Passali, M.D.
University degli Studi di Siena/Instituto di Discipline
    Otolarinolaringoliche

Francesco Maria Passali
ENT Department
University of Siena Medical School
Siena, Italy

Giulio Cesare Passali
ENT Department
University of Siena Medical School
Siena, Italy

Heinrich Rudert, M.D.
Department of Otolaryngology
University of Kiel

Barry M. Schaitkin, M.D., F.A.C.S.
Associate Professor
Department of Otolaryngology
University of Pittsburgh School of Medicine
Pittsburgh, Pennsylvania

Michael Schatz, M.D., M.S.
Chief
Allergy Department
Kaiser-Permanent Medical Center
And
Clinical Professor
Department of Medicine
University of California
San Diego School of Medicine
San Diego, California

Raymond Slavin, M.D.
Director
Division of Allergy and Immunology
Department of Internal Medicine
St. Louis University School of Medicine
St. Louis, Missouri

James Stankiewicz, M.D.
Professor
Department of Otolaryngology
Loyola University Medical Center
Chicago, Illinois

Todd W. Stultz
Consultant
Department of Dentistry
Acting Head
Dentomaxillofacial Imaging
Resident
Diagnostic Radiology
The Cleveland Clinic Foundation
Cleveland, Ohio

Lawrence W. C. Tom, M.D.
Associate Professor
Department of Otolaryngology
University of Pennsylvania School of Medicine
Children's Hospital of Philadelphia
Philadelphia, Pennsylvania

1

Surgical Anatomy of the Paranasal Sinus

M. PAIS CLEMENTE

The paranasal sinus region is one of the most complex areas of the human body and is consequently very difficult to study. The surgical anatomy of the nose and paranasal sinuses is published with great detail in most standard textbooks, but it is the purpose of this chapter to describe those structures in a very clear and systematic presentation focused for the endoscopic sinus surgeon.

A thorough knowledge of all anatomical structures and variations combined with cadaveric dissections using paranasal blocks is of utmost importance to perform proper sinus surgery and to avoid complications. The complications seen with this surgery are commonly due to nonfamiliarity with the anatomical landmarks of the paranasal sinus during surgical dissection, which is consequently performed beyond the safe limits of the sinus.

The sinus surgeon must be able to orientate himself or herself while looking through optical instruments that provide better illumination and a greater view of the delicate structures of the nose and paranasal sinus. The surgeon must also develop a mental three-dimensional anatomical image, allowing himself or herself to know the precise location, the relationships with vital structures, and especially where the danger points lie.

Besides clinical judgment and technical skills, a competent surgeon must also be a good anatomist. To achieve these goals, it is wise to perform a reasonable number of surgical dissections on cadaveric specimens, attend several dissection courses, and participate in many meetings. During the past years the author has organized international dissection courses on paranasal sinus surgery with limited numbers of participants. This is the best way to improve medical teaching, hospital practice, and patient care.

This chapter is divided into three sections: developmental anatomy, macroscopic anatomy, and endoscopic anatomy. A basic understanding of the embryogenesis of the nose and the paranasal sinuses facilitates comprehension of the complex and variable adult anatomy. In addition, this comprehension is quite useful for an accurate evaluation of the various potential pathologies and their managements. Macroscopic description of the nose and paranasal sinuses is presented through a discussion of the important structures of this complicated region. A correlation with intricate endoscopic topographical anatomy is discussed for a clear understanding of the nasal cavity and its relationship to adjoining sinuses and danger areas. A three-dimensional anatomy is complemented with schematic diagrams.

■ Developmental Anatomy

Nose Development

The embryogenesis of the nose and paranasal sinuses is related to the regional embryology of the cranial-oral-facial region. These primary events occur between the fourth and eighth weeks of fetal life. The first nasal structures are initially identifiable in the 5 mm, 4-week-old embryo.[1,2] At this point, there are three developing facial projections that contribute to the formation of the nose: the frontonasal process, the maxillary process, and the mandibular process.

The frontonasal process is ectodermally derived, and it develops independently over the forebrain giving rise to the forehead and the nasal olfactory placodes. A thickened plaque of ectoderm develops during the

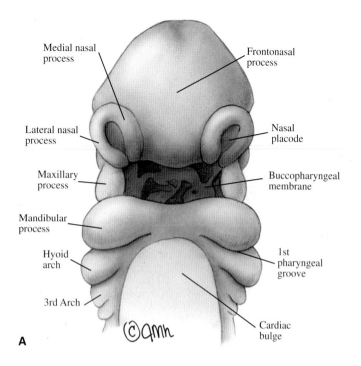

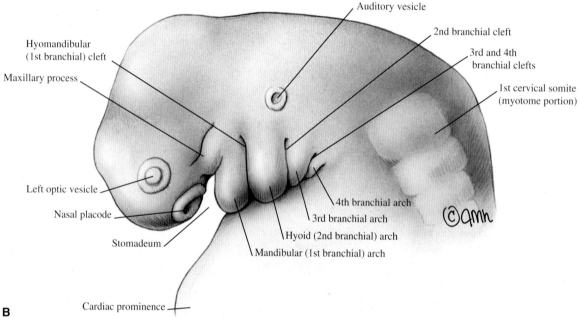

FIGURE 1–1 Embryo at 4 to 5 weeks. (A) Frontal view: Observe the branchial arch formation and the ruptured buccopharyngeal membrane. (B) Lateral view.

fourth intrauterine week on each side of the ventral surface of this frontonasal elevation. Within a few days these thickenings become paired lateral nasal placodes (Fig. 1–1). Initially the placodes have a convex external surface, but the unequal forward growth of the frontonasal swelling (particularly the medial and lateral sides of the nasal placodes) will transform these surfaces into concave nasal grooves. These grooves are well developed when the embryo is 32 to 34 days old. They are surrounded by the medial nasal swelling at the medial side of the nasal placode and the lateral nasal swelling at the lateral side of the nasal placode.[3]

Meanwhile, other outgrowths of mesenchymal origin called the maxillary processes grow ventrally from the dorsal ends of the mandibular processes (first visceral) arch. These maxillary swellings are located at the inferolateral border of the placodes. These three swellings are separated from each other by shallow depressions and continue to grow forward and downward. As they do so, the epithelial linings of the medial and lateral nasal swellings fuse inferiorly, and the nasal grooves become blind-ending tubes or pits, called the nasal pits, that will ultimately become the nares. The epithelium within the pits eventually develops neural processes that extend toward the brain to become the olfactory nerves. Thus, the development of the nasal pits is part of the cranial and neural tube formation.

The floor of each nasal pit is constituted by the fused medial and lateral nasal swellings and further anteriorly by the fused medial nasal and maxillary swellings. The epithelial lining in the contact plane is called the nasal fin and is disrupted anteriorly by the outgrowth of the surrounding tissues. Posteriorly, this epithelial band persists for a short period of time in the floor of the nasal

pit. As the nasal pit deepens, it becomes the nasal sac. As the cavity enlarges, the posterior limiting membrane (initially the nasal fin) becomes the oronasal membrane.

During the forward and downward growth of the various facial swellings, each swelling also increases its dimensions in a mediolateral direction. Thus, during the transformation of the nasal groove into the primary nasal cavity, the furrows between maxillary and lateral nasal swellings are increased, both on the external surface and on the internal surface of the lateral wall of the primary nasal cavity. The early structures responsible for the development of the eyes are visible at 28 days. Initially, the early eyes are oriented laterally (80 degrees to the neural axis), but during the next weeks the growth

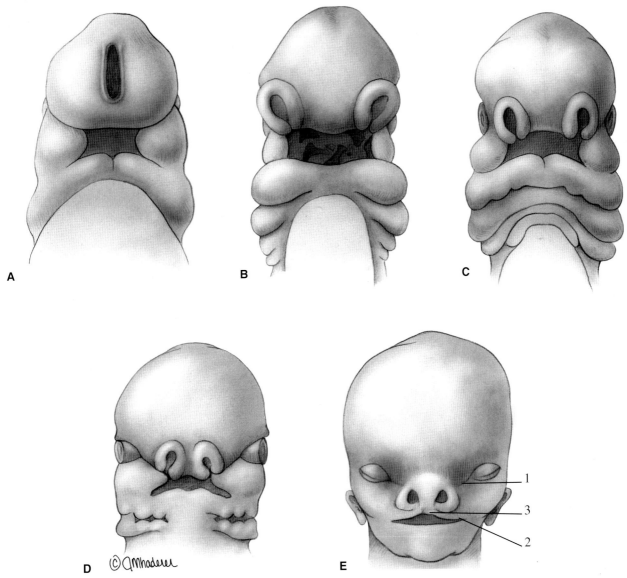

FIGURE 1–2 Developing face. (A) Fourth week. (B) Fourth to fifth week. (C) Fifth to sixth week. (D) Sixth to seventh week. (E) Eighth to tenth week. Note the orientation of the eyes forward and toward the midline, the nose development, the sealing of the nasolacrimal groove (1), and the formation of the upper lip (2) and the philtrum (3).

of the mesenchyme posterior to the eyes reorients the eyes forward toward the midline. The groove on the external surface is transformed into the nasolacrimal duct by the interposition of surface epithelium between the maxillary and lateral nasal swellings and by the loss of contact between this epithelium and the surface epithelium. It is like an infolded epithelial transformation. The groove on the inside surface will develop into the inferior meatus of the nasal cavity. The nasolacrimal duct connects the eye to the internal nasal cavity inferior to the attachment of the inferior turbinate. As the eye migrates from a lateral orientation relative to the developing nose, the nasolacrimal duct assumes a more oblique rather than horizontal direction (Fig. 1–2).

The rupture of the oronasal membrane in the 15 mm embryo takes place between days 42 and 44 in the posterior floor of the nasal pit, transforming this blind-ending cavity into a primary nasal cavity that communicates with the primary oral cavity through the newly formed opening, or primitive choana.[1–3] Lack of disintegration of the oronasal membrane results in choanal atresia. The part of the roof of the mouth in front of the

choana is the premaxilla (primitive palate). The external nares are widely separated by the remaining median frontonasal process, which gradually reduces, bringing the openings close together.

Simultaneously, other facial structures develop rapidly. The digestive tube is formed, and the cephalic opening of this tube, called the oral stoma, is found just caudal to the level of the nasal pits. The branchial clefts and

TABLE 1–1   Derivatives of Facial Components

Embryonic Part	Facial Derivatives	Skeletal Derivatives
Frontonasal process	Nasal bridge	Nasal bones
Median nasal process	Columella of nose	Perpendicular plate of the ethmoid bone
	Philtrum	Vomer
Lateral nasal process	Sides and ala of nose	
Maxillary process	Major portion of upper lip	Maxilla, zygoma, secondary palate
	Upper cheek	
Mandibular process	Lower lip, Lower cheek	Mandible

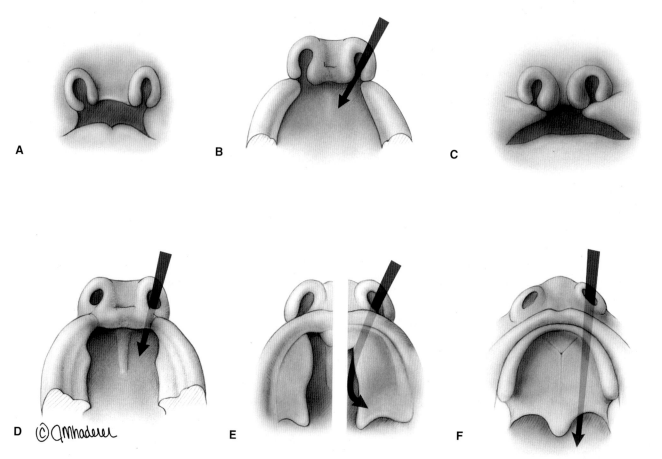

FIGURE 1–3 Development of the nose, mouth, and palate. (A–C) Formation of the nose, upper lip, and philtrum. (D–F) Different stages of palate formation and the separation of the nasal and oral cavities.

arches form ventral to the eyes and caudal to the oral stoma. The maxillary process, derived from the first branchial arch with part of the medial nasal process, becomes the upper jaw (Table 1–1).

From days 45 to 48 formation of the secondary palate begins, due to the separation between the nasal cavity and the oral cavity. By that time, vertical projections from the maxillary process, named palatal shelves, are identified. The palatal processes are located along the lateral aspect of the tongue, but as the tongue descends, they develop horizontally toward each other. The secondary nasal cavity is thus formed. The palatal closure progresses from anterior to posterior, and by days 63 to 70 the palatal shelves have fused along most of their length (Fig. 1–3). Only the area between the junction of the premaxilla and the palate remains incomplete during the prenatal life and thereafter. This persistent communication at the anterior palate is the incisive canal, which carries vessels and nerves between the nose and the mouth.[4]

The posterior choana is repositioned more posteriorly due to the development of the secondary nasal cavity and the formation of the palate. Also, the developing nasal septum fuses with the palatal shelves, creating two separate right and left nasal cavities. The precise timing of these events is subject to individual variations and possibly also to sexual and racial ones.[5] However, early in this stage the definitive nasal cavities are formed, and a cartilaginous frame begins to provide support to the nasal region as well as primary skeletal protection.

The nasal capsule is a cartilaginous envelope that encases the developing nasal structures and is part of the developing skull base (Fig. 1–4). This mesodermal structure forms a boundary to the nasal and paranasal sinus development. The paranasal cellular growth either is limited to the bounds of the perichondrium of the nasal capsule or extends beyond the borders of the perichondrium with reabsorption of the cartilaginous cells. This is the situation created by the development of the maxillary, frontal, and sphenoid sinuses beyond the ethmoid complex.

The developmental origin of the cartilaginous nasal capsule is unclear and subject to controversy.[6,7] It is possible that the mesenchyme (the loose embryonic mesodermal tissue) is directed by the neural crest cells, arising at the junction of the neural tube and ectoderm and streaming out into the mesoderm. The resulting mesoderm is then termed head mesenchyme.

The process of chondrification of the nasal capsule begins within the head mesenchyme with the lying down of chondroitin (the intercellular matrix). The fibrovascular tissue on the periphery of the nasal capsule is the perichondrium, which provides the nutrients to be diffused to the chondrocytes (cartilage cells). This induced process of chondrification starts in the cranial base at

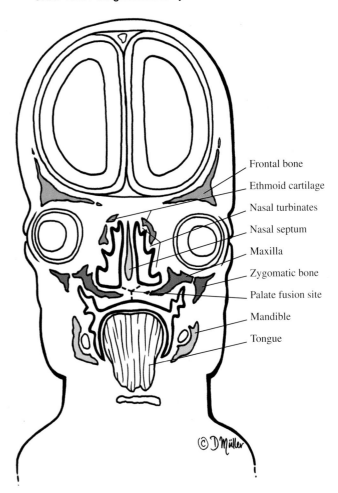

FIGURE 1–4 Eight- to 10-week embryo (coronal section) showing early development of the nasal capsule, including the lateral nasal wall and the turbinates.

the anterior aspect of the sphenoid bone. The nasal capsule begins to chondrify after the chondrocranium at the level of the nasal septum sometime during the middle of the third prenatal month. Cartilage formation in the lateral ethmoid bone starts in the fourth month and extends to the anterior or caudal area of the nose and septum, and subsequently to the dorsal part of the nasal capsule.

The process of ossification of the nasal capsule involves two mechanisms of bone formation: endochondral and membranous. Endochondral bone formation is related to the layered deposit of bone matrix along the perichondrial blood vessels that invade the cartilaginous tissue. Simultaneously, the cartilage is resorbed. The cells that form along these vessels are called osteocytes and have their own supply vessel. The compacted fibrovascular tissue at the periphery of this process of ossification becomes the periosteum. Membranous bone is the result of laying down bone matrix directly from periosteal cells without a preceding formation of cartilage.

The process of ossification of the nasal capsule includes both endochondral and membranous bone formation, although it is microscopically impossible to differentiate the two. There are a great number of centers of ossification, and it seems that they follow a predictable pattern. The first center is located at the anterior edge of what will be the sphenoid bone. This area is very important because it is considered the growth plate for the anterior skull base and face. The second center of ossification is in the lateral aspect of the nasal capsule. Multiple centers develop thereafter, each of the nasal and facial bones having at least one center of ossification.

Paranasal Sinus Development

The embryological development of the paranasal sinus is a very complex process, and its description varies among different authors. The growth pattern of the paranasal sinus is totally unpredictable and extremely variable from one individual to another, or even from side to side in the same person.[8]

The initial development of the nasosinus cavities takes place early in fetal life, occurring at the same time as the growth of the palate below, facial structures anteriorly, and the cerebral cranium above. The paranasal sinuses, with the exception of the sphenoid sinus, arise as evaginations from the lateral nasal wall.

At the begining, the lateral nasal wall is a smooth, undifferentiated structure, but during the seventh gestational week it starts to develop. A projection into the nasal capsule just superior to the palatal shelves appears first and is called the maxilloturbinal. It is followed by five other ethmoturbinals and the nasoturbinal. However, through reposition and fusion three to four ridges ultimately persist[4,9,10] (Fig. 1–5).

The maxilloturbinal forms the inferior turbinate, which is not considered ethmoid in its embryological origin. The first ethmoturbinal originates at either the superior aspect of the septum or the superior junction of the septum and the lateral nasal wall, and it gives rise to the middle turbinate. The furrow between the maxilloturbinal and the first ethmoturbinal eventually develops into the middle nasal meatus. It is at the primitive middle meatus that, during about the 13th week of development, an evagination of the lateral nasal wall produces a blind diverticulum: the embryonic infundibulum. The infundibulum is formed by a cord of epithelial cells that is surrounded by the underlying mesenchyme. On either side of this structure, the mesenchyme proliferates, deepening the infundibulum. The second ethmoturbinal develops shortly after the first ethmoturbinal and ultimately forms the superior turbinate. The furrow between the superior turbinate and the middle turbinate is the superior meatus. The third ethmoturbinal is the precursor of the supreme turbinate, which is present in only 26% of adults.[11] The supreme meatus is the furrow between the superior and the supreme turbinates. All of these structures are considered to be ethmoid in their origin.

The nasoturbinal is an additional prominence anterior and superior to the ethmoid furrow or middle nasal meatus and will develop into the agger nasi. At about the same time it is identified another mesenchymal ridge, called the uncinate process, develops on the superior and posterior border of the agger nasi. The uncinate

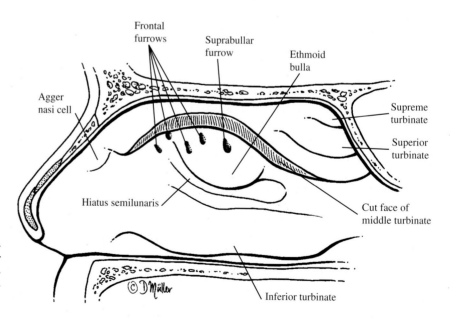

FIGURE 1–5 Right nasal wall of a neonate showing the turbinates and the agger nasi. The middle turbinate has been removed to present the anatomical structures of the middle meatus.

process may extend superiorly to the roof of the anterior ethmoid bone and posteriorly along the superior surface of the inferior turbinate.

During their development from the lateral nasal wall, the ethmoturbinals form bony structures that traverse the ethmoid complex to attach to the lamina papyracea of the orbit and skull base. The furrows continue to grow, developing evaginations that contribute to the extensive and complex pneumatization of the ethmoid bone.

All craniofacial structures (at first made of cartilage, then of bone) that are adjacent to the infundibular region are subject to penetration by the process of evagination and reabsorption. The maxillary bone, frontal bone, ethmoid bone, and nasoturbinate bone (agger nasi) are invaded and filled with air from the ethmoid cells. This process is called primary pneumatization. It is followed by secondary pneumatization, during which these epithelial-lined pockets expand into the adjacent bony structures for which the sinuses eventually will be named. Primary pneumatization occurs during the chondrocranial stage. Much of the secondary pneumatization takes place postnatally.

Generally, the sinuses are established in prenatal life, with the shape of each sinus being regular in appearance and somewhat "globular." The overall development of the paranasal sinuses is slow for the first 6 years of life, but after that age the speed of growth increases and the shape becomes irregular due to the distorting effects by the growing adjacent bony structures, including the other paranasal sinuses. By age 12 to 14, most of the sinuses have reached the adult size, but some sinuses continue to grow into late adulthood.[10,12]

Maxillary Sinus Development

The maxillary sinus is the first to develop during human fetal life, roughly during the 10th week. The maxillary sinus begins to form from an outpouching of the lateral wall of the ethmoid area of the nasal capsule within the infundibulum and immediately posterior to the developing uncinate process.[13,14]

This outgrowth enlarges slowly throughout fetal life due to the constriction by the perichondrium of the nasal capsule, limiting extension into the maxillary process (maxilla). Thus, the maxillary sinus appears as a slit, caught between the developing ethmoid cells, the inferior turbinate, and the bone of the maxilla. Only as the nasal capsule is resorbed during its ossification does the maxillary sinus have an opportunity to enter the developing maxillary process. As the maxillary sinus expands into the maxilla, it is restricted by dental development. Further growth of the maxillary sinus into the maxilla follows the development of the maxilla and the descent of the teeth (Fig. 1–6).

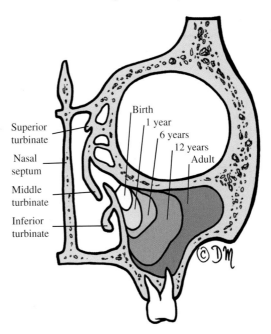

FIGURE 1–6 Developmental pattern of the maxillary sinus.

In the neonate, the largest sinus is represented by a small cavity whose lower border lies above that of the nasal floor and is encroached upon by the upper dentition. However, as the development of the mid-third of the face progresses and eruption of the permanent dentition occurs, the floor of the sinus migrates to a lower level than that of the nasal cavity (0.5–10 mm).[15]

Ethmoid Sinus Development

The earliest signs of development of the ethmoid sinus are seen during the fourth fetal month.[1-3] The ethmoid sinus has a multicentric origin. A great majority of the cells begin at the middle meatus as anterior ethmoid cells, and a minority develop from the superior and supreme meatus as posterior ethmoid cells. The anterior ethmoid cells appear as evaginations in the lateral nasal wall of the middle meatus. Somewhat later, the posterior cells evaginate the nasal mucosa in the superior meatus. All of these cells enlarge gradually throughout fetal life.

Other primitive structures called ethmoturbinals (middle, superior, and supreme), the uncinate process, the agger nasi, and the ethmoid bulla are medial extensions of the lateral wall of the nasal capsule. The attachments of these structures to the lateral nasal wall of the nasal capsule are the lamellae. There exist five lamellae with the following nomenclature (Table 1–2): first basal lamella (lateral extension of the uncinate process), second basal lamella (lateral extension of the ethmoid bulla), third basal lamella (attachment of the middle turbinate), fourth basal lamella (attachment of the supe-

TABLE 1–2   Classification of Lamellae

First basal lamella	Lateral extension of uncinate process
Second basal lamella	Lateral extension of ethmoid bulla
Third basal lamella	Attachment of middle turbinate
Fourth basal lamella	Attachment of superior turbinate
Fifth basal lamella	Attachment of supreme turbinate (when present)

rior turbinate), and fifth basal lamella (attachment of the supreme turbinate) when present (Fig. 1–7). The sinus cells during their development may stretch the lamellae but do not break through them, thereby retaining the integrity of each of the compartments.

During primary pneumatization, the rudiments of the ethmoid sinus consist of dimple-like depressions of the nasal mucosa into the nasal capsule. These depressions may originate from any of the mucosal furrows in the middle meatus or along the mucosa of the superior meatus, which is, itself, no more than a furrow at this time. The depressions gradually deepen and become globular air cells. As development progresses and these cells reach maximum growth and encroach on adjacent bony cells, they become flattened.

The ethmoid sinus is well developed at birth. During the second year after birth the air cells may grow beyond the confines of the ethmoid bone into the surrounding bones: maxilla, frontal, lacrimal, and sphenoid. The growth pattern of the ethmoid sinus is completely unpredictable, and development will continue until the ethmoid has reached almost adult size by the age of 12 years. Some further enlargements may take place in early adulthood.

The ethmoid sinus cells are divided into anterior and posterior groups based on their initial sites of pneumatization and the subsequent locations of their ostia (Fig. 1–8). Ethmoid cells may be further characterized on the basis of the skeletal structures they pneumatize. Thus, it is possible to define groups of cells as remaining within the ethmoid and others as lying beyond the ethmoid.

Ethmoid cells that belong to the ethmoid bone include the conchal, bullar, infundibular, and frontal recess cells. Among those that extend beyond the ethmoid bone are the agger nasi cells (anterior ethmoid cells that pneumatize the agger nasi on the medial surface of the frontal process of the maxilla and lacrimal bone),

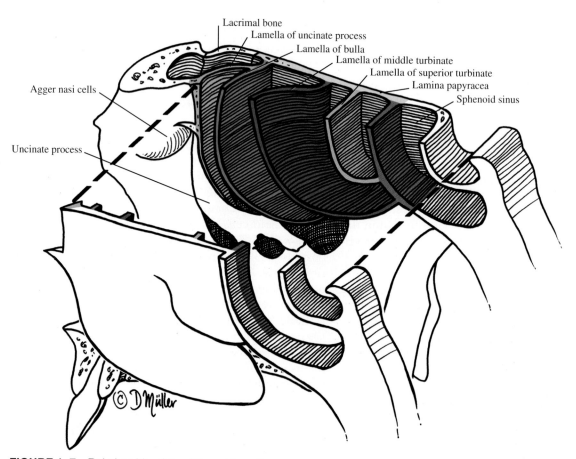

FIGURE 1–7   Relationship of the different lamellae.

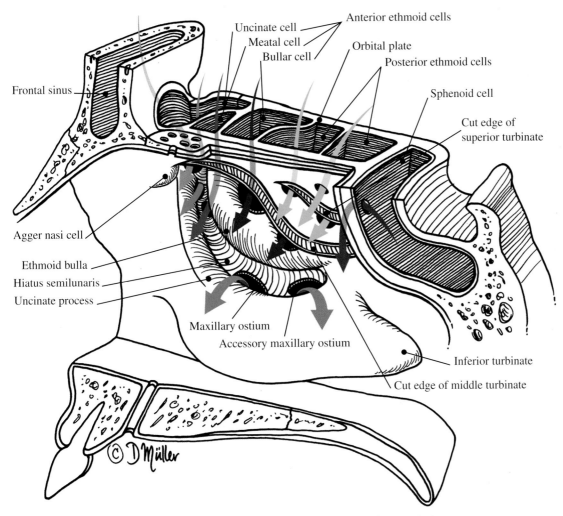

FIGURE 1–8   Bony anatomy of the various drainage systems of the paranasal sinuses.

frontal sinus cells (anterior ethmoid cells that pneumatize the frontal bone), orbital cells (anterior ethmoid cells that pneumatize the orbital roof), and palatine bone and sphenoid bone cells (posterior ethmoid cells that pneumatize these bones).

The ethmoid sinus is responsible for cellular colonization into the surrounding structures: anteriorly, the agger nasi; superiorly, the frontal sinus; posteriorly, the sphenoid sinus; inferiorly, the uncinate process; laterally, the orbital bony structures; and medially, the medial surface of the middle turbinate to produce a middle turbinate concha bullosa. This haphazard growth makes the ethmoid sinus different from one individual to another. The cells that are located within the ethmoid bone are termed intramural cells, whereas those whose development involves an adjacent bone such as the maxilla, lacrimal bone, frontal bone, or sphenoid bone are called extramural cells (Fig. 1–9). Regardless of their origins, the sinuses are named for the bone in

which they finally reside. For example, the frontal sinus is, in reality, often formed by displaced anterior ethmoid cells.

In the superior meatus there is a ridge in the lateral wall that is similar to the uncinate process. An accessory swelling is also seen there that resembles the ethmoid bulla of the middle meatus. A variety of structures of the superior nasal meatus are reminiscent of those that develop more completely in the middle meatus. The superior meatus is the origin of most of the posterior ethmoid air cells. These cells may also grow laterally into the junction of the nasal capsule and orbit posterior to the maxillary sinus cleft. Expansion of these cells into the posterior, lateral, and superior aspect of the maxilla is the usual origin of the ethmomaxillary cells (Haller's cells).[9,10,12] These cells may be small or even of significant size, and those of maximum development may give the appearance of an accessory maxillary sinus (Fig. 1–10).

FIGURE 1–9   Ethmoid Sinus Development

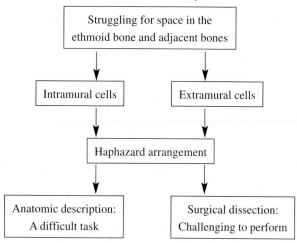

```
┌──────────────────────────────────────┐
│    Struggling for space in the       │
│  ethmoid bone and adjacent bones     │
└──────────────────────────────────────┘
        │                    │
        ▼                    ▼
┌─────────────────┐  ┌─────────────────┐
│ Intramural cells│  │ Extramural cells│
└─────────────────┘  └─────────────────┘
        │                    │
        ▼                    ▼
    ┌──────────────────────────┐
    │   Haphazard arrangement  │
    └──────────────────────────┘
        │                    │
        ▼                    ▼
┌──────────────────┐  ┌──────────────────────┐
│Anatomic          │  │ Surgical dissection: │
│description:      │  │ Challenging to perform│
│A difficult task  │  │                      │
└──────────────────┘  └──────────────────────┘
```

Frontal Sinus Development

The frontal sinus begins to develop during the fourth fetal month, after the development of the frontal recess. Initially, this recess is a pocket found medial to the very cephalic or superior aspect of the uncinate process and expands into the thick nasal capsule mesenchyme. The fetal frontal recess is found between the uncinate process and the anterior attachment of the middle turbinate. There are two or four furrows or pits within the frontal recess that can potentially form air cells.

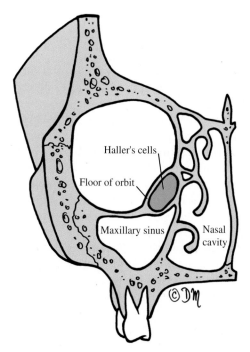

FIGURE 1–10   Haller's cells.

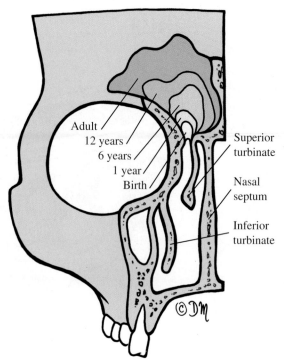

FIGURE 1–11   Developmental pattern of the frontal sinus.

The frontal sinus is described as developing in several ways:

1. by direct extension of the whole frontal recess
2. from the laterally placed anterior ethmoid cells within the frontal recess
3. from the ethmoid infundibular cells
4. from one or more of the anterior group of ethmoid cells arising in the frontal furrows

The great variation in the development of the frontal sinus accounts for the changes found in its drainage systems and for the presence or absence of a true frontonasal duct, the existence of which is the subject of some controversy.

The frontal sinus can therefore be formed by a direct extension of the whole frontal recess into the frontal bone or from the extension of anterior ethmoid cells within the frontal recess. A frontal sinus that develops from the ethmoid infundibulum or the first or second frontal furrows may have its drainage pathway restricted into a nasofrontal duct. The growth of the surrounding anterior ethmoid cells may also encroach on the proximal part of the frontal sinus, compressing it into a nasofrontal duct.[3,14] The diameter of this duct depends largely on the degree of encroachment by the surrounding ethmoid cells. This usually does not affect the frontal sinus, which develops directly from the wall of the frontal recess and has a distinct ostium named the

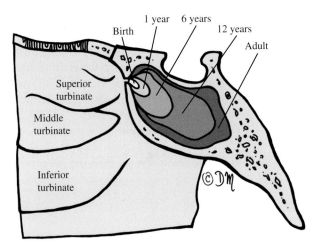

FIGURE 1–12   Developmental pattern of the sphenoid sinus.

primary frontal sinus ostium (the point of origin of the frontal sinus). Prenatally, the frontal sinus does not expand much further.

Secondary pneumatization occurs postnatally, generally beginning between the ages of 6 months and 2 years. Initially, the secondary pneumatization occurs laterally toward the orbital side of the frontal bone, but during the second year of life pneumatization has a more vertical direction. However, by definition, a frontal sinus is not present until the cell enters the vertical (ascending) portion of the frontal bone. During its development, the superior extremity of the frontal sinus reaches the midvertical height of the orbit at 4 years of age and the level of superior orbital rim at 8 years. It grows into the frontal squama at 10 years of age. The frontal sinus continues its growth at a slow rate into adolescence, when it may reach its final size (Fig. 1–11). The expansion into the vertical frontal bone occurs closer to the cranial cavity, and consequently the external table of the frontal bone is thicker than the inner table.

The development of the frontal sinus may be affected by the expansion of the surrounding anterior ethmoid cells. In this situation, one or more of these cells begin pneumatizing the frontal bone and may even exceed the primary frontal sinus outgrowth. The "true" sinus that is first present in such a case may encroach on the lumen of the second sinus by forming a bulbous projection (bulla frontalis) in the wall of the latter larger sinus. In these cases, a thin plate of bone separates the two sinuses.

The left and the right frontal sinuses develop independently, and asymmetry between the frontal sinus is more the rule than the exception, in contrast to the case with the maxillary sinus. Pneumatization may also extend as far laterally as the temporal bone, but this is unusual.

Sphenoid Sinus Development

The development of the sphenoid sinus is unique because of two factors: (1) It is the only sinus that does not arise as an outpouching from the lateral nasal wall and (2) there is no primary pneumatization, but rather a constriction of the developing presphenoid recess followed by secondary pneumatization.

During the third month of fetal development the nasal mucosa invaginates into the posterior portion of the cartilaginous nasal capsule. This primordium is only a small presphenoid recess within the posterior end of the cartilaginous nasal capsule. By the end of the third and early fourth fetal months the posterosuperior portion of the recess is separated incompletely from the nasal cavity by the development of a nasal mucosal fold, inferiorly based, curving upward and anterior to the body of the presphenoid. As the nasal capsule undergoes chondrification, a cartilaginous concha forms within this fold, developing cartilaginous concavities, which, by the fifth fetal month, enclose the presphenoid recess. This site of initial sinus rudiment and of

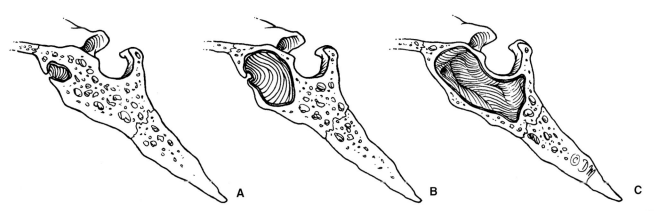

FIGURE 1–13   Anatomical variations of the sphenoid sinus pneumatization. (A) Conchal or fetal type. (B) Presellar or juvenile type. (C) Sellar or adult type.

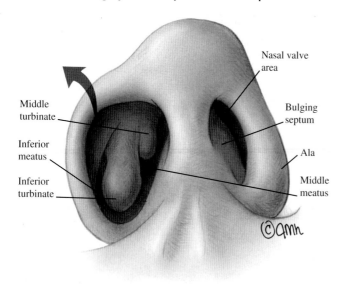

FIGURE 1–14 The nasal valve area. It is the area of peak restriction of nasal airflow.

initial constriction is preserved in adulthood as the location of the sinus ostium. The wall surrounding this cartilage is ossified in the later months of fetal development.

At birth the sphenoid sinus is no more than an encircled recess, located between the sphenoid concha and the presphenoid body. After birth, the sphenoid sinus primordium grows inferiorly and posteriorly. In the second and third years the intervening cartilage is resorbed, and part of the sphenoid concha fuses to the presphenoid body; the resulting cavity clearly becomes the sphenoid sinus. The presphenoid recess becomes the sphenoethmoid recess. Following this fusion, pneumatization of the sphenoid occurs with expansion into the presphenoid and, later, the basisphenoid parts of sphenoid bone, with the sphenoid concha remaining as the anterior sinus wall. By the age of 8 to 10 years a real sinus cavity may be observed, although the definitive form of the sinus is attained at puberty (Fig. 1–12). The origin of the sphenoid sinus from the posterior nasal cavity is always identified by the sinus ostium (the location where the sphenoid recess retained its continuity with the nasal cavity), which is located high on the anterior sinus wall, just a few millimeters below the sphenoethmoid recess.

The shape of the sinus is determined by the varying degrees of pneumatization that take place in the secondary pneumatization. The sphenoid sinus may pneumatize beyond the confines of the sphenoid body to the greater or lesser wings, the medial and lateral pterygoid plates, the palatine and basioccipital bones, or the ethmoid bone. The lateral expansion brings the sphenoid into contact with the second and third divisions of the trigeminal nerve as well as the nerve of the pterygoid canal (vidian nerve).

The sphenoid sinus may be classified according to its degree of pneumatization: (1) conchal or fetal-type sinus with minimal extension, which is relatively rare (2%); (2) presellar or juvenile-type sinus, expanding posteriorly to the anterior sellar wall, which occurs in ~10 to 24% of the adult population; and (3) sellar or adult-type sinus, extending below the sella or farther, which may be found in as many as 86% of all adults (Fig. 1–13).[3,10,14,16]

■ Macroscopic Anatomy

Nasal Cavity

The internal nose is constituted by two nasal cavities extending from the nares to the choanae and separated by the nasal septum. The nasal cavity is roughly a right triangle in outline, slightly wider toward its central position. The nares lead into the vestibule, the skin-lined part of the nasal cavity that contains the vibrissae (nasal hairs), the hair follicles, and the sebaceous glands.

The vestibule is limited above and behind by a curved ridge, the limen nasi. A recess of the vestibule reaches upward into the tip. The junction of the nasal skin and the mucous membrane of the nasal cavity occurs at a variable distance inside the nose, but it is clearly defined visually by the difference in color between skin and mucosa. The union of the skin-lined nasal vestibule with the mucosa-lined chamber of the nasal cavity has the shape of a triangular aperture, and it constitutes the narrowest area of the normal nasal airway called the nasal valve (Fig. 1–14). Its superior and lateral limits are formed by the upper lateral cartilage; its medial wall is represented by the nasal septum; and its base, by the floor of the nose. The nasal valve area marks the junction between the lower limit of the upper lateral cartilage and the upper portion of medial and lateral crura of the lower lateral cartilages.[17-22]

The mucosa of the nasal cavity has a pseudostratified ciliated columnar epithelium and communicates with the adjoining paranasal sinus and with the nasopharynx via the posterior choana. The nasal cavity has a roof, a floor, a medial wall, and a lateral nasal wall.[23-27]

ROOF

The upper zone of the nasal cavity is named the olfactory cleft. It is divided into a nasal part lying anteriorly, an ethmoid area centrally, and a sphenoid part posteriorly. The sloping anterior portion of the roof of the nasal cavity is formed by the nasal bones and the nasal spine of the frontal bone. The central segment of the roof is mainly defined by the cribriform plate of the eth-

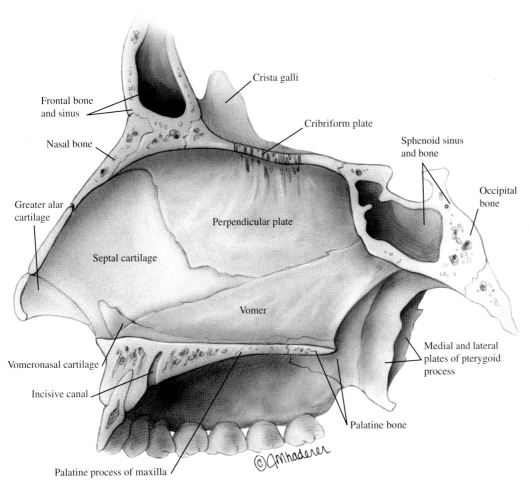

FIGURE 1–15 Nasal septum.

moid bone and is often referred to as the olfactory area. The descending posterior part of the roof of the nasal cavity is constituted by the anterior wall of the sphenoid sinus. The sphenoethmoid recess lies in this posterior segment. The junction between the vertical anterior wall and the horizontal floor of the sphenoidal sinus marks the end of the nasal cavity and forms the boundary of the choana.

FLOOR

The bony floor of the nasal cavity is formed by the premaxilla, the maxilla, and the horizontal plate of the palatine bone in the posterior portion. The floor is ~4.5 cm long and continues posteriorly into the soft palate. It extends laterally into the inferior meatus and medially to the nasal septum.

MEDIAL WALL

The medial wall of the nasal cavity is represented by the septum, which is composed of cartilaginous and bony segments (Fig. 1–15). The cartilaginous segment consists of the quadrilateral cartilage, with a contribution from the lower and upper cartilages. The upper margin of the septal cartilage is connected to the posterior border of the internasal suture and to the upper lateral cartilages. Anteriorly, this cartilage is related to the medial crura of the lower lateral cartilages at its superior level, and inferiorly, it rests on the anterior nasal spine. This spine is an extension of the maxillary crest, and it is positioned like the prow of a sailing ship. Also, inferiorly the quadrilateral cartilage sits in the groove of the maxillary crest. The bony elevation on the floor of the nose on which the entire cartilaginous septum sits is shaped much like the lines of a railroad track. The bony segment of the nasal septum includes the perpendicular plate of the ethmoid bone and the vomer. The perpendicular plate forms the upper and anterior part of the bony septum and is continuous above with the cribriform plate. The vomer is located below and behind the perpendicular plate of the ethmoid bone. The long anterior border of the vomer articulates with the perpendicular plate superiorly and with the quadrilateral cartilage inferiorly. The inferior border is related to the nasal crest formed by the maxillae and the palatine bones.

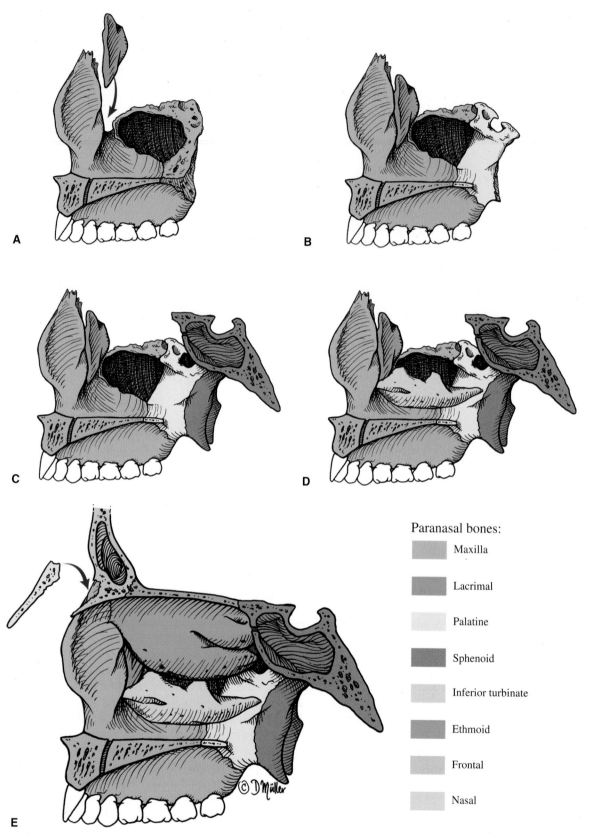

Paranasal bones:

Maxilla

Lacrimal

Palatine

Sphenoid

Inferior turbinate

Ethmoid

Frontal

Nasal

© D.Müller

FIGURE 1–16 Osteology of the right lateral nasal wall (medial view). (A) Articulation of the maxilla with the lacrimal bone. (B) Articulation of the maxilla with the palatine bone. (C) Articulation of the maxilla with the sphenoid bone. (D) Articulation of the maxilla with the inferior turbinate. (E) Articulation of the maxilla with the ethmoid labyrinth and nasal bone.

These structures of the nasal septum are covered by a mucosal envelope of mucoperichondrium and mucoperiosteum.

LATERAL NASAL WALL

The lateral nasal wall is a very complex anatomical structure and a very important area clinically. The lateral wall of the nasal cavity can be divided into three areas: Anteriorly, the lateral nasal wall consists of the frontal process of the maxilla and the lacrimal bone; the middle area is formed by the ethmoid labyrinth, the maxilla, and the inferior turbinate; and the posterior portion of the lateral nasal wall is represented by the perpendicular plate of the palatine bone and the medial pterygoid plate of the sphenoid bone. The osteology of the lateral nasal wall is complex and represented by eight bones, which are articulated in such a way as to build up a firm bony structure (Fig. 1–16).

The most important features of the lateral wall of the nasal cavity are the turbinates (Fig. 1–17). There are usually three (or rarely four), and they appear as delicate shelflike bony structures protruding from the lateral nasal wall covered by ciliated columnar mucous epithelium. The superior, middle, and inferior turbinates are present in almost all individuals, and a very small supreme turbinate may also occur. The supreme, superior, and middle turbinates are included in the ethmoid bone. The inferior turbinate is an independent bone. The air spaces below and lateral to the turbinates are named the superior, middle, and inferior meatus, respectively. They communicate with the common nasal cavity at the lower edge of each meatus (Fig. 1–18).

The inferior surfaces of the free-hanging portions of the turbinates are almost parallel to the nasal floor, but their supporting attachments usually are oriented diagonally from posterior-inferior to anterior-superior. Each supporting portion is called a primary lamella. There are five lamellae located from anterior to posterior: the uncinate process, the ethmoid bulla, the basal lamella of the middle turbinate, the basal lamella of the superior turbinate, and the fifth lamella of the supreme turbinates when present (Fig. 1–7). The superior and supreme turbinate lamellae are relatively horizontal.

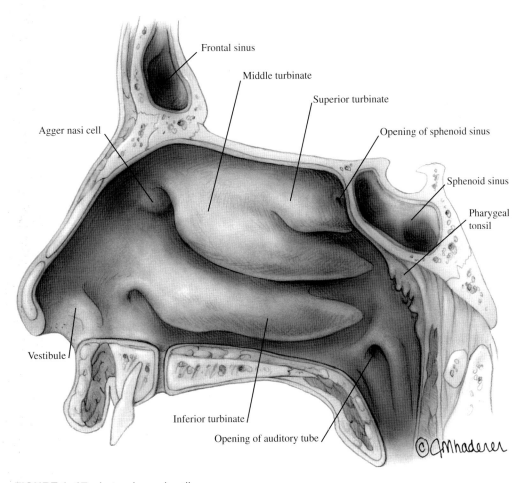

Frontal sinus
Middle turbinate
Superior turbinate
Agger nasi cell
Opening of sphenoid sinus
Sphenoid sinus
Pharygeal tonsil
Vestibule
Inferior turbinate
Opening of auditory tube

FIGURE 1–17 Lateral nasal wall.

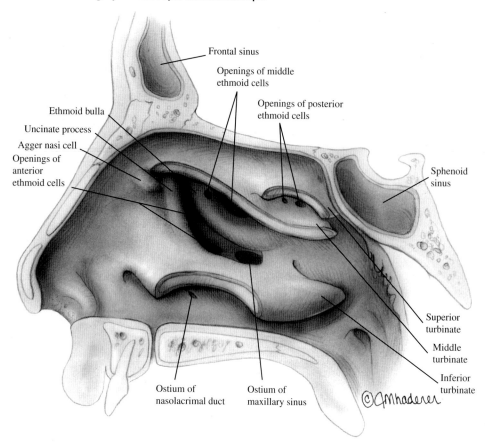

FIGURE 1–18 The turbinates are cut, and the meatus area is exposed.

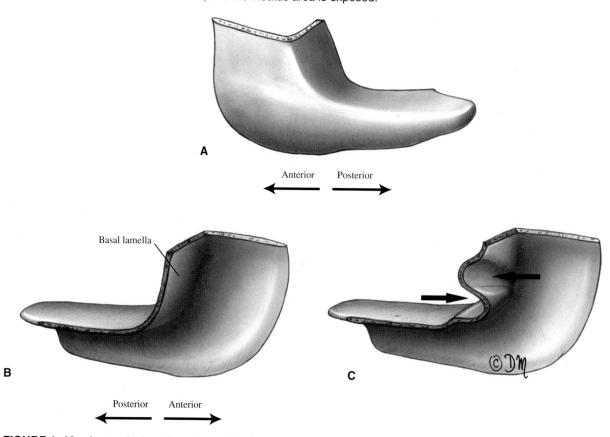

FIGURE 1–19 Anatomical configuration of the basal lamella of the right middle turbinate. (A) Medial view. (B) Lateral view. (C) Lateral view with distortion of the basal lamella by the ethmoid cells.

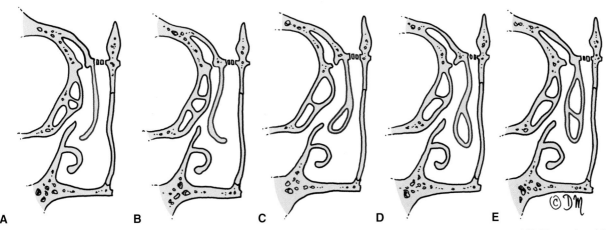

FIGURE 1–20 Anatomical variations of the middle turbinate. (A) Normal. (B) Paradoxical turbinate. (C) Normal turbinate with partial pneumatization. (D) Paradoxical turbinate with partial pneumatization. (E) Concha bullosa.

The superior turbinate belongs to the ethmoid bone, and it measures ~1.5 cm in length. The superior turbinate is attached to the lamina papyracea of the ethmoid bone by a thin bony partition. It is usually pneumatized, and it forms part of the posterior ethmoidal cells. The superior meatus lies between the middle and superior turbinates and contains the ostia of the posterior ethmoidal cells. Immediately behind the superior meatus is situated the sphenopalatine foramen. A small ridge, the supreme turbinate, is sometimes visible above the superior turbinate. If a supreme turbinate is present, a fifth basal lamella arises from it and extends laterally.

The middle turbinate is a portion of the ethmoid bone and is ~4 cm in length. The anterior end of the middle turbinate inserts into the ascending process of the maxilla and the posteromedial edge of the agger nasi. The superior attachment is in the paramedian sagittal plane and adheres to the lateral edge of the perforated portion of the cribriform plate along the ethmoid roof to a more vertical orientation along the lamina papyracea of the ethmoid bone. This twisting attachment of the middle turbinate bends within the middle third of the basal lamella, resulting in a prominent anterior vertical portion and a posterior descending horizontal plate (Fig. 1–19). The posterior portion of the insertion of the middle turbinate runs in a horizontal plane forming the roof of the posterior middle meatus. This posterior end is attached to the ethmoid crest of the perpendicular plate of the palatine bone. Pneumatization of the middle turbinate is frequent at its anterior end and in the main body mass. The pneumatized middle turbinate (also known as concha bullosa) is present in one-third of the population (Fig. 1–20). The middle turbinate is composed of a conchal bone, mucoperiosteum, a submucosal cavernous plexus, and respiratory mucous membrane.

The middle meatus lies between the middle and inferior turbinate attachments. The lateral wall of the middle meatus is the most important area of the lateral wall of the nasal cavity, as many of the paranasal sinuses open here. It houses several key anatomical structures: the uncinate process, the hiatus semilunaris, the ethmoid infundibulum, the ethmoid bulla, the lateral sinus, and the frontal recess. The term *ostiomeatal complex* is used to describe a group of anatomical structures belonging to the nasal lateral wall that are contributing to the final common drainage pathways of the anterior ethmoid, maxillary, and frontal sinuses. The ostiomeatal complex includes the middle meatus, the uncinate process, the hiatus semilunaris, the ethmoid infundibulum, the ethmoid bulla, the maxillary sinus ostia, and the frontal recess (Fig. 1–21).

Uncinate Process

The uncinate process (from the Latin *uncinatus*, meaning "hooked") is a thin, sagittally oriented lamella that runs anterosuperiorly to posteroinferiorly from the roof of the ethmoid bone to the perpendicular plate of the palatine bone and to the ethmoid process of the inferior turbinate. Three to five bony spicules unite the inferior convex border with similar structures of the ethmoid process of the inferior turbinate. The posterior end of the uncinate process curves laterally upward toward the roof of the maxillary sinus and may be continuous with the perpendicular plate of the palatine bone, or a complete bony absence may occur. This bony absence allows the mucosa of the maxillary sinus to contact the mucosa of the lateral nasal wall. This area is called the posterior fontanelle. A similar dehiscence in the uncinate process at its articulation with the inferior turbinate is termed the anterior fontanelle, and it is located anterior to the natural ostium of the maxillary

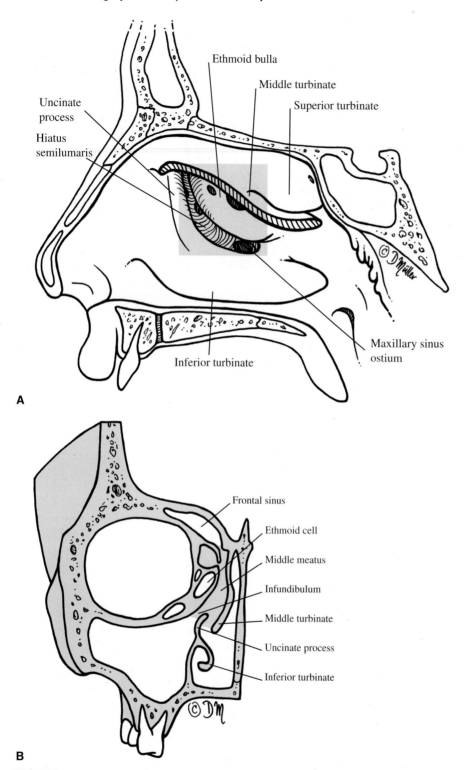

FIGURE 1–21 The ostiomeatal complex is illustrated after removing the middle turbinate (cut edge shaded). It includes the middle meatus, the uncinate process, the hiatus semilu-naris, the ethmoid infundibulum, the ethmoid bulla, the maxillary sinus ostia, and the frontal recess. (A) Lateral view after removing the middle turbinate. (B) Coronal section.

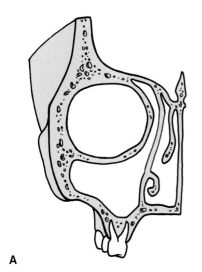 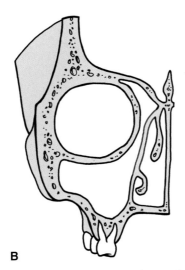 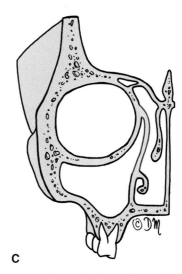

A   B   C

FIGURE 1–22   Anatomical variations of the uncinate process. Its superior portion may attach to the roof of the ethmoid bone centrally (A), to the middle turbinate medially (B), or to the lamina papyracea laterally (C).

sinus. Perforation of these membranes leads to openings of accessory ostia of the maxillary sinus. The upper portion of the uncinate process is hidden by the insertion of the middle turbinate, and it runs a variable course (Fig. 1–22). It may attach to the roof of the ethmoid bone, or it may also turn medially and fuse with the middle turbinate. When the uncinate process inserts laterally on the lamina papyracea, the ethmoid infundibulum is closed superiorly by a blind pouch named the recessus terminalis. In this situation, the ethmoid infundibulum and the frontal recess are separated from each other, and so the frontal sinus drains into the middle meatus medial to the infundibulum (Type I). When the uncinate process is inserted into the middle turbinate, the frontal recess and, consequently, the frontal sinus open directly into the ethmoid infundibulum (Type II) (Fig. 1–23).

The uncinate process may itself become pneumatized and provoke narrowing of the ethmoid infundibulum. Also, it can expand anteriorly and develop into infundibular cells. These cells may extend anteriorly and superiorly as far as the lacrimal bone, thereby creating the ethmolacrimal cells. The uncinate process can occasionally be absent and be replaced by a fibrous band.

Hiatus Semilunaris

The hiatus semilunaris is the two-dimensional space between the posterior edge of the uncinate process and the anterior wall of the ethmoid bulla. The hiatus semilunaris is usually hidden by the overhanging middle turbinate. It measures ~1.5 to 2 cm in length and runs from its inferior end in an anterosuperior direction. The hiatus semilunaris forms the doorway that leads to a lateral space called the ethmoid infundibulum.

Ethmoid Infundibulum

The ethmoid infundibulum is the three-dimensional space bounded by the uncinate process medially, the ethmoid bulla posteriorly, and the lamina papyracea laterally. The entire length of the ethmoid infundibulum may reach 4 cm, depending on the shape of the uncinate process. The ethmoid infundibulum can be entered through the hiatus semilunaris. The anterior end may extend to the posterior surface of the agger nasi cells or, in some cases, to the ascending process of the maxilla. The infundibular space is wider anterosuperiorly and narrower at its more posterior end because of the union of the uncinate process with the inferior turbinate and the membranous anterior fontanelle. The greatest width (free margin of the uncinate process to the lamina papyracea) is 5 to 6 mm, but in some cases it can be very shallow because the uncinate process runs close to the lamina papyracea (~1–1.5 mm away). The ethmoid infundibulum may be almost atelectatic according to anatomical variations of other structures such as paradoxical bending of the middle turbinate, a concha bullosa, or a hypoplastic maxillary sinus. In the most extreme conditions it may disappear if pathologic lesions compress the uncinate process laterally against the lamina papyracea.

The lateral surface of the ethmoid infundibulum leads to the medial wall of the maxillary sinus, where the ostium of the maxillary sinus resides. Its size is variable, with a diameter of 1 to 4 mm, and it can be round or elliptical or formed of two or three openings. An accessory maxillary opening is often found posterior to the true ostium.

Depending on the anatomical configuration of the uncinate process and the degree of pneumatization of the ethmoid bulla, the superior side of the infundibular

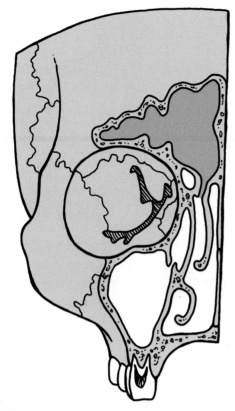 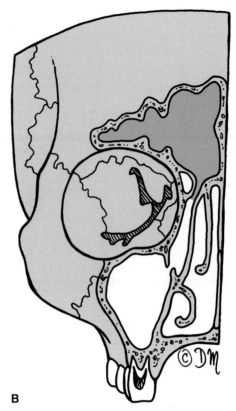

A   B

FIGURE 1–23 Frontonasal communication. (A) The frontal recess drains into the middle meatus (Type I). (B). The frontal recess opens directly into the ethmoid infundibulum (Type II).

space can communicate or not with the frontal recess. Normally, the frontal recess drains into the ethmoid infundibulum at its upper end if the anterior extremity of uncinate process has fused with the roof of the ethmoid or with the extension of the basal lamella of the middle turbinate. If the uncinate process inserts into the lamina papyracea, the ethmoid infundibulum is closed superiorly, creating a blind pouch called the recessus terminalis. In this situation, the frontal recess opens directly into the middle meatus medial to the ethmoid infundibulum.

Frontal Recess

The frontal recess is defined as the lower portion of the hourglass-shaped space above the level of the ethmoid infundibulum that gives access to the frontal sinus. The frontal recess represents the funnel-shaped lower part of the hourglass. Normally, the frontal sinus opens into the frontal recess through a channel that is less than 3 mm long, called the frontal ostium. The frontal ostium is usually found in the most anterosuperior part of the frontal recess.

The shape, dimensions, and limits of the frontal recess are determined by its surrounding structures. The agger nasi cells mark the anterior limit of the frontal recess. It is bounded above and in front by the floor of the

frontal sinus and its ostium. The fovea ethmoidalis creates the sloping posterosuperior boundary. The posterior wall of the frontal recess is variable, depending on the insertion of the ethmoid bulla. If the basal lamella of the ethmoid bulla ascends along its complete width and inserts into the roof of the ethmoid bone, it will form the posterior wall of the frontal sinus. However, this wall is often incomplete or absent, allowing the frontal recess to communicate with the space above, and occasionally behind, the ethmoid bulla, termed the lateral sinus. The posteroinferior part of the frontal recess is continuous with the infundibular cells and the ethmoid infundibulum. The medial boundary of the frontal recess depends on the anatomical configuration of the uncinate process and its superior attachment. If the attachment of the upper end of the uncinate process is the basal lamella of the middle turbinate, then the most anterosuperior part of the uncinate process becomes part of the medial wall of the frontal process also. In this situation, the frontal recess opens into the ethmoid infundibulum. The lateral wall of the frontal recess is formed mainly by the lamina papyracea. Sometimes the uncinate process inserts into the lamina papyracea instead of the middle turbinate, and in this case the uncinate process contributes to the lateral wall and to the floor of the frontal recess at its most anterior border. In this anatomical variation of the uncinate process the frontal recess opens directly into the middle meatus medial to the uncinate process.

The frontal recess communicates anteriorly with the pneumatized agger nasi cells. Occasionally the infundibular cells may extend posteriorly and laterally to the frontal recess and can reach as far as the fovea ethmoidalis. Also, a large cell in the head of the middle turbinate (concha bullosa) may open into the frontal recess from the medial side.

These and other anatomical variants, like the shape of the ethmoid bulla, may dictate the configuration of the frontal recess to a large extent. If the bulla is well pneumatized and extends far forward, the frontal recess will be narrowed. If there is also marked pneumatization of the agger nasi cells and the frontal ethmoid cells, the frontal recess may be reduced in volume and limited to a small tubular lumen. This anatomical variation probably gave rise to the term *nasofrontal duct*,[12] which has contributed to some confusing terminology presented in the past. For that reason, the nasofrontal duct is more appropriately named the frontal recess.

Ethmoid Bulla

The ethmoid bulla (also named bulla ethmoidalis) is a hollow bony protuberance situated in the lateral wall of the middle meatus behind the uncinate process. It is the most constant and largest of the anterior ethmoid air cells, with ~20 mm in length. There may be up to four cells pneumatizing the bulla, with the most common one being located superoposteriorly. It is pneumatized in 70% of all individuals, but, occasionally, the ethmoid bulla may not be pneumatized[12] and may even be absent.

Laterally, the bulla is attached to the lamina papyracea along its entire length from the upper to the posteroinferior end. Posteriorly, the ethmoid bulla may expand to the vertical portion of the basal lamella of the middle turbinate. Superiorly, the bulla may fuse with the roof of the ethmoid sinus, thereby forming the posterior wall of the frontal recess. If the bulla does not reach the roof of the ethmoid bone, the intervening space between it and the basal lamella is named the lateral sinus. A very large bulla may obliterate the space for the lateral sinus. On the contrary, a bulla that is wide open on its superior surface will make a large space for the lateral sinus and allow communication between the suprabullar ethmoid infundibulum and the sinus itself. The posterior wall of the bulla is incomplete in 25% of the population,[10] and this anatomical variant permits direct communication into the lateral sinus and/or suprabullar cells.

Lateral Sinus

The lateral sinus is a variable space not always present superior and posterior to the ethmoid bulla. This cleft is bounded by the ethmoid bulla anteriorly, the roof of the ethmoid superiorly, and the vertical portion of the basal lamella of the middle turbinate posteriorly. The lateral wall of the lateral sinus is the lamina papyracea, and, medially, this space faces the middle meatus. Depending on the configuration of the ethmoid bulla and the basal lamella of the middle turbinate, the lateral sinus may communicate with the frontal recess anteriorly, or it may be separated by the bulla inserting into the roof of the ethmoid bone. The lateral sinus drains into the middle meatus through a channel that runs posterior and superior to the ethmoid bulla if the anterior communication with the frontal recess is completely blocked. The lateral sinus may also communicate with the ethmoid bulla.

Agger Nasi

The agger nasi is a smooth bony swelling in the frontal process of the maxilla situated in front of the anterior insertion of the middle turbinate. Anteriorly, it can reach the bony nasal aperture. Superiorly, the agger nasi extends to the floor of the frontal sinus and contributes to the limitation of the frontal recess. Posteriorly, the agger nasi can reach the anterior attachment of the middle turbinate. The posterosuperior border is related to the anterior ethmoid infundibulum and lies along the inferior surface of the frontal recess. The medial wall of the agger nasi is attached to the anterosuperior portion of the uncinate process. The lateral wall can extend to the lacrimal bone and/or the orbital wall. Anterolateral to the agger nasi and running parallel to it is the nasolacrimal duct. The agger nasi, the frontal recess, and the nasolacrimal duct all lie in the same coronal plane. The opening of agger nasi is variable, but it drains into the anterior middle meatus and into the ethmoid infundibulum.

Inferior Turbinate

The inferior turbinate is an independent anatomical structure composed of the inferior conchal bone, mucoperiosteum, a submucosal cavernous plexus, and respiratory mucous membrane. The bone is scroll-shaped and attached to the conchal ridge of the medial process of the maxilla and the palatine bone (Fig. 1–24). It also articulates with the lacrimal bone by its lacrimal process and covers the lacrimal groove to form the bony canal for the nasolacrimal duct. The attachment of the inferior turbinate to the lateral nasal wall resembles a hockey stick with an angle between the short and the long process.

The surface of the bone is very irregular, perforated and grooved by many vessels, and covered by a strong attachment of the mucoperiosteum. The submucosal cavernous plexus of the inferior turbinate contains erectile tissue and responds to autonomic innervation and possibly endocrine influences. Consequently, the size of the turbinate may change significantly in response to

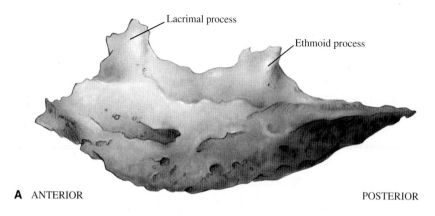

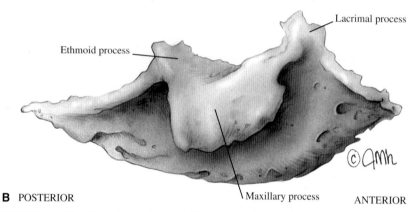

FIGURE 1–24   The right inferior turbinate. (A) Medial surface. (B) Lateral surface.

several different stimuli, decreasing the nasal airway. The respiratory mucous membrane here has a higher goblet cell density than that on the middle turbinate.

The inferior meatus lies inferolateral to the inferior turbinate. The nasolacrimal duct is the only structure that opens in this meatus. The duct opens close to the angle between the two attachment limbs of the inferior turbinate, which is situated anteriorly (Table 1–3).

TABLE 1–3   Drainage Areas of the Paranasal Sinus and Related Structures

Sphenoethmoid recess
• Sphenoid sinus
Superior meatus
• Posterior ethmoid cells
Middle meatus
• Ethmoid infundibulum
   – Frontal sinus
   – Maxillary sinus
   – Anterior ethmoid cells
   – Agger nasi cells
Inferior meatus
• Nasolacrimal duct (anterior third)

Vasculature, Innervation, and Lymphatic Drainage of the Nasal Cavity

The vascular supply of the nasal cavity is derived from three major arterial sources: the ophthalmic artery from the internal carotid artery, the internal maxillary artery, and the facial artery from the external carotid artery. The ophthalmic artery gives off the anterior and then the posterior ethmoid arteries along the medial wall of the orbit (Fig. 1–25). The anterior ethmoid artery supplies much of the blood flow to the nasal septum and anterior portion of the lateral nasal wall. The posterior ethmoid artery contributes to the arterial plexus of the posterior portion of the nasal septum and parts of the middle and superior turbinates. The internal maxillary artery gives off numerous branches, among them the greater palatine artery and the terminal division, the sphenopalatine artery (Fig. 1–26). The greater palatine branches irrigate the anterior floor and posterior region of the nasal fossa. The sphenopalatine artery vascularizes the posterior segment of the median nasal septum, as well as the lateral nasal wall, namely, the nasal turbinates and their meati. Terminal branches of these vessels form a rich anastomotic plexus in the mucope-

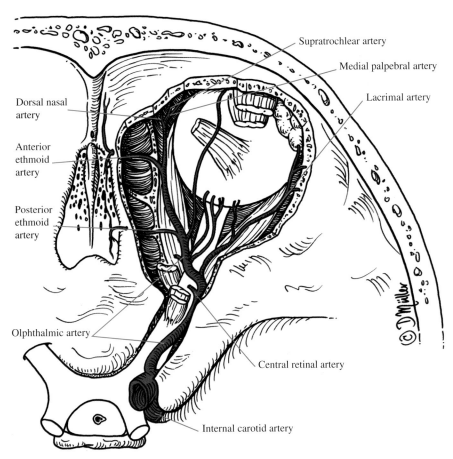

Dorsal nasal artery

Anterior ethmoid artery

Posterior ethmoid artery

Olphthalmic artery

Supratrochlear artery

Medial palpebral artery

Lacrimal artery

Central retinal artery

Internal carotid artery

FIGURE 1–25   The ophthalmic artery and its main branches, axial view.

riosteum. The facial artery divides into several branches, including the superior labial artery that supplies blood to the columella, nasal vestibule, and anterior lateral nasal wall (Figs. 1–27, 1–28). All of these vessels form a plexiform network in the mucosa and contribute to the Kiesselbach's plexus on the anterior septum, the most common site of epistaxis. The venous drainage of the nose is primarily from the anterior and posterior ethmoid veins through the ophthalmic vein and the sphenopalatine vein to the pterygoid plexus of veins. Because these venous structures usually do not possess valves, infection may be propagated throughout the entire septum, affecting the dural venous sinuses (especially the cavernous sinus) and resulting in severe, life-theatening complications.

The nasal cavity is supplied by a complex network of nerves that have different functions: sensory innervation, autonomic innervation, and olfaction. Sensory innervation of the nasal cavities is supplied by the branches of two divisions of the trigeminal nerve, the ophthalmic (V_1) and the maxillary nerves (V_2) (Fig. 1–29). The ophthalmic nerve (V_1) has several important branches: the nasociliary nerve and its terminal branches, the anterior and posterior ethmoid nerves. They supply the anterior part of the nasal septum and the anterior half of the lateral wall of the nose with a small contribution to the posterior nasal septum and superior turbinate through the posterior ethmoid nerve.

The second division of the trigeminal nerve, the maxillary nerve (V_2), gives off numerous branches, among them the nasopalatine, the anterosuperior alveolar, and the infraorbital nerves. The nasopalatine nerve innervates the posterior and inferior areas of the septum and the superior, middle, and inferior turbinates; the anterosuperior alveolar nerve supplies the most anterior and inferior portions of the nasal septum floor of the nasal cavities and lateral nasal wall; and the infraorbital nerve provides sensory innervation to the nasal vestibule, columella, nasal tip, and alar regions (Figs. 1–30, 1–31).

The autonomic innervation of the nasal cavities consists of sympathetic and parasympathetic systems. The sympathetic innervation to the nose and sinuses arises in the upper two thoracic segments of the spinal cord, ascending to the superior cervical sympathetic ganglion. Postganglionic sympathetic fibers course through

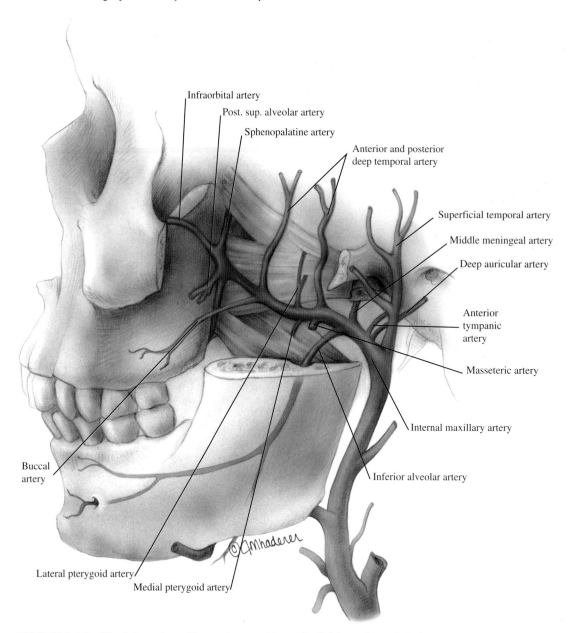

FIGURE 1–26   The internal maxillary artery and its main divisions, lateral view.

the carotid plexus and follow the internal and external carotid arteries to their final destination on small arterioles in the mucosa, where they provoke vasoconstriction (Fig. 1–32). The parasympathetic innervation for the nose and sinuses arises from the superior and inferior salivatory nuclei. These brain stem nuclei send off neurons that join the facial nerve. Some of the parasympathetic fibers branch off the facial nerve at the geniculate ganglion into the greater superficial petrosal nerve, ending at the pterygopalatine ganglion. Postganglionic parasympathetic fibers from this ganglion follow the sphenopalatine nerve through the sphenopalatine foramen into the posterior area of the nose to innervate the nose and the sinuses. These fibers terminate on blood vessels and mucous glands within the mucosa (Fig. 1–33). Stimulation leads to mucosal congestion due to dilatation of the blood vessels and increased production of mucous. The olfactory nerve, cranial nerve I, is the shortest of the 12 cranial nerves. The nerve fibers arise from the ciliated olfactory cells located in the olfactory epithelium covering the inferior surface of the cribriform plate, the superior turbinate region of the lateral wall of the nasal cavity, and the upper part of the septum. This is a region 2 to 5 cm² medial to lateral and 30 to 200 μm thick. The region may decrease and be replaced by respiratory epithelium with age. This

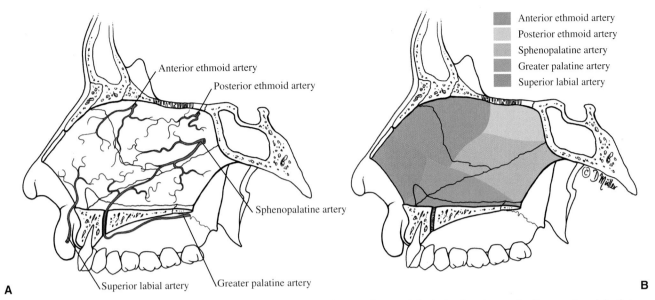

FIGURE 1–27   Blood supply to the nasal septum. (A) Four major arteries contribute to develop a plexiform network in the mucosa. (B) Areas of vascularization corresponding to the different vessels.

surface area, however, is considerably increased by the cilia of the olfactory receptor cells, which are thin (0.2 μm diameter) and nonmyelinated. The cells join together into about 20 olfactory nerve bundles, which pass through the foramina of the cribriform plate to reach the olfactory bulb. Each bundle carries a tubular sheath of dura and pia-arachnoid, which may pose a potential risk for cerebrospinal fluid leakage in injuries of the ethmoid roof. The olfactory bulbs sit over the cribriform plates and are situated on the undersurface of the

frontal lobe of the brain as swellings where the olfactory nerve fibers synapse in the glomeruli of the bulb (Fig. 1–30).

The resulting olfactory tracts pass back on the inferior surface of the frontal lobe to the olfactory trigone, from which diverging bundles establish a great number of connections with the hypothalamus, hippocampus, and other brain regions. These complex pathways are responsible for the difficult interaction of smell, taste, feeding behavior, and reproduction.

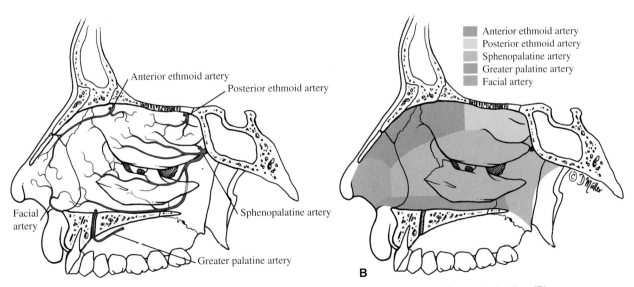

FIGURE 1–28   Blood supply to the lateral wall of the nose (A) showing its main areas of vascularization (B).

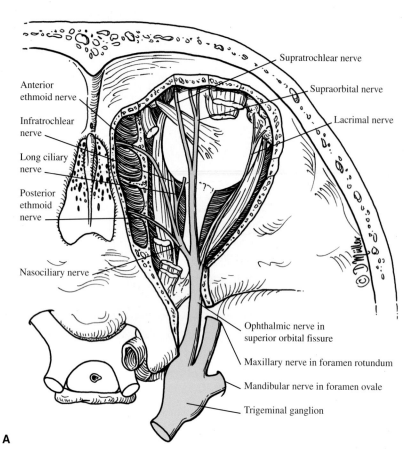

Supratrochlear nerve

Supraorbital nerve

Lacrimal nerve

Anterior
ethmoid nerve

Infratrochlear
nerve

Long ciliary
nerve

Posterior
ethmoid
nerve

Nasociliary nerve

Ophthalmic nerve in
superior orbital fissure

Maxillary nerve in foramen rotundum

Mandibular nerve in foramen ovale

Trigeminal ganglion

A

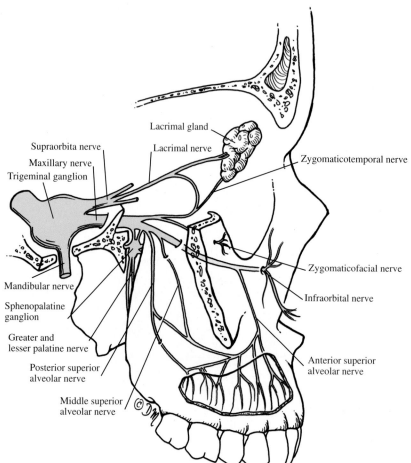

Lacrimal gland

Lacrimal nerve

Supraorbita nerve

Maxillary nerve

Trigeminal ganglion

Zygomaticotemporal nerve

Mandibular nerve

Sphenopalatine
ganglion

Greater and
lesser palatine nerve

Posterior superior
alveolar nerve

Middle superior
alveolar nerve

Zygomaticofacial nerve

Infraorbital nerve

Anterior superior
alveolar nerve

B

FIGURE 1–29 The trigeminal nerve. The three main branches are the ophthalmic (V_1), maxillary (V_2), and mandibular nerves. (A) Axial view. (B) Lateral view.

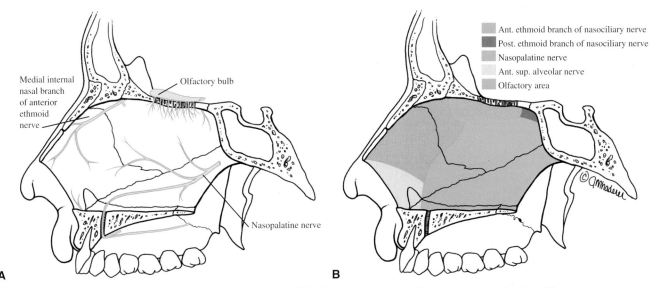

FIGURE 1–30   Sensory innervation of the nasal septum (A) with the corresponding areas of distribution (B).

The lymphatic drainage of the anterior part of the nasal cavities follows the vascular channels and joins those of the external nose to reach the submandibular nodes. Posteriorly, it drains into the retropharyngeal lymph nodes or passes directly to the deep cervical lymph chain. In addition, there are connections along the olfactory nerves draining into the subdural and subarachnoid spaces.

Paranasal Sinus

The paranasal sinuses are a group of pneumatic cavities surrounding the nasal cavity and lying immediatly

adjacent to the orbit, brain, and other vital neural and vascular structures. There are three paired paranasal sinuses on each side of the head—the maxillary, ethmoid, and frontal sinuses (Fig. 1–34)—and one single posterior midline sinus generally divided into two cavities, the sphenoid sinus.[28-37]

Maxillary Sinus

The maxillary sinus is a pyramidal-shaped cavity within the maxillary bone. This bone consists of a body and four processes that articulate with surrounding structures. The body has the configuration of a quadrilateral

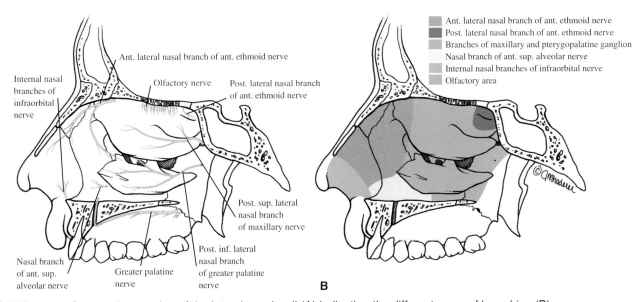

FIGURE 1–31   Sensory innervation of the lateral nasal wall (A) indicating the different areas of branching (B).

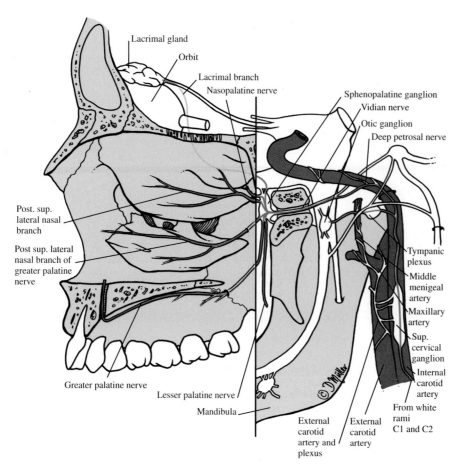

Lacrimal gland
Orbit
Lacrimal branch
Nasopalatine nerve
Sphenopalatine ganglion
Vidian nerve
Otic ganglion
Deep petrosal nerve
Post. sup. lateral nasal branch
Post sup. lateral nasal branch of greater palatine nerve
Tympanic plexus
Middle menigeal artery
Maxillary artery
Sup. cervical ganglion
Internal carotid artery
From white rami C1 and C2
Greater palatine nerve
Lesser palatine nerve
Mandibula
External carotid artery and plexus
External carotid artery

FIGURE 1–32 Sympathetic innervation of the nose and paranasal sinuses, lateral view. Preganglionic sympathetic fibers enter the superior cervical ganglion where they synapse. The resulting postganglionic fibers follow along the internal and external carotid arteries and branches to their destinations.

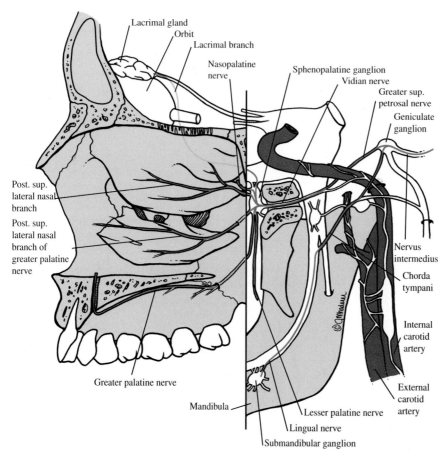

Lacrimal gland
Orbit
Lacrimal branch
Nasopalatine nerve
Sphenopalatine ganglion
Vidian nerve
Greater sup. petrosal nerve
Geniculate ganglion
Post. sup. lateral nasal branch
Post. sup. lateral nasal branch of greater palatine nerve
Nervus intermedius
Chorda tympani
Internal carotid artery
Greater palatine nerve
Mandibula
Lesser palatine nerve
Lingual nerve
Submandibular ganglion
External carotid artery

FIGURE 1–33 Parasympathetic innervation of the nose and the paranasal sinuses. Preganglionic fibers course along the facial nerve and then through the geniculate ganglion to the greater superficial petrosal nerve and vidian nerve to the sphenopalatine ganglion. Postganglionic parasympathetic secretomotor fibers pass to the blood vessels and mucous glands of the mucosa.

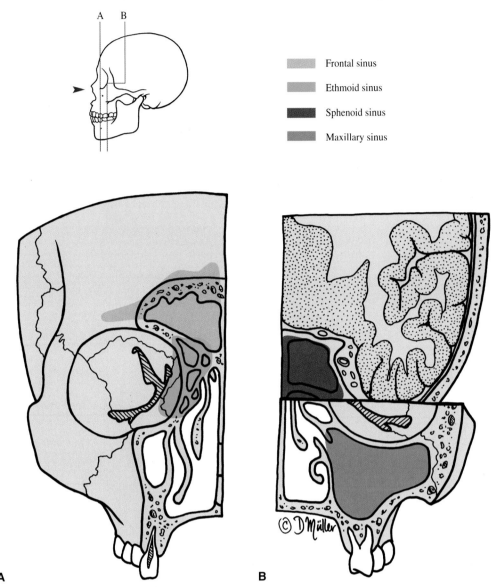

Frontal sinus

Ethmoid sinus

Sphenoid sinus

Maxillary sinus

FIGURE 1–34 Schematic drawing of the paranasal sinuses. (A) Coronal view along cut A. (B) Coronal view (at two different levels) correponding to cut B.

pyramid. The maxillary bone has four processes: The frontal process is articulated with the frontal bone and the nasal bone; the zygomatic process is connected with the zygomatic bone; the alveolar process is fused with the contralateral alveolar process, forming an alveolar arch containing the dentition; and the palatine process is linked with the palatine bone to constitute the roof of the mouth (Fig. 1–35).

The average adult dimensions of the sinuses are 36 to 45 mm in height, 38 to 45 mm in length, and 25 to 33 mm in width. The mean volume is 14.25 cc.

The quadrilateral pyramid of the maxillary sinus with its apex directed into the zygomatic process of the maxillary bone is limited by five walls: the medial, the ante-rior, the posterolateral, the superior, and the inferior walls.

The *medial wall* of the maxillary sinus (also considered the base of the pyramid) lies in juxtaposition to the lateral wall of the nasal cavity at the level of the middle and inferior meatus. The configuration of this medial wall is complex, and for descriptive purposes it may be divided into thirds vertically (Fig. 1–36).

The superior third is bony anteriorly and posteriorly. It is composed of the upper nasal surface of the body of the maxillary bone and a large opening that communi-cates with the maxillary sinus. This bony hiatus is re-duced in size by contributions from the lower border of the ethmoid labyrinth, the lateral wall of the ethmoid

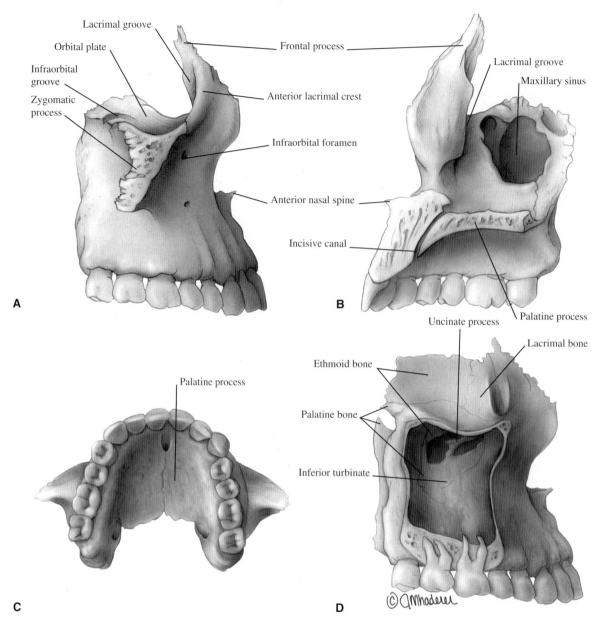

FIGURE 1–35   Bony anatomy of the maxilla. (A–C). Lateral, medial, and inferior views. The presence of the frontal, zygomatic, alveolar, and palatine processes. The maxilla contains the infraorbital foramen, the anterior portion of the spheno-palatine foramen, and the incisive canal. (D) Internal configuration of the maxillary sinus after removing part of the anterior, posterolateral, superior, and inferior walls to show the external view of the medial wall.

bulla above, the inferomedial descending process of the lacrimal bone as it forms part of the nasolacrimal duct anterosuperiorly, the maxillary process of the inferior turbinate below, and the perpendicular plate of the palatine bone posteriorly. In addition, the long arm of the uncinate process passes obliquely from anterosuperomedial to posteroinferolateral in the lateral wall of the middle meatus to connect with the inferior turbinate. It is the junction of the long and short arms of the J-shape of the uncinate process that articulates with the inferior

turbinate. The inferolateral edge of the uncinate process divides the upper anterior part of the maxillary hiatus into anteroinferior and posterosuperior areas. The remaining defect is closed by mucosa from both the nasal cavity and the maxillary sinus as it covers a thin fibrous layer (a continuation of the periosteum) to form two fontanelles, one anterior and one posterior, according to the divisions by the uncinate process.

The posterosuperior fontanelle contains the nasal opening of the primary maxillary ostium, which repre-

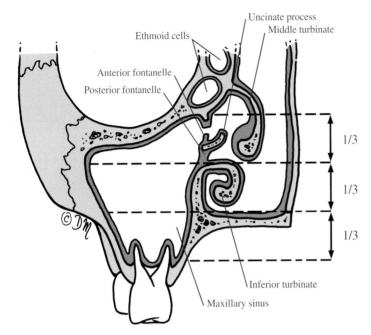

FIGURE 1–36 Coronal section passing halfway between the anterior and posterior boundaries of the maxillary sinus showing the vertical division of the sinus into thirds.

sents the point of embryological outpouching of nasal mucosa from the ethmoid infundibulum. In most instances, the ostium is located in the posterior third of the ethmoid infundibulum, in the superomedial aspect of the medial sinus wall. The ostium varies widely in size and shape, but the mean size is 2 to 3 mm, and it may be duplicated, but rarely. There are one to three accessory maxillary ostia usually found within the anteroinferior fontanelle. They are located below and in front of the primary maxillary ostium and sometimes behind it. The primary and accessory ostia may be united without a separating membranous ridge. Such a union forms an exceptionally large ostium within the ethmoid infundibulum.

The ridge created by the nasolacrimal duct courses in the anterior bony part of the medial wall in front of the maxillary hiatus. The duct passes from the anterosuperomedial corner of the maxillary sinus down and slightly backward to open in the inferior meatus at the junction of its anterior and middle thirds.

The middle third of the medial wall is situated below the inferior turbinate and forms the lateral wall of the inferior meatus. The inferior third of the medial wall is the alveolar process of the maxillary bone.

The *anterior wall* of the maxillary sinus is represented by the anterior wall of the maxilla. It extends from the pyriform aperture medially to the maxillozygomatic suture laterally, and from the infraorbital rim superiorly to the alveolus inferiorly. The anterior surface is directed forward and slightly laterally and contains several elevations on the inferior area over the roots of the teeth. Above the elevations are slight depressions, including the canine fossa, the thinnest region of bone, which lies

above the canine tooth. The lateral and central incisors are not part of the maxilla, and therefore the maxillary sinus does not relate to their dental roots. Above the canine fossa there is a funnel-shaped opening called the infraorbital foramen through which pass the infraorbital vessels and nerve. It lies ~5 mm below the inferior orbital ridge. The bone surrounding this foramen is quite thick. The anterior and lateral walls of the maxillary sinus are related to the soft tissues of the middle third of the face.

The *lateral and posterior walls* of the maxillary sinus are formed by the zygomatic bone and the greater wing of the sphenoid bone. These walls are formed by a curved plate of bone that is usually thick on the lateral side and quite thin on the medial aspect of the posterior portion. The posterosuperior and medial sides of the maxillary bone are related to the posterior ethmoid sinus and the ascending plate of the palatine bone. The maxillary tuberosity lies inferiorly and is often hollowed out by the sinus. The tuberosity articulates with the pyramidal process of the palatine bone and the lateral pterygoid plate of the sphenoid bone.

The lateral and posterior walls form the anterior boundary of the pterygopalatine fossa and the pterygomaxillary fissure. Entrance into the pterygopalatine fossa is gained through the pterygomaxillary fissure, which transmits the maxillary vessels. This fissure is situated on the medial wall of the infratemporal fossa and is represented by the space between the pterygoid process of the sphenoid bone and the convex posterior surface of the maxilla (Fig. 1–37).

The pterygopalatine fossa is pyramidal in shape and is formed by three bones: the maxilla, the palatine bone,

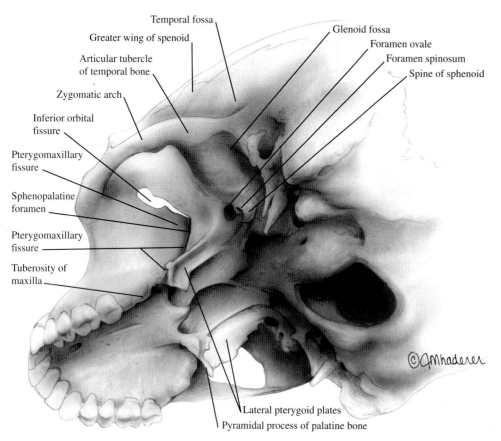

FIGURE 1–37   Osteology of the infratemporal fossa. Note that the anterior border of the lateral pterygoid plate forms the posterior limit of the pterygomaxillary fissure, which is the entrance to the pterygopalatine fossa.

and the pterygoid process of the sphenoid bone. It communicates with the interior of the skull through the foramen rotundum, which transmits the maxillary division of the trigeminal nerve, with the orbit via the inferior orbital fissure containing the infraorbital artery (a continuation of the maxillary artery), and with the nasal cavity by the sphenopalatine foramen, which carries the sphenopalatine artery. Extending posteriorly from this fossa is the pterygoid canal, which is crossed by the nerve of the pterygoid canal (also called the vidian canal).[38,39] Inferiorly, the fossa becames constricted and ends in the pterygopalatine canal, which conducts the greater palatine vessels and nerves.

The pterygopalatine fossa contains the pterygopalatine ganglion (a parasympathetic ganglion of the facial nerve carrying both postganglionic parasympathetic and sympathetic fibers), located high in the fissure. Postsynaptic parasympathetic fibers leave this ganglion and distribute with branches of the maxillary division of the trigeminal nerve. These fibers are secretomotor in function and provide parasympathetic innervation to the lacrimal gland and the mucosal glands of the nasal fossa, palate, and pharynx. The pterygopalatine ganglion is also a peripheral regulatory center for the innervation of the vessels of the nasal mucosa. The stimulation of this ganglion may produce redness, swelling, increased secretions from the nasal mucosa, and hyperemia of the orbital contents. This ganglion lies at a distance of 3 to 4 mm to the optic nerve and to the posterior ethmoid cells and also has a relationship with the maxillary and sphenoid sinuses. Inflammatory disorders of the nasal sinuses may produce pterygopalatine ganglion neuralgia after resolution of the inflammation. The pain radiates from the nose downward over the maxilla after inflammation of the maxillary sinus; backward toward the mastoid process to the parietal bone after inflammation of the posterior ethmoid cells; and to the occiput, the neck, and the scapula after inflammation of the sphenoid sinus.

The *superior wall* of the maxillary sinus represents the majority of the floor of the orbit. The orbital floor also includes the orbital process of the palatine bone posteromedially and the zygomatic bone anterolaterally. The orbital process of the palatine bone lies at the apex of the floor of the orbit and articulates posteriorly between the ethmoid bone and the maxilla (Table 1–4).

TABLE 1–4 Bones of the Orbit

Region	Maxilla	Frontal	Ethmoid	Lacrimal	Zygoma	Sphenoid	Palatine
Apex						Lesser wing, body	
Floor	Orbital plate				Orbital process		Orbital process
Roof		Orbital plate				Lesser wing	
Medial wall	Frontal process		Lamina papyracea	Orbital surface		Body	
Lateral wall					Orbital process	Greater wing (orbital surface)	
Base	Orbital rim	Orbital rim			Orbital rim		

The zygoma of the orbital floor thickens anteriorly to form part of the infraorbital rim, which is situated at a higher level than the orbital floor (Fig. 1–38). The superior wall of the maxillary sinus is very thin and has a somewhat triangular shape extending posterolaterally to the infraorbital fissure. This roof of the maxillary sinus slants inferiorly in a medial to lateral direction and slopes upward from anterior to posterior. The infraorbital fissure ends ~15 mm from the infraorbital rim. About 5 mm behind this point the infraorbital nerve (which has been traveling in the fissure) makes a right-angled bend medially and continues in a more inferior direction as it enters the infraorbital canal. This canal is often noted as a groove in the roof of the maxillary sinus containing the infraorbital vessels and nerve. It is occasionally absent, and in such cases the infraorbital vessels and nerve hang within the maxillary sinus and are more exposed to sinus infections and surgical trauma. The infraorbital canal exits the bone at the infraorbital foramen on the anterior wall of the maxilla. Near its midpoint this canal gives off a small canal for the anterosuperior dental vessels and nerve.

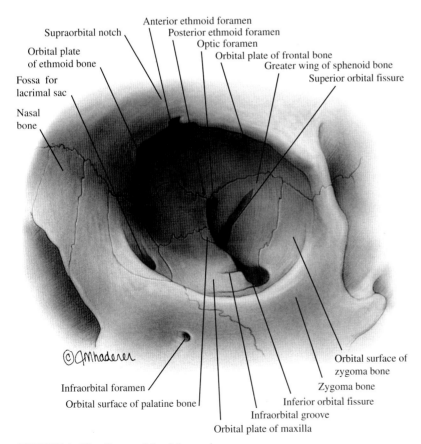

FIGURE 1–38 Bony orbit, oblique view.

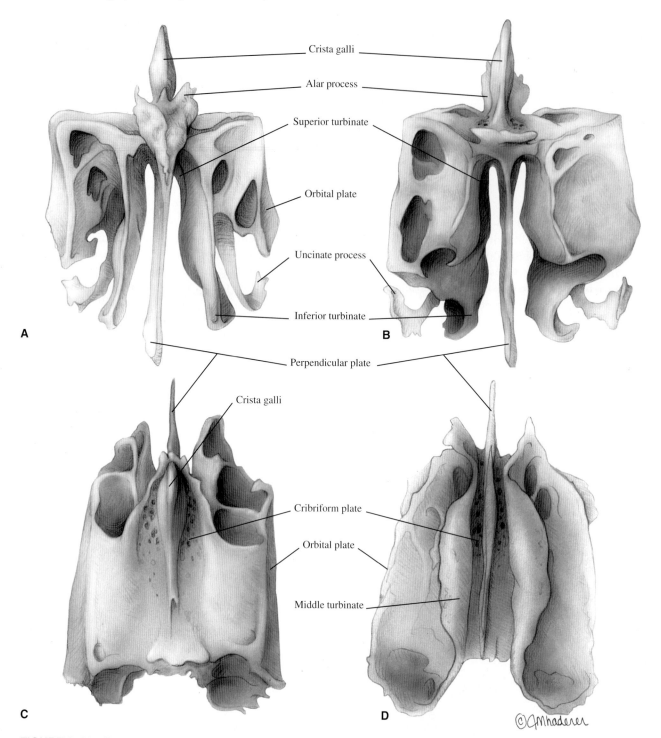

FIGURE 1–39   Bony anatomy of the ethmoid bone and its sinus. (A) Posterior view. (B) Anterior view. (C) Superior view. (D) Inferior view.

The *inferior wall or floor* of the maxillary sinus is curved rather than flat and is formed by the alveolar process of the maxilla. It extends inferiorly from the body of the maxilla and supports the teeth within bony sockets. Each maxilla contains a full quadrant of five deciduous or eight permanent teeth. The relationship of the maxillary teeth to the sinus varies according to the size of the sinus, the degree of pneumatization of the alveolar process, the dental age, and the state of preservation of the dentition. The roots of the premolars and the upper molars may ridge the floor of the sinus or project into it.

The floor may be divided by incomplete bony septa lying between the roots of the teeth (mainly in the posterior part of the sinus), which make the sinus floor irregular. The projecting roots are usually separated from the maxillary sinus by bone of variable thickness, but sometimes by mucosa alone. Periapical or periodontal inflammation of upper premolars and molars may therefore spread to the maxillary sinus, and endodontic treatment or extraction of these teeth may penetrate into the sinus.

The maxillary sinus may present anatomical variations related to the degree of pneumatization, its expansion to the surrounding structures, and the presence of septation. The maxillary sinus cavity may be so large that it extends into adjacent structures. This occurrence is recognized by recesses extending into the hard palate, the zygomatic bone, the alveolar process, regions around the infraorbital canal, the palatine bone, and the prelacrimal area. The cavity of the maxillary sinus may be divided either completely or partially by vertical, oblique, or horizontal bony or membranous septations. A separate or distinct duplication of the maxillary sinus may rarely occur on either side. The decreased development or lack of development of the maxillary sinus may occur alone or in association with other congenital anomalies such as cleft palate, choanal atresia, and mandibulofacial dysostosis. Hypoplasia of the maxillary sinus is observed in a small percentage of individuals, and total aplasia has been reported in rare cases.

Ethmoid Sinus

The ethmoid sinus is a complex group of small cavities located within the ethmoid bone, an unpaired bone situated in the median region above the level of the maxilla, between the floor of the anterior cranial fossa and the attachment of the uncinate process to the inferior turbinate. The ethmoid bone contributes to the floor of the anterior cranial fossa, the medial wall of the orbit, the nasal septum, and the lateral wall of the nasal cavity. It is ~3.3 cm × 2.7 cm × 1.4cm in size and contains 3 to 15 cells.

The ethmoid bone consists of five parts: a superior prominence (the crista galli), horizontal plate (the cribriform plate), a midline perpendicular plate (the perpendicular plate of the nasal septum), and two lateral masses or labyrinths suspended from the horizontal arms in the shape of a cross (Fig. 1–39).

The *crista galli* is the superior median projection of the ethmoid bone, which may vary in size and pneumatization.

The *perpendicular plate* is a central sagittal structure with a quadrilateral shape that forms the upper part of the bony nasal septum. It articulates anteriorly and superiorly with the nasal spine of the frontal bone and with the nasal bones, posteriorly with the sphenoidal crest and vomer, and inferiorly with the quadrilateral cartilage. Superiorly, it is attached to the cribriform plate.

The *cribriform plate* separates the anterior cranial cavity above from the nasal cavity below. It is composed of two narrow plates on either side perforated by olfactory nerve fibers, processes of dura, and ethmoid vessels and nerves. The cribriform plate lies at a lower level than the roof of the ajdacent ethmoid air cells and tends to slope downward as it passes posteriorly. The cribriform plate is divided into three parts: a thick horizontal medial portion that contains 20 or more foramina for the olfactory fibers; a lateral portion (also named lateral lamella) that arises from the horizontal segment at an angle to join the orbital plate of the frontal bone; and, the junction of the horizontal and lateral parts, which is the attachment point of the middle turbinate and superior turbinate to the ethmoid roof.

The lateral lamella can be thick, thin, or even absent. The angle at which it rises determines the height of the olfactory groove in the anterior cranial floor (Fig. 1–40). A more horizontal lateral cribriform plate produces a shallow olfactory groove. A lateral cribriform plate that rises almost perpendicular to join the ethmoid roof creates a narrow olfactory groove. In this second situation, the lateral edge of the middle turbinate is an extension of the lateral cribriform plate. In the same individual the cribiform plates of the two sides may be at different levels.

The *lateral ethmoid labyrinths* are found at the lateral side of the cribriform plate medial to each orbit and are constituted by thin, lightweight bony plate structures. The ethmoid labyrinth, as the name implies, is the most complex of all the sinuses and may be considered the pivotal sinus in the pathophysiology of the inflammatory sinus diseases. Each ethmoid labyrinth has the shape of a quadrilateral prism, measuring 4 to 5 cm in length and 2.5 to 3 cm in height. The bone is more narrow anteriorly (usually around 0.5 cm) and wider posteriorly (~1.5 cm). For the purposes of anatomical description, it is

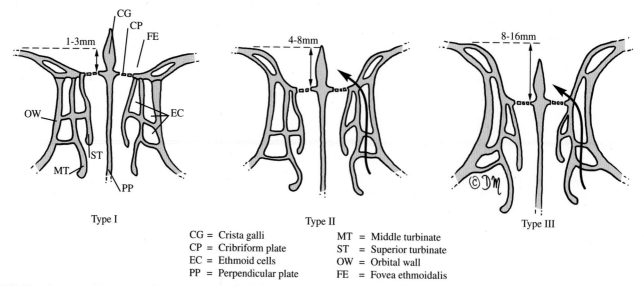

CG = Crista galli
CP = Cribriform plate
EC = Ethmoid cells
PP = Perpendicular plate

MT = Middle turbinate
ST = Superior turbinate
OW = Orbital wall
FE = Fovea ethmoidalis

FIGURE 1–40 The three variations of the olfactory fossa showing the thin lateral lamella of the cribriform plate and its increasing height from Type I to Type III.

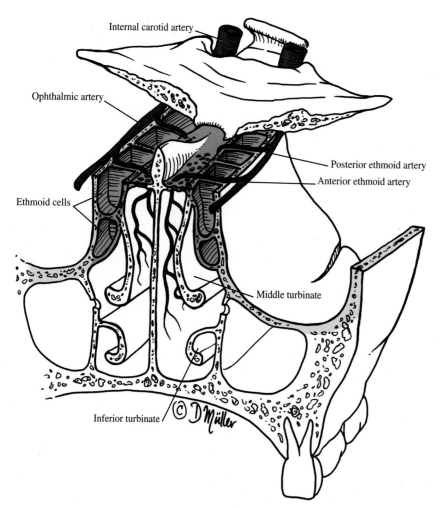

FIGURE 1–41 Schematic drawing of the course of the anterior ethmoid artery as it crosses three distinct cavities: the orbit, the ethmoid labyrinth, and the anterior cranial fossa.

best to consider the ethmoid labyrinth as a quadrilateral block with a roof and lateral, medial, inferior, anterior, and posterior walls.

The *roof of the ethmoid labyrinth* is thin and open, and it is closed by the stronger bony plates of the frontal bone. The junction of this structure with the lateral lamella of the cribriform plate defines the frontocribriform suture. This suture is situated in the medial wall of the ethmoid labyrinth above the level of the olfactory groove. The other bony plate of the frontal bone articulates with the lamina papyracea of the ethmoid bone to form the frontoethmoid suture and to close the roof of the ethmoid labyrinth. This suture is related to the medial orbital wall. The roof of the labyrinth is also known as the fovea ethmoidalis. The fovea is not a flat plate of bone but an undulating one because the domes of the most superior ethmoidal cells bulge into it, giving it such a contour. The anterior part of the fovea ethmoidalis lies more superiorly than the posterior one because the floor of the anterior cranial fossa descends 15 degrees from a horizontal plane as it passes posteriorly.

The *lateral surface of the ethmoid labyrinth* forms most of the medial wall of the orbit and is called the lamina papyracea. It is a thin, flat, smooth, rectangular bony plate that articulates with the frontal bone superiorly, the lacrimal bone anteriorly, the maxilla inferiorly, and the lesser wing of the sphenoid bone posteriorly. Along the frontoethmoid suture lie two foramina: the anterior and posterior ethmoid foramina.

The two foramina constitute very important landmarks, and they will be described in more detail.

The anterior ethmoid foramen is crossed by the anterior ethmoid artery, a terminal branch of the ophthalmic artery (Fig. 1–41). This foramen is located in the frontoethmoid suture ~25 mm posterior to the anterior rim of the lacrimal fossa. The anterior ethmoid artery traverses three distinct cavities: the orbit, the ethmoid labyrinth, and the anterior cranial fossa. It courses medially between the superior oblique and medial rectus muscles and turns posteriorly for a variable short distance to exit the orbit through the anterior ethmoid foramen. The artery enters the anterior ethmoid cana,l which passes in an anterior and medial direction from its opening either in the medial orbital wall or within the roof of the ethmoid labyrinth, where it crosses the ethmoid cells. The anterior ethmoid canal may be absent, and the artery and the nerve are then exposed to the ethmoid air cells. It then moves across the olfactory groove floor to the anterior base of the crista galli, where it gives off an important meningeal branch. At the level of the olfactory groove floor, at the side of the crista galli, the artery and the accompanying nerve pass through the cribriform plate to enter the nasal cavity at the upper nasal septum and lateral wall of the nose and sends a terminal branch to the dorsum of the nose

between the nasal bone and upper lateral cartilages. The anterior ethmoid artery, accompanied by the nerve, supplies the anterior and middle ethmoid cells and the frontal sinus.

The posterior ethmoid foramen is located within the frontoethmoid suture in the lateral ethmoid wall ~7 mm anterior to the anterior rim of the optic canal, although it may be absent. This foramen is the begining of the posterior ethmoid canal, which courses almost directly medial to its foramen. The smaller posterior ethmoid artery runs through the canal in the medial orbital wall to supply the posterior ethmoid cells, and also gives off a meningeal branch before terminating in nasal branches to the septum and lateral nasal wall that anastomose with the sphenopalatine artery.

The most critical area of the entire ethmoid region is the location where the anterior ethmoid artery enters the anterior cranial fossa through the lateral lamella of the cribriform plate.[40] This point is considered the area of least resistance because the lateral lamella is only one-tenth as strong as the roof of the ethmoid. This point of the lateral lamella can be extremely thin or even absent, and this is adjacent to the junction of the bony plate of the frontal bone with the lateral lamella of the cribriform plate.[41]

The *medial and inferior walls of the ethmoid labyrinth* must be considered together, for they comprise almost a slightly convex curved plane that bows into the nasal cavity. The medial wall of the ethmoid sinus forms part of the lateral wall of the nasal cavity, as has been described previously. The ethmoid bone is superior and medial to the maxillary bone, with the articulating line at the surface of the lamina papyracea of the ethmoid bone and the orbital surface of the maxillary bone.

The medial wall of the ethmoid labyrinth is composed of the superior turbinate, the middle turbinate, and sometimes the supreme turbinate. The supreme turbinate is inconstant. The spaces between these turbinates are the meati and are named for the turbinate that forms the superior aspect of the meatal space. Thus, there are supreme, superior, and middle meatues.

Anatomical variations are frequently noted in the turbinates. A pneumatization of the middle turbinate is called a concha bullosa. This aeration may involve only the vertical lamina or the inferior bulbous portion, or it may reach the entire turbinate.[42–44] The pneumatization expands from the superior aspect downward as an extension of ethmoid pneumatization crossing superiorly or through the region of the frontal recess. Its drainage may flow into the middle meatus directly, into the ethmoid infundibulum, or into the sinus lateralis. Other common variations of the middle turbinate are related with its paradoxical position with a lateral curvature. This curve is opposite the usual medial scroll curvature and so is named paradoxical turbinate. The superior turbinate may also be pneumatized, but this is very unusual.

The support for these structures is a bony septum known as the basal (or ground) lamella that continues from the base of the turbinate and crosses laterally through the mass of the ethmoid cells to attach to the medial side of the lamina papyracea. These basal lamellae are relative constant anatomical findings despite the degree of pneumatization of the ethmoid labyrinth and the extensive deformations of the air cells in response to pneumatization.[45-47] The lamellae of the uncinate process (ethmoid bulla, middle turbinate, superior turbinate, and occasionally the supreme turbinate) can be observed in an anteroposterior direction (Fig. 1–8).

The basal lamella of the uncinate process (oriented in a sagittal plane) divides the meatal space medially from the uncinate space laterally. The basal lamella of the ethmoid bulla lies anterior to the lamella of the middle turbinate as a frontally oriented plate. It can reach the roof of the ethmoid bone and thus forms the posterior wall of the frontal recess. This wall can be missing, and in this situation there is a direct communication between the frontal recess and the lateral sinus located above and behind the bulla.[48-50]

The basal lamella of the middle turbinate is composed of two segments: the anterior portion, lying almost in a frontal plane, and the posterior half, lying in a horizontal plane. The frontal plane of the anterior portion can be modified by a large anterior ethmoid cell, which may extend to the anterior wall of the sphenoid sinus. Conversely, the posterior ethmoid cells can displace the basal lamella anteriorly, giving an S-shaped aspect to the vertical portion of the lamella. The great variability of the shape of the insertion of the middle turbinate has a great surgical significance, and it is a very important radiological landmark on a computed tomography (CT) scan (Fig. 1–42).

The basal lamella of the middle turbinate divides the entire ethmoid labyrinth into an anteroinferior group and a posterosuperior group with different cell systems (Fig. 1–43). In general, the cells of the anterior ethmoid group are more numerous (two to eight) but smaller, whereas those of the posterior group are larger but fewer in number (one to seven). This is due to the primitive ethmoid capsule, which was much wider posteriorly than anteriorly. The anterior group drains into the anterior infundibulum of the middle meatus and the posterior cells into the superior meatus. The basal lamella is not a straight divider because the developing air cells push and distort what was its original linear position in the fetal ethmoid bone.

The anterior part of the ethmoid labyrinth may reach the lacrimal bone, the smallest of the facial bones. This bone is located between the frontal process of the maxilla anteriorly and the ethmoid block posteriorly. It is frequently pneumatized with the group of the anterior ethmoid cells termed the agger nasi cells. On its lateral side, the lacrimal bone forms the posterior half of the lacrimal fossa.

The posterior group of the ethmoid labyrinth comprises the cells between the basal lamella of the middle turbinate and the anterior wall of the sphenoid sinus. Frequently, a large ethmoid cell, called the cell of Onodi, encroaches on the sphenoidal sinus and shares a common osseous wall. This cell is a large posterior ethmoid cell that invades the anterosuperior aspect of the sphenoid sinus and may be duplicated. It is sometimes mistaken for the sphenoid cells itself, but there are sphenoid sinus cells below it. The Onodi cells may extend posterolaterally to embrace or even surround the optic nerve. These cells may migrate to the body of the sphenoid and even reach the anterior wall of the sella turcica.

The architecture of anterior ethmoid cells tends to be more complicated than the posterior ethmoid cells. The ethmoid sinus contains several groups of cells of different sizes and shapes according to the amount of air filling the ethmoid cavities. Much of the final configuration of the ethmoid labyrinth depends on its initial location, the degree of pneumatization, its air cells, its extension to other adjacent bony structures the cells can enter (cellular colonization), and the development of septation. These thin septa are bony septa that divide the ethmoid cells into compartments or cellular groups.

The classification of the ethmoid cell groups has been the subject of varying proposals by several authors regarding their location, ostium sites, and place of origin. A system of classification will be presented here based on their location in relation to fixed anatomical features.[51]

The anterior ethmoid cells comprise three cellular systems: the bullar system, the uncinate system, and the meatal system (Fig. 1–44). The bullar system is situated between the basal lamella of the bulla anteriorly and the basal lamella of the middle turbinate posteriorly. It consists of one to four cells, the intrabullar cells and the suprabullar cells. They all drain into the bullar groove. The largest and most constant ethmoid cell is named the ethmoid bulla (bulla ethmoidalis) of the intrabullar cells. The suprabullar cells lie on the top of the bullar system, spreading laterally and posteriorly. Sometimes, they may reach the sphenoid sinus, lying parallel to the posterior ethmoid cells. This posterior extension changes the shape of the basal lamella of the middle turbinate, producing an S-shaped deformity. Occasionally, the suprabullar system may extend anteriorly to the frontal sinus, and it may even form a posterolateral bulla in the posterior wall of the frontal sinus. The bullar cells cause the bulla to appear rounded in the middle mea-

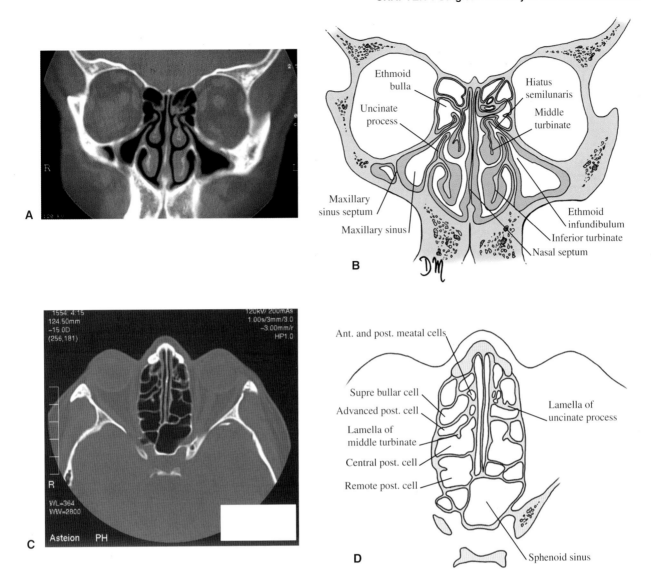

FIGURE 1–42 (A) Coronal CT scan of the nose and paranasal sinuses demonstrating the different anatomical structures. (B) Schematic diagram of the coronal CT scan. (C,D) Schematic diagram of the axial CT scan.

tus. It is usually these cells that expand in various directions and often account for the wide extramural ethmoid extensions. The uncinate system lies laterally to the basal lamella of the uncinate process, and its posterior limit is the basal lamella of the bulla. This system comprises three cells: the anterior, the superior, and the posterior, and sometimes one inferior. They all drain into the ethmoid infundibulum, above and behind the ostium of the maxillary sinus. The superior or terminal cell (Boyer's cell) may project superiorly and contributes to the formation of the frontal sinus. Sometimes this cell is autonomous, forming an external frontal bulla if it pneumatizes the frontal bone only partially. The anterior uncinate cell or agger nasi cell is not a constant finding, but when well pneumatized it produces a

smooth bony swelling on the lateral nasal wall in front of the anterior insertion of the middle turbinate. The word *agger* means "ridge," and some authors describe it as representing a vestigial turbinate. This cell may also pneumatize the frontal process of the maxilla, displacing the insertion of the uncinate process anteriorly. The posterior uncinate cell lies in front of the basal lamella of the bulla, but it is not common. The inferior uncinate cell is also described in the literature as Haller's cells. These cells can expand into the posterior, superior, and medial aspect of the maxillary sinus along the orbital floor. These cells may occur ocasionally (14% of cases),[52] but when present, their size can be impressive, and it may appear that they are a secondary or duplicated maxillary sinus. However, Haller's cells do not con-

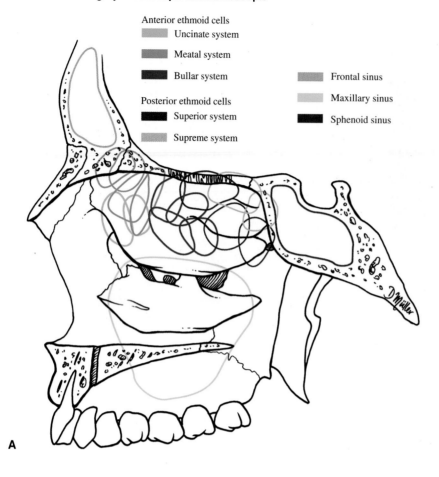

Anterior ethmoid cells
    Uncinate system
    Meatal system
    Bullar system

Posterior ethmoid cells
    Superior system
    Supreme system

    Frontal sinus
    Maxillary sinus
    Sphenoid sinus

A

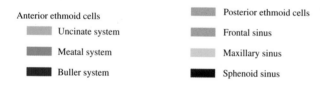

Anterior ethmoid cells
    Uncinate system
    Meatal system
    Buller system

Posterior ethmoid cells
Frontal sinus
Maxillary sinus
Sphenoid sinus

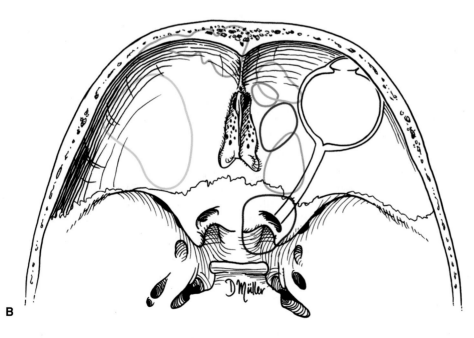

B

FIGURE 1–43 Schematic arrangement of the ethmoid labyrinth into anteroinferior and posterosuperior groups and its division in different cell systems. (A) Lateral view. (B) Endocranial projection of the ethmoid sinus and the other remaining paranasal sinuses.

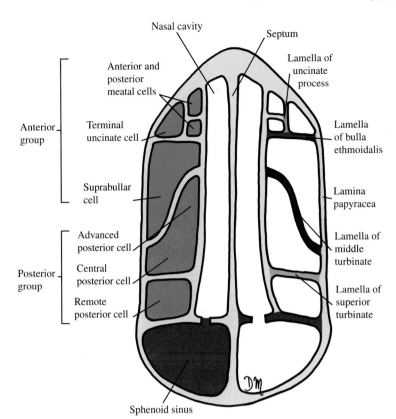

FIGURE 1–44 Basic cellular structure of the ethmoid labyrinth.

nect with the maxillary space, and they drain into the uncinate groove.

The meatal system is located medially to the basal lamella of the uncinate process, and its posterior limit is the basal lamella of the bulla. It is constituted by two cells: the anterior and the posterior meatal cells. The anterior cell has its origin in the fetal frontal recess and grows upward into the frontal bone, giving rise to the frontal sinus. The posterior meatal cell often protrudes into the posterior surface of the frontal sinus or may develop under the floor of the frontal sinus and bulge upward into it, creating a frontal bulla cell. All the meatal cells drain into the meatal groove.

For anatomical purposes, it is best to refer to two important landmarks for the anterior ethmoid group: (1) the most anterior smooth bony swelling represented by the agger nasi cells when well pneumatized in the frontal process of the maxilla and lacrimal bone located in front of the middle turbinate, and (2) the largest and most constant swelling designated by the ethmoid bulla and formed by the intrabullar cells.

The group of posterior ethmoid air cells are bounded by the basal lamella anteriorly and by the anterior wall of the sphenoid sinus posteriorly. Therefore, the posterior group of the ethmoid cells is above and behind the basal lamella, a very important landmark. The lateral wall of the posterior ethmoidal cells is formed by the lamina pa-

pyracea. The superior turbinate constitutes a major portion of the medial wall of this posterior group of ethmoid cells. Most of this space is occupied by a few large cells. The posterior ethmoid air cells are also characterized by incomplete septations. The posterior ethmoid group can be divided in two systems of cells: the superior (or central) and the supreme system of cells. The superior system is bounded by the basal lamella of the middle turbinate and the basal lamella of the superior turbinate posteriorly. It consists of the advanced posterior cell and the central posterior cell. The advanced posterior cell lies posterior to the basal lamella of the middle turbinate and often contributes to its twisting when the cell extends anteriorly and medially. The other central posterior cell is situated at the same level as the intrabullar cell of the anterior bullar system. Sometimes it is located between the advanced posterior and the remote posterior cell when it reaches the roof of the ethmoid bone. This superior or central group of cells drains into the superior meatus behind the advanced posterior cell. The supreme system of cells is located behind the basal lamella of the superior turbinate and is formed by the remote posterior cells. Usually these cells drain into the supreme meatus, but they may open into the superior meatus and thus should be considered as belonging to the superior system. This most posterior ethmoid air cell is in an upper position and may extend

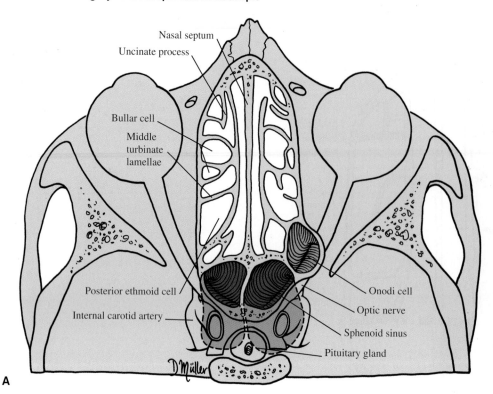

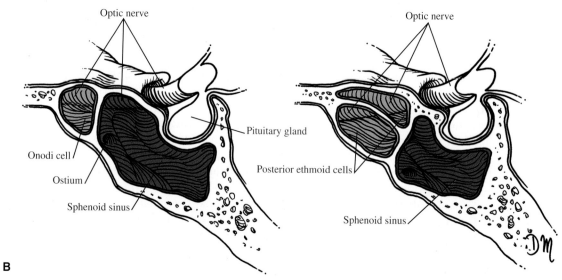

FIGURE 1–45   Sphenoid sinus. (A) Sagittal section showing its relationship with the optic nerve, internal carotid artery, and a posterior ethmoid cell (Onodi cell or sphenoethmoid cell). (B) Anatomical variations of the posterior ethmoid cells and their relationship with the sphenoid sinus and the optic nerve.

posterolaterally to embrace or even surround the optic nerve. It is called the sphenoethmoid or Onodi cell. It is present in 12% of individuals.[12] The bone surrounding the optic nerve at the posterosuperior corner of the ethmoid sinus is only 0.5 mm in thickness. However, the optic nerve is occasionally encountered bare, without

bony coverage in the Onodi cell or on the superolateral wall of the sphenoid sinus (Fig. 1–45). The Onodi cell is a very important anatomical landmark during the surgical approach to the posterior ethmoid cells and the lateral wall of the sphenoid sinus because of its relationship with the highly vulnerable optic nerve. The internal carotid artery may also project on the lateral wall of the posterior ethmoid cells. The posterior ethmoid cells may often expand beyond the confines of the ethmoid bone into the palatine bone, the maxilla, or the middle turbinate.

The remaining two basal lamellae are thin bony partitions. The basal lamella of the superior turbinate is attached to the lamina papyracea ~3 to 8 mm anterior to the optic nerve. This junction also marks the location of the posterior ethmoid artery. If a supreme turbinate is present, a fifth basal lamella arises from it and extends laterally to the lamina papyracea.

Frontal Sinus

The frontal sinus is contained within the frontal bone, one of the unpaired skull bones forming the anterior portion of the calvaria (Fig. 1–46). The frontal bone makes a major contribution to the floor of the anterior cranial fossa and, in doing so, forms the roof of the orbits. The frontal bone articulates with the ethmoid, sphenoid, parietal, and nasal bones, as well as with the zygoma and the maxilla (Fig. 1–47). The frontal bone occasionally presents a persistent midline metopic suture.

The frontal sinus is a triangular, pyramid-shaped cavity extending between the anterior and posterior tables of the ascending portion of the frontal bone. The apex

of the pyramid is superior, and the base lies inferiorly. The frontal sinus stretches superiorly into the superciliary region and posteriorly above the medial portion of the roof of the orbit, although it has been observed to extend as far as the sphenoid sinus. Its lateral extension has been reported to be well beyond the orbit and into the lateral portion of the frontal bone. The inferior extension may reach the nasal bone and the frontal process of the maxilla.

There are two frontal sinuses separated completely by a bony septum, which is located approximately in the midline. Bilateral asymmetry is a frequent anatomical finding, and the intersinus septum may be deviated as a result. Each sinus is further divided into incomplete chambers by a bony intrasinus septation, which creates deep recesses of the sinus, giving the sinus its scalloped configuration. Thus, the interior surface of the frontal sinus is often irregular because of the bony projections from the different walls. Ocasionally, accessory frontal sinuses are formed by the invasion of adjacent anterior ethmoid cells into the frontal bone. If an accessory frontal sinus is present before the definite frontal sinus is fully expanded, a bulla frontalis in the wall of the frontal sinus may signify the presence of a smaller accessory sinus (Fig. 1–48).

The two frontal sinuses are separated by a bony ridge, the crest of the frontal bone, in the midline on the intracranial surface. Also, at the midline and at the base of

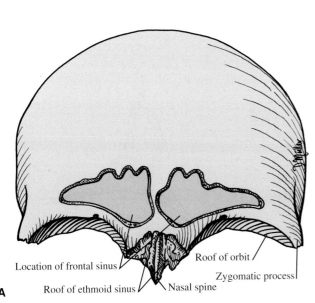

A

Location of frontal sinus *Roof of orbit* *Zygomatic process* *Roof of ethmoid sinus* *Nasal spine*

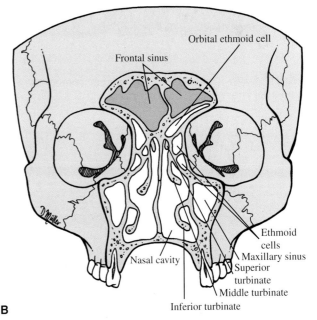

B

Orbital ethmoid cell *Frontal sinus* *Ethmoid cells* *Maxillary sinus* *Superior turbinate* *Middle turbinate* *Inferior turbinate* *Nasal cavity*

FIGURE 1–46 Bony anatomy of the frontal bone and its sinuses. (A) Frontal view. The anterior wall of the frontal bone has partially been removed to expose the sinus. (B) Coronal section. Orbital ethmoid cells often intrude between the orbit and the frontal sinus floor.

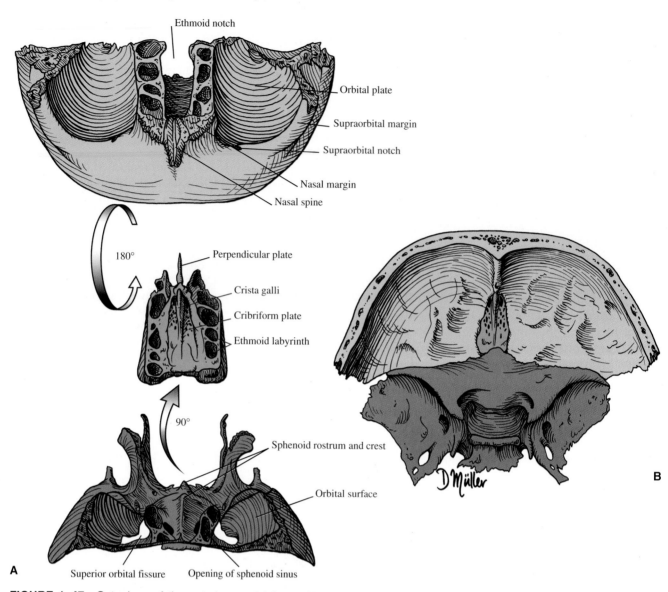

FIGURE 1–47 Osteology of the anterior cranial fossa. (A) Articulation of the frontal bone with the ethmoid and sphenoid bones. (B) The resulting bony structure of the anterior cranial fossa.

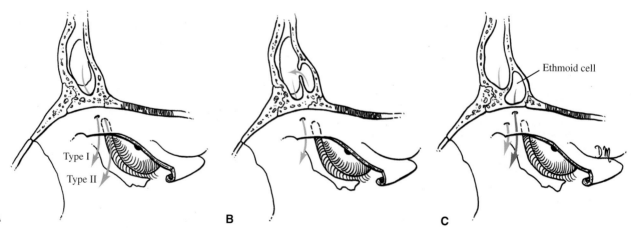

FIGURE 1–48 Anatomical variations of the frontal sinus, sagittal section. (A) Normal frontal sinus with Type I or Type II drainage systems. (B) Diverticulum of the frontal sinus with the same drainage system. (C) Ethmoid cell (frontal bulla) encroaching into the frontal sinus.

the frontal bone lies the foramen cecum, which is crossed by the emissary vein between the nasal cavity and the anterior extremity of the superior sagittal sinus.

The average frontal sinus measures 2.8 cm in height, 2.4 cm in width, and 2 cm in depth. The volume of the frontal sinus is highly variable, ranging form 0 to 37 cc, with a mean of 10 cc. The sinus cavity is deepest in the midline close to the floor of the frontal sinus at the level of the supraorbital ridge. The frontal sinus is bounded by anterior, posterior, medial, and inferior walls.[53–57] The inferior wall is the frontal sinus floor.

The *anterior wall* of the sinus forms the forehead and is by far the thickest of all sinus walls, measuring up to 12 mm. There is a definite trilayered bony structure identical to the rest of the calvaria with anterior and posterior tables and a middle diploë in all of the walls of the sinus, although the diploë is reduced in the posterior wall and floor of the sinus.

The posterior wall is a plate of thin, compact bone (1–2 mm) whose upper part is vertical. It gradually curves downward and posteriorly until it is almost horizontal (depending on the level of pneumatization of the orbital roofs that has occurred). The posterior wall of the frontal sinus is also the anterior wall of the anterior cranial fossa and can extend as far posteriorly as to the lesser wing of the sphenoid bone. The thin posterior wall of the frontal sinus is attached to the dura of the anterior cranial fossa; therefore, infections from the frontal sinus can spread through its posterior wall, resulting in an extradural abcess. The proximity of this sinus to the bone marrow of the frontal bone permits the spread of infection from the sinus directly into the bloodstream. This may explain the abcesses that develop elsewhere in the skull or even in a more distant site when an infection occurs within the sinus.

The *medial wall* of the frontal sinus is represented by the intersinus septum, the thin segment of bone that may occasionally have interruptions. This septum may be deviated so far laterally that it tends to lie over the contralateral sinus. However, the most inferior portion of this intersinus septum is always located in the same plane as the nasal septum and close to or at the midline. The frontal septum can become horizontal, with one sinus covering the other one.

The *inferior wall* of the frontal sinus is formed by the orbital roofs on the lateral side and the nasoethmoid floor on the medial side. The orbital roof is made of thin bone, as in the posterior wall of the frontal sinus. The floor of the sinus is convex above and inward and extends laterally over the orbital cavity, depending on the size of the sinus. The floor of the frontal sinus corresponding to the nasoethmoid floor is located near the midline and overlaps, in part, the fovea ethmoidalis and overlies the anterior ethmoid sinus. The most anterior area of the sinus floor is directly above the roof of the nose. It consists of a very thick bony mass of the nasal spinous process of the frontal bone, or internal nasal spine (spina nasalis interna), fused to the bones of the nose and to the frontal process of the maxilla.

At the frontal sinus floor close to the anteromedial aspect of the intersinus septum rests the frontal sinus ostium (Fig. 1–49). The frontal sinus ostium marks the site where pneumatization of the sinus began. It has a conical shape that leads to a narrow opening inferiorly called the frontal recess. The frontal sinus drainage pathway has an hourglass shape composed of three distinct segments: The top part of the hourglass is the frontal infundibulum, which is the inferior portion of the frontal sinus cavity narrowing like an upright funnel toward the second segment, the frontal ostium. The

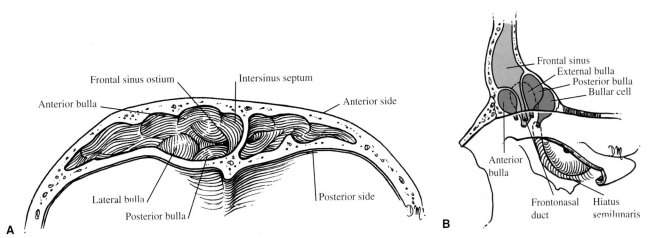

FIGURE 1–49 Location of the frontal sinus ostium (superior view) and its relationship with adjacent ethmoid cells at the nasoethmoid floor. (A) Axial view. (B) Sagittal view.

third segment is the inferior air chamber named the frontal recess. This functional unit for frontal sinus drainage has been referred to as the frontal sinus outflow tract. Thus, the drainage from the frontal sinus into the frontal recess is accomplished through the frontal sinus ostium, or, according to some authors,[12] through the nasofrontal duct, depending on the embryogenic origin of the frontal sinus. When the sinus develops directly as an extension of the frontal recess, it drains into the frontal recess through a short channel with a length less than 3 mm termed the frontal ostium. However, when the origin of the frontal sinus is from one of the cells of the ethmoid infundibulum, this canal is 3 mm or greater, resembling a tubular structure and named the nasofrontal duct. In this situation, the expanding anterior ethmoid cells of the frontal recess distort and displace with their growth the position of the canal, causing a serpentine course upward to the frontal sinus, thus giving rise to the nasofrontal duct. This duct leads from the anteromedial side of the frontal sinus floor into the infundibulum of the middle meatus. The term *nasofrontal duct* should be avoided because this structure lacks the tubular appearance the word *duct* implies. In reality, the walls and boundaries of the frontal recess belong to the adjacent structures, making the frontal recess a passive space and not a true duct.

Sphenoid Sinus

The sphenoid sinus is generally a set of paired, asymmetric cavities lying within the sphenoid bone. This bone is one of the most complex bones in the human body, forming the main part of the central skull base, a portion of the lateral skull, most of the apical component of the orbit, and the posterior wall of the nasopharynx. It is attached to the basiocciput, the petrous, and the squamous portions of the temporal bone. The sphenoid bone is the largest single bone in the skull base and is composed of a body that gives rise to the structures the sella turcica, the lesser wings (superiorly), the greater wings, the pterygoid plates (inferiorly), and the upper part of the clivus (Fig. 1–50). The sphenoid bone resembles a butterfly and contributes to the floor of the middle cranial fossa. The body of the "butterfly" is formed by the body of the sphenoid bone, and the wings are represented by the greater wings of the sphenoid bone. The remainder of the floor of the middle cranial fossa is formed by the petrous and squamous parts of the temporal bone.

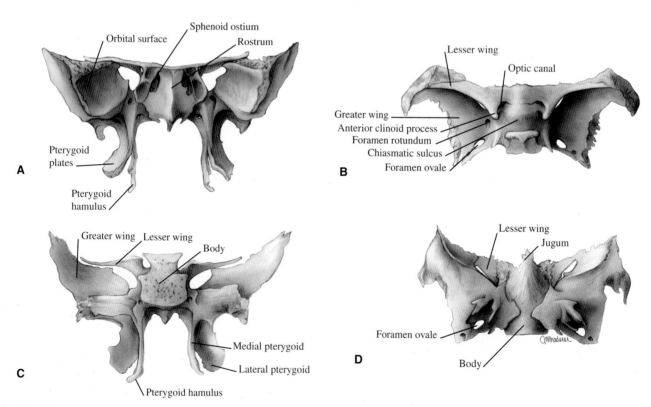

FIGURE 1–50   Bony anatomy of the sphenoid bone. (A) Anterior view. (B) Superior view. (C) Posterior view. (D) Inferior view.

The sphenoid sinus is located inside the body of the sphenoid bone. It has six sides toward the endocranial cavity and two sides toward the nasal cavity and nasopharynx.

The *superior wall or roof* of the sphenoid sinus is very thin and contributes to the anterior and middle floors of the base of the skull. It lies in direct contact, from front to back, with the olfactory nerves, the optic chiasm, and the hypophysis. The roof of the sphenoid sinus is in continuity with the roof of the ethmoid sinus, and this provides a useful landmark for surgical dissection. The bony walls of each lateral side are also very thin and composed of two areas: the orbital area in front and the cranial area behind. Depending on the degree of pneumatization of the sphenoid sinus, it is possible to see, immediately ajdacent to the lateral walls of the sphenoid bone, several very important structures: the internal carotid artery, the optic nerve, and, more posteriorly, the cavernous sinus and its contents.[58–61]

The *posterior wall* of the sphenoid bone forms the floor of the sella turcica, which is also known as the hypophyseal or pituitary fossa. It is composed of three parts: an olive-shaped swelling called the tuberculum sellae, a saddle-like depression called the hypophysial fossa, and posteriorly the dorsum sellae.

The *anterior wall* of the sphenoid bone faces the upper region of the nasal cavity and is connected to the perpendicular plate of the ethmoid and vomer in the midline and to the lateral masses of the ethmoid bone on each side. Between these attachments remains a free vertical surface above each nasal cavity on either side of the nasal septum. The anterior wall can be displaced by well-developed Onodi cells of the posterior ethmoid sinus. In this situation, the optic nerve is surrounded by the Onodi cells (Fig. 1–45). It is on this vertical surface that the sphenoethmoid recess is located above the choana and between the superior or supreme turbinates and the septum.

The *inferior wall or floor* of the sphenoid bone forms the dome of the choanae (posterior nares) and the nasopharynx. The junction of the anterior and inferior walls makes an obtuse, rounded angle called the choanal arch, which demarcates the border between the nasal cavity in front and the nasopharynx behind. The choana is limited laterally by the medial plate of the pterygoid process, medially by the posterior border of the septum, superiorly by the body of the sphenoid and by the posterior edge of the vomer, and inferiorly by the horizontal plate of the palatine bone (which also represents the posterior limit of the floor of the nasal cavity). The bony plate of this choanal arch is relatively thick, reinforced by the ala of the pterygoid plate and vomer. The nasopalatine artery runs along this arch toward the septum.

The lesser wing of the sphenoid bone forms the posterior lip of the anterior cranial fossa, part of the orbital wall that includes the optic canal and the anterior clinoid processes. The lesser wing is connected to the frontal bone along the posterior border of the anterior cranial fossa and to the cribriform plate of the ethmoid bone in the midline. It contributes to the posterior, apical area of the orbit, which includes the optic canal and the superior orbital fissure. The anterior clinoid process extends from the posterior border of the lesser wing laterally to the optic canal. This is a very important anatomical landmark for identifying the location of the optic chiasm.

The greater wing constitutes the largest portion of the sphenoid bone extending from the body of the sphenoid laterally to form part of the floor of the middle cranial fossa. More anteriorly, the greater wing forms the posterior wall of the orbit, including the inferior lip of the superior orbital fissure. Posteriorly, the greater wing creates the lateral side of the carotid canal.

Projecting off the inferior and most posterior portion of the greater wing is the spine of the sphenoid bone, an important landmark for identification of the foramina spinosum from which pass the middle meningeal vessels and the recurrent meningeal branch of the mandibular division of the trigeminal nerve. The greater wing of the sphenoid bone has two more foramina: the foramen rotundum (which is crossed by the maxillary branch of the trigeminal nerve) and the foramen ovale (which transmits an accessory meningeal artery and the mandibular division of the trigeminal nerve).

The medial and lateral pterygoid plates extend inferiorly from the body of the sphenoid and are attached to the posterior wall of the maxillary sinus on the medial surface. The medial pterygoid plate also forms the lateral wall of the nasopharynx superior to the eustachian tube. Between the base of the pterygoid plate and the vertical segment of the palatine bone is an opening called the sphenopalatine foramen (although not a true foramen), located 10 to 12 mm above the posterior end of the middle turbinate and in front of the choanae. This foramen transmits the sphenopalatine artery and the posterosuperior nasal branches of the maxillary nerve.

The clivus is the inferior projection of the body of the sphenoid and forms the posterior wall of the nasopharynx and part of the anterior wall of the foramen magnum.

The sphenoid sinus is formed by two generally asymmetric cavities in the body of the sphenoid bone. Asymmetry is caused by displacement of the median septum of the sphenoid sinus, which can take on a vertical, transverse, or oblique disposition. It may be in the midline, be S-shaped or C-shaped, be complete or incomplete, or even have an accessory septum. In some cases, the sphenoid bone can have three seemingly identical

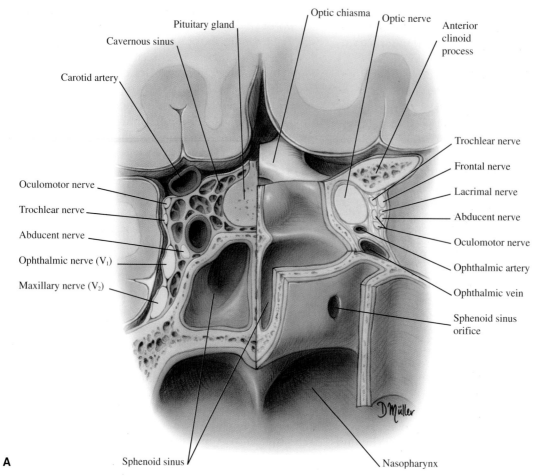

A

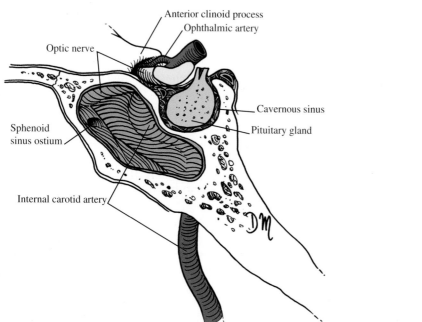

B

FIGURE 1–51 Sphenoid sinus. (A) Coronal section at various levels illustrating the relationship with surrounding vascular and neural structures. (B) Sagittal section showing the adjacent courses of the internal carotid artery and the optic nerve.

cavities. This anatomical variation combined with the degree of pneumatization and extension of the sphenoid sinus to other adjacent bony structures gives this sinus great variability in shape, size, and wall thickness even from one side to the other.

The average adult sphenoid sinus measures 20 mm × 23 mm × 17 mm, being smallest in the anteroposterior dimension. The size of the sphenoid sinus depends on the degree of intramural and extramural pneumatization. The intramural extension of the sinus is observed in the greater wings, lesser wings, and pterygoid plates of the sphenoid bone, whereas the extramural expansion is seen in the maxillary and ethmoid bones. Depending on the degree of pneumatization, the sphenoid sinus can be described as condral, presellar, or sellar (Fig. 1–13).

When the pneumatization of the sphenoid sinus is well developed, the surrounding vessels and nerves are in contact with the lateral wall of the sinus and are seen in the sinus cavity as ridges (Fig. 1–51). The internal carotid artery and the optic nerve are the two important anatomical structures seen on the lateral wall of the sphenoid sinus. Normally, a thin layer of bone covers these structures. However, in some individuals this bone may become very thin or completely disappear.

The internal carotid artery ascends from the carotid canal and courses vertically to cross posterior and lateral to the optic nerve. The optic nerve passes through the orbital apex transversely across the lateral wall of the sinus. Usually there is a depression in the lateral wall of the sinus called the optic recess just anterior and inferior to where the carotid artery and the optic nerve cross. This is a very important landmark identifying the sinus cell as the sphenoid sinus and indicating the position of the carotid artery and optic nerve. In addition, the bulging of the maxillary nerve may be seen on the lateral wall of the sinus. The canal for the vidian nerve may bulge on the floor of the sphenoid sinus. Thus, the carotid artery, optic nerve, ophthalmic or maxillary divisions of the trigeminal nerve, or the vidian nerve may be found immediately under the mucosa of the sphenoid sinus, without a bony covering. For this reason, any dissection should be carefully performed on the lateral wall of the sinus, taking into consideration the anatomical variation of the bony structures of the ethmoid and sphenoid bones and also from the internal carotid artery (Fig. 1–52). The cavernous sinus lies inferior to the location where the carotid artery and optic nerve cross on the lateral wall of the sphenoid sinus. This structure is usually separated from the sinus by a thick wall of bone.

Minor incomplete septations of the sphenoid sinus are also common. Removal of any sphenoid septations should be undertaken with great care, as the septations and the intersinus septum are sometimes attached off midline near or on the bony canal of the optic nerve and/or the internal carotid artery.

The ostium of the sphenoid sinus is usually located in the sphenoethmoid recess, medial to the superior or supreme turbinates and close to the nasal septum. It is a few millimeters below the cribriform plate, ~1 cm above the choana, and 5 mm lateral to the nasal septum. The shape of the sphenoid sinus ostium varies widely. It may be elliptical, oval, or round, with 2 to 3 mm in diameter. There may be two or more ostia on one side.

Vasculature, Innervation, and Lymphatic Drainage of the Paranasal Sinuses

The vascular supply to the maxillary sinus is derived from several sources: small branches from the facial, maxillary, infraorbital, and greater palatine arteries. Veins accompany these vessels and flow to the anterior

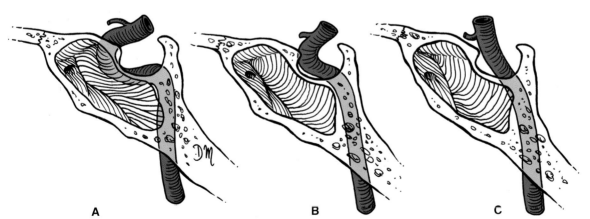

FIGURE 1–52 Anatomical variations in the course of the internal carotid artery in relation to the sphenoid sinus. A: exposed within the sphenoid sinus. B: covered by thin bone with minimal protection. C: extensive bony coverage and protection.

facial vein and pterygoid plexus. The maxillary sinus receives its innervation from branches of the maxillary division of the trigeminal nerve. The lymphatic drainage follows the vascular channels and is mainly directed to the submandibular nodes.

The vascularization of the anterior ethmoid sinus is provided by the anterior ethmoid artery (a branch of the ophthalmic artery) and the arteries of the middle meatus (branches of the sphenopalatine artery). The posterior ethmoid sinus is supplied by the posterior ethmoid artery (a branch of the ophthalmic artery) and the arteries of the superior turbinate (branches of the sphenopalatine artery). The venous drainage of the ethmoid sinus follows the arterial vessels, and the flow is directed to the facial vein, pterygomaxillary plexus, and cavernous sinus. The ethmoid sinus receives its innervation from the anterior and posterior ethmoid nerves (branches of the ophthalmic nerve V_1) and from nasal branches of the maxillary nerve, V_2. The lymphatic drainage follows the vessels and the lymphatic networks of the nasal cavity and the meninges.

Arterial supply of the frontal sinus is from the anterior ethmoid and the supraorbital arteries and from the arteries of the middle meatus. The venous drainage includes the anastomotic vein in the supraorbital notch, which connects the supraorbital and superior ophthalmic vessels, and also the diploic veins draining the superior sagittal and sphenoparietal sinuses.

Nerve supply comes from the anterior ethmoid nerve (V_1), the supraorbital nerve (V_1), and the lateral, posterior, and superior nasal branches of the maxillary nerve (V_2). The lymphatic system drains into the lymphatic network of the nasal cavity and the meningeal lymphatics.

Vascularization of the sphenoid sinus is received from branches of the ophthalmic artery (posterior ethmoid artery) and internal maxillary artery (artery of the pterygoid canal and sphenopalatine artery). Veins accompany these vessels to the sinuses surrounding the sella turcica, namely, the cavernous and sphenoparietal sinuses.

The sphenoid sinus receives its innervation from branches of the ophthalmic nerve, V_1, and from the maxillary nerve, V_2. The lymphatic drainage follows the vascular channels and the lymphatic networks of the nasal cavity and meninges.

■ Endoscopic Anatomy

Macroscopic anatomy of the nose and the paranasal sinus should be correlated with an endoscopic description of those structures.[62-65] The surgeon must develop a three-dimensional mental view of this complex region that allows him or her to know exactly the different anatomical structures, their relationships, and especially

the danger areas. Endoscopic topographical anatomy is presented by reviewing the most important landmarks of the nasal cavity.

Nasal Endoscopy

Nasal endoscopy is the examination of the nasal cavity using a rigid telescope or flexible fiberscope. The technique used to document nasal endoscopic findings is called videonasal endoscopy or videorhinoscopy. Its use has contributed tremendously to the improvement of medical care and to the quality of teaching by demonstrating anatomical relationships, revealing hidden structures, and presenting pathological conditions within the nasal cavity. Endoscopic examination of the nasal cavity should be performed routinely for better preoperative patient evaluation and postoperative care, for documentation of data, and for medicolegal purposes.

The microscope can also be used routinely to assess the nasal mucosa, the presence of secretions, structural changes (such as septal deviations), and other pathological alterations. Anatomical variations may influence the endoscopic examination and cause it to be more difficult (Table 1–5).

EQUIPMENT

The equipment required for nasal endoscopy includes 4 mm 0, 30, and 70 degree nasal telescopes for adults, 2.7 mm 0 and 30 degree nasal telescopes for children, a flexible fiberscope such as the Olympus ENFP₃, (Olympus Industrial America, New York, New York) and a light source.

For nasal endoscopy with video for viewing and recording a light source, a video camera, color monitor, and video recording system are necessary. There are different types of light sources available and in regular use in endoscopy. The choice is determined by the size and cost of equipment and by the brightness and whiteness of the light required for viewing and data documenta-

TABLE 1–5   Variations of Sinonasal Anatomy

Nasal cavity
  Septal deviation and spurs
  Concha bullosa
  Paradoxically curved middle turbinate
  Hypertrophic inferior turbinate
  Pneumatization of superior turbinate or vomer
  Choanal atresia
Middle meatus
  Prominent ethmoid bulla
  Pneumatization of uncinate process
  Hook-shaped/inverted/duplicated uncinate process
  Hypoplasia of maxillary sinus
Inferior meatus
  Pneumatization of inferior turbinate

tion. Video cameras are lightweight cubes 2 to 3 cm in size that produce computer-enhanced images of high-quality resolution with excellent color fidelity. There are several types of video cameras with special optical and electronic components. Three-chip cameras have individual chips for each of the primary colors and have the following features: video camera controller with automatic exposure and color control, automatic white balance, digital contrast enhancement, zoom lenses from 20 to 50 mm, and a built-in character generator. These cameras can be mounted on all telescopes and eyepieces and can be adapted to the operating microscopes. Documentation is easily performed using video recorders and the new single-image electronic processors that allow single images to be stored digitally and printed out later. In modern operating rooms, the entire endoscopic video system is assembled on a cart to eliminate the clutter of electric cords and interconnecting cables.

ENDOSCOPIC TECHNIQUE

Almost all of the anatomical structures of the nasal cavity can be examined using a 4 mm, 0 degree telescope or a 4 mm, 30 degree telescope. The lateral nasal wall requires an angled view, particularly when assessing the ostiomeatal complex area.

A mixture of topical anesthetic and vasoconstrictor is applied to the nasal mucosa in older children and adults. In infants and young children, general anesthesia allows a better and complete examination. The nasal cavity can be inspected through systematic examination generally by two observations or more if necessary (Table 1–6).

During the first observation the anatomical structures to be examined are the inferior turbinate, inferior meatus, floor of the nose, and nasal septum. By advancing the telescope into the posterior nasal cavity, the entire

TABLE 1–6   Endoscopic View of the Nasal Cavity

First observation	Floor of the nose
	Nasal septum
	Inferior turbinate
	Inferior meatus
	Choana
	Nasopharynx
	Eustachian tube orifice
	Rosenmüller's fossa
	Soft palate
	Middle turbinate and its contents
Second observation	Roof of the nasal cavity/superior turbinate/meatus
	Sphenoethmoid recess
	Sphenoid ostium

nasopharynx, soft palate, eustachian tube orifice, torus tubarius, and Rosenmüller's fossa can be visualized. A 4 mm, 0 degree telescope is routinely used for diagnostic purposes, although the 3 mm, 30 degree telescope can also be used.

When the 4 mm endoscope is introduced into the nose, it comes in contact with the vibrissae of the nasal vestibule obstructing the view of the nasal valve. The nasal valve is formed by the floor of the nose, the septum, and the lower edge of the upper lateral cartilage tilted inward, and it represents the first narrow point. Immediately behind the nasal valve lies the second narrow area of the nasal cavity formed by the anterior end of the inferior turbinate (Fig. 1–53). It may lie only 2 to 3 mm above the floor of the nose, so that an endoscope may only be introduced with difficulty beneath the inferior meatus. A retraction of the inferior turbinate may sometimes be needed to displace the turbinate medially and upward. The opening of the nasolacrimal duct is located in the anterosuperior part of the inferior meatus

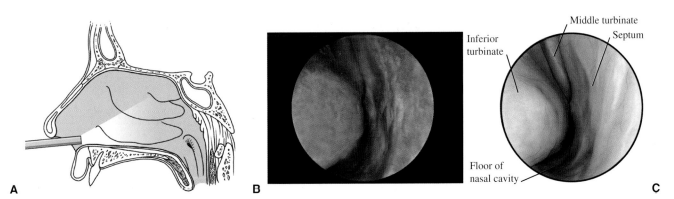

FIGURE 1–53   (A–C) Anterior endoscopic view of the right nasal cavity showing the nasal septum, the anterior end of the inferior turbinate, and the floor of the nasal cavity. (A) Sagital schematic view, (B) endoscopic view, (C) schematic view.

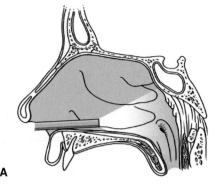
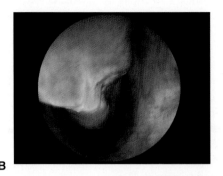
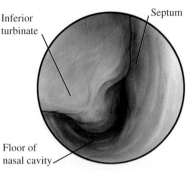

FIGURE 1–54 (A–C) Endoscopic view of the right inferior turbinate and part of the inferior meatus as a 4 mm, 0 degree telescope is passed along the floor of the nasal cavity. Note the nasal septum with inferior ridge and a septal division

A: sagital schematic view, B: endoscopic view, C: Schematic of endoscopic view illustrating floor of nose and medial surface of right inferior turbinate.

~1 cm behind the anterior end of the inferior turbinate. It is a slitlike opening, often recognized by a surrounding crescent of mucosal fold.

Access to the medial wall of the nasal cavity beyond the anterior insertion of the inferior turbinate is often hindered further by a ridge on the lower edge of the nasal septum (Fig. 1–54). This is formed by the premaxilla and the palatal ridge of the maxilla, from which is attached the lower edge of the septal cartilage. At a superior level the septal cartilage is widened, restricting the view of the nasal roof. More posteriorly the endoscopic examination is restricted sometimes by the oblique ascending septal ridge presented by the edge of the vomer and the end of the quadrilateral cartilage extending backward. This ridge may even touch the middle turbinate, obstructing the passage of the endoscope.

To visualize the posterior nasal region and the choana, the endoscope must be passed beneath, rather than over, the ascending septal ridge and along the floor of the nose. The choana is a very important posterior landmark of the nasal cavity and is 1.5 to 2.0 cm high in adults. The posterior end of the inferior turbinate protrudes into the lower part of the nasal choana from the lateral side, occupying up to half its height and narrowing this passage. By advancing the telescope into the posterior nasal cavity, it is usually possible to visualize the entire nasopharynx, soft palate, eustachian tube orifice, and Rosenmüller's fossa (Fig. 1–55).

The endoscope is partially withdrawn and redirected above the posterior end of the inferior turbinate, initiating the examination of the middle meatus through the posterior end of the middle turbinate. If this insertion is

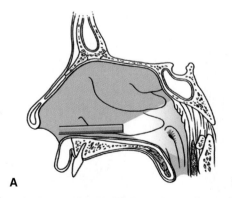
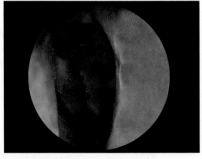
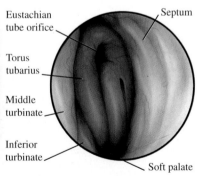

FIGURE 1–55 (A–C) Posterior endoscopic view of the right choana revealing the nasopharynx with the torus tubarius, and the eustachian tube orifice. The 4 mm, 0 degree telescope is placed between the inferior turbinate and the septum

along the floor of the nasal cavity. A: sagital schematic view. B:endoscopic view of posterior nasal cavity and nasopharynx. C: Schematic view.

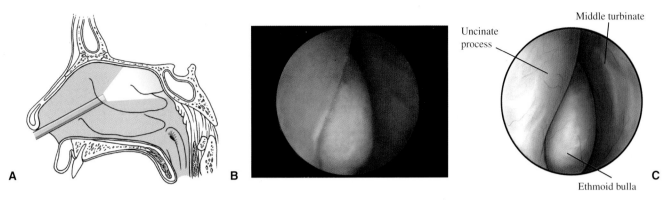

FIGURE 1–56   (A–C) Endoscopic view of the middle meatus with a 4 mm, 0 degree telescope presenting the middle turbinate, the uncinate process, and the ethmoid bulla. A: sag- ital schematic view. B: endoscopic view of right middle meatus showing uncinate process and ethmoid bulla. C: Schematic view.

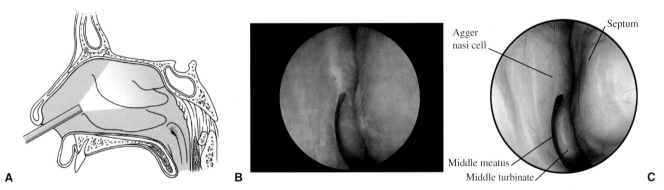

FIGURE 1–57   (A–C) Endoscopic view of the anterior inser- tion of the middle turbinate also exhibiting the smooth swelling of the agger nasi cells in front of the neck of the middle turbinate. A: sagital schematic view. B: endoscopic view of an- terior aspect of right middle turbinate. C: schematic view.

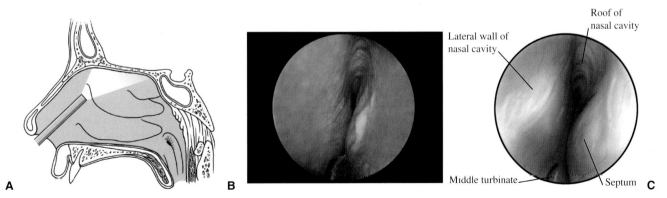

FIGURE 1–58   (A–C) Anterosuperior endoscopic view of the right nasal cavity showing the superior part of the nasal sep- tum and middle turbinate and the begining of the olfactory fossa (roof of nasal cavity). A: sagital view of right lateral nasal wall. B: endoscopic view of right superior nasal cavity. C: schematic view.

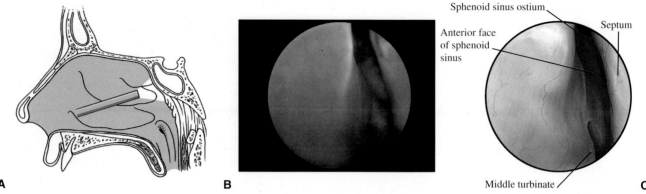

A   **B**   **C**

FIGURE 1–59 (A–C) Posterosuperior endoscopic view of the right nasal cavity revealing the anterior wall of the sphenoid sinus. Note that the posterior and of the middle turbinate is above the choanal opening. (A) sagital schematic view, (B) endoscopic view of the anterior wall of the sphenoid sinus, (C) schematic view.

difficult, the endoscope is removed and introduced through the anterior portion of the middle turbinate for evaluation of its lateral wall.

The middle turbinate is by far the most important landmark of the nasal cavity. The anterior attachment extends superiorly to articulate with the cribriform plate of the ethmoid bone. The middle meatus is the space underneath the middle turbinate. The middle meatus is the most important region for endoscopic nasal surgery because it is the normal pathway to the maxillary, ethmoid, and frontal sinuses and also provides surgical exposure to those sinuses. The middle meatus can only be examined properly after displacing the middle turbinate medially. The middle meatus extends over two-thirds of the length of the lateral nasal wall between the edge of the middle turbinate and the upper edge of the inferior turbinate. The endoscopic view shows the uncinate process, part of the ethmoid bulla, and the hiatus semilunaris (Fig. 1–56). The ethmoid infundibulum is usually not visible with the endoscope because this region is very narrow, and therefore the maxillary ostium cannot be inspected. The infundibulum may be quite shallow when the uncinate process is in close proximity to the lamina papyracea. Also, in the presence of a concha bullosa and/or paradoxical turbinate, the ethmoid infundibulum may be completely obliterated, resulting in recurrent sinus infections. Careful assessment of the mucosa of the middle meatus is essential because the mucosa may be a crucial factor in the persistence of disease and cannot be diagnosed radiographically. In narrower areas there is a greater chance of contact between the mucous surfaces, thereby giving rise to local mucosal edema or hyperplasia with the formation of small polyps.

Before removing the endoscope during the first observation, it is important to identify the agger nasi area, another useful landmark (Fig. 1–57). It is a smooth bony swelling extending superiorly from the nasal vestibule and lying in front of the anterior attachment of the middle turbinate. It may be pneumatized and thin walled, and contains the agger nasi cells, which are the most anterior ethmoid cells. It forms an intimate relation with the frontal recess. More often than not it has a thick bony wall.

In the same plane or 1 to 2 mm in front of the agger nasi area lies the nasolacrimal canal. It runs lateral to the lateral nasal wall and parallel to the agger nasi after descending medially under some ethmoid cells. The agger nasi, the frontal recess, and the nasolacrimal canal lie in roughly the same frontal plane. This proximity explains why the nasolacrimal canal is in danger in this area during endoscopic dissection, particularly in massive polyposis with bony erosion of the ethmoid cells. It is important to keep in mind that a significant number of failed endoscopic procedures are due to inadequate removal of disease in this area.

The second observation is directed toward the roof of the nasal cavity to examine the superior turbinate and meatus, the sphenoethmoid recess, and the sphenoid ostium. The endoscope is slowly withdrawn, and it is gently guided posteriorly to examine the upper level of the nose and its adjacent anatomical structures.

The superior turbinate can be visualized with the endoscope, but the superior meatus is very difficult to inspect, particularly if the septum is widened or deviated. Also, the superior meatus can be narrow if there is a supreme turbinate represented only by a smooth swelling. Posterior to the superior turbinate resides the downward-sloping anterior wall of the sphenoid sinus. The olfactory cleft, a narrow slit covered by olfactory mucosa and extending superiorly between the middle turbinate and the nasal septum to the roof of the nose, is visualized anteriorly (Fig. 1–58).

The attachment of the posterior insertion of the middle turbinate (situated in the upper third of the posterior choana just in front of its anterior edge) forms a landmark for the front wall of the sphenoid sinus (Fig. 1–59). It can also be palpated 1 cm above the dome of the choana paramedially. The location of the sphenoethmoid recess and the sphenoid ostium is higher somewhat more medially and posterosuperiorly to the superior turbinate. Often the natural sphenoid ostium cannot be recognized at endoscopy, but it has an oval or rounded shape when it is not covered by diseased mucosa.

The endoscopic findings can be recorded and stored for further analysis.

REFERENCES

1. Moore KL. *The Developing Human: Clinically Oriented Embryology.* 4th ed. Philadelphia: WB Saunders; 1988:170–205.
2. Hamilton WJ, Boyd JD, Mossman HW. *Human Embryology.* 4th ed. London: Williams & Wilkins; 1978:300–304.
3. Blitzer A, Lawson W, Friedman WH. *Surgery of the Paranasal Sinus.* Philadelphia: WB Saunders; 1991:1–24.
4. Anon JB, Rontal M, Zinreich SJ. *Anatomy of the Paranasal Sinus.* New York: Thieme Medical Publishers; 1996:3–10.
5. Burdia A, Silvey RG. Sexual differences in closure of the human palatal shelves. *Cleft Palate J.* 1969;6:1–7.
6. Bingham B, Wang RG, Hawke M, Kwok P. The embryonic development of the lateral nasal wall from 8 to 24 weeks. *Laryngoscope.* 1991;101:912–997.
7. Wang RG, Jiang SC, Gu R. The cartilaginous nasal capsule and embryonic development of human paranasal sinuses. *J Otolaryngol.* 1994;23:239–243.
8. Ritter FN, Fritsch MH. *Atlas of Paranasal Sinus Surgery.* New York: Igaku-Shoin; 1992:1–35.
9. Kennedy DW, Borger WE, Zinreich SJ. *Diseases of the Sinuses.* Hamilton, Canada: BC Decker Inc; 2001:1–11.
10. Schaeffer JP. The genesis, development and adult anatomy of the nasofrontal region in man. *Am J Anat.* 1916;20:125–146.
11. Zimmerman AA. Development of the paranasal sinus. *Arch Otolaryngol.* 1938;27:793–795.
12. Lang J. *Clinical Anatomy of the Nose, Nasal Cavity and Paranasal Sinuses.* New York: Thieme Verlag; 1989:1–5.
13. Libersa C, Laude M, Libersa JC. The pneumatization of the acessory cavities of the nasal fossae during growth. *Anat Clin* 1981;2:265–273.
14. Donald PJ, Gluckman JL, Rice DH. *The Sinuses.* New York: Raven; 1995:15–48.
15. McGowan DA, Baxter PW, James J. *The Maxillar Sinus.* Oxford: Wright; 1993:1–25.
16. Anand VK, Panje WR. *Practical Endoscopic Sinus Surgery.* New York: McGraw-Hill; 1993:1–15.
17. Tardy ME, Brown RJ. *Surgical Anatomy of the Nose.* New York: Raven 1990:55–97.
18. Larrabee WF, Makielski KH. *Surgical Anatomy of the Face.* New York: Raven; 1993:153–176.
19. McCollough EG. *Nasal Plastic Surgery.* Philadelphia: WB Saunders; 1994:147–212.
20. Tebbetts JB. *Primary Rhinoplasty: A New Approach to the Logic and the Techniques.* St. Louis: Mosby; 1998:99–132.
21. Toriumi DM, Becker DG. *Rhinoplasty: Dissection Manual.* Philadelphia: Lippincott, Williams & Wilkins; 1999:1–7.
22. Shaida AM, Kenyon GS. The nasal valves: changes in anatomy and physiology in normal subjects. *Rhinology.* 2000;38:7–12.
23. Levine HL, May M. *Endoscopic Sinus Surgery.* New York: Thieme Medical Publishers; 1993:1–28.
24. Stammberger H. *Functional Endoscopic Sinus Surgery.* Philadelphia: Becker; 1991:49–87.
25. Stammberger H, Hawke M. *Essentials of Functional Endoscopic Sinus Surgery.* St. Louis: Mosby; 1993:13–42.
26. Maran AGD, Lund VJ. *Clinical Rhinology.* Stuttgart: Thieme Verlag; 1990:1–32.
27. Gershwin ME, Incaudo GA. *Diseases of the Sinuses: A Comprehensive Textbook of Diagnosis and Treatment.* Totowa, NJ: Humana Press, Inc.; 1996:3–32.
28. Stamm AC. *Microcirurgia naso-sinusal.* Rio de Janeiro: Revinter; 1995:15–36.
29. Moore KL. *Clinically Oriented Anatomy.* 2nd ed. Baltimore: Williams & Wilkins; 1985:944–959.
30. Velayos JL. *Anatomía de la cabeza.* Madrid: Panamericana; 1994: 27–85.
31. Rice DH, Schaefer SD. *Endoscopic Paranasal Sinus Surgery.* 2nd ed. New York: Raven; 1993:3–50.
32. Navarro JAC. Cavidade do nariz e seios perinasais: anatomia cirúrgica. Brasil: All Dent;1997:27–116.
33. Marks SC. *Nasal and Sinus Surgery.* Philadelphia: WB Saunders; 2000:3–30.
34. Janfaza P, Nadol JB, Galla RJ, Fabian R, Montgomery WW. *Surgical Anatomy of the Head and Neck.* Philadelphia: Lippincott, Williams, & Wilkins; 2001:259–318.
35. McMinn RMH, Hutchings RT, Logan BM. *A Colour Atlas of Head and Neck Anatomy.* London: Wolfe Medical Publications; 1981: 65–73.
36. Hiatt JL, Gartner LP. *Textbook of Head and Neck Anatomy.* 2nd ed. Baltimore: Williams & Wilkins; 1987:225–234.
37. Netter FH. *Atlas of Human Anatomy.* Basle, Switzerland: Ciba-Geigy; 1989:32–44.
38. Prades J. *Microcirugia endonasal de la fosa pterigomaxilar y del meato medio.* Barcelona: Salvat Editores; 1980:11–22.
39. Daniels DL, Rauschning W, Lovas J, et al. Peterygopalatine fossa: computed tomographic studies. *Radiology.* 1983;149:511–516.
40. Rontal E, Rontal M, Guilford FT. Surgical anatomy of the orbit. *Ann Otol Rhinol Laryngol.* 1979;88:382–386.
41. Guerrier Y, Rouvier P. *Anatomie des Sinus EMC Oto-Rhino-Laryngologye.* 4e édition. Folder 202-66, A10 y 13.02, 20p. Paris: Editions Techniques.
42. Clark ST, Bagin RW, Salazar J. The incidence of concha bullosa and its relationship to chronic sinonasal disease. *Am J Rhinol.* 1989;3:11–12.
43. Zinreich SJ, Mattox DE, Kennedy DW, et al. Concha bullosa: CT evaluation. *J Comput Assist Tomogr.* 1988;12(5):778–784.
44. Yellin SA, Weiss MH, O'Malley B, Weingarten K. Massive concha bullosa masquerading as an intranasal tumor. *Ann Otol Rhinol Laryngol.* 1994;103:658–659.
45. Legent F, Perlemudter L, Vandenbrouck CL. Cahiers d'Anatomie ORL. 4e édition. Paris: Masson;1986:43–41.
46. Calhoun KH, Rotzler WH, Stiernberg CM. Surgical anatomy of the lateral nasal wall. *Otolaryngol Head Neck Surg* 1990;102:156–160.
47. Silva HF. *Conceitos actuais do tratamento cirúrgico das sinusites crónicas.* Porto. Thesis. 1992:49–74.
48. Ohnishi T. Bony defects and dehiscences of the roof of the ethmoid cells. *Rhinology.* 1981;19(4):195–202.
49. Bolafr E, Butzin CA, Parsons DS. Paranasal sinus bony anatomic variations and mucosal abornamalities: CT analysis for endoscopic sinus surgery. *Laryngoscope.* 1991;101:56–64.
50. Mattox DE, Delaney RG. Anatomy of the ethmoid sinus. *Otolaryngol Clin North Am.* 1985;18(1):3–14.

52. Stackpole SA, Edelstein DR. Anatomic variants of the paranasal sinuses and their implications for sinusitis. *Otolaryngol Head Neck Surg.* 1996;4:1–6.

53. Bent JP, Cuilty-Siller C, Kuhn FA. The frontal cell as a cause of frontal sinus obstruction. *Am J Rhinol.* 1994;8:185–191.

54. Shankar L, Evans K, Hawke M, Stammberg H. *An Atlas of Imaging of the Paranasal Sinuses.* Philadelphia: Lippincott; 1994:10–23.

55. Stammberger H, Kennedy DW. Paranasal sinuses: anatomic terminology and nomenclature. The Anatomic Terminology Group. *Ann Otol Rhinol Laryngol Suppl.* 1995;167:7–16.

56. Zeifer B. Update on sinosal imaging anatomy and inflammatory disease. *Neuroimaging Clin N Am.* 1958;8:607–614.

57. McLaughlin RB, Ryan RM, Lanza DC. Clinically relevant frontal sinus anatomy and physiology. *Otolaryngol Clin North Am.* 2001;34: 1–22.

58. Elwany S, Yacout YM, Tallaat M, et al. Surgical anatomy of the sphenoid sinus. *J Laryngol Otol.* 1983;97:227–241.

59. Hosemann W, Groß R, Göde U, Kühnel T, Röckelein G. The anterior sphenoid wall: relative anatomy for sphenoidotomy. *Am J Rhinol.* 1995;9:137–144.

60. Cheung DK, Attia EL, Kirkpatrick DA, Marcarian B, Wright B. An anatomic and CT scan study of the lateral wall of the sphenoid sinus as related to the transnasal transethmoid endoscopic approach. *J Otolaryngol.* 1993;22:63–68.

61. Kennedy DW, Zinreich SJ, Hassab MH. The internal carotid artery as it relates to endonasal sphenoidectomy. *Am J Rhinol.* 1990;4(1):7–12.

62. Wigand ME. *Endoscopic Surgery of the Paranasal Sinuses and Anterior Skull Base.* Stuttgart: Thieme Verlag; 1990:18–26.

63. Mehta D. *Atlas of Endoscopic Sinonasal Surgery.* Philadelphia: Lea & Febiger; 1993:11–28.

64. Klossek JM, Fontanel JP, Dessi P, Serrano E. *Chirurgie endonasale sous guidage endoscopique.* 2nd ed. Paris: Masson; 1995:2–23.

65. Bhatt NJ. *Endoscopic Sinus Surgery New Horizons.* San Diego: Singular; 1997:30–51.

2

Physiology of the Paranasal Sinuses

DESIDERIO PASSÀLI, GIULIO CESARE PASSÀLI, FRANCESCO MARIA PASSÀLI, AND L. BELLUSSI

Galen described the "porosity of the skull" for the first time in the second century A.D., but it was only later in 1489, with the work of Leonardo da Vinci, that we had a clear description of paranasal sinuses. In his anatomical tables Leonardo represented the frontal sinuses and maxillary ostium.[1]

The role of paranasal sinuses is largely unknown nowadays, even if a lot of interesting theories have been suggested. All the hypotheses that have been made, however, can be grouped under three main theories: the structural, the evolutionary, and the functional.

■ Structural Theory

Vesalio (1542) and Falloppio (1600) hypothesized that sinuses are just a way created by nature to make the bone structure lighter and thus diminish the work of the muscles of the neck. At the end of the 19th century Braune and Clasen[2] disproved that idea, because if sinuses had been full of cancellous bone, the total weight of the cranium would have increased by only about 1%. According to another hypothesis[3] belonging to the structural theory, paranasal sinuses contribute to the maintenance of equilibrium and the position of the head lightening the anterior portium of the cranium, but during the 1960s, this idea was proved not to be reliable through electromyographic studies of the muscles of the neck.

According to Flottes et al, paranasal sinuses would be the result of the development of the facial bones,[4] whereas, according to Proetz, they could have a function in remodeling facial bones.[5] However, changes in the morphology of sinuses do not seem to be related to changes of physiognomy.

■ Evolutionary Theory

The most innovative theory considers paranasal sinuses as the evolutionary response of anthropomorphic monkeys to the shift from the terrestrial environment to the aquatic one.

According to Hardy,[6] *Australopithecus* represents the link between *Homo habilis* and *Homo sapiens* and anthropomorphic monkeys. Our old ancestor would have gotten specific characteristics, such as bipedal gait, loss of down, the presence of subcutaneous fat, and a different production of sweat and tears to live in an aquatic environment.

About 6.5 millions years ago the African environment, where the *Australopithecus* lived, was invaded by the sea, which dissociated a piece of mainland that became an island. The monkeys that remained on the island, because they could not reach the mainland, had to learn to live in a different way, looking for food in the waters surrounding the island. Natural selection let them adapt to their new environmental condition by developing a floating mechanism as in the case of some aquatic amphibians and reptiles which have developed sacs of air to allow the floating of the cephalic part and the maintenance of the nasal cavities out of water. In the same way paranasal cavities, through hydrodynamic push, support the muscles of the neck and would have allowed *Australopithecus* to maintain airways out of the water. (It is interesting to underline how man, unlike other mammals, has another characteristic of aquatic reptiles, the membrane of Shrapnell, which diminishes the transmission of acoustic waves in water.[7])

According to the evolutionary theory, paranasal sinuses are now not only useless, they also represent a biological disadvantage, especially considering the diseases they frequently develop.

■ Functional Theory

Paranasal sinuses seem to have different functions. Bartholini[8] was the first to consider these cavities as important organs of resonance, and Howell[9] noted that the Maori of New Zealand have a particularly metallic voice because they do not have wide enough paranasal cavities. This theory was disproved by Proetz,[10] however, who stressed how animals with a strong voice, such as lions, do not have big sinuses. According to Proetz, paranasal sinuses work as a barrier for the vital organs against thermic and acoustic insults.

Cloquet[11] thought that in paranasal sinuses there was an olfactive epithelium. Even if this has been shown not to be completely true, however, the mucosa of paranasal sinuses represents in carnivorous mammals the residual aspects of the olfactory organ.

In our opinion, the most important function of paranasal sinuses is to improve the nasal function. The embryological origin as an invagination from the nose and the histological continuity of the respiratory mucosa covering the nasal fossae and the sinuses make these cavities an efficient mechanism in strengthening the defense function through the additional secretion of lythic enzymes and secretory immunoglobulins. The strict relationship of the paranasal sinuses with the nasal

cavities influences the functionality of the paranasal sinuses, and the center of the whole paranasal physiology is the patency of the ostia through which the sinuses ventilate, drain, and secrete mucus.

■ Ventilatory Function

We define sinusal ventilatory function as all gaseous exchanges between the nose and the paranasal sinuses and between the sinuses and the bloodstream through the mucosa.[12] The gaseous exchanges are determined by active phenomena, depending on nasal respiratory activity, and passive phenomena of passive diffusion.

During the act of breathing, the nasal valve transforms air into a laminar flow that, through the nasal cavities, spreads over the middle meatus, where it changes in microturbulences that lead to a uniform mixing of air. The alternation in expiration of every cycle creates a gradient of pressure between nasal and paranasal cavities, which causes airflow entering the sinuses at the end of every inspiration and at the beginning of the following expiration when a situation of hyperpressure exists inside the nasal cavities. This is inverted at the end of every expiration and at the beginning of the following inspiration when endonasal pressure reaches negative values (Fig. 2–1).

Only 1/1000 of the air volume of the sinuses is exchanged through a single respiratory act. (Actually, the exchange is faster, as demonstrated through O_2 microelectrodes placed in the maxillary sinus: 5 minutes is enough time to renew 90% of the gaseous content there.[13]) Therefore, even though the paranasal air exchange is 2 times faster during nasal versus oral breathing, the alternations of endonasal pressure do not

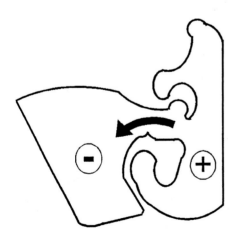
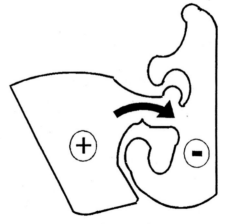

FIGURE 2–1 Sinonasal gaseous exchanges during inspiration and expiration. (A) At the end of inspiration, there is a positive pressure in the nasal cavity that determines airflow toward the sinus. (B) At the end of expiration, there is a negative pressure in the nasal cavity that determines airflow toward the nasal fossa.

influence the ventilation of paranasal sinuses very much. Pressure changes in nasal cavities contribute to ventilation of paranasal sinuses supplying only 1/10 of the total air. The other 9/10 depend on the processes of passive gaseous diffusion through the ostium.[14] In particular, the diameter of the ostium is affected by the speed of oxygenation in physiological conditions and by the efficiency of the drainage in pathological situations.[15]

All the studies on the patency of the ostia have been performed on the maxillary sinus, which is the most accessible one. Anatomical dimensions of the ostium are not related to the sinus volume and do not change because of gender. The anatomical diameter is different in every subject (mean values from 2 to 4 mm), reaching its final size and remaining stable at the end of the period of maxillofacial bone development. Because the mucosa that covers the wall of the ostium is rich with blood vessels and has the same histological characteristics as the nasal cavities, the diameter of the ostium can change following physiological events, such as the passage from standing to the supine position, physical exercise, and the phases of the nasal cycle. For example, when changing from standing to the supine position, the diameter is almost the same until the subject's inclination with the horizontal plane corresponds to an angle of 30 degrees., Then it rapidly decreases, reaching 70% of the starting value when in the supine position, because of the increase in hydrostatic pressure on the neck.

Functional changes in the diameter of the ostium play a fundamental role in the gaseous exchanges toward the sinus. When the ostium has a functional size of more than 2.4 mm, the oxygen contained in the sinus is adequate ($pO_2 = 116$ mm Hg), but when the size is less than 2.4 mm, pO_2 (oxygen partial pressure) decreases to 88 mm Hg when the ostium is closed. The value of 2.4 mm can be considered as critical for paranasal pathology. The anatomical integrity of the bone structure and of the mucosa is necessary but not sufficient for the efficiency of the ostiomeatal complex. Even when the diameter of the ostium is greater than the critical value, the presence of secretion can compromise its patency.

The patency of the ostium has been evaluated through the resistance values that the maxillary antrum has toward air introduced into it.[16] Through the evaluation of these resistances we can distinguish (1) subjects with patent ostium, (2) subjects with partially patent ostium, (3) and subjects with an obstructed ostium.[16] The level of O_2 in the first group is 16% of the gaseous content, 14% in the second and 11% in the third. Moreover, the ostium resistance is influenced by the presence of secretions showing a 20% decrease after irrigation.

The decrease of O_2 concentration, together with the stagnation of secretions, creates the ideal conditions for bacterial multiplication. The same bacteria, consuming oxygen, determine the decrease of the partial tension, potentiating the vicious cycle started with the obstruction of the ostium by mucosal edema and the increased production of mucus. Probably the relevant reduction of pO_2 depends only on the convergence of two factors: the obstruction of the ostium and bacterial superinfection.[17]

Gaseous exchanges between the sinuses and the bloodstream through the mucosa is another important part of the function of paranasal ventilation. To study that function, we have available to us specific techniques that use radioactive gaseous substances (e.g., xenon) whose time of washout is evaluated. It has been found that overall ventilation is not influenced by the ventilation of nearby sinuses, as demonstrated in patients with slow or absent air exchange in the sphenoid sinus, which can have a posterior ethmoid cell count of T 90% (time needed to eliminate 90% of a gaseous substance).[18]

■ Mucociliary Clearance

The nose and the paranasal sinuses represent the first line of defense of the lower airways against inert dangerous substances and microorganisms. They have specific and nonspecific means of defense. In the nose, the turbulences of air created by the nasal valve keep inhaled substances from having long contact with the nasal mucosa; in contrast, in the paranasal sinuses, this contact is prolonged and thus presents a risk for infectious processes.

Among the nonspecific mechanisms, mucociliary clearance plays an important role, as it happens in the nasal cavities. Its efficacy depends on the integrity of the mucociliary system, which consists of ciliated cells, goblet cells, and mucus. There are no structural and functional differences between paranasal ciliated cells and nasal ciliated cells. Goblet cells are remarkably more numerous in the maxillary sinus than in the other paranasal cavities.[19–22] The nasal mucus consists of water (95%), glycoproteins (2.5–3.0%), and electrolytes (1–2%) and depends on the activity of goblet cells, seromucosal glands of the chorion, lachrymal secretion, and aqueous vapor of inhaled air.

As regards the differences among the sinuses, glands are placed mostly in the ethmoid mucosa, then in the maxillary sinus, frontal sinus, and finally the sphenoid sinus.[19] The reason why the concentration of glands in the paranasal cavities is inferior to that in the nose is physiological: The production of mucus in the nose and in the paranasal sinuses is needed to prevent excessive dehydration of the epithelial cells. In closed cavities, as sinuses are, the mucus secreted by goblet cells is sufficient for this purpose and helps to create an adequate mucociliary transport.

The act of mucociliary transport (MCT) needs a continuous supply of O_2. Paranasal mucosa, like the mucosa of the middle ear, can take O_2 from metabolic activities or from sinusal atmosphere (whose composition is regulated by the gaseous exchanges through the ostia) or blood perfusion. O_2 mucosal absorption is 0.1 mL/min; this quantity is burned partially by the mucosa and partially enters the bloodstream. The hematic flow is 100 mL per 100 g of tissue (0.125 mm of mucosal thickness) in the maxillary sinus. We find the same value in the lungs; the flow is less in the kidneys and more in the brain and muscles.[16] O_2 absorption is made easier by the low perfusion, because it is higher when in the presence of inflammatory events.[23]

Different techniques are used to measure mucosal hematic perfusion of the paranasal cavities:

1. Insufflating xenon when the ostium is closed and evaluating, through a gamma camera, the gaseous washout in the cavity

2. Plethysmography: recording the internal pressure when the ostium is closed (it shows waves of pulsation that disappear, compressing the carotid artery and the jugular vein)

3. Doppler laser velocimetry: the hematic flow is evaluated by generating the ratio between diverted photons and nondiverted photons

MCT is influenced also by pCO_2 of atmosphere and blood.

In vitro studies have demonstrated that exposition to increasing quantities of CO_2 made MCT decrease at a concentration of 10 and 15 kPa (KiloPascal), while no change was noticed at a concentration of 5 kPa of pCO_2.[24] The change in the activity of MCT is due to the inhibition of cellular breathing that takes place when pCO_2 is more than 5 kPa.[25] On the other hand, the activity of respiratory mucosa produces CO_2 that is eliminated through a perfusion/diffusion and ventilation mechanism. The damage of one of these mechanisms causes an increase of pCO_2 in the sinuses and a decrease of velocity of clearance. The increase of pCO_2 over 10 kPa occurs also in inflammatory processes, with purulent secretion causing a decrease of MCT that makes the situation of the infected sinus get worse.

MCT has, on average, a 1 cm/min velocity. That value is actually quite variable. First of all, it changes because of the place of the respiratory epithelium; second, it is influenced by external factors (dimension, weight, and the chemical structure of the substances carried), environmental factors (e.g., temperature, humidity, contact with hypertonic or hypotonic solutions, and basic or acid substances), and internal factors. As regards internal factors, MCT is influenced by neuropeptides such as substance P or the flow of chlorine through mucosa that

causes the increase of the level of water in the sol phase. Finally, there is a long list of pollution substances (smoke, dusts, and chemical substances) that can influence the mucociliary system, directly damaging the epithelial cells or changing the physical and chemical characteristics of the secretions. All the factors that make MCT decrease also cause an increase in the individual's susceptibility to respiratory infections and neoplastic diseases.

Modern endoscopic techniques are able to give an adequate vision of MCT in vivo, particularly in the maxillary sinus. Typically, MCT follows specific and perhaps genetically determined paths for each sinus. In the maxillary sinus, mucus is carried along anterior, medial, posterior, and lateral walls and along the roof, creating, on each wall, a picture of a halo or of a star converging toward the ostium. That is the reason why the secretion is thicker near the ostium. However, the drainage seems to be faster at this level to favor ventilation and to avoid negative pressure and the development of infections. Little alterations of mucosa do not stop or change the transport, and mucus continues its "travels," passing over them. Only when secretions are thicker can they amass and stop where the defect is.

In the frontal sinus, MCT follows a spiral movement. Mucus is carried along the interfrontal septum, then along the roof, the lateral wall, and the inferior part of the anterior and posterior wall. The transport is also spiral in the sphenoid sinus and moves toward the ostium. In the ethmoid sinuses it can be rectilinear if the ostium is on the floor of the sinus or spiral if it is on one of the walls.[26]

The only way to determine the activity of MCT of the paranasal sinuses is to inject a tracing in the paranasal cavity and wait for clearance to examine the mucociliary transport time (MCTt). That is an invasive method, but it is the only one available to evaluate the changes of MCTt when changing the position of the head, doing physical exercises, and smelling, or in pathological conditions such as in changes of the dimensions of the ostium. There is an inverse proportion between the velocity of clearance and the diameter of the ostium: The smaller the ostium, the faster the transport. A wide ostium (5–6 mm) has an immediate clearance; an ostium with a diameter of 2 mm needs 3 to 4 days to have a complete clearance.[25]

■ Immune Defense

The immune system can be considered as a complex of different forms of defense: phylologically more ancient forms (non-specific immunity) and forms of selective defense (specific immunity). The aspecific, or natural, immunity plays its role in the paranasal sinuses through the production of particular factors such as

1. Lisozyme, which destroys the peptidoglycans of the cellular walls of bacteria and plays a useful role in this kind of infection;

2. Interferon, made by different cells (epithelial cells, macrophages, leukocytes, lymphocytes, and fibroblasts), with the activity of immune modulation;

3. Complement, which amplifies the immune response; and

4. Enzymes (peroxidase).

Macrophages and neutrophils also act to produce oxygen free radicals. Even though they are not able to get a selective response, they have an important role in activating the specific defense by producing mediators and cytokines that, in turn, activate lymphocytes. These cells produce more mediators and cytokines that activate other macrophages and neutrophils.[27] The specific immunity, however, is more precise and "cheaper" than aspecific defense.

Nasal-associated local immune tissue (NALT) has been studied only in the past two decades.[28,29] As in other areas, NALT is organized to make a barrier for antigens at the epithelial level, in the superficial and deep mucosal chorion.

Some cells (mastocytes, basophils, and rare lymphocytes) are present in the epithelium, but the main role in the immune response is played by the antigen-presenting cells (AP cells). Some studies[30] demonstrate the presence of dendritic cells in sinonasal mucosa that are similar to Langerhans' cells of the skin, marked by a particular arrangement of the histocompatibility system (HLA-DR) through which they can recognize the antigen and introduce it to macrophages and Th (T-helper) lymphocytes. The concentration of AP cells depends on the intensity of the antigenic stimulation.

As regards lymphocytes, T lymphocytes are more numerous than B lymphocytes: T helper type is the most represented in the epithelium and subepithelium, with a total concentration of 1000 cells per mm^2; their concentration decreases until 600 cells per mm^2 among the glands and in the deepest levels until 300 cells per mm^2 and the ratio Th:T goes from 2.5:1.00 to 1:1. This distribution has a precise sense: The prevalence of T cells (mostly Th in the epithelium) is fundamental for the collaboration with AP cells; epithelial and subepithelial T cells and T cells placed near the glands regulate the activity of the goblet cells and therefore SIgA (Secretory Immunoglobulin A) synthesis.[28]

Plasma cells, necessary for Ig synthesis in loco, are placed mostly in the lamina propria and represent 68% of the whole cellular population. They are the center of

the specific response and are represented mostly by plasma cells producing IgA (especially IgA$_2$) and, in an inferior quantity, IgG (Immunoglobulin G) and IgM (Immunoglobulin M). We do not find plasma cells producing IgE in physiological conditions.

IgG-positive subepithelial plasma cells represent 49% of the whole plasmacellular population in healthy people and only 11% in the periglandular zone; these values reach 68% and 24%, respectively, in the case of inflammation.[29] There are three different subclasses of IgG: G$_1$, G$_2$, and G$_3$, with a decreasing concentration.

If there is a deficiency of secretory IgA, there is an increased production of IgD (from 8% to 43%), while IgG remains very low. This particular behavior represents an advantage for the mucosa, because the low level of IgG limits the activation of complement and thus the afflux of inflammatory cells.

Rhinosinusal mast cells can be found in the secretions that cover the mucosa, mixed with epithelial cells in the superficial layers, and spread in a certain quantity in the lamina propria. This finding is important to explain the early phase of the allergic reaction with the immediate symptomatology in which only the mast cells in the secretion and in the epithelial and subepithelial layers are involved, releasing preformed mediators (histamine, tryptase, and heparin) and giving rise, after degranulation, to lipid mediators (prostaglandin and lymphotoxin). All these mediators induce nasal symptoms, such as itching, sneezing, nasal blockage, and discharge, through interaction with receptors present on both neural and vascular elements within the nasal mucosa.

As for fibroblasts, their role in the immune response is not yet well known; perhaps they participate in preparing an adequate environment for the growth of cells belonging to NALT, especially mastocytes. Eosinophils are not present in submucosal and nasal secretions in healthy conditions. They have a fundamental role in allergic inflammation and in nonallergic rhinitis.

If the main actors of the immune response are the above-mentioned cellular elements, the "telephone line" through which they communicate consists of soluble mediators (cytokines, chemotactic factors, and adhesion molecules). Cytokines are produced by numerous cells. The most relevant production belongs to T lymphocytes, but also to B lymphocytes; even macrophages and fibroblasts can produce them. Among different leukines, we must pay attention to IL4: It causes the switch of class toward the production of IgE. Additionally, IL2 and IL6 stimulate the increase of Th and the passage from B cells toward plasma cells producing Ig, and therefore have an important role in the immune response (Fig. 2–2).

In summary, the immune response of the mucosa of the sinuses does not differ from that in nasal mucosa as far as the cellular elements and mediators are

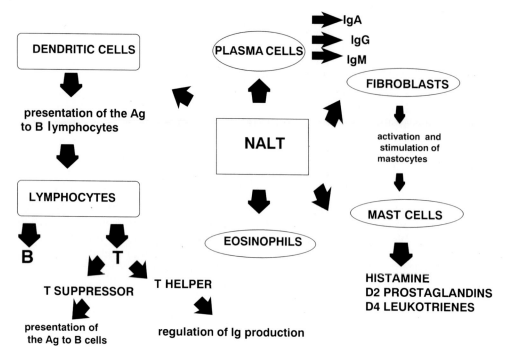

FIGURE 2–2 Cells involved in the immune defense. Ag, antigen; Ig, immunoglobulin; IgG, immunoglobulin G; IgM, immunoglobulin M; NALT, nasal-associated local immune tissue.

concerned. However, a balance between repeated antigenic stimuli and the activity of the specific and aspecific defense factors is easily reached in the nose, so that we can talk about a "physiological inflammation." In closed cavities, such as paranasal sinuses, the inflammatory mediators accumulate, transforming a defense mechanism in a pathologic event able to mantain itself.

■ Conclusion

In light of these considerations, it is difficult to consider paranasal cavities as "evolutionary residues." Even though this had been their role at the beginning of the human race, during the course of philogenesis they evolved and became, despite their relative accessibility, the "functional reserve" of the upper airways.

The real functions of the paranasal sinuses are not mysterious, although it may be difficult to understand them all. The sinuses, despite their anatomical "handicaps," (the small size and the upward position of the ostia) manage to renew rapidly their atmosphere and have a clearance rate that does not follow the rules of gravity or other physical laws; furthermore, they defend not only themselves but also nasal cavities. What we really are lacking here is a global vision that recognizes the unique aim of the entire structural complex.

If the paranasal sinuses exist only by chance, they have developed extraordinarily specialized functions, yet they have a fragile equilibrium that can be easily broken, giving way to a pathologic cycle in which only an impaired function determines the starting and the perpetuating of the whole process.

REFERENCES

1. Passali D, Bellussi L. La fisiologia dei seni paranasali. In: Antonelli AR, ed. *I tumori maligni dei seni paranasali. Relazione Ufficiale LXXXII Congresso Nazionale S.I.O.* Pisa, Italy: Pacini; 1995:31–56.
2. Braune W, Clasen FE. Die Nebenhohlen der Menschlichen Nase in ihre Bedeutung fur den Mechanismus des Riechens. *Zeit Ent.* 1877;2:S.1
3. Biggs NL, Blanton PL. The role of paranasal sinuses as weigth reducers of the head determinated by electromyography of postural neck muscles. *J Biomech.* 1970;3:255–262.
4. Flottes L, Clerc P, Devilla F. La physiologie des sinus. *Acta Otolaryngol Stockh.* 1977;83:16–19
5. Proetz AW. Observation upon the formation and function of the accessory nasal sinuses and mastoid air cells. *Ann Otol Rhinol Laryngol.* 1922;31:1083–1100.
6. Hardy A. Was man more aquatic in the past? *New Sci.* 1960;7: 642–645.
7. Evans PHR. The paranasal sinuses and other enigmas: an aquatic evolutionary theory. *J Laryngol Otol.* 1992;106:214–225.
8. Thomae Bartholini Casp. Fil. Anatomia, Caspari Bartholini ex parentis Iinstitutionibus, omniumque recentiorum et propriis observationibus tertùum ad sanguinis circulationem reformata; cum iconibus novis accuratisimis.additur & huic postremae editioni Th. Bartholini appendix de lacteis thoracicis & vasis lymphaticis. Amstelodami: sumptibus Sebastiani Combi & Joannis Lanou, 1669.
9. Howell HP. Voice production from the standpoint of the laryngologist. *Ann Otol Rhinol Laryngol.* 1917;26:643–655.

10. Proetz AW. *Applied Physiology of the Nose.* St. Louis: Annals Publishing Company; 1953.

11. Cloquet H. *A System of Human Anatomy* (1830). Robert Knox, trans. Edinburgh: Maclachlan and Stewart; 1838.

12. Aust R, Drettner B. The functional size of the human maxillary ostium in vivo. *Acta Otolaryngol Stockh.* 1974;78:432–435.

13. Aust R, Drettner B. The patency of the maxillary ostium in relation to body posture. *Acta Otolaryngol Stockh.* 1975;68:435–443.

14. Guerrier Y, Uziel A Exploration physique et functionnelle des fosses nasale. *Oto Rhino Llaryngol.* 1978;A-10:6–18.

15. Passàli D, Lauriello M. Le sinusiti. *Aggiorn Med.* 1990;14(9):600–609.

16. Drettner B, Aust R. Pathophysiology of the paranasal sinuses. *Acta Otolaryngol.* 1977;83:16–19.

17. Carenfelt C, Lundberg C. The role of local gas composition in the pathogenesis of maxillary sinus empyema. *Acta Otolaryngol.* 1978; 85:116–121.

18. Kalender WA, Rettinger G, Suess C. Measurements of paranasal sinus ventilation by xenon-enhanced dynamic computed tomography. *J Comput Assist Tomogr.* 1985;9:524–529.

19. Mogensen C, Tos M. Quantitative histology of the maxillary sinus. *Rhinology.* 1977;55:129–140.

20. Tos M, Mogensen C, Novontny Z. Quantitative histology of the normal ethmoidal sinus. *Oto Rhino Laryngol.* 1978;40:172–180.

21. Tos M. Mogensen C, Novontny Z. Quantitative histology of the normal frontal sinus. *Arch Otolaryngol.* 1980;106:143–150.

22. Tos M. Goblet cells and glands in the nose and paranasal sinus. In: Proctor D, Andersen J, eds. *The Nose: Upper Airway Physiology and the Atmospheric Environments.* Amsterdam: Elsevier; 1982: 99–140.

23. Rohr AS, Spector SL. Paranasal sinus anatomy and pathophysiology. *Clin Rev Allergy.* 1984;2:387–395.

24. Reimer A. The effect of carbon dioxide on the activity of cilia. *Acta Otolaryngol Stockh.* 1987;103:156–160.

25. Bicz W. The influence of carbon dioxide tension on the respiration of normal and leukemic human leukocytes: influence on endogenous respiration. *Cancer Res.* 1960;20:184–189.

26. Stammberger H. Endoscopic surgery: concepts in treatment of recurring rhinosinusitis: I. Anatomic and pathophysiologic considerations. *Otolaryngol Head Neck Surg.* 1986;94:147–156.

27. Mygind N, Winther B. Immunological barriers in the nose and paranasal sinuses. *Acta Otolaryngol Stockh.* 1987;103:363–368.

28. Korsrud FR, Brandtzaeg P. Immunology of human nasal mucosa. *Rhinology.* 1983;21:203–212.

29. Brandtzaeg P. Cells producing immunoglobulins and other immune factors in human nasal mucosa. *Protides Biol Fluids* 1985; 32:363–366.

3

Imaging of the Paranasal Sinuses

TODD W. STULTZ AND MICHAEL T. MODIC

Imaging of the paranasal sinuses has continued to evolve as treatment strategies and imaging technology have progressed. Cross-sectional imaging has proven to be a valuable tool for preoperative planning and has provided insight into the natural history of inflammatory sinus disease.[1] Although plain films once occupied a central role in the diagnosis and follow-up of sinus disease, they probably have no role at this point.[2] Uncomplicated sinusitis is a clinical diagnosis, and initial assessment of response to therapy is likewise clinical. A meta-analysis by Low et al[3] suggests that initial imaging is not helpful when the suspicion is high or low, but it is beneficial when the diagnosis remains in doubt. Advanced imaging modalities primarily assist in assessing complications of sinusitis, failure of response to therapy, surgical planning for functional endoscopic sinus surgery (FESS), and in some institutions provide data utilized for intraoperative surgical guidance.

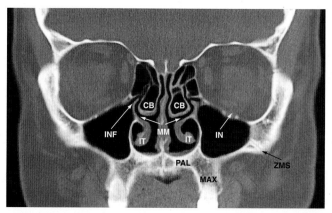

FIGURE 3–1 Direct coronal scan through the osteomeatal unit showing relevant anatomy. cb, concha bullosa of middle turbinate; IN, infraorbital nerve and canal; INF, infundibulum; IT, inferior turbinate; MAX, maxillary dentoalveolus (tooth-bearing area); MM, middle meatus (text label overlies the nasal septum); PAL, hard palate; ZMS, zygomaticomaxillary suture.

■ Imaging Modalities

Computed Tomography

Computed comography (CT) has become the primary imaging modality for assessing inflammatory sinus disease. Preoperative scanning is performed in the coronal plane, when possible, as this approximates the working plane during FESS and optimally displays the ostiomeatal unit (OMU) (Fig. 3–1). A cadaveric study by Melhem et al[4] demonstrated that a slice thickness of 3 mm and a scan plane within 10 degrees of perpendicular to the hard palate best display the OMU. CT provides excellent bony anatomical detail and, with the evolution of helical scanning, can rapidly acquire thin-slice axial data suitable for three-dimensional or multiplanar reformatting in sagittal, coronal, or oblique planes[5] (Fig. 3–2). Patients who cannot tolerate the neck hyperextension necessary for prone or supine coronal scanning (Fig. 3–3) and patients with extensive dental restorations (Fig. 3–4) are good candidates for thin-slice helical scanning with reformatting.[6] Helical scanning defines a combination of continuous rotational tube head motion about the patient, along with continuous feed of the patient through

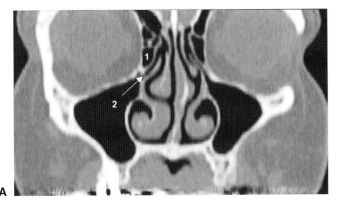

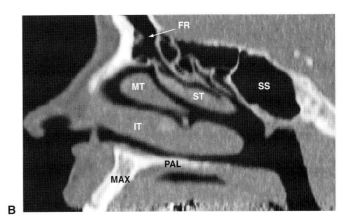

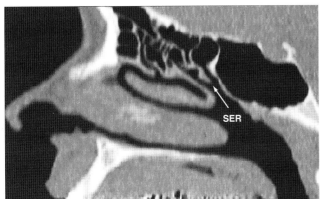

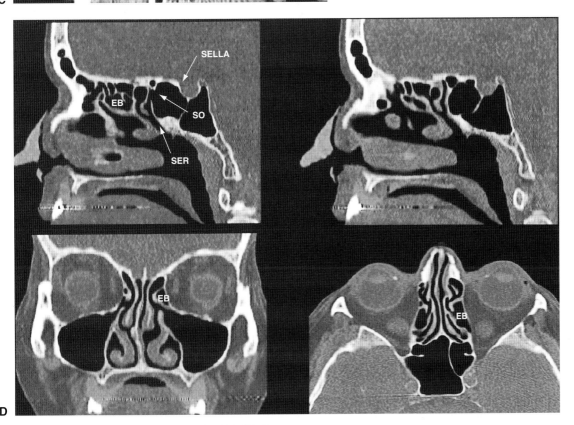

FIGURE 3–2 (A) Coronal reformat of axial CT data at approximately the same point as Figure 3–1. This permits a more direct coronal plane and avoids significant dental restoration artifact in the region of interest. (B) Sagittal reformat from the same axial dataset. The frontal recess is prominantly displayed, and is clearly an hourglass-shaped structure, not a duct. FR, frontal recess; IT, inferior turbinate; MAX, maxillary dentoalveolus; PAL, hard palate; MT, middle turbinate; SS, sphenoid sinus; ST, superior turbinate. (C) Sagittal reformat showing the sphenoethmoid recess (SER), as well as drainage pathways from posterior ethmoid air cells. (D) Direct axial and reformatted coronal and sagittal images showing the ethmoid bulla (EB), sphenoid ostium (SO), and SER.

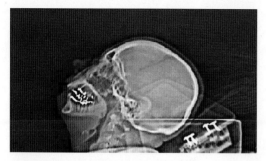

FIGURE 3–3 Topogram of patient in supine hyperextended position.

TABLE 3–1 Hounsfield Number for Various Tissues

Substance	Hounsfield Units
Air	−1000
Fat	−100
Infiltrated fat	−30 to + 20 (approx.)
Water	0
Simple fluid	0 to +20
Proteinaceous fluid	+20 to +50
Soft tissue	+30 to +50
Acute blood (normal hematocrit)	~ +80
Bone	+500 to +1000
Metal	> +1000

Normal hematocrit is approximately 80 HU. Hounsfield number decreases with decreasing hematocrit.

the scanner. This results in significantly shorter scan times, less motion artifact, and minimization of volume averaging artifact. Data for intraoperative guidance are always acquired as a thin section helical dataset to permit real-time multiplanar display in the operating room. Newer multidetector CT scanners allow acquisition of 4 to 32 slices with each scanner rotation. 64 slice units are in development. This degree of coverage dramatically reduces motion artifact, and in conjunction with 0.5 mm to 0.75 mm beam collimation permits very high-resolution multiplanar reformatted images.

The Hounsfield number or unit (HU) describes tissue density in CT (Table 3–1). Because the subcutaneous and intraorbital tissues contain substantial fat, there is usually sufficient contrast to recognize extension of disease to these areas from the sinuses. Diagnosis of subtle intracranial complications from sinus disease is more problematic with CT.[7] Iodinated intravenous (IV) contrast is not necessary in most routine or preoperative cases; however, it is very useful to demonstrate abnormal enhancement at the margin of an area of inflammation or abscess. This enhancement may be the only finding

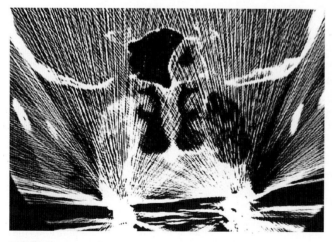

FIGURE 3–4 Severe dental artifact. When extensive restorations are present, thin section axial scanning with reformatting may be preferable.

in a situation such as an early subperiosteal postseptal abscess. Though relatively safe, use of IV contrast is not trivial, and a few simple points should be considered. Prior reaction to contrast should prompt brief questioning regarding its nature and whether the patient is aware if "ionic" (high osmolar) or "nonionic" (low osmolar) contrast was used. One or two hives with no therapy necessary should be noted but will probably not require a change in protocol for the scan. More significant reactions such as laryngeal or oropharyngeal edema and respiratory compromise will generally require rethinking the necessity for contrast, considering magnetic resonance imaging (MRI), or utilizing a steroid prep combined with low osmolar IV contrast. When considering contrast-enhanced CT, the radiologist at your institution should be contacted when confronted with a history of significant prior contrast reaction.

Renal dysfunction is a relative contraindication to iodinated contrast administration. At our institution, a baseline creatinine is not required for patients younger than 60 years with no history of renal compromise. We generally will not administer any iodinated contrast to patients with a creatinine greater than 2.0 mg/dL, unless they are undergoing regular dialysis. A diabetic with a creatinine of 1.4 to 2.0 mg/dL, where contrast-enhanced CT is essential, will be hydrated and receive low osmolar contrast. Again, if any questions arise regarding contrast administration for a patient at risk, discussion with the responsible radiologist is best prior to scheduling the scan.

Finally, a general discussion of CT would not be complete without addressing the issue of limited sinus CT as a substitute for plain films in the early workup of sinus disease. Often it seems these exams are done in an attempt to convince patients that their complaint is being investigated, while trying to limit the cost of the exam. The evaluation of an initial episode of acute sinusitis and the response to therapy is a clinical exercise. Subjective complaints by the patient correlate poorly with CT findings, as demonstrated by Bhattacharyya et al.[8] If the patient demonstrates persistent disease following therapy or complicated sinusitis or is deemed a candidate for

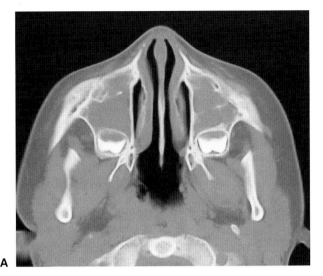

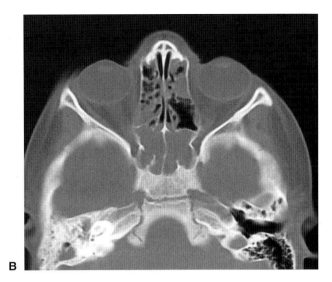

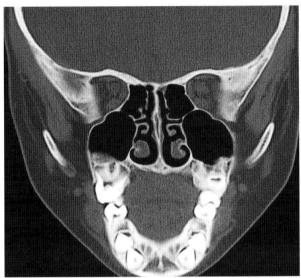

FIGURE 3–5 (A,B) Axial images pretreatment for acute sinusitis (simple CT protocol: thick sections, axial, five to nine images). (C) Coronal scan posttherapy.

surgical intervention, then complete coronal evaluation becomes the preferred option. Limited axial or coronal sinus CT probably adds little to patient management (Fig. 3–5). One exception to this may be patients about to undergo bone marrow transplantation. Oberholzer et al[9] studied 80 patients prior to bone marrow transplantation, revealing disease requiring therapy in 17 (21%). Patients with leukemia and non-Hodgkin's lymphoma were the most frequently affected. Given the profound immunosuppression these patients are subjected to, limited study to exclude significant sinus disease without complete evaluation of the OMU may be reasonable.

Magnetic Resonance Imaging

Magnetic resonance imaging also provides cross-sectional data and has been preferred over CT when coronal or sagittal imaging is desired. Helical CT with multiplanar reformatting has lessened the importance of this distinction. MRI utilizes the magnetic properties of protons in a strong magnetic field to generate weak radiofrequency signals that yield the diagnostic image. Unfortunately, from the perspective of sinus imaging, bony detail is more difficult to appreciate, as cortical bone has essentially no signal.[10] Additionally, the examinations are long compared with CT, and sedation may be required. MRI is probably superior to CT in most instances to assess potential intracranial complications of sinusitis or operative intervention.[10] One important point regarding MRI is that signal strength from the tissues, and hence image quality, is directly related to the strength of the scanner magnetic field. Most open MRI units operate at 0.3 to 0.5 Tesla (1 T = 10,000 × earth's gravitational field strength). High-field scanners operate at 1.5 Tesla. Subtle abnormalities may be missed in a low-field scanner. If medical conditions permit, claustrophobic patients will receive a higher quality study sedated in a high-field scanner rather than giving in to their request to be imaged in an open system.

Ultrasound

Ultrasound has been used recently for diagnosis of acute sinusitis in intensive care unit (ICU) patients[11] and has been investigated as a primary care screening tool,[12] but it has essentially no utility in presurgical imaging.

Nuclear Medicine

Nuclear imaging will generally be utilized for diagnosis of osteomyelitis in cases of complicated sinusitis. Intrathecal injection of tracer may be useful as a screening exam prior to CT cisternography when trying to identify cerebrospinal fluid (CSF) leaks.

■ Anatomy

Surgical anatomy has been covered previously. This discussion will focus on the radiologic appearance of normal and variant anatomy.

Normal Anatomy

A key concept underpinning functional endoscopic sinus surgery is that inflammatory sinus disease primarily results from impaired sinus drainage through the ostiomeatal channels. The goal of FESS is to restore physiologic drainage patterns. Radiologic examinations should be customized to optimally display the ostiomeatal channels that provide ventilation to and mucociliary clearance from the frontal, maxillary, ethmoid, and sphenoid sinuses. The term *ostiomeatal unit* defines air passages communicating between the frontal, anterior ethmoid, and maxillary sinuses, and is usually the main focus of FESS. Two other key areas to evaluate and describe are the frontal recess (FR) and the sphenoethmoid recess (SER).

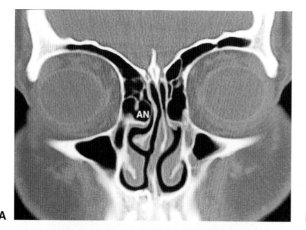

A

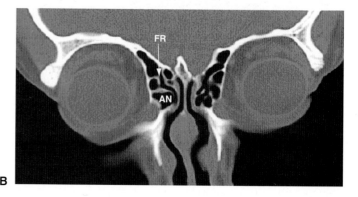

B

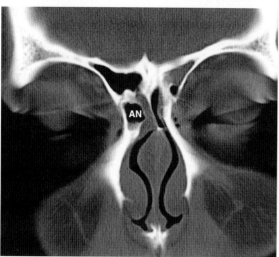

C

FIGURE 3–6 Agger nasi cells are distinguished from the ethmoid bulla by their more anterior location. They may impair drainage via the frontal recess. The term *anterior ethmoid air cell* may help avoid confusion. Images A–C show the appearance as one moves anteriorly. Note that the air cell is still visible with soft tissues of the eyelids and globes barely within the plane of imaging. AN, aggar nasi cells; FR, frontal recess.

Initial coronal CT images display the frontal sinuses. The FR is an hourglass-like narrowing between the frontal sinus and the anterior middle meatus. Sagittal images clearly demonstrate it is not a tubular structure, and therefore the term *frontal recess* is preferred over nasofrontal duct (Fig. 3–2B). Anterior, lateral, and inferior to the FR are the most anterior ethmoid air cells, usually referred to as agger nasi cells. (The nomenclature for these structures is undergoing modification to more directly reflect anatomical location, and so the term *anterior ethmoid air cell* is increasingly used.) They are usually immediately subjacent to the FR, and thus their size may directly influence drainage via the FR and the anterior middle meatus (Fig. 3–6) The frontal recesses are in actuality residual spaces remaining following pneumatization of the agger nasi cells and the ethmoid bulla more posteriorly. They are often fairly narrow and are common sites for inflammation and impaired mucociliary clearance.

The ethmoid infundibulum extends between the uncinate process and the inferomedial border of the orbit and is the primary drainage pathway from the maxillary sinus. The uncinate process of the ethmoid bone is a superomedial extension of the lateral nasal wall. Anteriorly, the uncinate process joins the medial wall of the agger nasi cells and the posteromedial wall of the nasolacrimal duct. The free edge of the uncinate process extends posterosuperiorly, and the lateral margin defines the superomedial aspect of the infundibulum. The ethmoid bulla is posterolateral to the free edge of the uncinate, usually the largest of the anterior ethmoid cells, and enclosed laterally by the lamina papyracea (Fig. 3–7). The ethmoid bulla represents a key surgical landmark, presenting a characteristic bulge in the superolateral nasal wall visible through the surgical endoscope. For this reason, it is considered separately from the other components of the ethmoid labyrinth, and it is referred to as though

it is a single structure even though it often contains more than one air cell. The hiatus semilunaris is defined as the gap between the ethmoid bulla and the free edge of the uncinate process, and it medially communicates with the middle meatus. Laterally and inferiorly, the hiatus semilunaris borders the infundibulum.

The lateral nasal wall is the origin of the superior, middle, and inferior turbinates. The turbinates divide the nasal cavity into the superior, middle, and inferior meati. The superior meatus drains the posterior ethmoid air cells, as well as the sphenoid sinus via the sphenoethmoid recess. The middle meatus drains the frontal sinus via the frontal recess, the maxillary sinus via the maxillary ostium leading into the ethmoidal infundibulum, and anterior ethmoid air cells via the ethmoid cell ostia. The inferior meatus receives drainage from the nasolacrimal duct, usually visible on three to four adjacent coronal sections through the anterior midface.

The middle turbinate attaches anteriorly to the medial wall of the agger nasi (anterior ethmoid) cells and the superior edge of the uncinate process. Superiorly, the middle turbinate adheres to the cribriform plate. Posteriorly, the middle turbinate connects to the skull base via the basal or ground lamella (Fig. 3–8) that fuses with the lamina papyracea just posterior to the ethmoid bulla. In most patients, the posterior wall of the ethmoid bulla is intact, and an air space is usually found between the ground lamella and the ethmoid bulla. This air space, the sinus lateralis, may extend superior to the ethmoid bulla, communicating with the FR. Dehiscence or absence of the posterior wall of the ethmoid bulla is not unusual and may permit

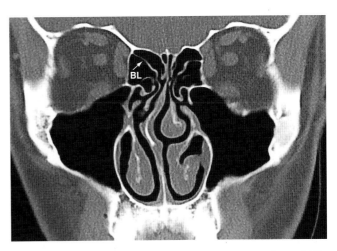

FIGURE 3–8 Basal lamella (BL) connecting the middle turbinate to the lamina papyracea. Damage may occur in this region from excessive traction during middle turbinectomy. Note the septal deviation and hypoplasia of the right middle turbinate (also the lack of any demonstrable sinus mucosal disease).

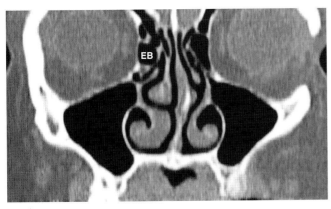

FIGURE 3–7 Reformatted axial scan showing the ethmoid bulla (EB). Note that it is more posterior, in the region of the uncinate and infundibulum.

communication between these two usually separated air spaces. The posterior ethmoid sinus consists of air cells between the basal lamella and the sphenoid sinus. The number, shape, and size of these air cells vary.

The sphenoid sinus is most posterior, contained within the clivus, lying anteroinferior to the sella turcica. Its ostium is usually in the superomedial portion of the anterior sinus wall and drains via the SER into the posterior aspect of the superior meatus. The SER is just lateral to the nasal septum and is best seen with axial or sagittal images (Fig. 3–2C,D).

The sphenoid sinus and posterior ethmoid air cells change in relation to one another as one moves from the midline laterally. Near the midline, the sphenoid sinus is the most superior aerated cavity, and laterally, the posterior ethmoid air cells become the most posterior and superior extent of the paranasal sinuses.

Anatomical Variations

The relation of a particular variation to inflammatory disease is related to its ability to narrow or obstruct the air passages of the FR, OMU, or SER. From a presurgical standpoint, important variants influence the risk to adjacent structures during specific operative maneuvers. Special note is made of encephalocele, which is a contraindication to all but the most limited endoscopic manipulation.

Septal Variants

Septal bowing may compress the middle turbinate laterally, narrowing the middle meatus. Bony spurs are often associated with septal deviation and may compromise the OMU (Fig. 3–9).

Middle Turbinate Variants

Concha bullosa defines a middle turbinate that is aerated, enlarges, and may obstruct the middle meatus or infundibulum (Fig. 3–10). Middle turbinate concha

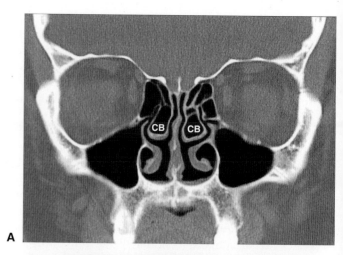
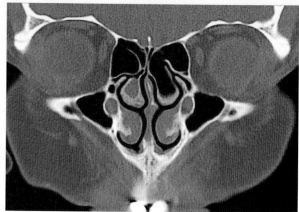

FIGURE 3–10   (A) Bilateral concha bullosa. (B) Bilateral concha bullosa with retained secretions versus mucosal thickening.

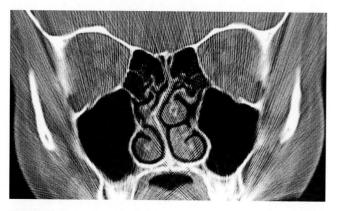

FIGURE 3–9 Septal deviation with spur. Again, note hypoplasia of the right middle turbinate.

bullosa may be unilateral or bilateral, superior turbinate involvement is less frequent, and inferior turbinate involvement is rare. The mucous membrane lining the concha bullosa is no different from the rest of the sinuses and may display inflammatory change, including development of air-fluid levels. In most people the major curvature of the middle turbinate is projected toward the septum. A paradoxical middle turbinate curves laterally (reverse scrolling) and may narrow the middle meatus (Fig. 3–11). A study by Lam et al[13] shows no specific relationship between concha bullosa and chronic sinusitis.

Uncinate Variants

The free edge of the uncinate process has a variable course. Lateral deviation narrows the infundibulum. Medial deviation may narrow or obstruct the middle meatus. Occasionally, the free edge of the uncinate is fused to the orbital floor or lamina papyrcea, described as an atelectatic uncinate process. Inflammation or hypoplasia of the ipsilateral maxillary sinus may be present

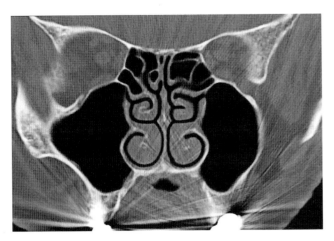

FIGURE 3–11   Paradoxical left middle turbinate curves laterally and may obstruct the middle meatus.

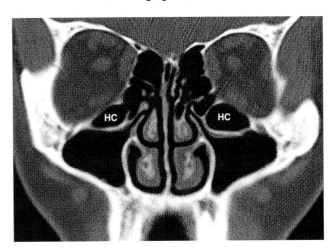

FIGURE 3–13   Large bilateral Haller's cells (HC). Again, nomenclature is shifting to more descriptive terminology, so the term *inferior ethmoid air cell* is increasingly used.

related to partial or complete obstruction of the infundibulum. Occasionally, the uncinate may be aerated (Fig. 3–12).

Ethmoid Variants

Haller's cells are ethmoid air cells that extend along the roof of the maxillary sinus and may contribute to narrowing of the infundibulum (Fig. 3–13). Again, nomenclature is shifting to more accurately describe anatomy, and so the term *orbital air cell* is frequently used. The ethmoid bulla may enlarge to narrow or obstruct the middle meatus and infundibulum. Large agger nasi cells can obstruct the frontal recess. Onodi cells are rare lateral and posterior extensions of the posterior ethmoid air cells, extending in close proximity to the optic nerves as they exit the orbits. Failure to recognize this variant may place the optic nerves at risk. Dehiscence of the lamina papyracea, either

congenital or post-traumatic, may increase the risk of orbital entry. An aerated crista galli may communicate with the frontal recess (Fig. 3–14). Obstruction of this ostium can lead to chronic sinusitis and mucocele formation. Although usually small, the presence of this variant may increase the risk of entry into the anterior cranial fossa.

Sphenoid Variants

Pneumatization of the sphenoid sinus can extend into the anterior clinoids or present as very large lateral recesses (Fig. 3–15). The former may place the optic nerves at risk; the latter may increase the risk of inadvertent perforation of the carotid artery. The septations of the sphenoid sinus are variable and may be incorporated in the bony wall covering the internal carotid artery. The margin of the carotid canal or optic canal adjacent to the sphenoid sinus may be dehiscent.

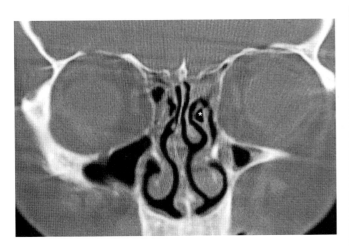

FIGURE 3–12   Aerated uncinate (*) is uncommon but may obstruct the infundibulum.

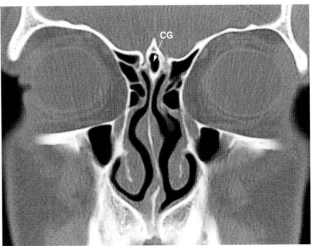

FIGURE 3–14   Aerated crista galli (CG).

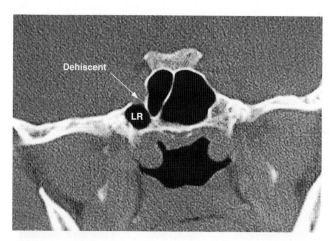

FIGURE 3–15 Large lateral recess (LR) of sphenoid. The presence of a dehiscence increases the risk of inadvertent carotid entry.

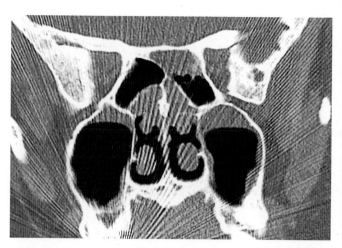

FIGURE 3–16 Dependent secretions in the maxillary sinuses (patient scanned supine hyperextended), as well as more foamy, inspissated secretions in the sphenoid sinus.

■ Inflammatory/Infectious Disease

Acute Sinusitis

Acute sinusitis is usually due to bacterial superinfection of an obstructed paranasal sinus. The specific bacteriology of acute sinusitis is covered in Chapter 2. The obstruction is usually the result of contact between edematous mucosal surfaces from a recent viral upper respiratory tract infection and most commonly involves a single sinus, typically the ethmoid. The edema disrupts the normal mucociliary drainage pattern of the sinus, and obstruction of the sinus ostium results. Scribano et al[14] showed that despite bony abnormality in the OMU, mucosal contact is the strongest predictor of maxillary inflammatory disease. The accumulated fluid within the sinus provides an ideal medium for bacterial superinfection. There is an increased risk of regional and intracranial complications with involvement of the frontal, ethmoid, and sphenoid sinuses due to proximity to the anterior cranial fossa, orbits, optic nerves, and cavernous sinus.

Normally, the sinus mucosa is imperceptible. Thickness greater than 4 mm is suggestive of pathology but may merely be a nonspecific finding. A notable example of this would be the alternating asymmetric thickening of the mucosa covering the turbinates seen as a manifestation of the nasal cycle. Traditionally, air fluid level has been considered the hallmark of acute sinusitis; however, the mere presence of an air-fluid level does not prove infection. Fluid from diagnostic or therapeutic lavage may remain for up to 2 weeks, and changes following a bout of acute sinusitis, even with successful therapy, may be seen for up to 6 to 8 weeks. CT findings in acute sinusitis may range from smooth or nodular mucosal thickening to complete opacification of the sinus (Fig. 3–16). The attenuation in these regions is typically that of water or low-density soft tissue. On MRI during acute sinusitis, the sinus contents display signal characteristics of free water with hypointense signal on T1-weighted images and hyperintense signal on T2-weighted images.

Chronic Sinusitis

Chronic sinusitis describes a patient who has repeated bouts of acute infection or persistent inflammation, with the anterior ethmoid air cells most commonly involved. Signs suggesting chronic sinusitis are mucosal thickening or opacification, bone remodeling and thickening related to osteitis from adjacent chronic mucosal inflammation, and polyposis. Even with these findings, however, diagnosing a current exacerbation of chronic sinusitis is clinical. Changes suggesting chronicity on a single scan may have been present for a long time and may not be related to the current episode (Fig. 3–17).

Thick secretions usually will not layer out and may form small droplike densities on CT as they progress along the medial wall of the maxillary sinus toward the ostium. Frothy secretions may also be seen, and sponge-like material usually suggests completely dessicated secretions. When sinus secretions are of low viscosity, the CT attenuation is on the order of 10 to 25 HU. When the secretions become thickened and concentrated, the CT attenuation increases with density measurements of 30 to 60 HU (Fig. 3–18).

MRI findings in chronic sinusitis are quite variable because of the changing concentrations of protein and free water protons. Initially, watery secretions are hypointense on T1-weighted images and hyperintense on

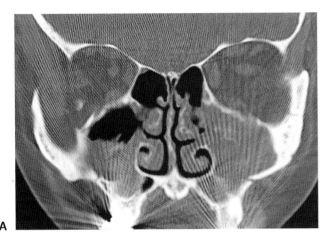
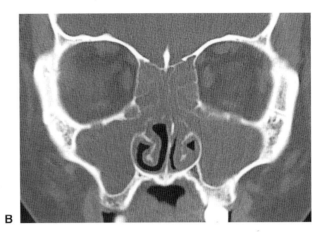

FIGURE 3–17   (A,B) Chronic polymicrobial sinusitis. The slightly heterogeneous wispy pattern in A should also raise suspicion for allergic fungal sinusitis with copious partially inspissated allergic mucin.

T2-weighted images. Som and Curtin[15] describe two important physiologic events when sinonasal secretions become obstructed: The number of glycoprotein-secreting goblet cells in the mucosa increases, and the mucosa resorbs free water. Over time, this causes a transition from a thin serous fluid to a thicker mucus and, ultimately, to a desiccated plug (Fig. 3–19). As the protein concentration increases, the signal intensity on T2-weighted images decreases. Cross-linking between glycoprotein molecules is believed to be responsible for these changes. Som and Brandwein[16] describe four patterns of MRI signal intensity that can be seen with chronic sinusitis: (1) hypointense on T1-weighted images and hyperintense on T2-weighted images, with total protein concentration less than 9%; (2) hyperintense on T1-weighted images and hyperintense on T2-weighted images, with total protein concentration increased to 20 to 25%; (3) hyperintense on T1-weighted images and hypointense on T2-weighted images, with total protein concentration

of 25 to 30%; (4) hypointense on both T1 and T2-weighted images, with protein concentration greater than 30% and inspissated secretions in an almost solid form. Inspissated secretions may occasionally be missed on MRI because the signal voids on T2-weighted images, and to a lesser degree T1-weighted images may be identical to normally aerated sinuses.

Anatomical variations have sometimes been suggested as causative factors in the presence of chronic inflammatory disease. Stammberger and Wolf[17] and Lidov and Som[18] found that a large concha bullosa could produce signs and symptoms by narrowing the infundibulum. Yousem et al,[19] however, found that the presence of a concha bullosa did not increase the risk of sinusitis. Similar findings were reported by Bolger et al,[20] who found that concha bullosa, paradoxical turbinates, Haller's cells, and uncinate pneumatization were not significantly more common in patients with chronic sinusitis than in asymptomatic patients. Yousem et al[19] found the

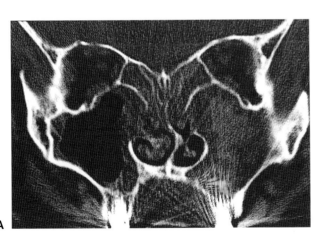
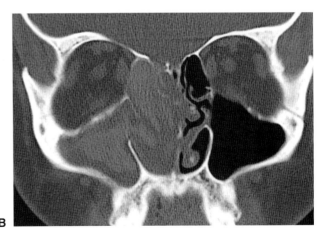

FIGURE 3–18   (A,B) High attenuation within the maxillary sinuses. Depending on the Hounsfield number, the differential for this appearance includes hemorrhage, inspissated secretions (high relative protein content), and allergic fungal sinusitis.

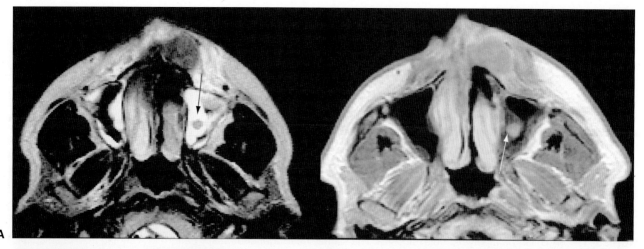

A

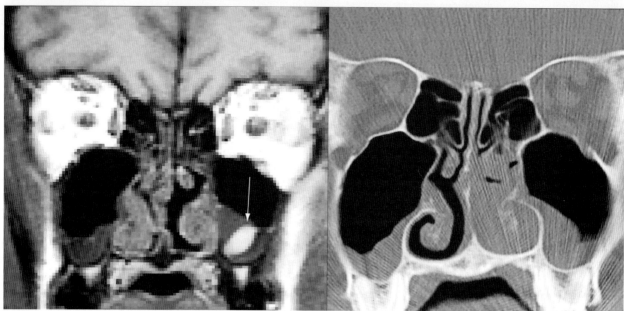

B

FIGURE 3–19 (A) Axial MRI (brain study for other reason) shows increased signal in a focus of left maxillary sinus mucosa on the T1-weighted image (arrow). The corresponding T2 image (left) shows decreased signal typical of high protein content. The sinus mucosa shows typical low signal on T1 and high signal on T2, typical for its usual high free water content. (B) Coronal T1 MR and corresponding CT in the same patient. Again seen is a focus of inspissated secretion in the left maxillary sinus mucosa, consistent with a mucous retention cyst. Note the near invisibility on CT.

presence of nasal septal deviation and a horizontally oriented uncinate process to be more common in patients with inflammatory sinusitis. In patients in whom the middle meatus was opacified, associated inflammatory changes were present in the ethmoid sinuses in 82% and in the maxillary sinuses in 84% of patients. Danese et al[21] studied 112 patients older than 16 years with chronic sinusitis. Dental, mycotic, traumatic, neoplastic, and postoperative cases were excluded. An association was found with ipsilateral septal ridges or spurs (33%), unusual deflections of the uncinate process (31%), and contralateral septal "watch glass" deviations (42%). As with other investigators,[22] no association with chronic sinusitis was found for concha bullosa, paradoxical middle turbinate, pneumatized uncinate process, hypertrophic ethmoid bulla, Haller's cell (orbital air cell), or accessory maxillary ostium. In general, simple opacification of the FR, OMU, or SER without coexistent sinus mucosal disease cannot be presumed significant.

Cystic fibrosis patients make up a distinct subset of patients with chronic sinusitis. A young patient displaying uncinate deossification, chronic mucosal thickening, and maxillary sinus mucocele should prompt consideration of this diagnosis.

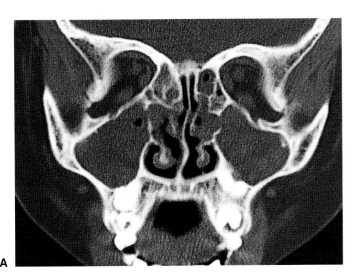

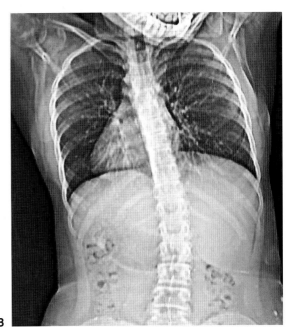

FIGURE 3–20   (A,B) Pansinusitis associated with Kartagener's syndrome. Note associated situs inversus totalis on the chest CT topogram.

Kartagener's syndrome patients also display chronic sinusitis that is often difficult to manage due to their nonfunctional cilia. Situs inversus totalis is an associated finding (Fig. 3–20).

Fungal Sinusitis

Fungal sinusitis is of concern when a patient fails to respond to standard antibiotic therapy. A thorough discussion of the microbiology of fungal sinusitis may be found in Chapters 9 and 20.

It is important to recognize that fungal sinusitis cannot be considered as a single entity. At least four distinct disease patterns exist, depending on the specific microbiology of the infection and the immune status of the patient. These are acute invasive, chronic invasive, mycetoma, and allergic. The maxillary and ethmoid sinuses are the most common sites of involvement.

Acute invasive disease occurs in the setting of significant immmunocompromise and is characterized by aggressive angioinvasive progression. This may manifest as direct intracranial or maxillofacial extension of disease or intracranial and extracranial thrombosis and infarction. Invasive *Aspergillus* in an immunocompromised patient and mucormycosis in a diabetic patient would be typical but by no means exclusive examples. CT will reveal intermediate to low attenuation progressing beyond the confines of the involved sinus, while T2-weighted MRI will usually demonstrate high signal due to the extensive edema in the region.

Chronic fungal sinusitis is seen in immunocompetent patients. This typically presents as a severe chronic granulomatous sinusitis that does not respond to standard antibiotic therapy. Dahniya et al[23] describe soft tissue mass within the paranasal sinuses, which is homogeneous with occasional lower attenuation components on CT. Erosion or expansion of the bony margins of the sinuses may occur, sometimes with intraorbital or intracranial extension (Fig. 3–21). If intracranial extension is suspected on CT, MRI will be beneficial to better characterize potential meningeal or brain involvement. This form of sinusitis is usually the result of inhalation of

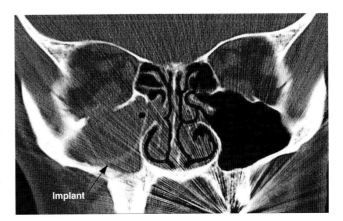

FIGURE 3–21   Right maxillary fungal sinusitis with displacement of a silastic implant for orbital floor reconstruction.

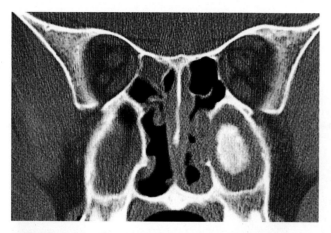

FIGURE 3–22 Sinonasal Wegener's granulomatosis with a calcified mycetoma in the left maxillary sinus.

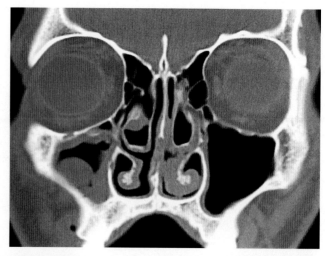

FIGURE 3–23 Polypoid mucosal thickening in a patient with allergic fungal sinusitis.

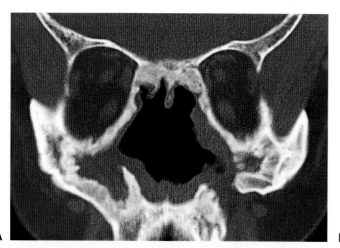

A

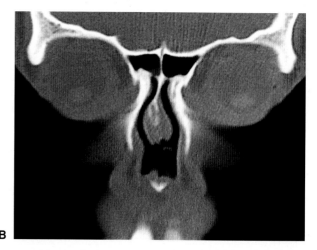

B

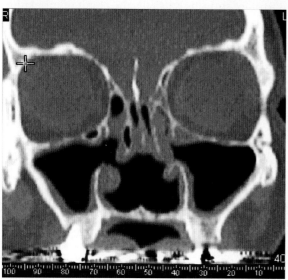

C

FIGURE 3–24 Wegener's granulomatosis. (A) Extensive destruction with severe chronic mucosal disease. (B) Typical early change consisting of cartilaginous destruction without bony involvement. (C) Reformatted axial CT demonstrating destruction secondary to cocaine abuse.

Aspergillus spores and is more commonly seen in the Middle East rather than in North America.

Mycetoma is most commonly seen in the maxillary sinus, in patients with normal immune status. Mucosal thickening is usually but not necessarily present. Thickening of the bony walls of the sinus may be related to prior disease with reactive osteitis, or it may be a more recent development. Comparison films are always helpful to make this distinction. CT usually demonstrates a focal hyperdense lesion with surrounding hypodense mucoid material. Flocculent calcification is described in up to 25% of cases evaluated with CT[24] (Fig. 3–22). On MRI, low-signal intensity on T1-weighted images and signal void on T2-weighted images have been found in a high proportion of patients with fungal sinusitis. The diminished signal is presumed to represent paramagnetic effects from iron and manganese within the hyphae. Even though a similar MRI appearance can be seen in chronic bacterial infection due to desiccated secretions, the decreased signal is not as pronounced as that found with fungal disease.

Allergic fungal sinusitis is analogous to allergic bronchopulmonary aspergillosis, described in the pulmonary medicine literature, and is seen in ~4 to 7% of the population.[25] Patients are usually atopic, with an exuberant immune response to the fungal colonization. Polypoid mucosal thickening is common (Fig. 3–23), and a large amount of mucus, referred to as "allergic mucin," may fill and at times significantly expand the involved sinuses (Fig. 3–18A). This material demonstrates fluid attenuation on CT, and although the expansion can be impressive, the involved sinuses are usually still identifiable. Erosion of the sinus wall is not a typical finding, until expansion is extreme. MRI usually demonstrates high to mixed signal on T2-weighted images. Wispy areas of low signal consistent with fungal elements are often seen within the high-signal mucoid material. Overall signal intensity on T2-weighted images will decrease as free water content decreases. Air-fluid levels are rare unless bacterial superinfection occurs.

Granulomatous Sinusitis

Many granulomatous diseases can involve the sinonasal cavity. Infectious causes include actinomycosis, aspergillosis, blastomycosis, leprosy, nocardiosis, rhinoscleroma, syphilis, and tuberculosis. Noninfectious causes include sarcoidosis and Wegener's granulomatosis. Foreign body granulomatous responses are seen with beryllium, chromate salts, and cocaine[16] (Fig. 3–24). These processes all have the potential to cause bone and cartilage destruction, but perforation of the cartilaginous nasal septum prior to bony destruction is a key finding.

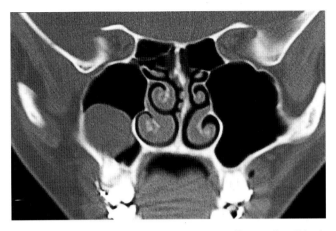

FIGURE 3–25 Mucous retention cyst. Generally, this is indistinguishable from a polyp on CT. The exception to this is infundibular widening, which is usually seen only with polyposis.

■ Specific Entities/Complications

Mucous Retention Cyst

Mucous retention cyst is a small cyst that most commonly occurs in the maxillary sinus floor in patients with previous inflammatory disease and is caused by inflammatory obstruction of a seromucinous gland within the sinus mucosal lining.[26] On CT, a mucous retention cyst will appear as a homogeneous, well-circumscribed low-attenuation to intermediate attenuation mass (Fig. 3–25). On MRI, it is usually hypointense on T1-weighted images and hyperintense on T2-weighted images owing to the large number of free water protons.

Mucocele

A mucocele is the result of a chronically obstructed sinus ostium, mucous secretions filling the sinus cavity with eventual expansion of the bony sinus walls.[15] Although most commonly caused by inflammatory obstruction of the ostium, a mucocele can be secondary to trauma, tumors, or surgical manipulation. Sixty-six percent of mucoceles occur in the frontal sinuses, with 25% and 10% occurring in the ethmoid and maxillary sinuses, respectively.[26] On CT, a mucocele is a hypodense, nonenhancing mass that fills and expands the sinus cavity (Fig. 3–26). On MRI, the appearance is variable owing to alterations in protein concentration of the obstructed mucoid secretions, as discussed previously. An infected mucocele, a mucopyocele, may demonstrate rim enhancement on contrast-enhanced CT.

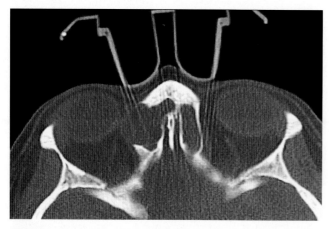

FIGURE 3–26   Right ethmoid mucocele. Note the preservation of the lamina papyracea with expansion. The patient was scanned with a stereotactic device for use with the Instatrak system.

Inflammatory Polyps

Paranasal sinus polyps result from a local upheaval of the sinus mucosa with mucous membrane hyperplasia secondary to chronic inflammation. This process often occurs in the setting of allergic sinusitis. Polyps can cause local problems if numerous, or large enough to obstruct the ostiomeatal channels, including the sinus ostia. On CT and MRI, polyps are often indistinguishable from mucous retention cysts, although widening of the infundibulum or SER may help in identifying polypoid disease (Fig. 3–27B,C). Very rarely, the stalk of a polyp may be visible, confirming the diagnosis. An antrochoanal polyp has a characteristic appearance, filling the involved maxillary sinus and extending posteriorly in continuity to the choanae (Fig. 3–27A).

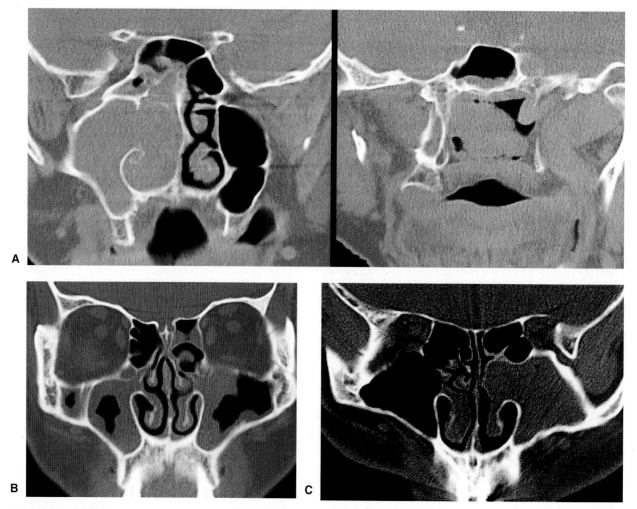

FIGURE 3–27   (A) Large antrochoanal polyp demonstrating infundibular widening and extension to the choanae. (B,C) Infundibular widening asociated with polypoid disease.

Orbital Complications

About 3% of patients with sinusitis develop some degree of orbital involvement. Children commonly display preseptal orbital manifestations early in the clinical course of a sinus infection. Complicated sinusitis is the most common cause of orbital infection, with 60 to 84% of cases attributed to it.[27] The ethmoid sinuses are the most common origin, followed by frontal, sphenoid, and maxillary sinuses in decreasing order of frequency. The ethmoid and maxillary sinuses are present at birth and responsible for orbital complications in younger children. The frontal sinuses are usually detectable radiographically after age 6 years but are not usually significant sources of infection until after 10 years of age. The sphenoid sinuses also develop late and are rarely implicated in the pediatric age group.

There is little argument about obtaining a CT scan when there is clinical evidence of postseptal infection or when there is failure to improve with antibiotics. Because the disease can be much more aggressive in the pediatric population, CT scanning should be considered when there is clinical evidence of preseptal inflammation.

When preseptal inflammation is present, CT reveals diffuse increased soft tissue density, fat infiltration, and thickening of the preseptal soft tissues. At this stage, there is swelling and redness of the eyelids but no proptosis or limitation of eye movement (Fig. 3–28). As infection spreads from the ethmoid sinus to the orbit, there is inflammation of the orbital periosteum. This tissue becomes thickened and elevated, with accumulation of an inflammatory collection. On CT, this reaction appears as an ill-defined, slightly enhancing mass on the sinus and orbital sides of the lamina papyracea. It is limited laterally by the periosteum, but in more advanced cases, it merges with a thickened and enhancing medial rectus muscle, which is displaced laterally. Subsequently, liquefaction may occur in the subperiosteal compartment to form an abscess. It is evident on CT as regions of low density, sometimes with an enhancing peripheral margin. The CT findings of low-attenuation material surrounded by an enhancing rim suggest the diagnosis of abscess rather than an inflammatory mass, although the distinction between them can be difficult, because they represent a continuum between these two states. Harris[28] demonstrated that CT cannot predict the exact nature of the material and that some enlargement of the subperiosteal collection is typical for the first few days of antibiotic therapy, regardless of the ultimate outcome. This early continued enlargement should not be construed as therapeutic failure.

Rare orbital complications of paranasal sinus infection include superior ophthalmic vein (SOV) thrombosis, cavernous sinus thrombosis, and blindness.[29] SOV thrombosis is suspected on CT scans when there is asymmetric enlargement of this vessel. This is most reliably seen on coronal scans, but occasionally it is well displayed on axial images that catch the vessel in-plane. Postcontrast images show minimal enhancement, although thrombus within the lumen can be hyperdense.

Cavernous sinus thrombosis is evident as fullness of the affected side with convexity of the lateral margin of

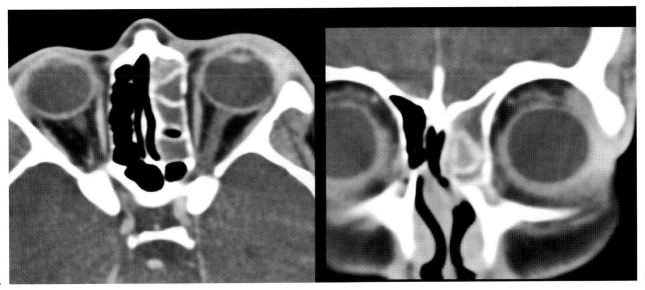

A
B

FIGURE 3–28 Left preseptal cellulitis associated with left ethmoid disease in a child displayed in the axial and coronal planes.

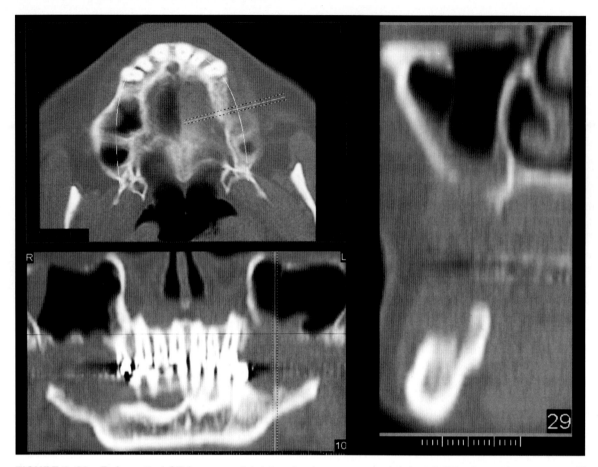

FIGURE 3–29 Reformatted CT from an axial dataset using a commercial dental CT reformatting program. There is left dentoalveolar osteomyelitis related to a prior dental abscess, now postextraction. Note the associated sinus mucosal thickening.

the cavernous sinus instead of the normal, slightly concave margin. Gadolinium-enhanced axial and coronal MRI in a high-field scanner with a targeted field of view (FOV) will display these changes more definitively than CT.

Permanent loss of vision is a rare complication of sinusitis, although rates as high as 10% have been reported in patients with postseptal Infection.[29] Possible mechanisms for loss of vision include optic neuritis as a reaction to adjacent infection, ischemia secondary to thrombophlebitis or arteritis, and pressure on the central retinal artery.

Osteomyelitis

Osteomyelitis may be seen as a complication of bacterial or fungal sinusitis. Alternatively, chronic sinus disease may be the result of osteomyelitis adjacent to a paranasal sinus (Fig. 3–29). Diagnosis of osteomyelitis in the maxillofacial region can be quite difficult, given the low-grade inflammation present in the periodontium of dentate patients. Bone scanning with planar imaging alone is often useless in pinpointing a focal abnormality. One approach involves an initial CT scan of the area in question. Dental CT reformatting is completed to maximize evaluation of the dataset if there is a question of odontogenic pathology or if the area in question is within the maxilla. If there is evidence of focal trabecular alteration, sclerosis, or lysis, bone scanning with technetium 99m pentetic acid (Tc 99m DTPA) is performed, including blood pool, and delayed single photon emission computed tomography (SPECT). At the same time as the initial injection of Tc 99m DTPA, indium 111 (In 111) labeled white blood cells (WBCs) from the patient are reinjected, and SPECT imaging of the maxillofacial region is completed at 24 hours (Fig. 3–30). SPECT imaging utilizes a rotating or multihead gamma camera to obtain multiple projections from the patient, yielding cross-sectional bone scan data. These images are then compared with the cross-sectional CT data. The blood pool portion of the exam reveals hyperemia in the area under scrutiny, delayed Tc 99m

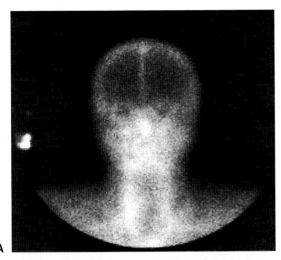

A

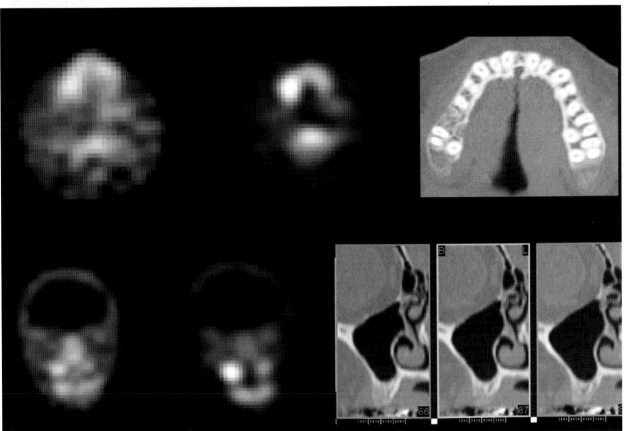

B

FIGURE 3–30 Dual injection Tc 99m and In 111 labeled WBC scan with SPECT. (A) No focal activity on blood pool image (planar). (B) Correlation of area of bone turnover where extraction was performed 4 months prior.

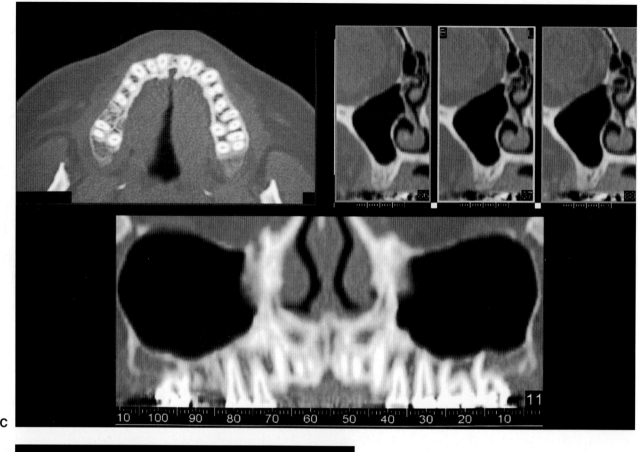

C

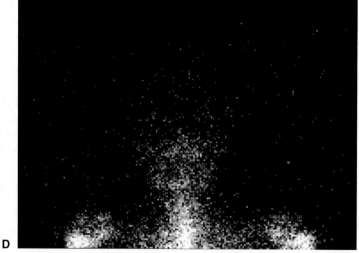

D

FIGURE 3–30 *(continued)* (C) Reformatted dental CT in area of interest. (D) No focal activity on WBC scan. This combination of findings would not be typical of osteomyelitis.

DTPA data reveal degree of bone turnover, and the delayed In 111 images identify areas of focal WBC chemotaxis. Positive Tc 99m DTPA and In 111 scans that correlate anatomically with one another and with the CT data are highly suggestive of osteomyelitis. Although this is much more involved than planar bone scanning, this correlative cross-sectional approach greatly improves spatial resolution in the maxillofacial region and permits more specific anatomical/physiologic correlation.

■ Unique Situations

Odontogenic pathology and a few oral and maxillofacial surgery procedures can affect the appearance of primarily the maxillary sinus on cross-sectional imaging. Thin-slice helical CT scanning with dental CT software reformatting is often helpful in evaluating the potential contribution of odontogenic pathology, as well as post-procedure changes to a particular presentation of maxillary sinus disease.

Odontogenic and Bone Pathology

Odontogenic-related sinus pathology typically would be inflammatory or infectious and manifest as failure of therapy in isolated maxillary sinusitis. The maxillary premolar and molar roots are in close approximation to the maxillary sinus floor, and pulpal inflammatory or infectious processes may act as a persistent nidus for sinus disease. Apical pulpal pathology of the incisors may violate the floor of the nasal cavity (Fig. 3–31). Although

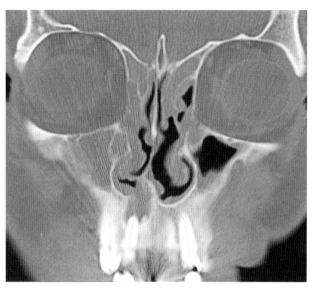

FIGURE 3–31 Periapical lesion of right incisor with secondary nasal mucosal disease and infundibular obstruction.

pulpal pathology is most common, advanced periodontal disease with vertical bony defects may cause focal sinus mucosal disease. Oral antral fistulae are most commonly postoperative sequelae, but they may occur in the setting of a perforated residual cyst that bridges the antral and oral mucosa. In dentate individuals, endodontic therapy of the involved tooth frequently removes the nidus for continued sinus disease, but in cases with combined periodontal involvement, failed endodontic therapy (Fig. 3–32), or root fracture, extraction

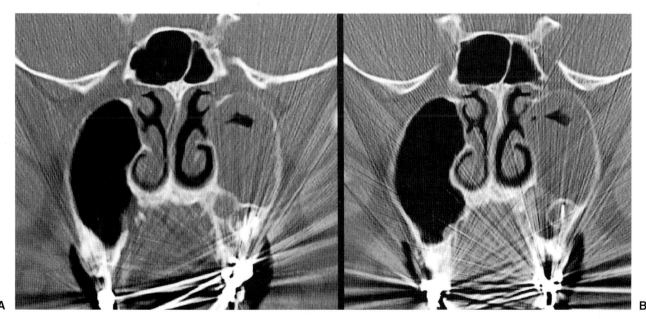

FIGURE 3–32 Persistent periapical pathology associated with an upper left molar postendodontic therapy. There is extensive associated maxillary sinus mucosal disease.

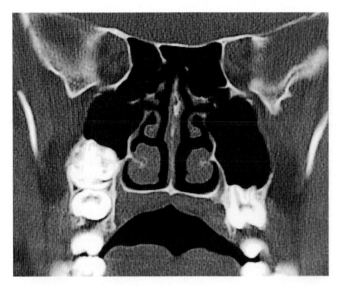

FIGURE 3–33 Complex odontoma on the floor of the right maxillary sinus. Occasionally these lesions will become large enough to obstruct the infundibulum.

may be necessary. In the case of an essential tooth for support of an existing prosthesis, apicoectomy with apical curettage may be attempted. Persistent infection or osteomyelitis following tooth extraction and, rarely, displacement of a root fragment into the maxillary sinus may also serve as a nidus for infection.[30]

Chronic sinus pathology can also be seen in the setting of an odontogenic cyst or odontoma (Fig. 3–33)

that causes obstruction at the infundibulum. In rare instances, the lesion becomes so large that the maxillary sinus is completely opacified.

Osteomas are most commonly found in the frontal sinus, vary in size, and may obstruct the FR or OMU (Fig. 3–34). Fibrous dysplasia may range from very small foci to extensive skull base expansion with compromise of physiologic sinus drainage (Fig. 3–35).

Dental Implants

Dental implants have come into wide use to support single-unit fixed prostheses (crowns), multiple-unit prostheses (bridges), and as fixtures for metal superstructure to attach implant-supported overdentures. When significant bony resorption has occurred in the maxilla, preimplant bone grafting is often undertaken using a "sinus lift" technique. During this procedure, a bony window is created in the lateral maxillary sinus wall, and the sinus membrane is gently lifted away from the bony antral floor. Imaging prior to this procedure focuses on septations in the floor of the maxillary sinus, as well as in the relationship of the apices of any remaining teeth to the sinus floor that may impede raising a mucosal flap. Once the flap is elevated, autogenous bone or various allogenic-bone combinations are inserted in this pocket to provide additional bone for implant osseointegration. Disruption of the sinus mucosa during this procedure may lead to sinusitis, graft infection, migration or extrusion of graft material, and in extreme cases oral antral communication.

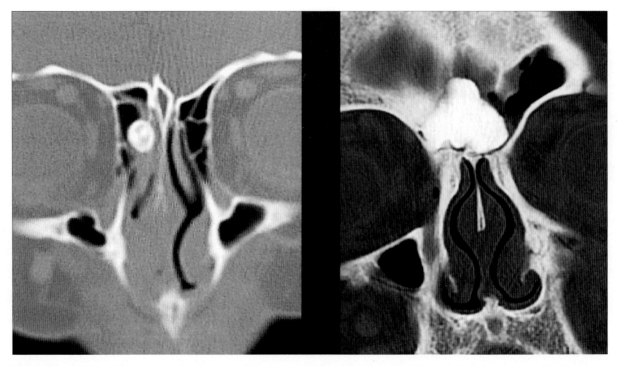

A   B

FIGURE 3–34   (A) Small right ethmoid osteoma. (B) Large right frontal osteoma with associated sinus opacification.

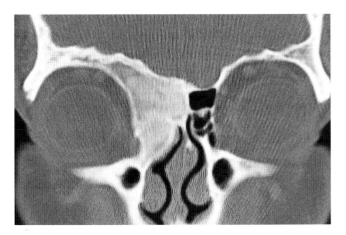

FIGURE 3–35 Right ethmoid fibrous dysplasia.

Unusual bony thickness along the maxillary sinus floor or unusual configuration of the bone with or without dental implants should alert the observer to the possibility of prior grafting within the maxillary sinus[31] (Fig. 3–36).

■ Nasal Masses

A complete discussion of congenital and acquired nasal masses is beyond the scope of this review, but there are several important points to consider. In general, when a mass is suspected, MRI with a targeted FOV to maximize spatial resolution will clarify whether changes seen on CT are manifestations of a mass or inflammatory sinus disease. Schneiderian papilloma (inverting papilloma) often causes obstruction at the maxillary sinus ostium, with secondary opacification (Fig. 3–37). Early in the

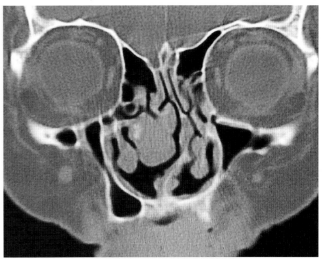

FIGURE 3–37 Inverting papilloma. Note the lack of infundibular widening as the lesion grows medially from the region of the infundibulum.

disease process, mass effect and bony erosion may be limited, but later the degree of expansion and bony destruction will suggest a mass. T2-weighted MRI will usually display the frondlike folds of this lesion as folded areas of intermediate signal within the high signal of thickened mucosa and mucus. Squamous cell carcinoma also presents as a mass and on MRI will tend to display a more disorganized "whirling" pattern of predominantly high signal with interspersed low signal on T2-weighted images. Lymphoma often extends beyond the confines of the involved sinus, with an attenuated ghost image of the sinus wall visible on CT (Fig. 3–38).

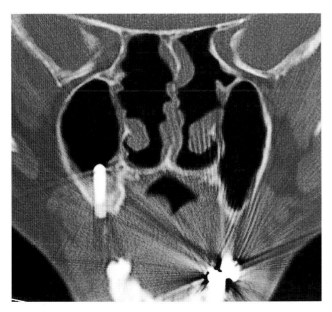

FIGURE 3–36 Maxillary dental implant with focal mucosal disease and poor incorporation of bone graft.

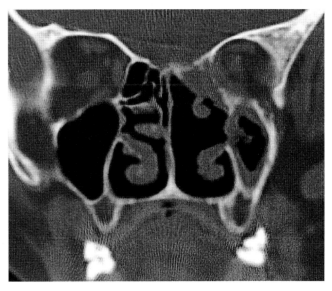

FIGURE 3–38 Recurrent ethmoid lymphoma. Note the ghostlike preservation of the medial orbital wall, although orbit invasion had already occurred.

Osteosarcoma is sometimes seen in the setting of pre-existing fibrous dysplasia or Paget's disease, but if bone expansion with osseous matrix and significant periosteal reaction is present, this should always be considered. Approximately 7% of osteosarcomas occur within the face and jaws.

Nasal masses in children typically reflect congenital processes. Meningocele, lipomeningocele, encephalocele, and combined variants are common examples. Nasal congestion may also be on the basis of pyriform aperture stenosis, midnasal stenosis, or variations of choanal atresia. Schwannoma, juvenile nasal angiofibroma (JNA), and lymphoma are usually easily distinguished based on their history, appearance on exam, and imaging characteristics. CT generally will provide detailed sinonasal anatomy, and MRI will clarify the nature and extent of an associated mass if present. An exception to this is JNA, which demonstrates intense enhancement on postcontrast CT, making determination of extent fairly straightforward when combined with a review of bone windows.

■ Postoperative Imaging

Imaging of the paranasal sinuses postsurgically is also best accomplished by complete coronal or axial CT with reformatting (Fig. 3–39). The type and extent of surgery should be assessed, noting areas of resection, persistent ostiomeatal obstruction, or inadvertent postsurgical changes. Panje and Anand[32] have developed a classification system for FESS, briefly outlined below.

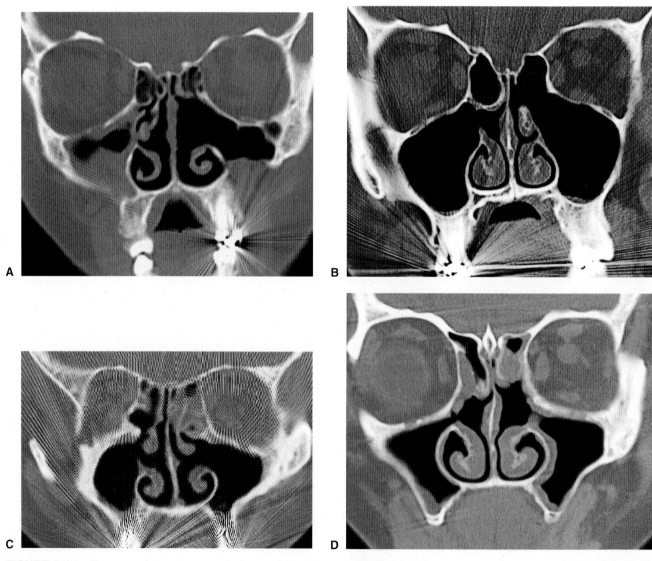

FIGURE 3–39 Postoperative appearance in four patients following FESS procedures. (A) Type III. (B) Type IV. (C) Type III. (D) Type III.

Type I: Uncinatectomy with or without agger nasi cell exenteration

Type II: Uncinatectomy, bulla ethmoidectomy, removal of sinus lateralis mucous membrane, and exposure of the frontal recess or frontal sinus

Type III: Type II plus maxillary sinus antrostomy through the natural ostium

Type IV: Type III plus complete posterior ethmoidectomy

Type V: Type IV plus sphenoidectomy and stripping of the mucous membrane

Postoperatively, the frontal recesses should be identified to determine their patency, as recurrence of disease is often due to persistent obstruction in this area. For example, a persistent agger nasi cell may continue to narrow the frontal recess.

Observe the extent of the uncinatectomy and removal of the ethmoid bulla if performed. The outline of the middle turbinate should be examined to determine whether a middle turbinectomy has been performed. Traction applied during the course of middle turbinectomy can inflict damage at the cribriform plate and the attachment of the basal lamella to the lamina papyracea.

Inspection of the entire course of the lamina papyracea should be performed to evaluate the integrity of this structure. Postoperative dehiscences are commonly found just posterior to the nasolacrimal duct, at the level of the ethmoid bulla and basal lamellar attachment.

The margins of the sphenoid sinus should be evaluated for bony dehiscence or cephalocele, particularly in the region of the optic nerves, maxillary division of the trigeminal nerve, and carotid canal.

■ Operative Complications

The field of view during FESS is quite small, and variant anatomy can make surgical landmarks difficult to identify. All patients scheduled to undergo FESS should have a preoperative coronal CT scan. Many practitioners now perform operative localization CT scans for direct interactive operative guidance at surgery.

In general, complications can be divided into minor and major. Minor complications include periorbital emphysema, epistaxis, postoperative nasal synechiae, and odontalgia. Although common, fortunately they are usually self-limited and do not require postoperative radiologic evaluation. Major complications are rare, but they can be catastrophic or fatal.

If the anterior ethmoid artery is severed during surgery, it often retracts onto the orbit, preventing immediate control of the hemorrhage and resulting in very rapid formation of an intraorbital hematoma. If intraorbital and intraocular pressure builds up because of an expanding hematoma or from forcing of air into the

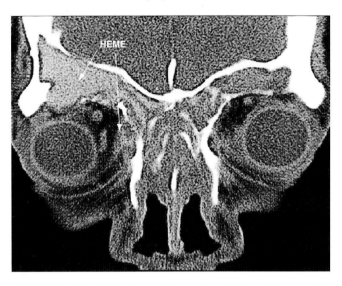

FIGURE 3–40 High attenuation in the right frontal sinus following mucocele resection consistent with hemorrhage. Note the subtle insinuation into the medial orbit.

orbit from the nasal cavity via a dehiscent lamina papyracea, visual impairment or blindness secondary to ischemia can result. In a patient with a normal hematocrit, concentrated acute blood such as that within a hematoma will have HU from 55 to 75 and should be readily visible on a noncontrast CT scan of the orbits (Fig. 3–40).

Massive hemorrhage can occur from direct injury to major vessels. Laceration of the internal carotid artery can occur in the setting of a dehiscent carotid canal and is often fatal. Emergent carotid ligation or angiography with balloon occlusion of the lacerated artery may be necessary. Patients who report severe postoperative headache or photophobia should have a noncontrast CT scan of the head followed by cerebral angiography to detect vascular injury if subarachnoid blood is found.

Postoperative cerebrospinal fluid leak is another major complication of FESS. These leaks occur following inadvertent penetration of the dura. The injury may involve the cribriform plate, fovea ethmoidalis, anterior cranial fossa, or skull base. Deep penetration may cause cerebral contusion, laceration, or cephalocele. A CSF leak may not become clinically apparent for up to 2 years after surgery and will often close spontaneously with conservative measures such as a lumbar drain.[33] Persistent signs require radiologic work-up.

A radionuclide CSF study was often utilized as the initial radiologic screening examination in such patients. Even though images of the head and neck are obtained, it is unusual to actually see evidence of the leak on these images. With wider availability of high-resolution helical CT with reformatting, noncontrast CT and CT cisternography are increasingly used as first-line examinations (Fig. 3–41).

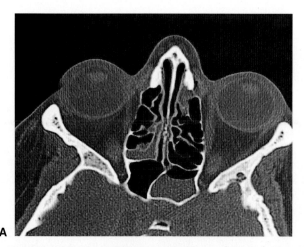

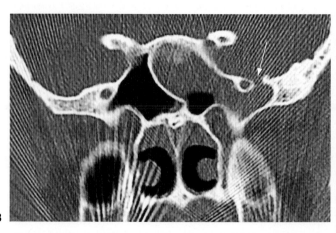

FIGURE 3–41   (A,B) CT cisternography showing fluid in the sphenoid sinus. Although not visually apparent, examination of the Hounsfield number of this fluid revealed increased den-sity consistent with contrast-enhanced CSF reaching the sinus cavity. The coronal image suggests a dehiscence at the superior aspect of the lateral recess (arrow).

■ Intraoperative Computer-Assisted Guidance

Even though CT provides a "road map" for the surgeon, the information that is provided is remote. The surgeon must mentally transfer information from the image to the operative site. Various intraoperative guidance devices have been developed, with a common theme of referencing a sensor on a suction device or instrument to the patient, and simultaneously to a thin-section axial CT dataset identical to those used for multiplanar refor-matting. Sensor types employed have included light-emitting diode, sound, and magnetic devices.[34] Real-time multiplanar reformatting of the CT dataset shows the position of the operative sensor as intersecting crosshairs on simultaneously displayed axial, coronal, and sagittal images.

Initially, there is a substantial learning curve to deal with this additional equipment, both from a technical perspective and additional visual information external to the patient. The division of concentration may be ameliorated somewhat by the use of a video display as the primary visualization during the procedure. With this approach, the monitors can be brought together and the visual data integrated more easily.

■ Conclusion

Computed tomography remains the workhorse modality for cross-sectional imaging of the paranasal sinuses. Scanners with helical capability, as well as multidetector-multislice scanners are pushing data acquisition times into the 10 to 15 second range. This reduces motion artifact, decreases patient radiation dose, and expands the capacity within imaging departments to provide state-of-the-art imaging to a larger number of patients. The bone detail afforded by CT is unsurpassed as a surgical planning tool, and with the current state of multidetector CT and multiplanar reformatting available, offers many of the advantages previously available only with MRI. Real-time referencing of a three-dimensional CT dataset now per-mits image-assisted endoscopic surgery, although there is a technical learning curve for successful implementation.

MRI has selected indications, most notably assessment of suspected sinonasal masses, skull base, and intracra-nial complications of inflammatory sinus disease.

Coordinated use of cross-sectional nuclear imaging in a correlative fashion with cross-sectional CT or MRI should make diagnosis of complex maxillofacial infec-tions more reliable.

Imaging for uncomplicated acute sinusitis is still a controversial topic, but the practice is probably unwar-ranted. Ultrasound has yet to prove any significant util-ity in the assessment of inflammatory sinus disease.

REFERENCES

1. Jorlssen M. Recent trends in the diagnosis and treatment of sinusitis. *Eur Radiol.* 1996;6:170–176.
2. Goldstein J, Phillips C. Current indications and techniques in evaluating inflammatory disease and neoplasia of the sinonasal cavities. *Curr Probl Diagn Radiol.* 1998;27:41–71.
3. Low D, Desrosiers M, McSherry J, et al. A practical guide for the diagnosis and treatment of acute sinusitis. *CMAJ.* 1997;156(suppl 6): S1–14.
4. Melhem E, Olivero P, Benson M, et al. Optimal CT evaluation for functional endoscopic sinus surgery. *AJNR Am J Neuroradiol.* 1996;17:181–188.
5. Bernhardt TM. Rapp-Bernhardt U, Fessel A, et al. CT scanning of the paranasal sinuses: helical CT with reconstruction in the coronal direction versus coronal helical CT. *Br J Radiol.* 1998;71:846–851.

6. Klevansky A. The efficacy of multiplanar reconstructions of helical CT of the paranasal sinuses. *AJR Am J Roentgenol.* 1999;173:493–495.

7. Conlon B, Curran A, Timon C. Pitfalls in the determination of intracranial spread of complicated suppurative sinusitis. *J Laryngol Otol.* 1996;110:673–675.

8. Bhattacharyya T, Piccirillo J, Wippold F. Relationship between patient-based descriptions of sinusitis and paranasal sinus computed tomographic findings. *Arch Otolaryngol Head Neck Surg.* 1997;123:1189–1192.

9. Oberholzer K, Kauczor H, Heussel C, et al. Clinical relevance of CT of the paranasal sinuses prior to bone marrow transplantation [German]. Rofo. *Fortschritte auf dem Gebiete der Roentgenstrahlen und der Neuen Bildgebenden Verfahren.* 1997;166:493–497.

10. Hahnel S, Ertl-Wagner B, Tasman A, et al. Relative value of MR imaging as compared with CT in the diagnosis of inflammatory paranasal sinus disease. *Radiology.* 1999;210:171–176.

11. Lichtenstein D, Biderman P, Meziere G, et al. The sinusogram, a real time ultrasound sign of maxillary sinusitis. *Intensive Care Med.* 1998;24:1057–1061.

12. Laine K, Maatta T, Varonen H, et al. Diagnosing acute maxillary sinusitis in primary care: a comparison of ultrasound, clinical examination and radiography. *Rhinology.* 1998;36:2–6.

13. Lam WW, Liang EY, Woo JK, et al. The etiological role of concha bullosa in chronic sinusitis. *Eur Radiol.* 1996;6:550–552.

14. Scribano E, Ascenti G, Loria G, et al. The role of the ostiomeatal unit anatomic variations in inflammatory disease of the maxillary sinuses. *Eur J Radiol.* 1997;24:172–174.

15. Som P, Curtin H. Chronic inflammatory sinonasal diseases including fungal infections: the role of imaging. *Radiol Clin North Am.* 1993;31:33–44.

16. Som P, Brandwein M. Sinonasal cavities: inflammatory diseases. In: Som P, Curtin H eds. *Head and Neck Imaging.* 3rd ed. St. Louis: CV Mosby; 1996:126–185.

17. Stammberger H, Wolf G. Headaches and sinus disease: the endoscopic approach. *Ann Otol Rhinol Laryngol Suppl.* 1988; 134:3–23.

18. Lidov M, Som P. Inflammatory disease involving a concha bullosa (enlarged pneumatized middle nasal turbinate): MR and CT appearance. AJNR *Am J Neuroradiol.* 1990;11:999–1001.

19. Yousem D, Kennedy D, Rosenberg S. Ostiomeatal complex risk factors for sinusitis: CT evaluation. *J Otolaryngol.* 1991;20:419–424.

20. Bolger W, Butzin C, Parsons D. Paranasal sinus bony anatomic variations and mucosal abnormalities: CT analysis for endoscopic sinus surgery. *Laryngoscope.* 1991;101:56–64.

21. Danese M, Duvoisin B, Agrifoglio A, et al. Influence of nasosinusal anatomic variants on recurrent, persistent or chronic sinusitis. x ray computed tomographic evaluation in 112 patients. *J Radiol.* 1997;78:651–657.

22. Jones NS, Strobl A, Holland I. A study of the CT findings in 100 patients with rhinosinusitis and 100 controls. *Clin Otolaryngol.* 1997;22:47–51.

23. Dahniya M, Makkar R, Grexa E, et al. Appearances of paranasal fungal sinusitis on computed tomography. *Br J Radiol.* 1998;71:340–344.

24. Zinreich SJ, Kennedy DW, Rosenbaum AE, et al. Paranasal sinuses: CT imaging requirements for endoscopic sinus surgery. *Radiology.* 1987;163:769–775.

25. Corey J, Delsupehe K, Ferguson B. Allergic fungal sinusitis: allergic, infectious or both? *Otolaryngol Head Neck Surg.* 1995;113:110–114.

26. Laine F, Smoker W. The ostiomeatal unit and endoscopic sinus surgery: anatomy, variations, and imaging findings in inflammatory diseases. AJR *Am J Roentgenol.* 1992;159:849–857.

27. Osguthorpe J, Hochman M. Inflammatory sinus diseases affecting the orbit. *Otolaryngol Clin North Am.* 1993;26:657–671.

28. Harris G. Subperiosteal abscess of the orbit: computed tomography and the clinical course. *Ophthal Plast Reconstr Surg.* 1996;12:1–8.

29. Patt B, Manning S. Blindness resulting from orbital complications of sinusitis. *Otolaryngol Head Neck Surg.* 1991;104:789–795.

30. Abrams JJ, Glassberg RM. Dental disease: a frequently unrecognized cause of maxillary sinus abnormalities? AJR *Am J Roentgenol.* 1996;166:1219–1223.

31. Zimbler MS, Lebowitz RA, Glickman R. Antral augmentation, osseointegration, and sinusitis: the otolaryngologist's perspective. *Am J Rhinol.* 1998;12:311–316.

32. Panje W, Anand V. Endoscopic sinus surgery indications, diagnosis, and technique. In: Anand VK, Panje WR, eds. *Practical Endoscopic Sinus Surgery.* New York: McGraw-Hill; 1993:68–86.

33. Hudgins P. Complications of endoscopic sinus surgery—the role of the radiologist in prevention. *Radiol Clin North Am.* 1993;31:21–31.

34. Fried MP, Kleefield J, Ghopal H. Image-guided endoscopic surgery: results of accuracy and performance in a multicenter clinical study using an electromagnetic tracking system. *Laryngoscope.* 1997; 107:594–601.

4

Diagnosis and Management of Rhinosinusitis

HOWARD L. LEVINE

Prior to considering management of rhinosinusitis, the physician must be certain about the diagnosis. Proper diagnosis is achieved only with thorough knowledge about the pathophysiology and etiology of the disease. Accurate diagnosis and subsequent treatment are achieved by complete understanding of the symptoms and signs of the disease, the ability to perform an accurate head and neck examination, and understanding of the subtle significance of findings seen on computed tomography scans and nasal endoscopic examination. Once the disease is certain, treatment options need to be available that include both medical and surgical options.

In the United States, rhinosinusitis is an extremely common disease and is increasing in prevalance. There were over 32 million cases of sinusitis reported and 11.6 million patient visits, mostly to primary care physicians. Since 0.5% to 5% of viral upper respiratory tract infections result in rhinosinusitus, it is estimated that from the 1 billion viral infections there would be about 20 million cases of acute bacterial rhinosinusitis.[3,4] Not only is acute sinusitis common, but it is also costly, with approximately $3.5 billion spent each year in the United States.[5] The cost of management of sinusitis in 1994 to the U.S. health care system was $2.4 billion, and this does not include diagnostic evaluation, such as adiology, or surgery.

Restricted activity days are the number of days a person is away from customary activities. From 1986 to 1988, there were 50 million such days. From 1990 to 1992, there were 73 million restricted activity days, which is almost a 50% increase in the number of days compared with the period 1986 to 1988. These numbers suggest that sinusitis is increasing in frequency or severity.

Although the majority of those afflicted with rhinosinusitis have self-limited disease or are managed easily by their primary care physicians, there are those with difficult and frustrating problems who eventually make their way to the otolaryngologist. It is then the subspecialist otolaryngologist who must be adequately armed to diagnose and manage the disease so that the patient may reasonably and efficiently return to work, family, school, social encounters, and activities of enjoyment.

Poor air quality in spite of improved automobile, bus, truck, and industrial emissions may be one of the reasons for the increase in the frequency and/or severity of sinusitis (Fig. 4–1). In the Great Lakes area of the United States, for example, there are many manufacturing, steel, and automotive industries. In 1993, the Environmental Protection Agency measured air quality and pollution in the United States. The 8-hour carbon dioxide concentration in the Steubenville-Weirton area (~75 miles southwest of Cleveland, Ohio) was fifth highest. The average particulate count in Cleveland and the cities around Cleveland was fourth highest. Sulfur dioxide content was the highest in the United States in the Steubenville-Weirton area, seventh highest in Youngstown and Warren, Ohio (smaller communities between Cleveland and Pittsburgh, Pennsylvania), and tenth highest in Cleveland. Many people refer to this part of the United States as the "sinus belt," and it may very well be so, just because of the air quality and pollution.

Evaluation begins with the patient history. A good history is dependent upon knowledge of the etiology and pathophysiology of the disease. If the etiology is understood, then the treatment is usually easier and more suc-

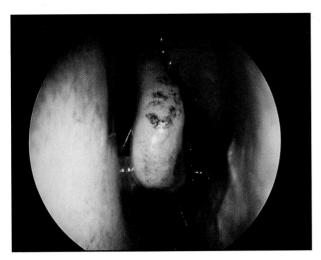

FIGURE 4–1 Air pollution causing particulate matter to lodge on the middle turbinate, creating irritation and edema.

cessful. Most physicians agree about the common causes and predisposing factors for sinusitis. These include upper respiratory infections, allergic rhinitis, asthma, day care centers, environment such as cigarette smoke (both active and passive), air pollution, structural abnormalities such as deviated nasal septum, and nasal polyps. Less common predisposing factors are immunodeficiency, swimming, adenoiditis, foreign body, cystic fibrosis, substance abuse, and neoplasm.

A few general comments are needed about some of these etiologic and predisposing factors.

It may be difficult to differentiate infectious rhinosinusitis from a common self-limited viral upper respiratory infection, allergic rhinitis, or vasomotor rhinitis. The ability to determine this may be clearer with the more recent definitions of rhinosinusitis (see below). If allergic rhinitis is present, then sinusitis is generally preceded by the typical allergic symptoms of itchy eyes, itchy nose, watery eyes, and sneezing fits. Mucus tends to be thin and watery in allergic rhinitis and thick and purulent in infectious rhinosinusitis. Vasomotor rhinitis generally has symptoms of watery nasal drainage and nasal obstruction that alternates from one side of the nose to the other. Some factors that incite vasomotor rhinitis are perfume, cigarette smoke, light, cold, foods (especially beer and wine), pregnancy, certain medications, and stress.

If asthma is present and out of control, sinusitis may be the cause, and evaluation is needed. There may be associated aspirin or nonsteroidal anti-inflammatory drug sensitivity. This is often called triad asthma, Samter's triad, or Fernand Widal triad and is an abnormality in the arachidonic acid metabolic cycle. It most commonly affects young adults ages 20 to 40. Triad asthma is often

a frustrating management problem for the patient, primary care physician, and otolaryngologist because of repeated rhinosinusitis, sinus and nasal polyps, and asthma out of control. These patients require ongoing medical management for their pulmonary problems, infectious rhinosinusitis, and nasal polyps, and often frequent surgery to remove polyps and relieve obstruction.

Day care centers commonly have been places where young children go while parents are at work. They also can be places where respiratory disease is transmitted because of close and direct contact. However, day care centers are no longer limited to just children. In addition to the pediatric day care centers, there is an increasing number of adult day care centers because of the growing aging population in the United States. Anytime there are centers where people come together of any age, there is a greater chance that they will contract an upper respiratory tract infection and develop sinusitis.

Although immunodeficiency syndromes are uncommon, they must be looked for when there are recurrent episodes of respiratory tract infection and the traditional management has failed. Whether it is an adult or a child, immunodeficiency should be considered if a patient is experiencing frequent upper respiratory tract infections, sinusitis, otitis media, pneumonia, or bronchitis. If the patient has frequent, severe, or resistant disease, the immune system should be evaluated.

It is not clear whether swimming causes or worsens rhinosinusitis. Although there is no scientific evidence, some physicians feel that there are increased symptoms of sinusitis if there is frequent swimming in polluted water or when diving water is forced into the nasal and sinus cavity and becomes trapped.

In children, adenoiditis must be considered as an etiology for rhinosinusitis. Tonsillitis is frequently considered as part of the cause of upper respiratory tract disease, but adenoiditis is infrequently considered. In the pediatric patients adenoiditis may cause sinusitis, or sinusitis may cause adenoiditis. This is not clear. Enlarged adenoids may become infected and seed the sinuses or may merely obstruct the flow of secretions from the nasal and sinus cavities into the throat, causing stasis of secretions and subsequent infection. In a child who has repeated and medically unresponsive sinusitis and adenoid hypertrophy, an adenoidectomy is often performed before surgical intervention for sinus disease and is successful. It is less invasive, more conservative, and often can rid the sinus disease by managing the infectious source, the adenoids.

A foreign body within the nose should be considered, especially in the pediatric patient, as well as a patient who may have an emotional or mental disorder or who is institutionalized. A foreign body may obstruct the flow of secretions from the sinuses and create infection.

Cystic fibrosis is considered in all pediatric and young adult patients with sinus and/or nasal polyps.

Substance abuse, especially of cocaine and marijuana, can alter the ciliary function of the nose and predispose to sinusitis. General active and passive cigarette smoke is part of exposure to substance abuse. Smoke is particulate matter inhaled and is an irritant to the respiratory tract, specifically the nasal and sinus ciliary function.

When there is unilateral sinus disease, it is important to have follow-up for the patient with repeated examinations and/or imaging to be sure that a neoplastic process is not the etiology. When unilateral sinus disease does not resolve, consider neoplasm and obtain proper imaging, nasal endoscopic examination, and biopsy as needed.

Although sinusitis is one of the most common disease entities, it has been poorly defined. The American Academy of Otolaryngology Head and Neck Surgery Paranasal Sinus Committee has attempted to define sinusitis.[6] This committee agreed that as part of the description and definition of the disease, the term *rhinosinusitis* should now be used. In general, sinusitis does not occur without rhinitis, and rhinitis does not occur without sinusitis. This is similar to what occurs in the ear. Otologists understand that patients with acute otitis media will often have roentgenographic appearance of mastoiditis without a clinical mastoid infection. This is because of the communication between the middle ear and the mastoid air cells. The same is true in the nose and sinus with the interconnection between the spaces of the nasal sinus cavities. For this reason, rhinitis and sinusitis most often exist together, and therefore the term *rhinosinusitis* is appropriate.

Major and minor symptoms and signs of rhinosinusitis were defined by the committee and used as criteria to determine the diagnosis of rhinosinusitis. These criteria are symptoms and signs and are used to define five different types of rhinosinusitis: acute, recurrent acute, subacute, chronic, and acute exacerbation of chronic. From these criteria and definitions, a clinician should be able to diagnosis most cases of rhinosinusitis by history.

Major criteria associated with rhinosinusitis are facial pain and pressure, facial congestion and fullness, nasal obstruction, nasal discharge that is a purulent postnasal drip, change in sense of smell, and purulence on nasal endoscopic examination. Minor criteria are headache, fever, halitosis, fatigue, dental pain, cough, ear pain, pressure, and fullness.

There can be a strong suspicion of rhinosinusitis if there are two major criteria, or one major and two minor criteria, or there is purulence on examination. There is a suggestion of rhinosinusitis if there is one major criterion or two minor criteria.

Acute rhinosinusitis will last for less than 4 weeks. Fever or facial pain alone does not constitute a history of rhinosinusitis unless there are other symptoms. It may be difficult to differentiate a common cold or viral upper respiratory infection from acute rhinosinusitis. A bacterial infection is probable if the symptoms are worse after 5 days. If the symptoms are present for more than 10 days, a bacterial infection is probable. Also, a bacterial infection is suspected if the symptoms are greater than expected for viral disease (more than just myalgias and hoarseness).

Subacute rhinosinusitis is a natural progression of acute rhinosinusitis and lasts 4 to 12 weeks, with complete resolution after medical management. This is the patient whose nasal endoscopic examination typically reveals edema and some mucoid or mucopurulent secretion in the middle meatus.

Recurrent acute rhinosinusitis is defined as four or more episodes of rhinosinusitis in a year, each lasting 7 to 10 days, and an absence of intervening signs and symptoms between episodes. This patient typically goes to the otolaryngologist or primary care physician and is treated with antibiotics and decongestants and gets better. A few weeks later the patient calls and says, "My disease has come back, and I need more medicine." The patient often receives a "stronger" antibiotic or a longer course and once again gets better. A few weeks later, though the disease comes back. Typically such patients have some anatomical abnormality obstructing the outflow from the sinus into the nose, such as a choncha bullosa of the middle turbinate or uncinate process, deformed uncinate process, large ethmoid sinus bulla, or Haller's cells. A minor upper respiratory infection will cause enough edema in the ostiomeatal complex around these anatomical abnormalities to worsen the obstruction and cause the recurrent infection.

Chronic rhinosinusitis lasts for more than 12 weeks. Facial pain does not constitute a suggestive history in the absence of other signs and symptoms.

There can be acute exacerbation of chronic rhinosinusitis. The symptoms of chronic rhinosinusitis may worsen, but the patient may return to the baseline after treatment.

Medical management of rhinosinusitis includes use of the correct antibiotics, topical and/or systemic decongestants, and mucolytics. If polypoid or edematous mucosa or nasal or sinus polyps are present, topical and/or systemic steroids are used. Antihistamines are not used because they may dry already thick, purulent secretions.

When examining the patient with suspected rhinosinusitis, it is important to do a complete head and neck examination. An anterior rhinoscopic examination with a nasal speculum and headlight should be done before and after decongesting the nose to get an overview of the nasal cavity, the middle turbinate, the inferior turbinate, and their relationship to the nasal septum.

A nasal endoscopic examination is performed on all patients with nasal and/or sinus symptoms. The nose is

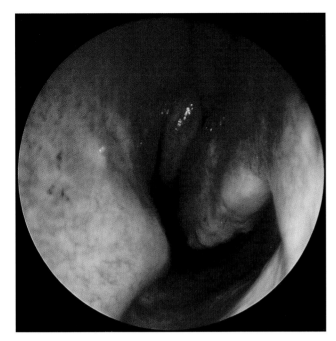

FIGURE 4–2 Nasal endoscopic view of the nasal floor showing the relationship between the inferior nasal turbinate and the nasal septum.

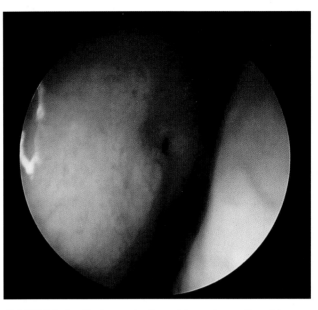

FIGURE 4–4 Endoscopic view of the sphenoethmoid recess, also known as the posterior osteomeatal complex, revealing the superior turbinate and meatus.

anesthetized and decongested using Boyette's solution. (Boyette's solution contains 4% lidocaine, phenylephrine, and sodium chloride; sterile water is added to make 200 mL. A touch of peppermint oil is used to mask the bitter taste of the lidocaine.) This solution provides comfort in adults and most children and permits complete nasal endoscopic examination.

A television monitor is used in the author's clinic so that the patients can see their nose and sinus cavity to better help them understand their pathology and the etiology of their disease. Nasal endoscopy is performed in a consistent manner. The floor of the nose is examined, looking at the relationship between the inferior turbinate and the nasal septum (Fig. 4–2). The endoscope is passed back along the floor of the nose into the nasopharynx (Fig. 4–3). The nasopharynx is examined

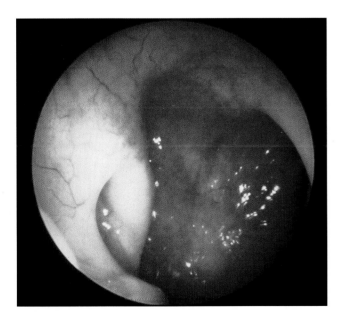

FIGURE 4–3 Nasal endoscopic view of the nasopharynx demonstrating adenoid hypertrophy possibly contributing to rhinosinusitis.

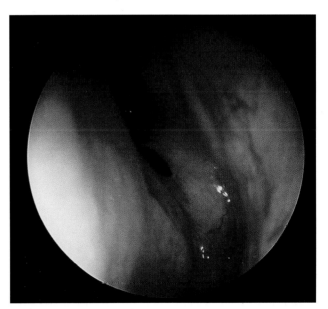

FIGURE 4–5 The posterior osteomeatal complex (sphenoethmoid recess) and the ostium of the sphenoid sinus.

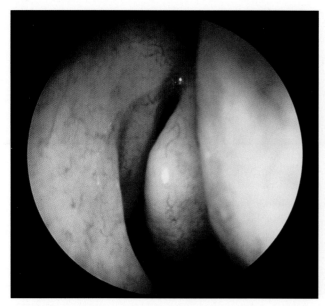

FIGURE 4–6   The middle turbinate is examined to determine its shape and relationship to the anterior osteomeatal complex and nasal septum.

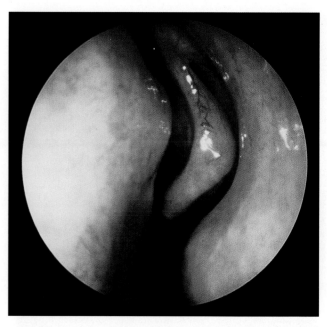

FIGURE 4–8   A paradoxically bent middle turbinate may obstruct outflow from the middle meatus into the nasal cavity.

for lymphoid hypertrophy or neoplasm. The endoscope is withdrawn slightly into the posterior nasal cavity and rotated superiorly to view the sphenoethmoid recess (posterior ostiomeatal complex) (Figs. 4–4, 4–5). This can often be seen, but at times the space between the middle and/or superior turbinate and the nasal septum is so narrow that the region cannot be adequately evaluated. The endoscope is brought forward, and the mid-

dle turbinate is examined (Fig. 4–6). Its shape is assessed, looking at whether it is bulbous (and may have a concha bullosa within it) or paradoxically bent, narrowing the outflow from the middle meatus (anterior ostiomeatal complex) into the nose (Figs. 4–7, 4–8,

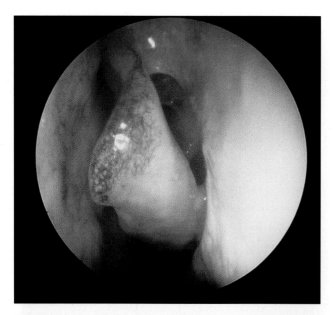

FIGURE 4–7   Small polyps on the anterior aspect of the middle turbinate may obstruct airflow and/or the outflow from the osteomeatal complex into the nasal cavity.

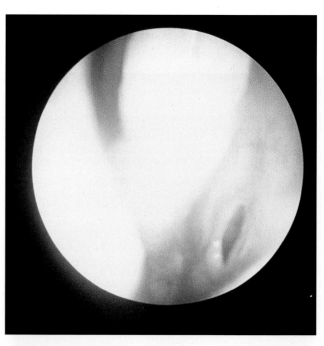

FIGURE 4–9   An accessory ostium from the maxillary sinus into the nasal cavity may be a sign of repeated infection. Mucus may flow from the maxillary sinus out through the natural ostium only to reenter the sinus through the accessory ostium, creating stasis of secretions and subsequent rhinosinusitis.

and 4–9). An attempt is made to rotate the endoscope into the middle meatus and assess the uncinate process, its shape and degree of rotation, its relationship to the ethmoid bulla, and whether accessory ostia exist. A 30-degree 2.7 mm endoscope or 0-degree 4 mm endoscope is used. When infection is seen, an endoscopic guided culture is obtained from the posterior or anterior ostiomeatal complex. Most children can be examined endoscopically in the outpatient clinic. A few children require nasal endoscopic examination under anesthesia.

There have been many other techniques to evaluate the sinuses that have been tried over the years, such as palpation, transillumination, and ultrasound. Because of the great variability and inconsistency of the methods of evaluation, the sophisticated nasal sinus physician rarely uses these. Occasionally, cytology can help in looking for eosinophilia or inflammation, but for the most part even this is not generally helpful.

Allergy testing is important when there are clinical symptoms, such as itchy nose, itchy eyes, thin watery nasal drainage, and sneezing. Allergic rhinitis may be the etiology of rhinosinusitis, as the edematous, inflamed mucosa creates congestion in an already narrowed and compromised ostiomeatal complex. This obstructs the outflow from the sinus into the nasal cavity.

Nasal function testing using rhinomanometry is important for some rhinologists in assessing obstructive nasal sinus problems. Its role in the diagnosis and management of sinusitis is unclear.

An office biopsy may be important if neoplasm is seen or suspected. This may help in the planning of further diagnostic testing and management.

Roentgenographic examination of the sinuses has long been an important part of the diagnostic evaluation of sinusitis. Traditionally, plain sinus roentgenography (Caldwell, Waters, and anteroposterior) views have been the main roentgenographic method of examination. Today, these have limited use in evaluation of rhinosinusitis except perhaps in some cases of acute or recurrent acute disease. There is certainly no value in chronic rhinosinusitis. Plain sinus films often mistake overlying structures or a congenital hypoplastic sinus as an opacified sinus (Figs. 4–10, 4–11).

A CT scan of the sinuses shows critical detail and pathology. It is most valuable for patients with subacute, recurrent, and chronic sinusitis. It is also valuable when either the patient history or physical findings present a diagnostic dilemma. A CT scan of the sinuses should be obtained when patients are at their best. This is often ~4 weeks after medical therapy. This allows the sinusitis to resolve or become quiescent, fluid to disappear, and mucosal thickening to lessen. At that time the site of pathology is often apparent and the nature of treatment more obvious. Even though a patient may feel better within a few days or a week after treatment, the CT scan will not improve until several weeks later. The CT scan resolves very slowly even though the patient's symptoms go away quickly.

Two types of CT scans are used: a screening or limited scan and a full CT scan. The screening or limited scans can be either five axial views (Fig. 4–12), replacing the

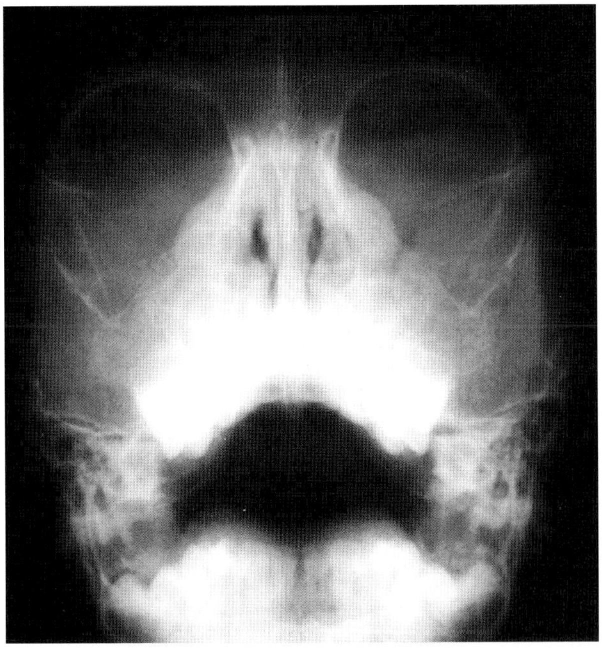

FIGURE 4–10 Plain sinus x-ray appearing to demonstrate an opacified maxillary sinus. However, CT scan shows a congenital hypoplastic sinus.

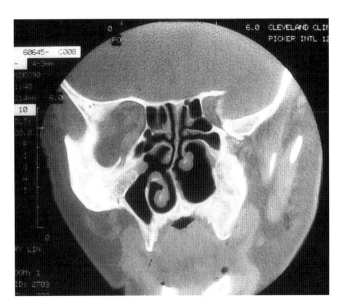

FIGURE 4–11 CT scan of hypoplastic maxillary sinus.

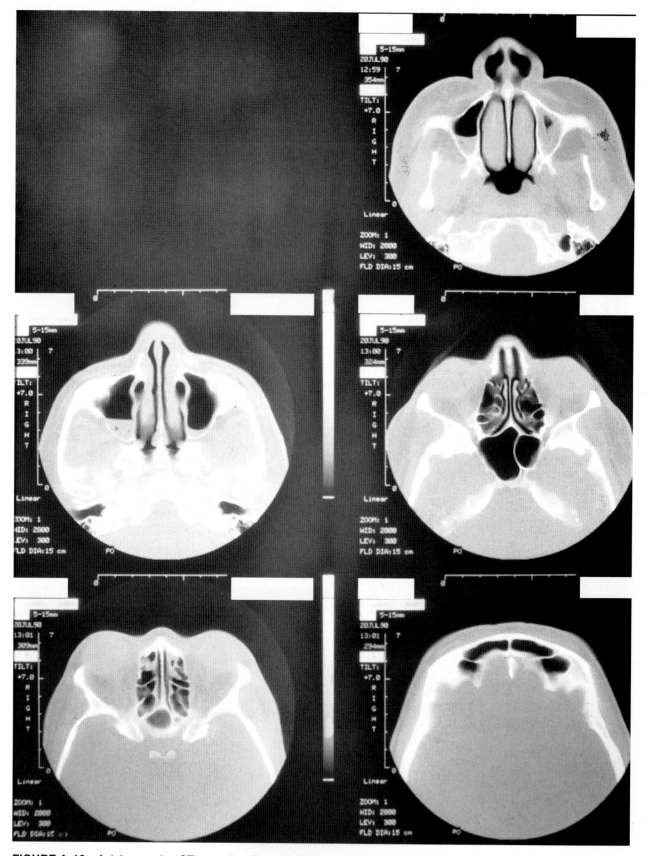

FIGURE 4–12   Axial screening CT scan visualizes all of the sinuses efficiently.

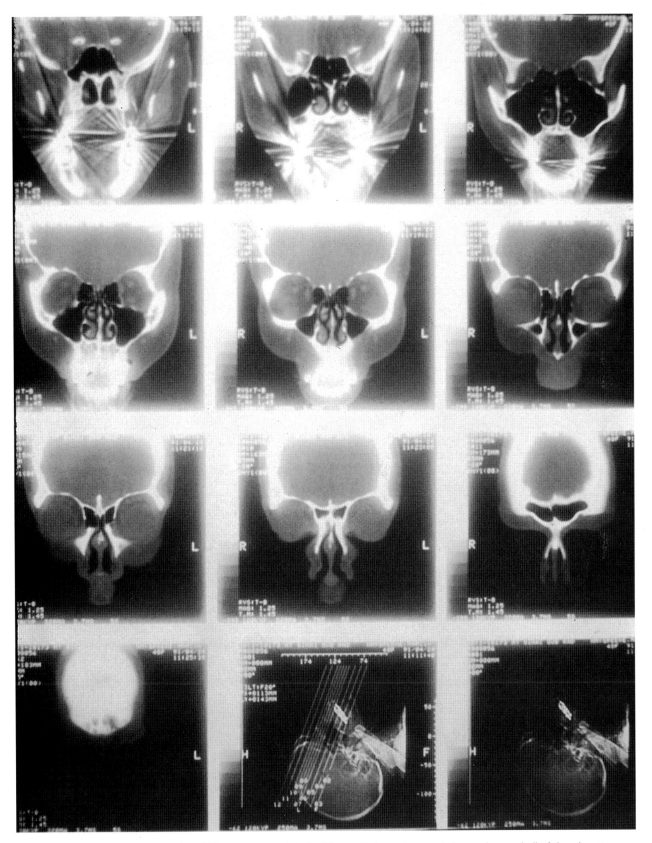

FIGURE 4–13   Coronal screening CT scan shows detail of the anterior osteomeatal complex and all of the sinuses.

TABLE 4–1   Causes of Acute Rhinosinusitis

Cause	Percent of Patients
Haemophilus influenzae	38
Streptococcus pneumoniae	37
Other *Haemophilus* species	8
Streptococcus pyogenes	6
Moraxella catarrhalis	5
Alpha streptococci	3
Gram-negative bacilli/mixed anaerobes	3

plain sinus films, or a coronal scan (Fig. 4–13). Usually, the coronal scan has a greater number of cuts in the region of the ostiomeatal complex and shows greater detail in this region.

The bacteriology of rhinosinusitis varies depending on whether the rhinosinusitis is acute or chronic. The bacteriology of rhinosinusitis in the United States has remained fairly unchanged over the years. For acute rhinosinusitis, the causative organisms are *Haemophilus influenzae* (38%) and *Streptococcus pneumoniae* (37%)[7] (Table 4–1).

For chronic rhinosinusitis, *Staphylococcus aureus* is the most common organism. Seventeen percent of patients will have *S. aureus*. The literature states that the next most common organisms are *Streptococcus viridans* (14%) and *H. influenzae* (10%)[7] (Table 4–2).

Most of the endoscopic-guided cultures obtained in my own office reveal *S. aureus* and/or *Pseudomonas* in a large number of patients with chronic sinusitis. Anaerobic organisms are also common and important pathogens.

Some patients with rhinosinusitis may have a viral agent as the cause. If the secretions are thick and purulent, all that is needed for treatment is a decongestant and mucolytic. Guaifenesin is the most common mucolytic to thin the mucus. A dosage of 2400 mg per day is generally needed. A decongestant will help improve drainage. If the secretions are thin and watery, a decongestant and antihistamine are used.

TABLE 4–2   Causes of Chronic Bacterial Rhinosinusitis

Aerobic

Type	Percent of Patients
Staphylococcus aureus	17
Streptococcus viridans	14
Haemophilus influenzae	10
Neisseria species	8
Staphylococcus epidermidis	7
Streptococcus pneumoniae	5
E. coli	4

Anaerobic

Peptostreptococci	34
Corynebacteria	23
Bacteroides species	23
Veillonella	17

It is common for patients to call the physician's office with the earliest symptoms of an upper respiratory tract infection. Many of these patients demand an antibiotic, believing that this is the only way to get relief. However, most of these infections are self-limited and require only a decongestant and/or mucolytic. It becomes the physician's responsibility to understand the natural history of upper respiratory tract infections and rhinosinusitis and treat the patient appropriately. In the United States and now increasingly around the world there is an antibiotic crisis. There are bacteria that are becoming resistant and therefore becoming more difficult to treat. This is making the problems for physicians and patients more difficult. But as physicians we must educate our patients that they do not need antibiotics for a common cold and that there are potential problems from taking antibiotics needlessly. Amoxicillin prophylaxis for otitis media will cause a 45% increase in the incidence of β-lactamase *H. influenzae*. One week later 45% of family members will be colonized with β-lactamase-producing bacteria.

There are several ways to think about the best choice of an antibiotic for rhinosinusitis. The choice can be based on what has worked traditionally, the use of approved antibiotics, antibiotics based on extent of disease, or antibiotics based on endoscopic-guided culture and sensitivity.

There are some antibiotics, proven to be historically effective, that are well tolerated and relatively inexpensive. Amoxicillin, doxycycline, and trimethoprim sulfate were commonly used and are effective antibiotics for rhinosinusitis.

The U.S. Food and Drug Administration has approved the following antibiotics for the management of acute rhinosinusitis: amoxicillin clavulanate (Augmentin), cefprozil (Cefzil), cefuroxime axetil (Ceftin), ciprofloxacin (Cipro), clarithromycin (Biaxin), loracarbef (Lorabid), levofloxacin (Levaquin), and trovafloxacin (Trovan). There are no approved antibiotics for chronic rhinosinusitis.

Severity of disease is another way to choose an antibiotic. If the disease is mild (based on signs and symptoms), amoxicillin is the first drug of choice. It is inexpensive, well tolerated, and effective. Although this still should be considered a first-line drug, a different antibiotic may need to be chosen if patients are at high risk for resistance to amoxicillin. These are patients who have had frequent respiratory infections, adults or children in day care centers, or those with any of other predisposing factors. All of these patients have a greater chance of having a resistant organism (especially β-lactamase-producing *H. influenza*, *M. catarrhalis*, or *S. aureus*).

If the rhinosinusitis is moderately severe, then amoxicillin clavulanate (Augmentin), cefuroxime axetil (Ceftin), ciprofloxacin (Cipro), or levofloxacin (Levaquin) is chosen. These antibiotics are generally used for 10 days for patients who have acute rhinosinusitis, subacute rhinosinusitis, and recurrent acute rhinosinusitis. For those who have chronic rhinosinusitis, treatment is generally for at least 21 days and occasionally for 4 to 6 weeks. An endoscopic-guided culture will often help determine the choice of antibiotic.

When there is severe disease or a complication of sinusitis such as orbital cellulitis or abscess, meningitis or brain abscess, or osteomyelitis, intravenous antibiotics are used. The chosen antibiotic may be a combination of vancomycin plus ceftriaxone (Rocephin), trovafloxacin (Trovan), or ciprofloxacin (Cipro) administered intravenously. Depending on the severity of the illness, these antibiotics may be administered in the hospital or as home parental antibiotics.

Although their primary care physicians manage the majority of patients with rhinosinusitis, there are those patients who require referral to the otolaryngologist. Referral should be considered for the patient with an impending complication or severe disease. This may be manifest by skin erythema, severe facial pain, suspected orbital or intracranial complication, symptoms in spite of two antibiotic trials, recurrent acute rhinosinusitis, chronic symptoms in spite of 8 weeks of nasal corticosteroid, decongestants, and/or antibiotics, frontal sinusitis, and sphenoid sinusitis.

Patients with rhinosinusitis generally have thick and tenacious secretions. To help reduce the viscosity and promote drainage, all patients with rhinosinusitis should maintain adequate hydration and use mucolytics.

Successful management of rhinosinusitis depends on proper diagnosis, understanding the pathophysiology of disease, a thorough head and neck and nasal sinus evaluation, complete nasal endoscopic examination, and proper choice of treatment regimen.

REFERENCES

1. Benninger MS, Hlozer SE, Lau J. Diagnosis and treatment of uncomplicated acute bacterial rhinosinusitis: summary of Agency for Health Care Policy and Research evidence-based report. *Otolaryngol Head Neck Surg* 2000;122:1–7.
2. Agency for Health Care Policy and Research. Diagnosis and treatment of acute bacterial rhinosinusitis. *Evid Rep Technol Assess (Summ)* 1999;9:1–5.
3. Gwaltney JM Jr. Acute community-acquired sinusitis. *Clin Infect Dis* 196;23:1209–1223.
4. Berg O, Carenfelt C, Rystedt G, et al. Occurrence of asymptomatic sinusitis in common cold and other acute ENT infections. *Rhinology* 1986;24:223–225.
5. Ray NF, Baraniuk JN, Thamer M, et al. Healthcare expenditures for sinusitis in 1996: contributions of asthma, rhinitis, and other airway disorders. *J Allergy Clin Immunol* 1999;103:403–414.
6. Adult rhinosinusitis defined: report of the Rhinosinusitis Task Force Committee Meeting. *Otolaryngol Head Neck Surg.* 1997;117:S4–S5.
7. Sydnor A Jr, Gwaltney JM Jr, Cocchetto DM, Scheld WM. Comparative evaluation of cefuroxime axetil and cefaclor for treatment of acute bacterial maxillary sinusitis. *Arch Otolaryngol Head Neck Surg.* 1989;115:1430–1433.

5

The Relationships of Allergy and Asthma to Rhinosinusitis: Epidemiological, Mechanistic, and Clinical

MICHAEL SCHATZ AND RAYMOND G. SLAVIN

Sinusitis frequently coexists with allergy and/or asthma. The simultaneous occurrence of these illnesses has potential pathogenetic as well as clinical implications. This chapter will review the many-faceted interfaces between allergy, asthma, and sinusitis. First, the etiology, diagnosis, and therapy of allergic rhinitis will be presented. The interrelationships between allergy and sinusitis will then be explored, including potential mechanistic as well as diagnostic and therapeutic aspects. Next, a specific allergy-sinus interface, allergic fungal sinusitis, will be described. Finally, the mechanistic and clinical interrelationships between asthma and sinusitis will be reviewed.

■ Allergic Rhinitis

Allergic rhinitis affects between 20 million and 40 million people in the United States annually, including 10 to 30% of adults and up to 40% of children.[1,2] Moreover, the prevalence appears to be increasing.[2] Several recent reviews regarding the pathogenesis, diagnosis, and treatment of allergic rhinitis have been published.[2–5] This section will summarize clinically relevant information about this common entity.

Etiology/Pathogenesis

Allergic rhinitis is caused by an intranasal IgE-mediated reaction to inhalant antigens. Recent concepts of pathogenesis suggest that IgE-mediated reactions are promoted by Th2 helper lymphocytes, which synthesize interleukins (IL) 4, 5, 6, and 13.[6] In contrast, Th1 helper lymphocytes, which promote delayed-type hypersensitivity,

produce IL-2, interferon γ, tumor necrosis β, and IL-12,[6,7] while both Th1 and Th2 cells express IL-3, -10, and granulocyte-macrophage colony–stimulating factor (GM-CSF).[6,7]

The combination of antigen with nasal mast cell– or basophil-fixed specific IgE leads to the release of vasoactive and pro-inflammatory mediators and cytokines. The effects of these mediators and cytokines on blood vessels, mucus-secreting cells, nerves, and inflammatory cells lead to the eosinophilic inflammation, typical symptoms, and nasal hyperreactivity associated with allergic rhinitis. Histamine, the most well known mediator derived from mast cell degranulation, accounts for approximately half of the symptoms of allergic rhinitis.[3]

Allergic rhinitis may be perennial or seasonal, depending on the primary antigens involved. Perennial allergic rhinitis is caused by inhalant allergens such as house dust mites, animal dander, and indoor molds. Such perennial allergic rhinitis may be worse in the winter when the home is closed up and forced air heating systems are operating. Seasonal allergic rhinitis is usually due to tree pollen (early spring), grass pollen (late spring), or weed pollen (fall). In addition, outdoor mold spores may cause seasonal allergic rhinitis, especially during the spring and fall. Although grass pollen may be more perennial in subtropical climates, springtime exacerbations are usually still present.

Recently, an alternative clinical classification for allergic rhinitis has been proposed.[5] Intermittent allergic rhinitis was suggested to describe symptoms that are present less than 4 days per week for less than 4 weeks per year, and persistent allergic rhinitis was suggested to describe symptoms that are present more than 4 days a week for more than 4 weeks per year. Moderate-severe (vs. mild) allergic rhinitis was considered to be present when one or more of the following symptoms occur due to the untreated illness: sleep disturbance, impairment of daily activities (leisure and/or sport), impairment of school or work, or troublesome symptoms.

Clinical Findings/Diagnosis

The diagnosis is usually strongly suspected on the basis of the history. Sneezing, clear rhinorrhea, nasal itching, and eye itching are usually prominent. A seasonal pattern may be noted, as described above. Allergic triggers (cleaning house, animal dander exposure, freshly cut grass) may be identified. Physical examination of the nose (pale edematous mucosa) and eyes (palpebral inferior conjunctival injection) may support the diagnosis, although the absence of these findings does not exclude the diagnosis of allergic rhinitis. Nasal eosinophilia also supports the diagnosis, although the presence of nasal eosinophila may be due to other causes (eosinophilic nonallergic rhinitis, nasal polyps), and nasal eosinophilia may be absent in some patients with definite allergic rhinitis.

The definitive diagnosis of allergic rhinitis is made with the demonstration of specific IgE against antigens to which the patient is exposed and that correlate temporally with the patient's nasal symptoms. Skin testing is the most sensitive technique to demonstrate specific IgE, although in vitro tests (radioallergosorbent test [RAST], Enzyme Linked Immunosorbent Assay (ELISA) may be considered if skin testing is not available, if the patient cannot stop antihistamines, for patients with diffuse skin disease, and for pregnant women.

Management

Potential management of allergic rhinitis involves antigen avoidance, pharmacological therapy, and immunotherapy. More complete antigen avoidance information may be found elsewhere.[2] The most important aspects of dust mite control involve obtaining plastic or synthetic encasings for the pillows, mattress, and box springs and washing the bedclothes in hot water weekly. Mold avoidance involves reduction of the conditions that promote mold growth (moisture, warmth, and darkness) and the use of a fungicide where mold is growing. Although elimination of an animal from the home is the best form of avoidance for dander-induced disease, washing the pet weekly and an air purifier with a high-energy particulate air (HEPA) filter may provide some reduction in airborne animal dander antigen. Avoidance of outdoor pollen and mold spore exposure when the patient is outdoors is difficult, although air-conditioning and HEPA filters may minimize the indoor concentrations of these outdoor allergens.

Antihistamines are particularly helpful for the sneezing, itching, and runny nose associated with allergic rhinitis. The second-generation antihistamines (Table 5–1) generally may be preferred due to the absence or reduction of important side effects, such as anticholinergic effects, sedation, and performance impairment. Desloratadine, fexofenadine, and loratadine are classified by the U.S. Food and Drug Administration (FDA) as nonsedating because standard doses result in no greater incidence of sedation than that seen with placebo. The incidence of sedation with cetirizine at a standard adult dose of 10 mg is higher than with placebo, although it is significantly less sedating than most first-generation antihistamines.[2] Azelastine is a topical antihistamine with efficacy that appears comparable to oral antihistamines. However, ~20% of patients in clinical trials complain of bitter taste, and 11.5% report somnolence.[2]

Although earlier second-generation antihistamines (terfenadine, astemizole) were rarely associated with serious cardiovascular effects (ventricular tachyarrythmias, cardiac arrest, or sudden death associated with prolonged QT interval), cetirizine, desloratadine, fexofenadine, and loratadine have not been shown to be associated with QT interval changes or rhythm disturbances.[2]

Oral decongestants (pseudoephedrine, phenylpropanolamine, phenylephrine) are α adrenergic agonists

TABLE 5–1   Second-Generation Oral Antihistamines*

Agent	Usual Adult Dosing	Available with Decongestant	Reduced Dose with Liver Disease	Reduced Dose with Renal Impairment	Pregnancy Category
Cetirizine (Zyrtec)	5–10 mg daily	No	5 mg daily	5 mg daily	B
Desloratadine (Clarinex)	5 mg daily	No	Start at 5 mg every other day	Start at 5 mg every other day	C
Fexofenadine (Allegra)	60 mg bid	Yes	60 mg daily	No change	C
Loratadine (Claritin)	10 mg daily	Yes	Start at 10 mg every other day	Start at 10 mg every other day	B

* Modified from Dykewicz MS, Fineman S, eds. Diagnosis and management of rhinitis: parameter documents of the Joint Task Force on Practice Parameters in Allergy, Asthma and Immunology. *Ann Allergy.* 1998;81:463–518.

that may be used as a supplement to antihistamines when nasal congestion is prominent. These drugs may be administered alone or as combination products with several antihistamines. Side effects from oral decongestants may include insomnia, loss of appetite, and excessive nervousness. In addition, because of their pharmacological effects, these drugs should be avoided or used with caution in patients with cardiac arrythmias, angina pectoris, hypertension, hyperthyroidism, glaucoma, and urinary dysfunction. Pseudoephedrine appears to be less likely than phenylpropanolamine to cause elevated blood pressure.[2] Antihistamines and/or decongestants may be used as needed for intermittent symptoms and regularly for mild to moderate daily symptoms.

Nasal cromolyn has an excellent safety profile and may be considered, especially for children and pregnant women with mild to moderate daily symptoms. Nasal cromolyn may also be used 15 minutes prior to predictable intermittent allergen exposure (e.g., going to a house with a pet) to prevent allergy symptoms. The disadvantages of nasal cromolyn include its frequent dosing requirements (qid) and its lack of efficacy in 30 to 40% of the population, despite strict adherence to the frequent dosing regimen.[5]

Intranasal corticosteroids are the single most effective medication for the treatment of allergic rhinitis. A recent meta-analysis confirms that they are more effective than oral antihistamines in the treatment of allergic rhinitis.[8] Several intranasal corticosteroid preparations are available (Table 5–2). They are particularly useful in patients with daily moderate or severe symptoms, and they work best when administered regularly. The available data suggest that intranasal steroids (except for dexamethasone) are not associated with clinically significant systemic effects in adults.[2] However, the FDA has recently presented data suggesting that some nasal corticosteroids may slightly (but statistically significantly) reduce the growth rate in children, although the overall significance of these observations, especially regarding

an effect on ultimate height, is unclear.[2] Because of this concern, the FDA recommends that (1) intranasal steroids should be used in children at the lowest effective dose, (2) height should be monitored routinely, and (3) other therapeutic approaches should be appropriately used so that intranasal steroid doses may be minimized.

Montelukast, a leukotriene receptor antagonist, was approved by the FDA for the treatment of seasonal allergic rhinitis. The use of leukotriene receptor antagonists for the pharmacotherapy of allergic rhinitis has been reviewed.[9] The studies published to date demonstrate that leukotriene receptor antagonists are sometimes more effective than placebo, are no more effective than second-generation antihistamines, and are less effective than intranasal steroids in the treatment of allergic rhinitis.[9] The exact role for leukotriene receptor antagonists in the treatment of allergic rhinitis remains to be determined.

Intranasal ipratropium may be useful for patients with allergic rhinitis who experience prominent watery rhinorrhea. Finally, regarding pharmacological therapy, a short (5–7 days) course of oral corticosteroids may be required occasionally for severe allergic rhinitis. Intraturbinate injection of corticosteroids is not recommended for treatment of rhinitis because the possible benefits do not outweigh the potentially serious side effects of cavernous vein thrombosis and blindness, especially because alternatives such as intranasal or oral steroids are available.[2]

Allergen immunotherapy may be considered for patients with clear-cut allergic rhinitis that is not adequately controlled by other means.[2] Because of potentially life-threatening allergic reactions, it should be performed only by specialists trained in its use. Immunotherapy should be given for a 12-month trial, and, if effective, continued for 3 to 5 years and then evaluated for trial discontinuation. The clinical benefit derived from immunotherapy can be measured in symptom and/or medication reduction, but not usually eradication or cure.

TABLE 5–2   Nasal Corticosteroid Sprays*

Agent	Trade Name(s)	Dose per Inhalation	Base Initial Adult Dosage
Beclomethasone dipropionate	Beconase AQ	42 mcg	1–2 sprays per nostril 2x/day
Budesonide	Rhinocort AQ	32 mcg	1 spray per nostril 2x/day or 2 sprays per nostril 1x/day
Flunisolide	Nasarel Nasalide	25 mcg	2 sprays per nostril 2x/day
Fluticasone propionate	Flonase	50 mcg	2 sprays per nostril 1x/day or 1 spray per nostril 2x/day
Mometasone	Nasonex (AQ)	50 mcg	2 sprays per nostril 1x/day
Triamcinolone acetonide	Nasacort Nasacort AQ	55 mcg	2 sprays per nostril 1x/day
Dexamethasone Sodium phosphate	Dexacort	84 mcg	2 sprays per nostril 2–3x/day

* Modified from Dykewicz MS, Fineman S, eds. Diagnosis and management of rhinitis: parameter documents of the Joint Task Force on Practice Parameters in Allergy, Asthma and Immunology. *Ann Allergy.* 1998;81:463–518.

■ Allergy and Sinus Disease

Epidemiological Observations

Sinus disease has been reported to occur in 53 to 63% of allergic subjects,[10-13] and allergy has been reported to be present in 20 to 56% of patients with sinusitis.[11,14-23] However, whether this represents a true association between allergy and sinus disease or just the frequent coexistence of two common conditions is not totally clear. Savolainen[14] studied 225 patients with documented acute maxillary sinusitis and 103 age-matched controls. Allergy was diagnosed on the basis of history, skin tests, and nasal smear. A statistically significant increase in definite (25% vs. 16.5%) or probable (6.5% vs. 3%) allergy was found in the subjects with sinusitis compared with controls. In a national survey of chronic sinusitis in Korea,[24] in which chronic sinusitis was diagnosed based on symptoms and endoscopic examination, symptoms of allergic rhinitis (not specifically defined in the article) were 10 times more likely in patients with chronic sinusitis than in subjects without chronic sinusitis ($p < 0.05$). Berrettini et al[25] found abnormal sinus CTs in 67.5% of 40 mite-sensitive patients with perennial allergic rhinitis, compared with 33.4% of controls undergoing cranial CTs for dizziness. In contrast, the incidence of radiologically diagnosed sinusitis was not increased in allergic versus nonallergic subjects in 91 children with chronic respiratory symptoms,[11] 445 children and adults with chronic nasal symptoms,[13] or 270 patients with asthma and/or rhinitis.[10]

One longitudinal study has also provided evidence against a specific association between allergy and sinusitis. In this study,[26] 64 patients with allergic rhinitis and 23 nonallergic individuals were followed for 11 months. During the period of observation, the subjects with allergic rhinitis did not experience more frequent or longer lasting upper respiratory infections or sinusitis than did nonallergic subjects.

Although the above studies have not supported a clear-cut relationship between the frequency of sinusitis and the presence of allergy, several studies have noted a relationship between the severity of sinusitis and the presence of allergy. In these studies[15,16,27] correlations were reported between the extent of sinus disease, as determined by sinus CT scan, and the presence of specific IgE, as determined by RAST testing. Extensive disease in these studies was also correlated with the presence of asthma, peripheral eosinophilia, sinus tissue eosinophilia, and total serum IgE level.

Mechanistic Considerations

If allergy predisposes to more severe sinusitis, if not more frequent disease, what might the mechanism(s) be?

Three potential mechanisms have been considered: (1) an IgE-mediated reaction occurring in the sinuses themselves, (2) allergic rhinitis-induced ostial obstruction, and (3) a constitutional predisposition to sinus mucosal inflammation in allergic patients.

Pelikan et al[28] evaluated sinus radiology at baseline and then either 6 or 12 hours after allergen challenge in 37 patients with chronic sinusitis who were studied at a time of minimal symptoms. Forty-one positive nasal allergen challenges were observed in 29 of 37 patients. In 32 of the 41 positive nasal responses, a positive maxillary sinus response was also observed (>3.0 mm increased thickening and/or increased opacification or decreased aeration). In contrast, a positive sinus response occurred in only 3 of 21 negative nasal challenges ($p < .01$). These data would be consistent with either a local sinus IgE-mediated reaction occurring coincident with the nasal allergic response or sinus changes occurring secondary to allergy-induced ostial obstruction. However, this study is weakened by the fact that the radiographs were apparently not interpreted in a blinded fashion and definitive criteria for a positive sinus response were apparently not established a priori.

Three studies argue against a local IgE-mediated reaction occurring in the sinus. In the first study,[29] five nonatopic subjects inhaled technetium-labeled ragweed. Intense reactivity was detected in the nasal cavity, but none was detected in the sinuses, suggesting that the antigen does not penetrate into sinus tissue. In the second study, Liu et al[30] evaluated tissue-specific mite IgE in the sinus mucosa and nasal turbinates of 60 patients with sinusitis. Although specific mite IgE was elevated in the turbinate tissue of atopic patients, mite IgE was not found to be elevated in sinus mucosa. Finally, Slavin et al[31] studied five highly symptomatic ragweed-sensitive adults during the ragweed season. Using three different sinus imaging modalities, no sinus inflammation was demonstrated in these patients.

Melen et al[32] evaluated ostial diameter on entry and during the peak of the pollen season in 20 patients with seasonal allergic rhinitis treated with intranasal budesonide or placebo. Ostial diameters were normal at both time periods and were not different in budesonide-versus placebo-treated subjects, even though budesonide-treated patients reported significant symptomatic improvement. Consistent with these observations, sinus CT scan–defined ostiomeatal unit abnormalities did not correlate with sinus mucosal changes or with clinical status in 10 patients with ragweed allergic rhinitis.[33] These data do not support the concept that allergy-induced ostial obstruction leads to sinusitis in allergic subjects.

Finally, several studies have evaluated immunohistochemical markers of inflammation in sinus biopsies from allergic versus nonallergic subjects with chronic sinusitis. Although tissue eosinophilia appears to be prominent in both allergic and nonallergic subjects,[34–36] it may be more prominent in allergic subjects.[15,37–39] An increase in macrophages[34] and polymorphonuclear leukocytes[38,39] has also been reported in the sinuses of both allergic and nonallergic patients with chronic sinusitis.

Cells expressing receptors for IL-5, GM-CSF, IL-6, and IL-13 appear to be increased in both allergic and nonallergic subjects with sinusitis compared with controls,[36,40–43] although IL-5 appears to be more prominent in allergic subjects,[39,41,44,45] whereas GM-CSF appears to be more prominent in nonallergic subjects.[40,41] Both allergic and nonallergic patients have been reported to manifest increased total (CD3)[36] and helper (CD4)[36,46] sinus T cells, and suppressor/cytotoxic (CD8) T cells have been reported to be decreased in allergic subjects but increased in nonallergic subjects compared with controls.[36] In addition, only allergic subjects have been reported to have increased mast cells,[34] CD20+ B cells,[47] and IgE-producing B cell precursors in sinus biopsies,[47] and allergic subjects exhibited a higher proportion of CD30 positive mononuclear cells (presumably Th2 cells) in sinus mucosa than nonallergic subjects.[43] These data suggest that Th2 cytokines and their receptors are important in the eosinophilic inflammation of sinusitis in both allergic and nonallergic subjects, but that involvement of somewhat different cytokine pathways and effector cells may lead to increased inflammation in allergic subjects.[40] The putative antigen that is stimulating the apparent immunological inflammatory response in the sinuses remains unknown, but microbial superantigens appear to be one possibility.[48]

Diagnostic Considerations

Regardless of the mechanisms involved, the frequent coexistence of allergy and sinus disease demands a high index of suspicion for the presence of allergy in patients with sinus disease and for sinus disease in patients with allergic rhinitis. In patients with chronic sinusitis, the presence of asthma,[15] increased total serum IgE level,[15,37,49] and more prominent nasal eosinophilia[49] may suggest an allergic component. However, as discussed above, the definitive diagnosis of allergic rhinitis in patients with chronic sinusitis entails identification of antigen-specific IgE that correlates with symptoms upon exposure to the antigen(s).

The presence of sinus disease in patients with allergic rhinitis may be difficult to predict on clinical ground alone. However, the following findings have been reported to correlate with significant radiologic sinus abnormalities in patients with underlying allergic rhinitis: cough,[12,50] purulent mucus,[50] thick posterior nasal drainage,[12] and a negative nasal smear for eosinophils.[12,50] In addition, in a study of 91 children with chronic respiratory symptoms, 59% of whom were atopic, the triad of rhinorrhea, cough, and the absence of sneezing was strongly correlated ($r = 0.49$) with abnormal sinus CT scans.[11]

Therapeutic Considerations

The diagnosis of sinusitis in patients with known allergic rhinitis has obvious treatment implications. Antibiotics are often effective,[45,50] and other appropriate medical and surgical management would be dictated by the severity and responsiveness of the sinus disease. The implications of a diagnosis of allergy in patients with chronic sinusitis are less certain. Avoidance of antigens to which the patient is sensitive would be recommended, although there are no studies that evaluate the response of sinus disease to antigen avoidance in allergic individuals.

There are some data regarding the effects of nasal steroids in allergic patients with sinusitis. Two studies[36,41] report decreased expression of interleukins (IL-4, IL-5, IL-13) in the sinus biopsies of allergic subjects with chronic sinusitis treated with intranasal steroids in comparison to allergic subjects with sinusitis not receiving intranasal steroids. The exact clinical significance of these findings is not clear. However, in conjunction with observations that intranasal steroids are the most effective pharmacological agents for the management of allergic rhinitis,[2] these data suggest that patients with allergic rhinitis and chronic sinusitis generally should receive intranasal steroids. In addition, two studies[51,52] suggest that the addition of intranasal steroids to antibiotic treatment of acute sinusitis in patients with a history of recurrent sinusitis or chronic rhinitis reduces symptoms of acute sinusitis and improves clinical success rates. In one of these studies,[51] patients were excluded for "active seasonal allergic rhinitis," and atopic status (any RAST score >3), which was present in 38% of subjects, did not predict responsiveness to nasal steroid therapy.

Inhalant antigen immunotherapy has been clearly shown to be effective in patients with allergic rhinitis.[2] However, its efficacy specifically for sinus manifestations in allergic patients with chronic sinusitis is less well documented. Schlenter and Mann[53] reported an improved prognosis in 15 allergic patients with relapsing sinusitis treated with immunotherapy compared with 16 atopic patients with sinusitis not so treated. However, only the abstract of this study is in English, and we cannot therefore evaluate the details of this study. Lehrer et al[54] reported a decrease in sinusitis episodes during 12 to 27 months of follow-up in four allergic subjects treated with immunotherapy, but these observations in this small sample are uncontrolled.

The largest study of immunotherapy in allergic patients with sinusitis was reported by Asakura et al.[55]

These authors studied 37 allergic subjects with sinusitis. Skin tests were positive to *Candida*,[9] dust,[32] and bacterial vaccine[5] in these 37 subjects. Twenty of the subjects were treated with immunotherapy (19 to dust, one to *Candida*), and 17 received medical therapy only; treatment was not randomized. A third group of 15 nonallergic patients with sinusitis was treated medically. Treatment was apparently given for 2 to 3 months, and symptoms, signs, and x-rays improved in all groups. However, after treatment, the immunotherapy group manifested decreased symptoms and signs and better x-rays than the nonimmunotherapy-treated group. Although possibly indicating that immunotherapy benefits sinus disease in allergic patients, we believe that more definitive and better designed studies will be required before immunotherapy can be routinely recommended for the treatment of sinus manifestations in allergic subjects.

Allergic status may also influence the responsiveness to surgical therapy for sinusitis. It is known that patients with extensive hyperplastic sinus mucosal thickening have a poorer outcome with sinus surgery.[56] In addition, allergic subjects with perennial rhinitis may have less benefit from surgical procedures for chronic rhinosinusitis compared with those without allergies.[57] In a study of 15 allergic patients with diffuse sinus disease but without nasal polyposis, more than 50% did not improve after sinus surgery.[57] An increased number of cells expressing IL-5 messenger RNA (mRNA) was found in the ethmoid sinuses at the time of surgery in patients who did not respond to the surgical intervention. Further studies of allergy and the immunologic characteristics of the sinus mucosal inflammation as potential sinus surgery prognostic factors appear warranted.

■ Allergic Fungal Sinusitis

The first case of allergic fungal sinusitis (AFS) was probably described in 1976 in a patient with allergic bronchopulmonary aspergillosis with nasal obstruction, nasal polyps, and aspergillus-positive sinus culture.[58] Subsequently, "allergic aspergillosis of the maxillary sinuses" was described in five patients,[59] and "allergic *Aspergillus* sinusitis" was reported in seven patients.[60] In 1989, Robson et al[61] introduced the term AFS after it was recognized that fungal species other than *Aspergillus* could be grown in sinus cultures from these patients.

In the past 10 years, AFS has been increasingly recognized,[62–65] and specific diagnostic criteria have been proposed.[62,64] It is estimated that AFS can be diagnosed in 4 to 8% of patients undergoing surgery for chronic sinusitis.[60,65] Although substantial consensus exists regarding appropriate therapy,[62,63,65–67] no double-blind, randomized, controlled clinical therapeutic trials have been reported to date.

Etiology/Pathogenesis

AFS has been thought to be due to an IgE- and an IgG-mediated immune response to fungal antigens residing in the sinuses, analogous to allergic bronchopulmonary aspergillosis.[64,66] The most common fungus involved appears to be *Bipolaris*.[62,64] Other dematiaceous molds (*Alternaria, Curvularia lunata*, and *Pseudallescheria boydii*)[62,68] and *Aspergillus*[62,63] have also been relatively frequently reported. It is hypothesized that atopic, immunologically competent patients exposed to appropriate fungi in the sinuses for prolonged periods of time develop intense sinus mucosal immunologically induced inflammation and hypertrophy, functional ciliary impairment, and the entrapment and sequestration of an expanding allergic mucin mass (see below) that leads to the characteristic clinical manifestations.[64] Although noninvasive, this allergic mucin mass may expand into the orbit, the cranium, or both.[64]

Diagnosis

Recently proposed criteria for the diagnosis of AFS are summarized in Table 5–3.[62,64] AFS needs to be differentiated from other fungal sinus diseases: sinus mycetoma, acute invasive fungal sinusitis, chronic invasive fungal sinusitis, and granulomatous invasive fungal sinusitis[68] (Tables 5–4 and 5–5). Based on a literature review of 99 case reports,[62] a Mayo Clinic series of 44 cases,[65] and a recent consecutive series of 67 patients with AFS,[64,66] characteristic clinical manifestations can be described.

Patients are typically relatively young (mean age 26–42)[62,64,65] and often have a history of intractable sinus disease, in spite of frequent antibiotics and multiple previous surgeries.[64,65,68] Nasal polyps have been reported in 80 to 100% of patients and asthma in 54 to 64%.[62,64,65] Three-fourths of patients in one series[64] reported expelling nasal casts (dark green, rubbery formed elements) from the nose. Proptosis was reported in 4 of 11 patients in one small series,[63] and orbital symptoms were described in 7 of 42 patients in the Mayo Clinic series.[65]

All patients have radiologic evidence of sinusitis, usually pansinusitis.[68] Sinus CTs characteristically reveal hyperplastic sinusitis[64] involving three or more sinuses,[65] frequently with demonstrable hyperattenuating extramucosal

TABLE 5–3 Diagnostic Criteria for Allergic Fungal Sinusitis[64,68]

1. Radiologic evidence of sinusitis of one or more paranasal sinuses
2. Allergic mucin in the sinus
3. Fungal hyphae in the mucin or positive sinus fungal culture
4. Absence of diabetes, immunodeficiency or immunosuppressive therapy
5. Absence of fungal invasion

TABLE 5–4   General Features of Noninvasive and Invasive Fungal Sinusitis*

Syndrome	Common Causes	Geographic Distribution	Characterisitics of Host	Associated Conditions
Allergic fungal sinusitis	Bipolaris species, Curvularia lunata, and Aspergillus fumigatus	Humid areas, especially coastal United States	Immunocompetent, frequently atopic	Chronic sinusitis, nasal polyps
Sinus mycetoma (fungus ball)	A. fumigatus and dematiaceous fungi	Humid areas, especially coastal United States	Immunocompetent, sometmes atopic	Chronic sinusitis, nasal polyps
Acute (fulminant) invasive fungal sinusitis	Fungi of the order Mucorales and A. fumigatus	No specific geographic location	Immunocompromised; rarely immuno-competent	Diabetes mellitus, malignant conditions, immunosuppressive therapy
Chronic invasive fungal sinusitis	A. fumigatus	No specific geographic location	Immuncompromised	Diabetes mellitus
Granulomatous invasive fungal sinusitis	A. flavus	Predominantly North Africa	Immunocompetent	None

* Reprinted with permission from deShazo, RD, Chapin K, Swain RE. Fungal sinusitis. *N Engl J Med.* 1997;337:254–259.

material, which reflects allergic mucin with fungal elements.[62,64] Loss of bony sinus margins has been reported in 23 to 33% of patients.[62,65]

The diagnostic allergic mucin is grossly seen as brown or green-black material with peanut butter or cottage cheese consistency.[68] Histologically, it consists of clumps of intact and necrotic eosinophils, Charcot-Leyden crystals, cellular debris, and fungal hyphae within a background of pale, eosinophilic to basophilic amorphous mucin.[60,68] Additional histological findings on hematoxylin and eosin stains are sinus mucosal changes indistinguishable from the mucosal infiltrate of bronchial asthma: eosinophils, plasma cells, and small lymphocytes; absence of necrosis, granuloma formation, or giant cells; stromal edema; thickened respiratory epithelial basement membrane; partially desquamated respiratory epithelium; and distended mucus glands.[64] Demonstration of fungal elements in the allergic mucin requires the use of a methenamine silver stain.

Atopy has been reported in 76 to 100% of patients[50,52] and an elevated total IgE level in 67 to 74% of patients.[62,64] In addition, similar to allergic bronchopulmonary aspergillosis, the IgE level has been shown to correlate with disease activity (see below).[66] Positive skin

TABLE 5–5   Pathology, Clinical Features, Treatment, and Prognosis of Noninvasive and Invasive Fungal Sinusitis*

Syndrome	Histopathological Findings	Clinical Presentation	Treatment	Prognosis
Allergic fungal sinusitis	Sparse fungal elements in dense, eosinophil-rich mucoid material ("allergic mucin") containing rare hyphae; lymphoplasmocytic and eosinophilic response in adjacent mucosa	Chronic pansinusitis, nasal polyps, calcification within sinus on CT, proptosis or eye muscle entrapment in children	Debridement, aeration, oral and topical corticosteroids, and allergen immunotherapy	Recurrence common
Sinus mycetoma (fungus ball)	Dense accumulation of fungal elements in a mucoid matrix forming an expansile mass; low-grade chronic inflammatory response in adjacent mucosa	Rhinosinusitis (often unilateral), nasal obstruction, green-brown nasal discharge, calcification in sinus on CT	Debridement, aeration; antifungal agents not required	Excellent
Acute (fulminant) invasive fungal sinusitis	Fungal elements in mucosa, submucosa, blood vessels, or bone, with extensive tissue necrosis and neutrophilic inflammation	Fever, cough, crusting of nasal mucosa, epistaxis, headache, mental status changes	Radical debridement until histopathologically normal tissue is evident, antifungal agents, treatment of underlying conditions	Fair when disease is limited to sinus; poor with intracranial involvement
Chronic invasive fungal sinusitis	Necrosis of mucosa, submucosa, bone and blood vessels, with low-grade inflammation	Orbital apex syndrome	Radical debridement, antifungal agents	Poor
Granulomatous invasive fungal sinusitis	Granuloma with multinucleated giant cells and palisading histiocytes	Unilateral proptosis	Debridement, aeration, and itraconazole therapy	Good, but disease can recur

* Reprinted with permission from deShazo, RD, Chapin K, Swain RE. Fungal sinusitis. *N Engl J Med.* 1997;337:254–259.

tests to the cultured fungi have been reported in 58 to 100% of patients.[62,64,65,69] Although precipitating antibodies against the involved fungi were reported in 89% of 27 patients in the earlier literature series,[62] only 8% of patients in the recent consecutive case series had demonstrable fungal precipitins.[64] However, 67% of patients in this series did demonstrate fungal-specific IgG that also correlated with disease activity, although less strongly than total IgE.[66] In addition, serum *Bipolaris*-specific IgG antibodies were reported to be present in all eight patients with *Bipolaris* AFS in one series.[69] Although peripheral eosinophilia was reported in 65% of patients in the Mayo Clinic series,[65] it was less common (38.5%) in a series of 17 AFS patients[69] and uncommon in another series of patients, with a mean eosinophil count of 4.5%.[64]

Ponikau et al[70] have described a much higher incidence than in prior reports of AFS diagnosed on the basis of radiologically documented sinusitis, allergic mucin, and fungal organisms within that mucin. In 101 consecutive surgical cases, these diagnostic criteria for AFS were met in 93% of patients. One reason for the high incidence may have been the use of a novel culturing technique that resulted in positive nasal fungal cultures in 96% of 210 consecutive patients with chronic rhinosinusitis (including the 101 surgical cases) and in 100% of 14 controls with no evidence of nasal or sinus disease.

Treatment

Although sinus surgery alone is not usually adequate, it is still necessary to remove polyps, accumulated inspissated allergic mucin, and hypertrophic sinus mucosa.[62,66–68] Recent articles do not recommend antifungal agents, based on their lack of efficacy.[62,63,65–68] Intranasal steroids have been recommended as concomitant therapy,[67] although no specific data on their efficacy in patients with AFS are available.

Although oral corticosteroids have also been recommended,[62] only recently is there definitive evidence of their efficacy. Schubert and Goetz[66] have reported that the severity of clinical rhinosinusitis 2 months after surgery was significantly worse in subjects not treated with oral corticosteroids compared with those who received oral corticosteroids. Moreover, patients receiving ≥2 months of oral corticosteroids demonstrated longer times between surgeries. In addition, at 12 months, clinical outcomes were better in those continuing oral corticosteroids compared with those who did not continue them. The recommended oral corticosteroid regimen is 0.5 mg/kg daily for 14 days, then 0.5 mg/kg every other day, tapered over 3 months to 5 mg every other day for at least 12 months postoperatively. Intercurrent acute rhinosinusitis should be treated with short "bursts" of prednisone and with antibiotics if indicated.[67]

Schubert and Goetz[66] reported another interesting and clinically important observation regarding the course and response to treatment of AFS. Similar to allergic bronchopulmonary aspergillosis, serum total IgE level could be used to monitor disease activity. An increase of ≥10% in total IgE level during follow-up was found to be 79% sensitive and 77% specific in predicting the need for repeat surgical intervention. Although the positive predictive value of such a rise was only 48%, the negative predictive value was 93%. Thus, changes in IgE level <10% over time are very likely to reflect a lack of disease progression.

Although Schubert and Goetz[66] used immunotherapy to relevant aeroallergens as part of their therapy, they did not include the AFS organism in their immunotherapy extracts. However, results from a nonblinded study suggest that 1 to 3 years of immunotherapy with fungal and nonfungal antigens to which hypersensitivity was demonstrated had a positive impact on the disease in 11 subjects.[71] No repeat surgeries for recurrent AFS were required in these patients, and only three of them received a short course of oral steroids on one occasion each. Further experience and controlled observations will be necessary before a definitive recommendation regarding fungal antigen immunotherapy in the management of AFS can be made.

■ Relationship between Sinusitis and Asthma

General Considerations

Sinusitis is an extremely common disorder that extracts a significant price both directly and indirectly. It is the most commonly reported chronic disease in the United States, affecting 14.7% of the population.[72] It accounts for 11.6 million physician office visits per year and for the fifth highest antibiotic use of all diseases.[73]

The frequent association of paranasal sinus disease and bronchial asthma has been noted for a great many years. Several clinical studies in the 1920s and 1930s emphasized the importance of sinusitis as a trigger for asthma.[74–76] However, the relationship between sinusitis and asthma then seemed to fall into disrepute, and little was written about this relationship for the next several decades. One prevailing thought was that sinus changes simply reflected a disease of the entire respiratory membrane. Therefore, management of sinusitis per se would be expected to have little effect on the courses of lower respiratory tract disease. In the last two decades, the relationship of sinusitis and asthma has been revived.[77–79]

There is no question that a high incidence of radiographic evidence of sinusitis is present in both children and adults with asthma. One study from Los Angeles

Children's Hospital showed that 75% of pediatric patients admitted with status asthmaticus had abnormal sinus x-rays.[80] An adult study from Finland reported abnormal sinus radiographs in 87% of patients with an exacerbation of asthma.[81]

A more recent study looked at 35 patients with mild to moderate asthma. The authors found that all the subjects with severe asthma had abnormalities in the CT scans of the sinuses compared with 88% of the individuals with mild to moderate asthma.[82] There has been a suggestion that the association between chronic sinusitis and asthma was strong only in the group of sinusitis patients with extensive disease.[15]

It appears that the peripheral blood eosinophil level is a good marker for extensive rhinosinusitis. In one study, 104 patients undergoing sinus surgery had CT scans reviewed for extent of disease, total serum IgE, and specific IgE antibodies to common inhalant antigens and a peripheral blood eosinophil count. The authors found that among the patients with peripheral blood eosinophilia, 87% had extensive sinus disease as seen by CT scan.[15]

A recent study showed that the vast majority of patients with severe asthma not only had sinus CT abnormalities, but that the extent of sinus disease was positively related to airway inflammation. This was reflected by increased eosinophils in induced sputum and peripheral blood, as well as increased levels of NO in exhaled air. This is indicative of an association between sinonasal and lower airway inflammation in patients with severe asthma.[83]

The overriding question is whether this association represents an epiphenomenon; that is, are sinusitis and asthma manifestations of the same underlying disease process in different parts of the respiratory tract, or is there a causal relationship? Can sinusitis trigger bronchial asthma?

Although more objective evidence is needed, there are data to indicate that difficult-to-control asthma will improve when coexistent sinusitis is cleared by medical and/or surgical treatment. This can be considered as strong suggestive evidence for an etiologic role of sinusitis in lower airway disease. Before examining this evidence, let us explore the possible mechanisms relating sinusitis to asthma.

Potential Mechanisms Relating Sinusitis to Asthma

THE EOSINOPHIL

The eosinophil is known to play an important role in mediating injury to bronchial epithelium in chronic asthma. In one study, researchers assessed the role of the eosinophil in chronic inflammatory disease of the paranasal sinuses by examining tissue from patients who

underwent surgery for chronic sinusitis.[37] Sinus tissue from patients with sinusitis and concomitant chronic asthma and/or allergic rhinitis was extensively infiltrated with eosinophils. In contrast, sinus tissue from patients with chronic sinusitis alone had no eosinophils. Immunofluorescent studies demonstrated a striking association between the presence of extracellular deposition of major basic protein and damage to sinus mucosa. The histopathology of the paranasal respiratory epithelium also appeared similar to that described in bronchial asthma.

The marked tissue eosinophilia associated with chronic hyperplastic sinusitis has been shown to be strongly correlated with local cytokine production, particularly GM-CSF and IL-2. Interestingly, IL-5 mRNA expression was not a prominent feature.[44] The suggestion is that the eosinophil acts as an effector cell in chronic inflammatory disease of the paranasal respiratory epithelium. This points to the possibility that sinus disease in patients with asthma may be caused by the same mechanisms that cause damage to bronchial epithelium.

NEURAL REFLEXES

The postulated neuroanatomical pathways that could connect the paranasal sinuses to the lungs are as follows[84]: Receptors in the nose, pharynx, and presumably the paranasal sinuses give rise to afferent fibers that, in turn, form part of the trigeminal nerve. The trigeminal nerve passes to the brainstem, where it can connect via the reticular formation with the dorsal vagal nucleus. From the vagal nucleus, parasympathetic efferent fibers travel in the vagus nerve to the bronchi. The cholinergic parasympathetic nervous system plays a role in maintaining resting bronchial muscle tone as well as in mediating acute bronchospastic responses. The vagus nerve provides the cholinergic motor supply to airway smooth muscle.

INFLAMMATORY MEDIATORS

Another proposed mechanism whereby sinusitis may act as an aggravator of asthma is local stimulation of irritant receptors by inflammatory mediators produced by the sinuses with resultant reflex bronchospasm. Inflammatory mediators, including leukotrienes, prostaglandin D_2 (PGD_2), and histamine were measured in maxillary sinus lavage fluid obtained during surgery for chronic sinusitis.[83] The findings were compared with levels of mediators in nasal lavage fluid from a group of allergic rhinitis subjects. The results indicated that the levels of leukotrienes, histamine, and PGD_2 in sinus fluid were significantly elevated over those of the control nasal lavage fluid and were in the range associated with local inflammation and irritant receptor stimulation.[85]

In a study utilizing radionucleotide techniques, pulmonary aspiration of upper airway secretions could not be demonstrated.[86] The authors concluded that seeding of the lower airways by mucopurulent secretions is unlikely to account for coexistent pulmonary disease. It also seemed unlikely that locally produced inflammatory mediators would be aspirated into the lung.[86] The possibility exists, however, that sinus secretions could set off reflexes in other parts of the respiratory tract that might result in worsening of asthma.

In a study[87] of 106 patients with chronic sinusitis, histamine challenges to the lower airway before and after medical treatment of sinusitis were performed. Forced expiratory volume in 1 second (FEV_1) was measured as an index of bronchial narrowing, and midinspiratory flow (MIF_{50}), as an index of extrabronchial airway narrowing. After treatment, both intrabronchial and extrabronchial hyperreactivity decreased, with the reduction in extrabronchial hyperreactivity being more pronounced and preceding the intrabronchial hyperreactivity decline. The changes in intrabronchial and extrabronchial reactivity were strongly associated with the degree of pharyngitis as determined by history, physical examination, and nasal lavage. The authors propose that airway hyperresponsiveness in sinusitis might depend on pharyngobronchial reflexes triggered by seeding of the inflammatory process into the pharynx through postnasal drip of mediators and infected material from affected sinuses.

These authors have followed up this study with observations demonstrating actual damage of the pharyngeal mucosa in patients with chronic sinusitis.[88] Marked thinning of the epithelium was seen with a striking increase in pharyngeal nerve fiber density. This would favor increased access of irritants to submucosal nerve endings inducing the release of sensory neuropeptides via axon reflexes with activation of a neural arc, resulting in reflex airway constriction. As previously noted, the extent of sinus disease seen on CT was correlated with peripheral blood and sputum eosinophilia. This suggests not simply a local phenomenon, but rather a systemic process. Patients with chronic hyperplastic rhinosinusitis have an intense inflammatory process of the upper airway. It could be hypothesized that the inflamed sinus tissue not only releases mediators and cytokines into the circulation, which would directly affect the lower airways, but also releases chemotactic factors that recruit eosinophils from the bone marrow and direct them to the upper and lower airways.[89]

With this mechanistic background, let us turn to the clinical effects of sinusitis therapy on the asthmatic state.

Results of Therapy of Sinusitis on Asthma

MEDICAL THERAPY

A study by Rachelefsky and associates[78] demonstrated that children with combined sinusitis and lower airway hyperreactivity showed significant improvement of the

TABLE 5–6 Disease Characteristics before and after Treatment for Sinusitis in 48 Children*

Characteristic	Before	After
Cough	100%	29%
Wheeze	100%	15%
Normal pulmonary function tests	0	67%
Bronchodilator treatment	100%	21%

* Data from Rachelefsky, GS, Katz RM, Siegel SC. Chronic sinus disease with associated reactive airway disease in children. *Pediatrics.* 1984;73:526–532.

asthmatic state when they received appropriate medical treatment for their sinusitis. Disease characteristics before and after treatment for sinusitis in those 48 children with hyperreactive airway disease are demonstrated in Table 5–6. Only seven of the children required sinus lavage; the remainder received appropriate medical therapy. As shown in the table, 79% of the children were able to discontinue bronchodilator therapy after resolution of the sinusitis. Pulmonary function tests showed normal results in 67% of those with pretreatment abnormalities. Similar results were reported in another group of children with asthma and sinusitis from the University of Pittsburgh.[90] Another similar study done by Oliveira and Sole[91] looked at improvement of bronchial hyperresponsiveness (BHR) in children treated for sinusitis. The authors studied 46 atopic and 20 normal children. Methacholine challenges were done both before and 30 days after the sinusitis was treated with nasal saline, antibiotics, antihistamine, or decongestant and 5 days of prednisone. The authors found that the only patients who showed a decrease in their sensitivity to methacholine after treatment were patients with rhinitis and asthma with opacified maxillary sinuses at entry and those who had normal sinus radiographs at 30 days into the study. Therefore, the authors concluded that children with allergic rhinitis and sinusitis with asthma improved their BHR to methacholine and decreased their symptoms with appropriate response of their sinuses to medical therapy.[91]

There are no similar studies on adults showing the beneficial effect on asthma by appropriate medical therapy of sinusitis.

SURGICAL THERAPY

There is evidence that patients with medically resistant rhinosinusitis demonstrate improvement in their asthma after definitive nasosinus surgery.

One study[92] reported results from a trial involving 205 adult patients with the aspirin triad, that is, nasal polyps, asthma, and aspirin sensitivity, all of whom were steroid-dependent. After functional endoscopic sinus surgery (FESS), 40% were able to discontinue steroids; another 44% were controlled on alternate day or bursts of steroids. This is particularly notable because patients with the aspirin triad have asthma that is notoriously difficult to control. Another study[93] looked at 20 patients with chronic sinusitis and asthma, age 16 to 72 years. Following FESS, 70% reported the frequency of asthma to be much less, and 65% reported significantly less severe asthma. Of particular interest was a 75% reduction in hospitalization and an 81% reduction in emergency department/urgent office visits in the year following FESS.[93]

The effect of FESS on chronic sinusitis and concomitant childhood asthma is also promising. Parsons and Phillips[20] reported findings from a series of 52 children (average age 7.4 years; range 7 months–17 years). After FESS, chronic cough resolved or improved in 84% of the patients, and 96% of the subjects reported a decreased frequency of asthma episodes. The average number of exacerbations per month fell from 6.7 to 2.5, and emergency department visits decreased 79%.[20] Manning et al[94] studied 14 steroid-dependent childhood asthmatics, 6 of whom had primary immunodeficiency. After FESS, 11 showed improvement in their asthma. There was a decrease in lost school days from 22.3 to 14.5 and in-hospital days from 21.4 to 6.5.[94]

A study by Dunlop et al[95] looked at 50 patients with asthma who had endoscopic surgery. A total of 20% had reduction in the amount of inhaled corticosteroids required, and there were significant decreases in the use of oral corticosteroids and hospitalizations in the year after the surgery. Similarly, Dhong et al[96] observed 19 patients who underwent endoscopic sinus surgery for rhinosinusitis. These patients demonstrated significant improvements in diurnal and nocturnal asthma symptoms and had improvements in asthma medication scores. No changes were noted in pulmonary function tests. In an adult outcome study by Gliklich and Metson,[97] it was noted that patients with preexisting asthma had the greatest improvement in overall health measures after sinus surgery. However, Goldstein et al[98] did a retrospective medical record analysis on 13 patients with asthma who underwent FESS for medically refractory chronic rhinosinusitis and found no significant change in group mean asthma symptoms, asthma medication usage, pulmonary function test results, and number of emergency room visits or hospitalizations.

Okayama et al[99] looked at 42 patients with chronic rhinosinusitis, 50 patients with stable asthma, 50 patients with chronic bronchitis, and 40 patients with allergic rhinitis and compared methacholine BHR. They found that BHR in subjects with chronic rhinosinusitis was less than that of the subjects with asthma but was similar to those with chronic bronchitis or allergic rhinitis in both its prevalence and degree. The authors then further examined patients with chronic rhinosinusitis and bronchial asthma who underwent endoscopic surgery. They noted that after the surgical treatment for chronic

rhinosinusitis, the patients had a significant decrease in their BHR with improvements in both nasal symptoms and sinus lesions. Therefore, adequate therapy of chronic rhinosinusitis appeared to reduce BHR.

Conclusion

Direct evidence linking the processes of sinusitis to asthma mechanistically is lacking.[94] Basic mechanisms need to be investigated further by establishing experimental animal models and by appropriate human studies. However, the studies described above indicate that proper treatment of rhinosinusitis by medical and/or surgical means frequently results in significant improvement of asthma symptomatology in both children and adults. These studies provide strong suggestive clinical evidence that rhinosinusitis not only occurs in association with bronchial asthma but also may play a role in its pathogenesis.

REFERENCES

1. Malone DC, Lawson KA, Smith DH, et al. A cost of illness study of allergic rhinitis in the United States. *J Allergy Clin Immunol.* 1997;99:22–27.
2. Dykewicz MS, Fineman S, eds. Diagnosis and management of rhinitis: parameter documents of the Joint Task Force on Practice Parameters in Allergy, Asthma and Immunology. *Ann Allergy.* 1998;81:463–518.
3. Baraniuk JN. Pathogenesis of allergic rhinitis. *J Allergy Clin Immunol.* 1997;99:S763–S772.
4. Rachelefsky G. Pharmacologic management of allergic rhinitis. *J Allergy Clin Immunol.* 1998;101:S367–S369.
5. Bousquet J, van Cauwenberge PB, Khaltaev N, et al. Allergic rhinitis and its impact on asthma: ARIA workshop report. *J Allergy Clin Immunol.* 2001;108(suppl):S147–S333.
6. Abbas AK, Murphy KM, Sher A. Functional diversity of helper T lymphocytes. *Nature.* 1996;383:787–793.
7. Rogge L, Barberis-Maino L, Biffi M, et al. Selective expression of an interleukin-12 receptor component by human T helper 1 cells. *J Exp Med.* 1997;185:825–831.
8. Weiner JM, Abramson MJ, Puy RM. Intranasal cortiosteroids versus oral H₁ receptor antagonists in allergic rhinitis: systematic review of randomized controlled trials. *BMJ.* 1998;317:1624–1629.
9. Nathan RA. Pharmacotherapy for allergic rhinitis: a critical review of leukotriene receptor antagonists compared with other treatments. *Ann Allergy Asthma Immunol.* 2003;90:182–191.
10. DeCleyn KM, Kersschot EA, DeClerck LS, et al. Paranasal sinus pathology in allergic and non-allergic respiratory tract disorders. *Allergy.* 1986;41:313–318.
11. Nguyen K-L, Corbett ML, Garcia DP, et al. Chronic sinusitis among pediatric patients with chronic respiratory complaints. *J Allergy Clin Immunol.* 1993;92:824–830.
12. Rachelefsky GS, Goldberg M, Katz RM, et al. Sinus disease in children with respiratory allergy. *J Allergy Clin Immunol.* 1978;61:310–314.
13. Iwens P, Clement PAR. Sinusitis in allergic patients. *Rhinology.* 1994;32:65–67.
14. Savolainen S. Allergy in patients with acute maxillary sinusitis. *Allergy.* 1989;44:116–122.
15. Newman LJ, Platts-Mills TAE, Phillips CD, et al. Chronic sinusitis: relationship of computed tomographic findings to allergy, asthma and eosinophilia. *JAMA.* 1994;271:363–367.

16. Hoover GE, Newman LJ, Platts-Mills TAE, et al. Chronic sinusitis: risk factors for extensive disease. *J Allergy Clin Immunol.* 1997; 100:185–191.

17. Bertrand B, Eloy P, Rombeaux P. Allergy and sinusitis. *Acta Otorhinolaryngol Belg.* 1997;51:227–237.

18. Davis WE, Templer JW, Lamear WR, et al. Middle meatus antrostomy: patency rates and risk factors. *Otolaryngol Head Neck Surg.* 1991;104:467–472.

19. Orobello PW, Park RI, Belcher LJ, et al. Microbiology of chronic sinusitis in children. *Arch Otolaryngol Head Neck Surg.* 1991; 117:980–983.

20. Parsons DS, Phillips SE. Functional endoscopic surgery in children: a retrospective analysis of results. *Laryngoscope.* 1993;103:899–903.

21. Shapiro GG, Virant FS, Furakawa CT, et al. Immunologic defects in patients with refractory sinusitis. *Pediatrics.* 1991;87:311–316.

22. Benninger MS, Mickelson SA, Yaremchuk K. Functional endoscopic sinus surgery: mortality and early results. *Henry Ford Hosp Med J.* 1990;38:5–8.

23. van Dishoeck H. Allergy and infection of the paranasal sinuses. *Fortschr Hals Nasen Ohrenheilkd.* 1961;10:1–29.

24. Min Y-G, Jung H-W, Kim H-S, et al. Prevalence and risk factors of chronic sinusitis in Korea: results of a nationwide survey. *Eur Arch Otorhinolaryngol.* 1996;253:435–439.

25. Berrettini S, Carabelli A, Sellari-Franceschini S, et al. Perennial allergic rhinitis and chronic sinusitis: correlation with rhinologic risk factors. *Allergy.* 1999;54:242–248.

26. Hinriksdotter I, Melen I. Allergic rhinitis and upper respiratory tract infection. *Acta Otolaryngol Suppl.* 1994;515:30–32.

27. Baroody FM, Suh S-H, Naclerio RM. Total IgE serum levels correlate with sinus mucosal thickness on computerized tomography scans. *J Allergy Clin Immunol.* 1997;100:563–568.

28. Pelikan Z, Pelikan-Filipek M. Role of nasal allergy in chronic maxillary sinusitis–diagnostic value of nasal challenge with allergen. *J Allergy Clin Immunol.* 1990;86:484–491.

29. Adkins TN, Goodgold HM, Hendershott L, Slavin RG. Does inhaled pollen enter the sinus cavities? *Ann Allergy Asthma Immunol.* 1998;81:181–184.

30. Liu C-M, Shun C-T, Song H-C, et al. Antigen-specific IgE antibody and cytogram in mucosa of the nose and sinus. *Am J Rhinol.* 1993;7:111–115.

31. Slavin RG, Leipzig JR, Goodgold HM. Allergic sinusitis revisited. *Ann Allergy Asthma Immunol.* 2000;85:273–276.

32. Melen I, Ivarrson A, Schrewelius C. Ostial function in allergic rhinitis. *Acta Otolaryngol.* 1992;492(suppl):82–85.

33. Naclerio RM, deTineo ML, Baroody FM. Ragweed allergic rhinitis and the paranasal sinuses: a computerized tomographic study. *Arch Otolaryngol Head Neck Surg.* 1997;123:193–196.

34. Demoly P, Crampette L, Mondain M, et al. Assessment of inflammation in noninfectious chronic maxillary sinusitis. *J Allergy Clin Immunol.* 1994;94:95–108.

35. Baroody FM, Hughes CA, McDowell P, et al. Eosinophilia in chronic childhood sinusitis. *Arch Otolaryngol Head Neck Surg.* 1995;21:1396–1402.

36. Al Ghamdi K, Ghaffar O, Small P, et al. IL-4 and IL-13 expression in chronic sinusitis: relationship with cellular infiltrate and effect of topical corticosteroid treatment. *J Otolaryngol.* 1997;26:160–166.

37. Harlin SL, Ansel DG, Lane SR, et al. A clinical and pathological study of chronic sinusitis: the role of the eosinophil. *J Allergy Clin Immunol.* 1988;81:867–875.

38. Demoly P, Sahla M, Campbell AM, et al. ICAM-1 expression in upper respiratory mucosa is differentially related to eosinophil and neutrophil inflammation according to the allergic status. *Clin Exp Allergy.* 1998;28:731–738.

39. Suzuki M, Watanabe T, Suko T, Mogi G. Comparison of sinusitis with and without allergic rhinitis: characteristics of paranasal sinus effusion and mucosa. *Am J Otolaryngol.* 1999;20:143–150.

40. Kotsimbos TC, al Ghamdi K, Small P, et al. Upregulation of Th-2 cytokine receptors in atopy- and nonatopy-associated chronic sinusitis. *J Otolaryngol.* 1996;25:317–321.

41. Wright E, Frenkiel S, Al-Ghamdi K, et al. Interleukin-4, interleukin-5 and granulocyte-macrophage colony-stimulating factor receptor expression in chronic sinusitis and response to topical steroids. *Otolaryngol Head Neck Surg.* 1998;118:490–495.

42. Ghaffar O, Lavigne F, Kamil A, et al. Interleukin-6 expression in chronic sinusitis: co-localization of gene transcripts to eosinophils, macrophages, T lymphocytes, and mast cells. *Otolaryngol Head Neck Surg.* 1998;118:504–511.

43. Suzuki H, Goto S, Ikeda K, et al. IL-12 receptor β_2 and CD30 expression in paranasal sinus mucosa of patients with chronic sinusitis. *Eur Respir J.* 1999;13:1008–1013.

44. Hamilos DL, Leung DYM, Wood R, et al. Chronic hyperplastic sinusitis: association of tissue eosinophilia with mRNA expression of granulocyte-macrophage colony-stimulating factor and interleukin-3. *J Allergy Clin Immunol.* 1993;92:39–48.

45. Goldenhersch MJ, Rachelefsky GS, Dudley J, et al. The microbiology of chronic sinus disease in children with respiratory allergy. *J Allergy Clin Immunol.* 1990;85:1030–1039.

46. Driscoll PV, Naclerio RM, Baroody FM. CD4+ lymphocytes are increased in the sinus mucosa of children with chronic sinusitis. *Arch Otolaryngol Head Neck Surg.* 1996;122:1071–1076.

47. Ghaffer O, Durham SR, Al-Ghamdi K, et al. Expression of IgE heavy chain transcripts in the sinus mucosa of atopic and nonatopic patients with chronic sinusitis. *Am J Respir Cell Mol Biol.* 1998;18:706–711.

48. Schubert MS. A superantigen hypothesis for the pathogenesis of chronic hypertrophic rhinosinusitis, allergic fungal sinusitis and related disorders. *Ann Allergy Asthma Immunol.* 2001; 87:181–188.

49. Liu C-M, Shun C-T, Song H-C, et al. Investigation into allergic response in patients with chronic sinusitis. *J Formos Med Assoc.* 1992; 91:252–257.

50. Rachelefsky GS, Katz RM, Siegel SC. Chronic sinusitis in children with respiratory allergy: the role of antimicrobials. *J Allergy Clin Immunol.* 1982;69:382–387.

51. Meltzer EO, Charous BL, Busse WW, et al. Added relief in the treatment of acute recurrent sinusitis with adjunctive mometasone furoate nasal spray. *J Allergy Clin Immunol.* 2000;106:630–637.

52. Dolor RJ, Witsell DL, Hellkamp AS, et al. Comparison of cefuroxime with or without intranasal fluticasone for the treatment of rhinosinusitis. *JAMA.* 2001;286:3097–3105.

53. Schlenter WW, Mann WJ. Operative therapie der chronischen sinusitis—Erfolge bei allergischen und nictallergischen patienten. *Laryngol Rhinol Otol.* 1983;62:284–288.

54. Lehrer JF, Majid A, Silver J, Cordes B. Recognition and treatment of allergy in sinusitis and pharyngotonsillitis. *Arch Otolaryngol.* 1981;107:543–546.

55. Asakura K, Kohma T, Shirasaki H, Kataura A. Evaluation of the effects of antigen specific immunotherapy on chronic sinusitis in children with allergy. *Auris-Nasus-Larynx (Tokyo).* 1990;17:33–38.

56. Kennedy DW. Prognostic factors, outcomes and staging in ethmoid sinus surgery. *Laryngoscope.* 1992;102:1–18.

57. Lavigne F, Nguyen CT, Cameron L, et al. Prognosis and prediction of response to surgery in allergic patients with chronic sinusitis. *J Allergy Clin Immunol.* 2000;105:746–751.

58. Safirstein BH. Allergic bronchopulmonary aspergillosis with obstruction of the upper respiratory tract. *Chest.* 1976; 70:788–790.

59. Millar JW, Johnston A, Lamb D. Allergic aspergillosis of the maxillary sinuses. *Prod Scot Thor Soc.* 1981;36:710.

60. Katzenstein ALA, Sale SR, Greenberger PA. Allergic *Aspergillus* sinusitis: a newly recognized form of sinusitis. *J Allergy Clin Immunol.* 1983;72:89–93.

61. Robson JMB, Benn RAV, Hogan PG, et al. Allergic fungal sinusitis presenting as a paranasal sinus tumour. *Aust N Z J Med.* 1989; 19:351–353.

62. deShazo RD, Swain RE. Diagnostic criteria for allergic fungal sinusitis. *J Allergy Clin Immunol.* 1995;96:24–35.

63. Chhabra A, Handa KK, Chakrabarti A, et al. Allergic fungal sinusitis: clinicopathological characteristics. *Mycoses.* 1996;39:437–441.

64. Schubert MS, Goetz DW. Evaluation and treatment of allergic fungal sinusitis: I. Demographics and diagnosis. *J Allergy Clin Immunol.* 1998;102:387–394.

65. Cody DT, Neel HB, Ferreiro JA, Roberts GD. Allergic fungal sinusitis: the Mayo Clinic experience. *Laryngoscope.* 1994;104:1074–1079.

66. Schubert MS, Goetz DW. Evaluation and treatment of allergic fungal sinusitis: II. Treatment and follow-up. *J Allergy Clin Immunol.* 1998;102:395–402.

67. Schubert MS. Medical treatment of allergic fungal sinusitis. *Ann Allergy Asthma Immunol.* 2000;85:90–101.

68. deShazo RD, Chapin K, Swain RE. Fungal sinusitis. *N Engl J Med.* 1997;337:254–259.

69. Manning SC, Holman M. Further evidence for allergic pathophysiology in allergic fungal sinusitis. *Laryngoscope.* 1998;108:1485–1496.

70. Ponikau JU, Sherris DA, Kern EB, et al. The diagnosis and incidence of allergic fungal sinusitis. *Mayo Clin Proc.* 1999;74:877–884.

71. Mabry RL, Marple BF, Folker RJ, Mabry CS. Immunotherapy for allergic fungal sinusitis: three years' experience. *Otolaryngol Head Neck Surg.* 1998;119:648–651.

72. Benson V, Marons MA. Current estimates from the National Health Interview Surgery, 1993. *Vital Health Statitics.* 1993;10(182).

73. McCuig LF, Hughes JM. Trends in antimicrobial drug prescribing among office based physicians in the United States. *JAMA.* 1995;273:214–219.

74. Gottlieb MS. Relation of intranasal sinus disease in the production of asthma. *JAMA.* 1925;85:105–109.

75. Bullen SS. Incidence of asthma in 400 cases of chronic sinusitis. *J Allergy.* 1932;4:402–408.

76. Weille FL. Studies in asthma: XIX. The nose and throat in 500 cases of asthma. *N Engl J Med.* 1936;215:235–238.

77. Phipatanakul CS, Slavin RG. Bronchial asthma produced by paranasal sinusitis. *Arch Otolaryngol.* 1974;100:109–115.

78. Rachelefsky GS, Katz RM, Siegel SC. Chronic sinus disease with associated reactive airway disease in children. *Pediatrics.* 1984; 73:526–532.

79. Slavin RG. Relationship of nasal disease and sinusitis to bronchial asthma *Ann Allergy.* 1982;49:76–79.

80. Fuller CG, Schoettler JJ, Gilsanz V, et al. Sinusitis in status asthmaticus. *Clin Pediatr.* 1994;33:712–719.

81. Rossi OVJ, Pirila T, Laitinen J, et al. Sinus aspirates and radiographic abnormalities in severe attacks of asthma. *Int Arch Allergy Immunol.* 1994;103:209–216.

82. Bresciani M, Paradis L, DesRoches A, et al. Rhinosinusitis in severe asthma. *J Allergy Clin Immunol.* 2001;107:73–80.

83. tenBrinke A, Grootendorst D, Schmidt JT, et al. Chronic sinusitis in severe asthma is related to sputum eosiniophilia. *J Allergy Clin Immunol.* 2002;109:621–626.

84. McFadden ER. Nasal-sinus-pulmonary reflexes and bronchial asthma. *J Allergy Clin Immunol.* 1986;78:1–3.

85. Georgitis JW, Matthews BL, Stone B. Chronic sinusitis: characterization of cellular influx and inflammatory mediators in sinus lavage fluid. *Int Arch Allergy Immunol.* 1995;106:416–421.

86. Bardin PG, Van Heerden BB, Jourbert JR. Absence of pulmonary aspiration of sinus contents in patients with asthma and sinusitis. *J Allergy Clin Immunol.* 1990;86:82–88.

87. Bucca C, Rolla G, Scappaticci E, et al. Extrathoracic and intrathoracic airway responsiveness in sinusitis. *J Allergy Clin Immunol.* 1995; 95:52–59.

88. Rolla G, Colorgrande P, Scappaticci E, et al. Damage of the pharyngeal mucosa and hyperresponsiveness of airway in sinusitis. *J Allergy Clin Immunol.* 1997;100:52–57.

89. Denburg J, Sehmi R, Saito H, et al. Systemic aspects of allergic disease: bone marrow responses. *J Allergy Clin Immunol.* 2000; 196(suppl):242–246.

90. Friedman R, Ackerman M, Wald E. Asthma and bacterial sinusitis in children. *J Allergy Clin Immunol.* 1984;74:185–189.

91. Oliveira C, Sole D. Improvement of bronchial hyperresponsiveness in asthmatic children treated for concurrent sinusitis. *Ann Allergy Asthma Immunol.* 1997;79:70–74.

92. English GM. Nasal polypectomy and sinus surgery in patients with asthma and aspirin idiosyncracy. *Laryngoscope.* 1986;96:374–380.

93. Nishioka GJ, Cook PR, Davies WE, et al. Functional endoscopic sinus surgery in patients with chronic sinusitis and asthma. *Otolaryngol Head Neck Surg.* 1994;110:494–500.

94. Manning SC, Wasserman RL, Silver R, Phillips DL. Results of endoscopic sinus surgery in pediatric patients with chronic sinusitis and asthma. *Arch Otolaryngol Head Neck Surg.* 1994;120:1142–1145.

95. Dunlop G, Scodding GK, Lund VJ. The effect of endoscopic sinus surgery on asthma: mangement of patients with chronic rhinosinusitis, nasal polyposis, and asthma. *Am J Rhinol.* 1999;13:261–265.

96. Dhong H, Jung YS, Chung SK, Choi DC. Effect of endoscopic sinus surgery on asthmatic patients with chronic rhinosinusitis. *Otolaryngol Head Neck Surg.* 2001;124:99–104.

97. Gliklich R, Metson R. Effect of sinus surgery on quality of life. *Otolaryngol Head Neck Surg.* 1997;117:12–17.

98. Goldstein M, Grundfast S, Dunsky EH, et al. Effect of functional endoscopic sinus surgery on bronchial asthma outcomes. *Arch Otolaryngol Head Neck Surg.* 1999;125:314–319.

99. Okayama M, Lijima H, Shimura S, et al. Methacholine bronchial hyperresponsiveness in chronic sinusitis. *Respiration (Herrlisheim).* 1998;65:450–457.

6

Rhinosinusitis in Immunocompromised Hosts

DESIDERIO PASSÀLI, MARIA LAURIELLO, GIULIO CESARE PASSÀLI, FRANESCO MARIE PASSÀLI, AND L. BELLUSSI

Immunity is the result of the interaction of different and numerous mechanisms that involve some specific and nonspecific factors, whose integrity is essential for an efficient and prompt answer. We define a subject as immunocompromised when any immune factors are altered in quality or in quantity.

Immunodeficiency can be classified as (1) primary or congenital and (2) secondary or acquired. Both types can be due to defects of the nonspecific or specific immune response. Table 6–1 lists some of the primary immunodeficiencies classified on the basis of the immune defect. The current names of the related syndromes are also reported.

Acquired immunodeficiency is gaining interest in the research community because there are many paraphysiological and pathological conditions that can cause it. It is difficult to find a classification similar to the one suggested for primary immunodeficiency because the etiologic factors (viral or bacterial infections, tumors, drugs, etc.) interact in different ways with the mechanism of the immune response that is differently influenced, either in its humoral or its cellular arm. Briefly, the main responsible factors for acquired immunodeficiency are premature birth, pregnancy, old age, viral infections, bacterial or helminthic infections, malnutrition, toxic factors (impaired renal or hepatic function, long treatment with corticosteroids or cytostatics, long antibiotic therapy), organ transplants, myelopathies, and lymphoid and nonlymphoid tumors.

The most common causes of immunodeficiency associated with chronic recurrent sinusitis are immunoglobulin deficiencies, including IgG subclass deficiencies. Human IgG consist of four subclasses based on antigenic differences in their heavy polypeptide chain. The IgG subclasses are found in normal serum in the following relative proportions: IgG1 (60–70%), IgG2 (14–20%), IgG3 (4–8%), and IgG4 (2–6%). IgG1 and IgG3 are thought to be the subclasses preferentially produced in response to protein antigen in adults, and IgG2 and IgG4 have been associated mostly with responses to carbohydrate antigens.

In particular, the IgG1 subclass is responsible for antibody response to bacterial protein antigens such as tetanus toxoid and diphtheria. If there is a deficiency of IgG1, a functional assessment of antibody titers should be performed before and after the administration of tetanus and diphtheria toxoid. IgG2 is responsible for antibodies directed against polysaccharide capsules such as *Haemophilus influenzae* and *Streptococcus pneumoniae*. The IgG3 subclass plays an important role in the primary response to *Moraxella catarrhalis* and the M component of *Streptococcus pyogenes*. The significance of IgG4 remains unclear.

Chronic or recurrent chest infections may be associated with IgG2 deficiency, with or without absent IgG4 and/or low IgA levels.[1] Scadding et al[2] demonstrated that in patients with chronic rhinosinusitis the subclass of IgG that was defective was IgG3.

The incidence of IgA deficiency is 1 case per 600 to 800 in the general population. This is the predominant subclass of immunoglobulin on mucosal surfaces. Selective deficit of IgA is the most frequent primary immunodeficiency, and it is often associated with infections of the upper airways. Patients with IgA deficiency often have a coexisting IgG subclass deficiency or an autoimmune disorder.

TABLE 6–1 Primary Immunodeficiencies

| | | Primary Immunodeficiencies | | |
T Lymphocytes	B Lymphocytes	Combined	Phagocytosis	Complement
Congenital thymic agenesis	Sex-related agammaglobulinemia (Bruton's syndrome)	Ataxia-telangiectasia (Luis-Barr syndrome)	Giobbe syndrome	Deficiency of the Cs1 inhibitor or hereditary angioneurotic edema
Immunodeficiency with thymoma	Transitory hypogammaglobulinemia	Wiskott-Aldrich syndrome	Chronic granulomatous disease	
	Common variable hypogammaglobulinemia Selective deficiency of IgM, IgG and subclasses, and IgA		Chédiak-Higashi syndrome	

■ General Considerations Regarding HIV Infection

Among the acquired immunodeficiencies, human immunodeficiency virus (HIV) is increasingly widespread and no longer confined to risk categories (intravenous drug users, homosexuals, and blood recipients). Heterosexual contacts are becoming an important path of diffusion.

The ear, nose, and throat (ENT) manifestations of HIV infection are well known, and the findings in acquired immunodeficiency syndrome (AIDS) patients have been described.[3] To understand why and how people suffering from AIDS are susceptible to ENT pathologies, in particular rhinosinusitis, it is useful to remember the characteristics of HIV virus and the means of defense of the nasal mucosa.

HIV is a retrovirus that attacks the immune system. The infection develops in four phases. In the initial stage, the virus colonizes helper T lymphocytes and macrophages and replicates unchecked.[4] This phase is called primary acute infection; during this phase, from 30 to 70% of infected people develop a clinical syndrome marked by fever, pharyngitis, headache, and retro-orbital pain.[5] Also during this phase the virus spreads and colonizes the lymphoid organs. The immune answer appears generally in 3 weeks and is associated with a decrease of viremia and the absence of symptoms.

The second phase, referred to as the asymptomatic stage, is variable in duration and is marked by the progressive depletion of T and B lymphocytes and the deterioration of the function of monocytes and macrophages. The third phase develops when the patient presents with persistent generalized lymphadenopathy. The fourth phase is the symptomatic, or AIDS, stage. Symptoms during this phase include persistent fever, diarrhea, a loss of weight (more than 10%), polyadenopathy, tumors, and opportunistic infections (Table 6–2).

Various studies have evaluated the manifestations of HIV in the head and neck. It appears that up to 84% of infected individuals have either symptoms or signs that may involve otolaryngologists.[3] Initial infection may manifest itself as an acute seroconversion illness with an acute mononuclease-like syndrome. Thus, the symptoms that may be presented to the ENT specialist are odynophagia, retro-orbital pain, headache, and oral ulceration.

Numerous aspects of manifested AIDS also involve the otolaryngologist. For example, the most common neoplastic conditions associated with HIV are Kaposi's sarcoma and lymphoma. Kaposi's lesions are commonly found in the mucosa of the oral cavity, especially in the palatal and gingival areas.

The main nonspecific defense of the nose, paranasal sinuses, and upper airways is the integrity of physical and chemical barriers: anatomical integrity of skin and mucosa, efficiency of mucociliary clearance, normal

TABLE 6–2 Classification of HIV Infection*

Group 1	Group 2	Group 3	Group 4
Acute HIV infection	Asymptomatic phase	Persistent generalized lymphadenopathy	Subgroup A: constitutional diseases Subgroup B: neurologic diseases Subgroup C: infectious diseases Subgroup D: secondary cancers Subgroup E: other diseases

Source: Centers for Disease Control. Classification system for human T-lymphotropic virus type III/lymphadenopathy-associated virus infections. *MMWR* 1986; 35:334–339.

microbial flora, and correct pH. Milgrim[6] studied the correlation between HIV-positive status and alterations of mucociliary transport time. Through the saccharin clearance test a significant increase of MCTt was found in HIV-positive subjects. This alteration could contribute to the development of rhinosinusitis, even though it is not the main responsible factor.

Another important element involved in nasal immune response is the inflammatory response, which depends on many elements, among them neutrophils. When the level of neutrophils dips below 100/mm³, there is an increasing incidence of bacterial and fungal infections.[7] The most important causes of neutrophilic loss are the alteration of their production in bone marrow and their destruction in the splenic site.

Neutrophilic loss is not a common aspect of AIDS. Instead, the loss of lymphocytes is the most relevant aspect of this disease. The decrease of lymphocytes is remarkable when these cells fall under 1000/mm³.

During HIV infection, there is a constant alteration in quantity and quality of T helper CD4. The virus links to this type of lymphocyte through a particular glycoprotein (p120) that is on its external membrane.

After that linkage, through fusion with the membrane of the T cell, the virus goes into the cytoplasm. Its RNA is then transcribed into DNA through inverse transcriptase so that the DNA of the virus becomes part of the cellular DNA. Because of the viral activation, new viral units are formed that leave the cell through a process called gemmation, destroying the cellular membrane. As the infection goes on, the number of lymphocytes decreases. When the level is below 200/mm³, the possibility of opportunistic infections is high.

Moss et al[8] hypothesized that quantitative defects in immune cells of the nasal mucosa of HIV-positive subjects could mirror those in the peripheral blood and explain a predisposition to sinus disease in this population. To prove their idea, Moss et al analyzed nasal mucosa biopsies from AIDS patients, demonstrating a low level of CD3+ and CD4+ lymphocytes not only in the peripheral blood.

In conclusion, HIV infection creates the immunologic premise to develop nasal and paranasal diseases. Two predictors have been asssociated with a higher probability of rhinosinusitis: bilateral absence of maxillary infundibular patency and low total count (odds ratio 0.99; 95% CI = 0.99 − 1.00) and percentage of CD4+ (odds ratio 0.93; 95% CI = 0.88 − 1.00).[9]

■ HIV and Rhinosinusitus

Rhinosinusitis represents one of the expressions of manifested AIDS, set in group 4, subgroup C (Table 6–2), where we can find the secondary infectious diseases.

Recurrent sinusitis has an incidence varying from 25 to 30% to 60% in HIV-infected patients.[10,11,12] Godofsky et al[13] found that the incidence of rhinosinusitis shows a direct relationship with the decrease of CD4+ lymphocytes.

Two kinds of rhinosinusitis should be described in AIDS patients: allergic and infective.

Regarding allergic rhinosinusitis, HIV-positive subjects have a greater susceptibility than HIV-negative patients. Small et al[14] showed that IgE-mediated nasal allergy is more common in patients infected with HIV who have higher levels of IgE and a smaller quantity of IgG. Garcia-Rodriguez et al[9] reported that atopy was present in 18% of patients, according to the expected prevalence in their geographic area, and that most patients were severely immonosuppressed. They concluded that rhinosinusitis in HIV-infected individuals does not appear to be related to IgE-related immediate hypersensitivity. However, we have not found much literature on this topic; moreover, allergic rhinosinusitis in immunocompromised hosts does not seem to have any particular characteristics if compared with the aspects of this disease in normal subjects.

In contrast, infective rhinosinusitis is frequent and particular in AIDS patients. Among the differences between sinusitis in HIV- and non-HIV-infected patients, we must include pathogenesis, bacteriology, and management. The etiologic factors can be divided into two categories: (1) common and (2) opportunistic ones that are rare in normal subjects but frequent in immunocompromised patients. Among the common agents we can include *Streptococcus pneumoniae*, *Haemophilus influenzae*, *Moraxella catarrhalis*, and *Escherichia coli*.

Regarding opportunistic infections, several agents have been reported: virus (*Cytomegalovirus*), bacteria (*Staphylococcus epidermidis*, *Pseudomonas aeruginosa*, *Mycobacterium tubercolosis*, *Mycobacterium kansasii*, *Mycobacterium avium* complex, *Veillonella parvula*), fungal agents (*Candida albicans*, *Aspergillus flavus*, *Pseudallescheria bodyii*, *Cyiptococcus neoformans*), and protozoa belonging to the order Microsporida. The first described case of *Arthrographis kalrae* pansinusitis was reported by Chin-Hong et al.[15] *Arthrographis kalrae* can be isolated from soil and compost, but only rarely has it been described as a pathogen in dorsal hand, lung, and corneal ulcers. The case reported demonstrates that *Arthrographis kalrae* has the potential to cause invasive sinusitis in AIDS patients.

Regarding viruses, the first manifestation of cytomegalovirus (CMV) sinusitis in patients suffering from AIDS was described in 1996 by Marks et al.[16] *Cytomegalovirus* was cultured from the sinuses of four patients who were positive for HIV. The infection was documented as invasive. We found only six cases of CMV sinusitis in the literature. Jutte et al[17] reported the first case of CMV sinusitis leading to the diagnosis of HIV.

Regarding bacterial and fungal agents, recent years have seen a large increase in the number of patients with impaired host defense mechanisms. Improved antimicrobial therapy, improvement in the care of patients suffering from cancer, and the prolonged survival of high-risk individuals have created the potential for infection by almost any opportunistic agent.

In terms of bacterial infection, some cases of infection with *Bordetella bronchiseptica* have been diagnosed.[18] *B. bronchiseptica* is a pleomorphic gram-negative coccobacillus, which is a common cause of respiratory tract infection in dogs and may also infect cats. This germ, in HIV-infected people, may cause a range of illnesses from mild to severe sinusitis, bronchitis, and pneumonia. No clear association with contact with dogs or cats was evident in the patients who were studied.

Bacterial agents can become multiresistant to antibiotics. Therefore, the immunocompromised host develops a persistent septic state from sinus diseases.

Regarding fungal infections, the systemic form is caused by fungi that are either primary pathogens or opportunistic agents. Normal, healthy individuals can be infected by any pathogenic fungus.

Host defenses limit infection with these pathogens to the subclinical or chronic course; immunosuppresive or other predisposing factors can lead to a more fulminant and serious infection with fungal agents. There are a lot of factors predisposing to fungal sinusitis[19]: traumatized skin or burn injuries, patients with a qualitative or quantitative alteration of neutrophils, chronic granulomatous disease, ketoacidosis, therapy with deferoxamine, intravenous drug abuse, malnutrition, patients treated with broad-spectrum antibiotics, high-dose corticosteroids, and impaired cell-mediated immunity (AIDS).

Fungal sinusitis is classified as invasive or noninvasive on the basis of the clinical setting, histopathologic findings, and clinical course[20,21] (Table 6–3). According to the majority of reports, the immunocompromised host is frequently affected by invasive fungal rhinosinusitis.

TABLE 6–3 Fungal Infections in Immunocompromised and Nonimmunocompromised Patients

Immunocompetent Patient Noninvasive Forms	Immunocompromised Patient Invasive Forms
Mycetoma	Mucor/Rhizomucor/R. pusillus
Allergic sinusitis	Candida sp.
	Aspergillus sp.
	Fusarium sp.
	Scedosporium sp.
	Alternaria
	Bipolaris
	Cladosporium
	Curvularia
	Drechslera

The type of immunodeficiency is predictive of the fungal infection.[22] Opportunistic infection with *Candida* sp. and *Aspergillus* sp. is a frequent consequence of neutropenia or of a congenital defect in neutrophilic function. Mucormycosis is an important opportunistic infection in patients with neutropenia, traumatized skin, treatment with deferoxamine, and malnutrition. This is a general term to indicate a group of fungal agents belonging to the class Zygomycetes that can lead to an acute rhinosinusitis with a progressive mucosal necrosis and eventual extension to the orbit or the frontal lobe and possible impairment of the V, VI, and VII cranial nerves[23] (Figs. 6–1, 6–2). *Fusarium* is a frequently involved agent in sinusitis in neutropenic patients. *Candida, Aspergillus, Alternaria, Cryptosporidium, Cryptococcus, Histoplasma,* and *Coccidioides* are the most frequent etiologic agents in patients with cell-mediated loss, such as AIDS patients. *Candida* sinusitis can occur in diabetic ketoacidosis.

Mycotic rhinosinusitis caused by *A. flavus* can develop following four different paths: colonization by *Aspergillus* of a sinus already suffering from a phlogosis, allergic aspergillosis of sinuses, invasive subacute or chronic rhinosinusitis, and fulminant invasive rhinosinusitis. The most important risk factor for this kind of rhinosinusitis is a prolonged defect of neutrophils or previous upper respiratory tract infections.

Fungal infection in immunocompromised patients often begins with sinus involvement. In fact, the sinuses seem to be a portal of entry for fungal infection.

A rare but lethal cause of sinusitis in AIDS patients is *Acanthamoeba* infection. Current therapeutic regimens have not been successful for most of the reported cases of *Acanthamoeba* sinusitis with subsequent dissemination, and the prognosis is poor.[24]

Microsporidia, which are obligate intracellular protozoa seen in AIDS patients with diarrhea, have only recently been identified in sinonasal tissue. Rossi et al[25] presented case reports of five AIDS patients with microsporidian sinusitis, manifested by congested, edematous, and polypoid mucosa with a superimposed bacterial infection. Microsporidia are missed on routine histopathology, and electron microscopy of sinonasal tissue is mandatory for a correct diagnosis and appropriate management of refractory sinusitis. Moreover, the otolaryngologist is consulted by other specialists when patients are suspected of having fungal dissemination with an immunocompromised status. Early detection is important for the outcome.

As usual, anamnesis is a very important aid for the doctor. The ENT specialist is often consulted to evaluate a pathology in an immunocompromised host who does not know he or she is HIV positive. The otolaryngologist must be the first to suspect it, following not only the indications given by the examination of the typical symptoms presented by HIV patients, but also the data

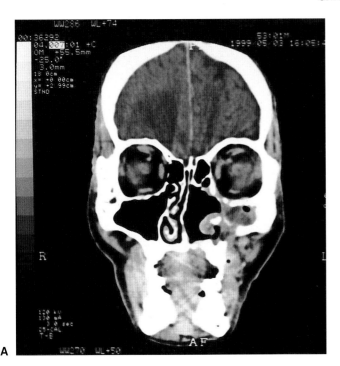

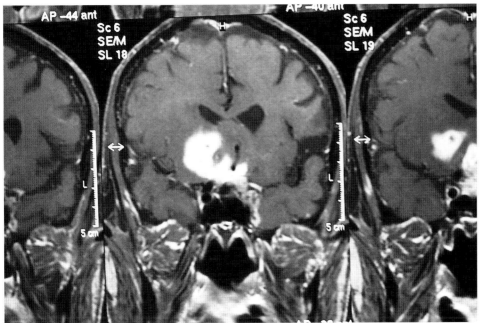

FIGURE 6–1   (A) CT scan of the nose and paransal sinuses (coronal section) in a patient affected by mucormycosis. The patient was suffering from diabetes and was also traumatized by a cow kick in the face; he arrived at our observation after previous surgery (Caldwell-Luc technique) for a severe, mycotic maxillary sinusitis that was not responsive to the convential medical therapy. (B) CT scan (coronal section) in the same patient who later developed a cerebral abscess in the cranial base through a thrombophlebitis of the cavernous sinus.

collected through the patient's history. In the cross-sectional epidemiological study performed by Porter et al,[12] sinonasal disease severity was higher than the self-reported severity of mouth/throat disease ($p = .001$), ear disease ($p = .003$), and neck/salivary disease ($p = .001$). Additionally, the severity of sinonasal symptoms was not associated with CD4+ count ($p = .93$), whereas the over-all health status was associated with CD4+ count ($p -.02$). Therefore, sinonasal disease severity did not improve as general health status improved.

All the risk factors for AIDS must be examined. Therefore it is important to ask patients about their

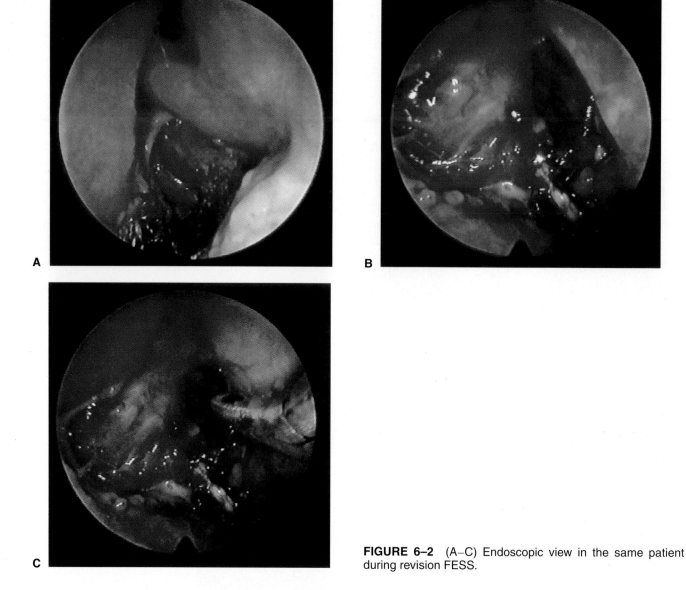

FIGURE 6–2 (A–C) Endoscopic view in the same patient during revision FESS.

sexual behavior, whether they use intravenous drugs, or if they have undergone blood transfusions. It is fundamental to suspect an HIV infection to initiate a prompt treatment because, as it has already been emphasized, this kind of rhinosinusitis can become disseminated and be lethal.

Regarding the symptoms of sinusitis by opportunistic agents, the most frequent clinical characteristics of bacterial or fungal sinusitis in an immunodeficient host are fever without any evident infective cause, facial pain or headache, purulent rhinorrhea, high fever (100.4–104°F), facial edema, sometimes hyposmia, and cacosmia. According to the clinical study by Hunt et al,[26] invasive fungal sinusitis can present as either an indolent or a fulminant process in individuals with CD4 lymphocyte count less than 50 cells/mm³, absolute neutrophil count

less than 1000 cells/mm³, subtle radiographic evidence suggesting invasion, and indolent clinical course.

In cases of intracranical extension, orbital involvement is very common: orbital cellulitis, palpebral ptosis, proptosis, subconjuctival bleeding, and/or amaurosis can appear.

Of course, locally invasive infections have a different clinical picture from disseminated fungal infections. In this case, other organs are involved by the necrotic fungal infection, such as lungs, spleen, kidneys, liver, gastrointestinal tract, and skin. Patients with disseminated fungal infection often have more than one location or organ involved in association with more than one positive culture.[27]

An objective evaluation is very important in diagnosing infective rhinosinusitis, especially in the early phase of the pathology. Areas of pale mucosa can be considered as one of the first signs of bacterial or fungal invasion of capillary vessels. Osteolysis and chondrolysis of the septum are pathognomonic and underline the importance of nasal culture and biopsy. Culture on Sabouraud's medium sometimes provides an accurate diagnosis and enables antifungal drugs to be tested. Histological studies are positive in the majority of the cases, whereas the cultural examination can sometimes be negative. X-ray is a cheap method to diagnose sinusitis in some patients, but because we dispose of CT and MRI, it is not usually performed.[28]

CT is the main tool for evaluating sinus pathology, because it allows for the analysis of the anatomy and pathology of the bone. Donato et al,[29] however, emphasized that CT scanning of the nose and the paranasal sinuses is not specific in the differential diagnosis between fungal lesions and other etiologic factors. The main alterations found in immunocompromised patients are sinus opacities, pseudocystic images within the sinus, and bone erosion.

MRI can better evaluate the pathology of the soft tissues and is more useful in making a differential diagnosis between neoplastic and inflammatory pathology. CT and MRI are complementary when performed together, especially in immunodeficient people, who are more susceptible to developing tumors of the sinuses, such as lymphoma. However, CT can be considered the "gold standard" in the diagnosis of sinusitis in AIDS patients, just as in immunocompetent people.[30,31]

In the end, we must not forget laboratory exams, not only to be sure of the diagnosis of AIDS but also to evaluate the rate of CD4+ lymphocytes and to monitor the progression and stability of the pathology.

■ Treatment

To conclude the analysis of rhinosinusitis in the immunocompromised host, a look at the recommended therapy is necessary.

Rhinosinusitis is essentially a medical problem.[32] The management of fungal sinusitis remains controversial, with many advocating combined therapy (antifungal chemotherapy and surgical drainage). Antibiotic therapy is the first treatment to be followed by the patient. The empirical therapy for the habitual germs involved in the sinusal pathology includes stable β-lactamase.

Topical and systemic decongestants can also be used during antibiotic therapy. If the patient does not react to a 2-week treatment, a culture must be prepared, and antibiotic therapy for *Pseudomonas* should be started. Sinus evaluation should be done through endoscopy; this allows a culture to be prepared from the middle meatus. Following the results of the culture, an adequate

antibiotic therapy should be started and continued for 2 to 6 weeks.[33] CT should be performed when patients do not respond to one cycle of antibiotic therapy and before starting a surgical treatment.

Asymptomatic patients should undergo endoscopic sinus surgery, and sinus tissue should be used for cultures to start a new and specific antibiotic treatment. A new endoscopy with a sinus cleaning should be performed every 2 to 3 days until there is no evidence of pathology.

Sinusitis in immunocompromised patients is a potentially life-threatening disease, when resistance antibiotherapy is observed. For this reason, it requires particular attention from the ENT specialist. Sinusitis is one of the main risk factors for pyogenic bacterial pneumonia in HIV-infected patients.[34]

Disseminated fungal infection with sinus involvement is perhaps the form with the most severe prognosis. Two exams should be requested promptly: nasal culture and sinonasal biopsy obtained by an endoscopic approach. Medical therapy with antibiotics is necessary, and when it fails, endoscopic sinus surgery is necessary.

Regarding the prognosis of sinusitis in individuals infected with HIV, in the multivariate analysis performed by Belafsky et al,[35] older age and a lower CD4 cell count were associated with death. We agree with the conclusion by Tarp et al[36] that the high occurrence of sinusitis in HIV-infected patients and the high rate of atypical agents should lead to a search for sinusitis and the etiology to ensure the correct treatment.

In conclusion, the correct approach for this pathology is multidisciplinary: Oncologists, hematologists, infectiologists, ENT specialists, and sometimes neurosurgeons and ophthalmologists must be involved.

REFERENCES

1. Stanley PJ, Corbo G, Cole PJ. Serum IgG subclasses in chronic and recurrent respiratory tract infections. *Clin Exp Immunol.* 1984; 58:703–708.
2. Scadding GK, Lund VJ, Darby YC, Navas-Romero J, Seymour N, Turner MW. IgG subclasses levels in chronic rhinosinusitis. *Rhinology.* 1994;32:15–19.
3. Barzan L, Tavio M, Tirelli U, Comoretto R. Head and neck manifestations during HIV infection. *J Lar Otol.* 1993;107:133–136.
4. Nowak MA, McMichael AJ. How HIV defeats the immune system. *Sci Am.* 1995;271(8):42–49.
5. Cooper DA, Gold G, Maclean P, Donovan B, Finlayson R, Barnes TG. Acute IDS retrovirus infection: definition of a clinical hillness associated with seroconversion. *Lancet.* 1985;1:537–541.
6. Milgrim LM. Mucociliary clearance abnormalities in the HIV-infected patients: a precursor to acute sinusitis. *Laryngoscope.* 1995; 105:102–108.
7. Stammberger H. Endoscopic surgery for mycotic and chronic recurring sinusitis. *Ann Otol Rhinol Laryngol.* 1985;94(119):1–11.
8. Moss RB, Scott TA, Goldrich M, et al. Nasal mucosa cells in human immunodeficiency virus type-1 seropositive patients with sinusitis. *J Clin Lab Anal.* 1996;10(6):418–422.

9. Garcia-Rodriguez JF, Corominas M, Fernandez-Viladrich P, Monfort JL, Dicenta M. Rhinosinusitis and atopy in patients infected with HIV. *Laryngoscope.* 1999;109(6):939–944.

10. Mafeson LM. Sinusitis in children infected with HIV: clinical characteristic, risk factors and profilaxis. *Clin Infect Dis.* 1995; 21:1175–1181.

11. Belafsky P, Kissinger P, Davidowitz SB, Amedee RG. HIV sinusitis: a rationale for a treatment algorithm. *J La State Med Soc.* 1999; 151(1):11–18.

12. Porter JP, Patel AA, Dewey CM, Stewart MG. Prevalence of sinonasal symptoms in patients with HIV infection. *Am J Rhinol.* 1999;13(3):203–208.

13. Godofsky EW, Zinreich J, Armstrong M, Leslie JM, Weikel CS. Sinusitis in HIV-infected patients: a clinical and radiographic review. *Am J Med.* 1992;93:163–169.

14. Small CB, Kaufman A, Armenaka M, Rosenstreich DL. Sinusitis and atopy in human immunodeficiency virus infection. *J Infect Dis.* 1993;167:283–290.

15. Chin-Hong PV, Sutton DA, Roemer M, Jacobson MA, Aberg JA. Invasive fungal sinusitis and meningitis due to *Arthrographis kalrae* in a patient with AIDS. *J Clin Microbiol.* 2001;39(2):804–807.

16. Marks SC, Upadhyay S, Crane L. Cytomegalovirus sinusitis: a new manifestation of AIDS. *Arch Otolaryngol Head Neck Surg.* 1996; 122(7):789–791.

17. Jutte A, Fatkenheuer G, Hell K, Salzberg B. CMV sinusitis as the initial manifestation of AIDS. *HIV Med.* 2000;1:123–124.

18. Dworkin MS, Sullivan PS. *Bordetella bronchiseptica* in HIV-infected persons (Abstract 13223). *Int Conf AIDS.* 1998;12:130.

19. Rombaux Ph, Bertrand B, Eloy Ph. Sinusitis in the immunocompromised host. *Acta Otorhinolaryngol Belg.* 1997;51:305–313.

20. Hora JF. Primary aspergillosis of the paranasal sinuses and associated areas. *Laryngoscope.* 1965;75:768–773.

21. Rispal D, Jarry DT, Tomas C, Jarry DM. Mycoses sinusiennes. *Cahiers Oto-Rhino Laryngol.* 1997;31:459–467.

22. Levitz SM. Overviews of host defences in fungal infection. *Clin Infect Dis.* 1992;14:37–42.

23. Vangehuchten S, Coeckelenbergh A, Verbeurgt L. Le SIDA et les manifestations ORL. *Acta Otorhinolaryngol Belg.* 1994; 48:81–86.

24. Kim SY, Syms MJ, Holtel MR, Nauschuetz KK. Acanthamoeba sinusitis with subsequent dissemination in an AIDS patient. *Ear Nose Throat J.* 2000;79(3):68,171–174.

25. Rossi RM, Wanke C, Federman M. Microsporidian sinusitis in patients with the acquired immunodeficiency syndrome. *Laryngoscope.* 1996;106(8):966–971.

26. Hunt SM, Miyamoto RC, Cornelius RS, Tami TA. Invasive fungal sinusitis in the acquired immunodeficiency syndrome. *Otolaryngol Clin North Am.* 2000;33(2):335–347.

27. Rombaux Ph, Eloy Ph, Bertrand B, Delos M, Doyen C. Lehtal disseminated infection with sinus involvement in the immunocompromised host: case report and review of the literature. *Rhinology.* 1996;34:237–241.

28. Sarter E. Radiographic evaluation of the paranasal sinuses. *Curr Probl Diagn Radiol.* 1985;14:27–39.

29. Donato V, Capua A, Cardello P, Pompili E, Tombolini V, Maurizi R, Martino P. The radiology of cerebral and paranasal sinus fungal lesions. *Radiol Med Torino.* 1994;88(5):559,563.

30. Klossek JM, Serrano E, Peloquin L, Percordani J, Fontanel JP, Pessey JJ. Functional endoscopic sinus surgery and 109 mycetomas of paranasal sinuses. *Laryngoscope.* 1997;107:112–117.

31. Stammberger H, Jakse R, Beaufort F. Aspergillosis of the paranasal sinuses: x-ray diagnosis, histopathology and clinical aspects. *Ann Otol Rhinol Laryngol.* 1984;93:251–256.

32. Milgrim LM, Rubin JS, Rosenstreich DL, Small CB. Sinusitis in human immunodeficiency virus infection: typical and atypical organisms. *J Otolaryngol.* 1994;23:450–453.

33. Josephson GD, Stern J. Chirurgia sinusale nel paziente immunocompromesso. In: Schaefer SD, ed. *Patologia Sinusale.* Mosby Italia; 1998:20–25.

34. Baril L, Astagneau P, Nguyen J, et al. Pyogenic bacterial pneumonia in human immunodeficiency virus-infected inpatients : a clinical, radiological, microbiological, and epidemiological study. *Clin Infect Dis.* 1998;26(4):964–971.

35. Belafsky PC, Amebee R, Moore B, Kissinger PJ. The association between sinusitis and survival among individuals infected with the human immunodeficiency virus. *Am J Rhinol.* 2001;15(5):343–345.

36. Tarp B, Fiirgaard B, Moller J, et al. The occurrence of sinusitis in HIV-infected patients with fever. *Rhinology.* 2001;39(3):136–141.

7

Pediatric Rhinosinusitis

KEN KAZAHAYA AND LAWRENCE W. C. TOM

Upper respiratory tract infections (URIs) are the single most common disorders seen by primary care physicians. Children usually have six to eight URIs annually.[1] Symptoms include cough, nasal obstruction, rhinorrhea, low-grade fever, and sore throat. Most conditions resolve with conservative management.[2] It has been estimated that 5 to 10% of URIs are complicated by rhinosinusitis.[3]

Chronic rhinosinusitis is becoming an increasingly common diagnosis in children and can be a frustrating problem.[4] Several factors may contribute to this trend. More young children are attending day care centers, increasing the transmission of URIs. Environmental pollutants and allergens predispose children to rhinosinusitis. There is also heightened awareness and improved ability to diagnose sinus disease with recent advances in imaging technology and fiberoptic instrumentation.[2]

■ Definition and Clinical Presentation

The spectrum of pediatric nasal and paranasal infections ranges from acute viral rhinitis to chronic rhinosinusitis. The viral URI is the most common infection, and its incidence peaks during early childhood. The usual pathogens include rhinovirus, adenovirus, coronavirus, influenza virus, parainfluenza virus, respiratory syncytial virus, and coxsackievirus. During the winter months, an increased incidence of viral URIs is common, but the peak month, September, coincides with the beginning of school. Clinically, patients experience a sudden onset of nasal congestion with clear or mucoid rhinorrhea, usually accompanied by fever. Symptoms resolve within 10 to 14 days with symptomatic treatment.[5]

Acute rhinosinusitis is defined by the persistence of URI symptoms for more than 10 days and less than 6 weeks, with fewer than four episodes a year. Typically, the symptoms are more severe than with those of a URI. Treatment requires antibiotics, and the condition resolves without permanent mucosal changes.[6]

In younger children the clinical presentation is less obvious, and only older children and adolescents present with adultlike symptoms. Symptoms often associated with acute adult rhinosinusitis, such as fever and purulent nasal discharge, are often absent in young children.[4] Rhinorrhea and daytime cough are present in 80% of children with acute rhinosinusitis. Acute rhinosinusitis is the second most common cause of cough in children. The cough is present during the day and may worsen at night.[6] Fatigue, behavioral changes, and increased irritability are also frequently noted. In infants, irritability may be the only presenting symptom.[7] Less frequently, acute rhinosinusitis may manifest as a severe URI with a fever greater than 39°C, facial pain, periorbital swelling, and copious, purulent rhinorrhea. Other symptoms, such as fetid breath and dental pain, may also be present.[8]

Recurrent acute rhinosinusitis is defined as more than four episodes of acute rhinosinusitis a year. These episodes resolve with medical treatment. Between episodes, there is an absence of the signs and symptoms of acute rhinosinusitis.[9]

Subacute rhinosinusitis is defined by the persistence of symptoms lasting longer than 6 weeks but less than 3 months. It represents a continuum between acute and chronic rhinosinusitis. The nasal discharge may be of any quality, and low-grade fevers may also be present.[8]

Chronic rhinosinusitis has symptoms persisting longer than 12 weeks. In contrast to acute rhinosinusitis, radiographic evidence of mucosal thickening or opacification of the paranasal sinuses is present even after appropriate medical management.[6]

■ Differential Diagnosis

Rhinorrhea and nasal congestion in children may be a result of multiple causes, including foreign bodies, enlarged and/or infected adenoids, allergic rhinitis, choanal atresia, hypothyroidism, congenital syphilis, and masses.[10] Other causes of chronic rhinitis include rhinitis medimentosa and vasomotor rhinitis.[11] Rhinorrhea in neonates is frequently misdiagnosed as rhinosinusitis. This condition is more appropriately named rhinitis of infancy.[12]

Chronic cough is caused most frequently by reactive airway disease. Other etiologies include gastroesophageal reflux, cystic fibrosis, pertussis, mycoplasma bronchitis, and tuberculosis.[8]

■ Developmental Anatomy

The growth of the individual sinuses varies with age and affects the clinical presentation of paranasal sinus disease. An understanding of the developmental anatomy of the nose and paranasal sinuses is important for the management of pediatric rhinosinusitis.

In utero, the maxillary sinuses develop early in the second trimester as lateral buds within the ethmoid infundibulum at the posterior aspect of the middle meatus. The anterior and posterior ethmoid sinuses originate during the third and fourth months of gestation, respectively. An anterosuperior ethmoid infundibulum expansion becomes the fetal frontal recess. The development of the sphenoid sinuses is unique, as they do not originate from the lateral nasal wall. They begin as recesses within the posterior aspect of the cartilaginous nasal capsule around the fourth month.[13]

In the newborn, the paranasal sinuses are small and contribute very little to the nasal-paranasal volume. The turbinates are extremely bulky, and their respective meatus are excluded from the functional airway. The ethmoid sinuses and bulla, the uncinate process, and the hiatus semilunaris are already well developed. The maxillary sinus is a shallow sac. The frontal sinus presents as a small cell in the anterosuperior portion of the infundibulum. The sphenoid sinus is a blind mucosal sac in the sphenoethmoid recess.[14]

Wolf et al[14] reviewed the growth of the paranasal sinuses from birth to age 12. In children from age 1 to 4 years, the ethmoid sinuses expand in all directions.

They are more developed than the other sinuses and can be the origin of orbital complications. The maxillary sinus enlarges laterally to the infraorbital canal and inferiorly to the level of the attachment of the inferior turbinate. The frontal sinus expands slowly and begins pneumatizing the frontal bone. The sphenoid sinus is 4 to 8 mm in diameter at age 4.

From 4 to 8 years, the development of the paranasal sinuses slows, but they continue to expand in all directions. The ethmoid air cells enlarge more slowly than the frontal and maxillary sinuses. The frontal sinus expands laterally into the frontal bone. The maxillary sinus floor descends to the level of the middle of the inferior meatus, and the lateral wall expands past the infraorbital canal. At this time the tooth buds of the secondary teeth are at greater risk during surgery involving the maxilla.[14]

Between 8 to 12 years, the growth of the paranasal sinuses accelerates, and pneumatization progresses rapidly. The maxillary sinus continues to grow, especially after the secondary dentition has erupted. The maxillary sinus floor reaches the level of the nasal cavity floor. The ethmoid sinuses are almost completely pneumatized. The sphenoid sinuses have reached their permanent size and position but will continue to undergo alterations in shape. The frontal sinuses become clinically significant in size between age 8 to 10 years. By 12 years, the nasal cavity and paranasal sinuses have nearly completed their development.[14]

The adult paranasal anatomy is reached during the second decade of life. The ethmoid sinuses attain their final form between 12 and 14 years. By 14 to 16 years, the sphenoid sinus has completed its development. The maxillary sinus continues to grow until 14 to 18 years. The frontal sinus usually reaches its final size by age 15, but in some individuals growth may continue until age 21.[13]

Developmental variations exist. The frontal sinuses are present bilaterally in 80% of patients but are often asymmetric. Unilateral frontal sinus hypoplasia is reported in 3.0 to 7.4% of patients and bilateral agenesis in 1 to 4.8%. The sphenoid sinus has wide variation in shape, size, symmetry, intersinus septum position, and wall thickness. The sphenoid sinus may also pneumatize areas outside the body of the sphenoid bone. Careful inspection of the sphenoid anatomy is recommended prior to any surgery. There is a 1.0 to 1.5% incidence of bilateral agenesis of the sphenoid sinuses.[13]

■ Pathogenesis and Predisposing Factors

Normal paranasal physiology requires patency of the ostia, normal mucociliary clearance, and normal secretions. When any one of these changes, ostial obstruction, retention of secretions, and infection can occur.[15]

Factors that predispose to changes can be divided into systemic and local conditions. Systemic factors include URIs, allergies, immunodeficiencies, mucociliary dysfunction, and diseases, such as cystic fibrosis. Local factors include structural abnormalities, adenoid hypertrophy and infection, trauma, and irritants.[16]

Viral URIs are the most common predisposing factor of rhinosinusitis. Rhinosinusitis develops in 10% of URIs. The infection causes mucosal edema and impairment of ciliary function, causing both ostial obstruction and mucous stasis.[6]

Mucosal swelling is commonly caused by allergy. Fifty-eight to 81% of all patients treated for chronic rhinosinusitis have a positive allergy evaluation.[17] Children should be evaluated for the signs and symptoms of allergy, such as itchy and watery eyes, itchy palate, sneezing, clear rhinorrhea, allergic shiners, allergic salute, and mucosal hyperemia. An allergy evaluation should be considered in any child with significant sinus disease. Allergies to food, particularly milk proteins, are the most common allergies in young children.[18]

Children have a physiologic delay in the development of their immune system. A 2-year-old child's immune system is ~50% of the adult level and does not reach adult level until age 10. This diminished immune competence increases the potential for infection. Pathologic abnormalities in the immune system also occur. Infants may have hypogammaglobulinemia, and young children more commonly have Ig subclass deficiencies. The most common immunodeficiencies in children with chronic rhinosinusitis are IgG3 deficiency and poor humoral antibody response to pneumococcal antigen (Ag) 7. Quantitative Ig measurements should be considered in the evaluation of children with chronic rhinosinusitis.[19,20]

Ciliary dysfunction leads to stasis of secretions within the paranasal sinuses, providing an environment for infection. Structural abnormalities affect ciliary function in disorders such as Kartagener's or immotile cilia syndrome. Ciliary function may be affected temporarily by viral infections and exposure to irritants and pollutants.[15] Assessing ciliary function in vivo with a saccharin clearance test or examining the ultrastructure of the cilia by electron microscopy can be used to diagnose ciliary dyskinesis.[21,22]

Cystic fibrosis is an autosomal-recessive disorder with widespread exocrine gland dysfunction. Abnormalities in the mucus prevent the movement of secretions.[15] Bacteria, especially *Pseudomonas*, and fungi, can colonize these inspissated secretions.[23] Ten to 30% of patients with cystic fibrosis have nasal polyps, and 70% of children with polyps have cystic fibrosis.[24,25] A sweat test or genetic testing should be performed on any child with nasal polyps.[24,26]

Although asthma does not cause rhinosinusitis, it has been associated with chronic rhinosinusitis. Parsons and Phillips[7] reported that 46% of children with rhinosinusitis had asthma. In older children and adolescents, asthma is associated with nasal polyps.

Abnormalities may block the sinus ostia and predispose to disease. Some conditions include foreign bodies, septal deviations, polyps, neoplasms, congenital or craniofacial anomalies, meningoceles, and encephaloceles.[4] Imaging of any intranasal mass should be performed prior to a biopsy to determine its origin and extent.

Adenoid hyperplasia and infections may predispose a child to rhinosinusitis. Large or infected adenoids may produce nasal obstruction and symptoms of rhinosinusitis.[26] The adenoids may serve as a reservoir for pathogenic bacteria.[27]

Other local predisposing factors include irritants such as air pollution and tobacco smoke.[15] Abuse of topical decongestants can cause mucosal swelling and rhinorrhea. This condition is termed *rhinitis medimentosa*.[4]

■ Diagnosis

History

The diagnosis of pediatric rhinosinusitis may be challenging. Although a thorough history is important, most children are poor historians and frequently cannot accurately describe their symptoms. Children under 5 years of age are less verbal, and their symptoms are usually nonspecific. Older children can usually be questioned more successfully. Information from the parents and the referring physicians is invaluable.[28]

Questions regarding cough and rhinorrhea, the most common symptoms of pediatric rhinosinusitis, must be asked. The history should also include details pertaining to the presence, duration, and quality of other symptoms, such as fever, nasal obstruction, headaches, facial pressure and pain, behavioral changes and irritability, fetid breath, otalgia, and periorbital edema. Precipitating events should be investigated. A history of day care, smoke exposure, and siblings' health should be obtained.

Physical Examination

The physical exam of a child can be difficult. During the evaluation, observations concerning cough, hyponasality, allergic salute or shiners, rhinorrhea, and other signs should be noted. Younger children usually tolerate only limited anterior rhinoscopy with an otoscope. Older children may allow the use of a headlight and nasal speculum or a fiberoptic nasopharyngoscope, which can also inspect the nasopharynx and adenoids. Adolescents may tolerate rigid endoscopy after being topicalized with a decongestant and local anesthetic.

During the examination of the nasal cavity, purulence, crusting, and mucus should be noted and characterized. The mucosa, turbinates, meatus, and septum should be inspected.[26] Rhinosinusitis is confirmed by the presence of mucopurulence in the middle meatus.[4] Purulent postnasal drainage and enlarged or inflamed lymphoid tissue in the oropharynx are common but nondiagnostic signs.[15] Unilateral purulent rhinorrhea may suggest a mass, foreign body, or unilateral choanal atresia.[4]

Cultures of nasal secretions may be warranted if symptoms persist even with conventional medical management or if the symptoms return within 1 week after cessation of antibiotics. Cultures of secretions from the middle meatus or ethmoid bulla provide the best bacterial yields in chronic rhinosinusitis.[29] In children, the variable size and position of the developing maxillary sinus make a sinus puncture unsafe.[14]

Transillumination has little value in young children. The increased thickness of the bone and soft tissues limits its effectiveness. It may be useful in the adolescent whose paranasal sinuses are nearly completely developed.[16]

Imaging

Plain lateral neck radiographs can help in diagnosing enlarged adenoid tissue.[15] Plain sinus films are readily available and inexpensive but are not specific or sensitive, especially for chronic disease. They can help diagnose acute rhinosinusitis and are most accurate with well-developed maxillary and frontal sinuses.[30]

McAlister et al[31] and Lazar et al[32] compared computed tomography and plain films. Plain films under- and overestimated the degree of chronic disease and were not a reliable screen for chronic rhinosinusitis. What appeared to be mucosal thickening on plain films was not reliably confirmed by CT and should not be used as diagnostic criteria for rhinosinusitis. For unilateral, recurrent, or chronic rhinosinusitis, CT is the imaging study of choice. Axial CT is excellent for demonstrating the sphenoid sinus and the surrounding anatomy. Coronal CT is useful in demonstrating all the paranasal bony anatomy and the relationship of relevant structures.

The timing of the CT is critical. The child should be maximally medically treated prior to the study. This usually implies treatment with at least 3 to 4 weeks of appropriate oral antibiotics, nasal saline, and steroid sprays. CT should be performed in children who remain symptomatic after medical therapy and who are likely to undergo surgery.

The CT findings should be correlated with clinical findings. Up to 45% of asymptomatic patients may have incidental maxillary or ethmoid opacification. In addition, patients with resolving URIs may have persistent CT findings for up to 2 weeks after resolution of the infection.[33]

Magnetic resonance imaging is useful for demonstrating soft tissue structures. It can help evaluate fungal sinusitis and extension of sinus tumors.[15] Compared with CT, MRI tends to overemphasize mucosal disease, leading to a higher false-positive rate.[34]

■ Microbiology

Acute and subacute pediatric rhinosinusitis pathogens are similar to those reported for otitis media and acute adult rhinosinusitis.[35–37] The most common pathogens are *Streptococcus pneumoniae* (25–30%), *Moraxella catarrhalis* (15–20%), and *Haemophilus influenzae* (15–20%). Anaerobes were isolated from only ~2 to 5% of aspirates. Adenovirus, parainfluenza, and several other viruses were cultured in 3 to 15%.

Chronic pediatric rhinosinusitis is considered a polymicrobial infection. In addition to the pathogens isolated in acute rhinosinusitis, *Staphylococcus aureus* and anaerobes, particularly *Bacteroides* species, have been cultured.[6,38] Muntz and Lusk[29] described cultures from 204 ethmoid bulla and found a predominance of α-hemolytic *Streptococcus* and *Staphylococcus aureus*, with a high incidence of β-lactamase producing organisms and anaerobes in only 7% of cases. Brook,[39] however, reported a 92% incidence of anaerobic infection.

Systemic conditions may alter the pathogenic flora. Patients with cystic fibrosis have a higher incidence of *Pseudomonas* infections. Immunocompromised patients may have fungal infections with *Aspergillus* species, *Rhizopus* species, and *Fusarium* species.[40] Invasive fungal rhinosinusitis must be considered in severely immunocompromised children.

■ Medical Treatment

Acute pediatric rhinosinusitis resolves spontaneously in 40% of cases and therefore should be treated conservatively.[41] The goals of therapy are the control of infection, reversal of mucosal pathology and tissue edema, facilitation of sinus drainage, and reestablishment and maintenance of ostial patency.[42]

Children with chronic rhinosinusitis frequently have concurrent allergy, lower airway disease, and systemic diseases, requiring multiple medications and therapeutic interventions. It is essential that these children be treated in consultation with pulmonologists, allergists, and immunologists.[42]

The mainstays of medical treatment of pediatric rhinosinusitis are antibiotics and steroids. Adjunctive medical treatment such as mucolytic agents, nasal irrigations, anticholinergic agents, antihistamines, and mast-cell stabilizers may also be instituted. Other therapeutic interventions such as immunotherapy or Ig replacement therapy may be required.[42]

Analgesia and patient comfort are important and should not be overlooked. Acetaminophen and sometimes a narcotic may be necessary to temporarily control pain until medical therapies become effective or drainage of the obstructed sinus is achieved.

It is important to assess and define the caretakers' expectations of treatment. Information concerning the effect of the disease on the child and family should be obtained. Patient and family education about the nature of the disease, treatment options, and expectations are important in the management of rhinosinusitis.[28]

Antimicrobials

Antibiotics should be chosen to cover the usual pathogens (*S. pneumoniae, M. catarrhalis,* and *H. influenzae*), taking into consideration local resistance patterns. In the past, amoxicillin for at least 3 to 4 weeks has been commonly used as the initial antibiotic. With the emergence of more β-lactamase-producing strains of *M. catarrhalis* (75%) and *H. influenzae* (50%) and the increasing prevalence of multiple drug-resistant strains of *S. pneumoniae,* alternatives to amoxicillin should be considered.[6,16,26] If a child is referred for treatment of refractory rhinosinusitis, an additional course of antibiotics should be given irrespective of any prior treatment. Another option for treatment duration has been to extend antibiotics 1 week past the resolution of symptoms.[16] Failure of clinical improvement after 48 to 72 hours suggests a resistance organism or complication, and clinical reevaluation is warranted.[43]

Commonly, amoxicillin-clavulanate has been recommended in regions where there is a high incidence of β-lactamase-producing organisms or for prior treatment failure. Other choices include loracarbef, cefuroxime axetil, and trimethoprim-sulfamethoxazole.[26]

Clindamycin is particularly effective against anaerobes and resistant strains of pneumococci. It should be considered for patients who have failed to respond to augmented penicillins or cephalosporins. It is also useful for patients with multiple drug allergies.[26]

As of January 1997, the U.S. Food and Drug Administration had approved amoxicillin-clavulanate, clarithromycin, cefprozil, cefuroxime axetil, loracarbef, and levofloxin for the treatment of rhinosinusitis. Other effective antibiotics include trimethoprim-sulfamethoxazole, cefaclor, cefixime, cefpodoxime proxetil, erythromycin-sulfisoxazole, and clindamycin. Penicillin, erythromycin, cephalexin, and tetracycline should be avoided because they do not cover the major pathogens in acute rhinosinusitis.[44]

In chronic rhinosinusitis, cultures from a sinus aspirate or the middle meatus can help guide therapy. A prolonged treatment of 4 to 6 weeks may be required.[43] As an empiric choice, a β-lactamase-resistant antistaphylococcal antimicrobial with anaerobic coverage is recommended.[38]

Some children may have recurrent bouts of acute rhinosinusitis that are commonly due to frequent viral URIs, often propagated by day care. If mechanical factors and other predisposing conditions are eliminated as etiologic factors, prophylactic antibiotics may be considered.[1] Although there has been no systematic evaluation of antibiotic prophylaxis, this modality has been extrapolated from treatment of recurrent otitis media. Amoxicillin and sulfisoxazole have been used at one-half the therapeutic dose once a day. If several episodes still occur during prophylaxis, a broader spectrum antibiotic should be considered.[45]

Steroids

Topical nasal steroids are used as an adjunctive to antibiotic therapy. They inhibit early- and late-phase allergic responses and IgE-mediated release of histamine and reduce the inflammatory response.[46] Multiple preparations and delivery methods are available. They have no significant systemic effects when properly dosed. They help improve symptoms, decrease inflammatory responses, and aid in the regression of radiological abnormalities.[44]

The FDA has approved topical nasal steroids for pediatric use. Currently, fluticasone is approved for children 4 years and older; budesonide, beclomethasone, flunisolide, and triamcinolone are approved for those over 6 years. Mometasone is approved for use in children 12 years or older.[47] Fluticasone has a higher topical potency, receptor binding affinity, and half-life of receptor binding than budesonide, beclomethasone, flunisolide, and triamcinolone acetonide.[48]

Systemic steroids are effective in treating inflammatory conditions. They reduce tissue edema, allowing for better penetration of topical steroids into the nasal cavity and promoting sinus drainage. They can also play a significant role with nasal polyps, Sampter's triad (asthma, aspirin sensitivity, and nasal polyps), or extensive generalized mucosal edema.[42]

Systemic corticosteroids have potential side effects and should not be used routinely. Their long-term use can also cause adrenal suppression, and sudden withdrawal can result in adrenal insufficiency. If steroids are used longer than 1 or 2 weeks, doses should be tapered.[44]

■ Surgical Management

Sinus surgery is indicated for patients with rhinosinusitis complications, chronic disease despite maximal medical therapy, or aggravation of disease states such as cystic fibrosis and asthma.[1] Prior to surgery, a CT should be performed to evaluate the anatomy and extent of disease. Patients who fail medical therapy and whose CT demonstrates significant ostiomeatal obstruction, paranasal disease, or spread outside the paranasal sinuses are surgical candidates.[17]

Surgery for Acute Rhinosinusitis

Surgery for acute pediatric rhinosinusitis is uncommon but performed to drain a sinus when infection fails to resolve or a complication arises.[43] Procedures considered for the treatment of severe acute pediatric rhinosinusitis include inferior meatal antrostomy, external ethmoidectomy, frontal sinus trephination, and endoscopic sinus surgery (ESS).

The inferior meatal antrostomy had been popularized as a less aggressive and more effective alternative to the Caldwell-Luc procedure.[49,50] The antral window procedure was thought to provide more lasting drainage and ventilation. Muntz and Lusk[51] noted that inferior meatal antrostomies were not effective in treating chronic rhinosinusitis in children. They and others have also reported a high rate of antrostomy closure.[52] The frequency of Caldwell-Luc procedures is decreasing. In children, it can result in sinus hypoplasia, impaired maxillary growth, and injury to the unerupted tooth buds.[1] Inferior antral windows may have a place in the treatment of patients with cystic fibrosis or ciliary dysfunction by providing a route for gravity-dependent drainage.[43] External ethmoidectomy requires a skin incision and typically requires longer hospitalization than ESS.[53]

Inferior meatus antrostomies have potential complications. The short medial to lateral distance in the developing pediatric maxillary sinus increases the risk of injury to the lateral wall of the maxillary sinus. Teeth may be injured because of the relatively high floor of the maxillary sinus in younger children. In creating the inferior antral window, the inferior turbinate and the attached lateral nasal wall may outfracture, leading to the lateral displacement of the uncinate process and further obstruction of the ostiomeatal complex.[14]

With the increasing use and proficiency of ESS techniques in children, severe acute rhinosinusitis requiring surgical intervention is probably best treated with an endoscopic procedure. Except in adolescents, pediatric acute rhinosinusitis is typically limited to the anterior ethmoid and maxillary sinuses. It is often sufficient to perform a middle meatal antrostomy and an anterior ethmoidectomy.[1] Surgery should be tailored to the extent

of the disease, with maximal preservation of mucosa, periosteum, and bone.[54]

In children, the orbit may be at increased risk because of the close relationship between the uncinate process and lamina papyracea. The inferior turbinate may be located more superiorly along the lateral nasal wall, making the anterior margin of the uncinate process closer to the lamina papyracea. Additionally, the lamina papyracea is thinner in children.[14]

Surgical Management of Chronic Rhinosinusitis

The surgical procedures for chronic pediatric rhinosinusitis can be divided into indirect and direct procedures.

INDIRECT PROCEDURES

The goal of the indirect procedures is to improve the health and function of the paranasal sinuses by addressing local predisposing factors. This includes adenoidectomy, septoplasty, removal of foreign bodies, repair of choanal atresia or stenosis, turbinectomy, and polypectomy.[1]

The adenoids should always be assessed by radiography or nasopharyngoscopy. Enlarged and/or infected adenoids can obstruct the nasopharynx and posterior nasal choanae, causing obstruction, rhinorrhea, and other symptoms similar to rhinosinusitis. An adenoidectomy can be performed to relieve this obstruction.[28]

The role of adenoids in the pathogenesis of pediatric rhinosinusitis has not been established. Adenoid hypertrophy or infection probably adversely affects sinonasal pathology and may contribute to chronic rhinosinusitis.[17] Takahashi et al[55] reported an improvement in rhinosinusitis by plain films in young children age 6 months after adenoidectomy. Lee and Rosenfeld[27] concluded that the adenoids might act as a reservoir of bacteria and cause sinonasal symptoms much like the relationship with otitis media. The improvements seen after adenoidectomy may reflect a physiologic effect on the nasopharyngeal microflora by creating a smooth posterior pharyngeal wall and decreasing pathogenic bacteria.[56] Adenoidectomy should be considered before sinus surgery. During the adenoidectomy, diagnostic nasal endoscopy can be performed.

■ Direct Procedures

If the symptoms of chronic rhinosinusitis persist after medical management and indirect procedures, direct procedures should be considered. The primary direct procedure is ESS. Other interventions have included maxillary sinus lavage, inferior meatus antrostomy, Caldwell-Luc procedure, external ethmoidectomy, and frontal sinus obliteration.

Only a fraction of children with refractory rhinosinusitis undergo ESS. Lusk[43] reported that of 1254 children referred for management of rhinosinusitis, 420 (33%) underwent ESS. In Stammberger's series of more than 9000 patients who have undergone ESS, less than 2% were children under 16 years.[52]

ESS is an effective procedure that avoids external incisions, allows for visualization of the nasal and paranasal anatomy, and restores normal paranasal physiology. The goals of ESS include elimination of foci of residual disease, relief of ostiomeatal obstruction, and correction of anatomical abnormalities.[28,57]

Most children have disease limited to the anterior ethmoids and the middle meatus; therefore, a maxillary antrostomy and the anterior ethmoidectomy may be sufficient to restore normal physiology.[1] ESS should be performed with conservatism, gentle tissue handling, and preservation of normal mucosa. It is imperative to minimize mucosal abrasions and tissue trauma and preserve the middle turbinate.[58] Parsons and Phillips[7] performed a partial middle turbinectomy to decrease synechiae formation but discovered that significant scarring between the middle turbinate remnant and the lateral nasal wall developed. Furthermore, the middle turbinate remnant contracted obscuring anatomical landmarks and obstructing the nasofrontal duct. It is typically unnecessary to enter the frontal and sphenoid sinuses in children, and manipulation of these areas should be avoided to reduce the risk of synechiae formation and subsequent disease.[59]

The postoperative care of children differs from adults. Children are given oral antibiotics, nasal steroids, and nasal saline. Antibiotics are continued until there is no further intranasal crusting.[60] Office endoscopies with debridements in children are difficult, if not impossible. Children often require debridement under general anesthesia 2 to 4 weeks after the initial procedure. The common findings at the second procedure are adhesions and granulation tissue.[15] Stankiewicz[19] reported 50% of patients who underwent a second procedure had closure of the maxillary antrostomy. He proposed that part of the problem with healing after pediatric ESS is because postoperative debridements and examinations are often difficult to perform, and therefore the tissues heal without monitoring. Judicious removal of the granulation tissue and lysis of adhesions should be performed.

The incidence of revision ESS in children seems to correlate with adults. Lusk[61] reported the overall incidence for revision ethmoid surgery as 11%, and Lazar et al[62] reported 8 and 7.6% in children. Willner et al[15] noted that the most common findings at revision were significant adhesions between the lateral nasal wall and the middle turbinate and narrowing of the ostia. Children with allergies, cystic fibrosis, and immunodeficiencies have compromised healing and a higher incidence of revision surgery.[19]

Faust and Rimell[4] reported a 2% complication rate for pediatric ESS. The most common complications were synechiae, persistent or recurrent polyps, and bleeding.[15] Other complications include orbital hematoma and ecchymosis, dacrocystorhinitis, blindness, epiphora, extraocular muscle injury, cerebrospinal fluid rhinorrhea, otalgia, meningitis, and recurrence of disease.[60,63] By maintaining excellent visualization with meticulous hemostasis and having a thorough understanding of the anatomy, the risk of complications, especially involving the orbit or skull base, can be minimized.

There has been controversy over the possible effects of ESS on facial growth. Although there have been several reports that demonstrated that sinus surgery may cause midface growth abnormalities in animal models, there is no evidence that any significant craniofacial anomalies have resulted from ESS in children.[4,52]

Most parents with realistic expectations believe that their children have significant improvement after ESS. Lusk and Muntz[59] reported that 80% of patients without systemic diseases were improved following surgery. Gross et al[17] reported that patients and parents believed ESS was helpful, with 64% improved and 28% resolved, and 88% stated they would undergo surgery again.

■ Complications of Pediatric Rhinosinusitis

The incidence of complications from pediatric rhinosinusitis is greater than in adults.[64] Complications are usually related to the region of the involved sinus and can be divided into intrasinus, orbital, intracranial, and lower respiratory. In children, the risk of complications increases because of thinner bony septa, larger vascular foramina, more porous bones, and open suture lines. Periorbital cellulitis is the most common pediatric complication.[65]

Intrasinus/Local Complications

Intrasinus complications of pediatric rhinosinusitis include mucoceles and osteomyelitis. Mucoceles are mucus-filled cystic lesions caused by chronic obstruction of the sinus ostia. Ostial obstruction is usually caused by an inflammatory process but may be a result of trauma, tumors, or surgical manipulation. In the presence of obstruction, the continued production of mucus results in chronic elevated pressure within the sinus. Over a period of years, the sinus enlarges as the pressure from the mucocele causes bony resorption and remodeling.[66]

Sixty-six percent of mucoceles occur in the frontal sinus. The ethmoids are involved in 25% of cases, and 10% develop in the maxillary sinus. Mucoceles of the sphenoid sinus are rare but are the most common space occupying lesions of the sphenoid. Patients with frontal mucoceles most commonly present with frontal headaches and displacement of the globe. Diplopia and deep nasal or periorbital pain may also occur. Sphenoid mucoceles present with occipital or vertex headaches, visual symptoms, or proptosis. Treatment consists of providing wide-open drainage of the mucocele and affected sinuses.[67]

Osteomyelitis is a complication of acute rhinosinusitis. The most commonly affected sites are the maxillary and the frontal bone. The anterior face of the maxilla can be affected by a staphylococcal infection of the sinus. Children present with tenderness and erythema over the anterior cheek. Frontal bone osteomyelitis is not uncommon and usually occurs in older children with developed frontal sinuses. Associated periosteal edema can result in a soft, doughy feeling over the affected area, known as Pott's puffy tumor. Frontal bone osteomyelitis may also be associated with subdural or brain abscesses. Early and widespread use of antibiotics has reduced the incidence of osteomyelitis.[64] The treatment of osteomyelitis is aggressive with intravenous antibiotics, drainage of the affected sinus, and debridement of diseased bone. Postoperative IV antibiotics should be continued at least 2 to 3 weeks followed by 6 weeks of oral antibiotics or until a gallium scan is negative.[68] Extended IV antibiotics may be necessary in severe cases.[69]

Periorbital Complications

Orbital complications are the most common problem associated with rhinosinusitis and have the highest incidence in children. Reviewing 134 patients with orbital complications of rhinosinusitis, Schramm et al[70] found that 75% of patients were under 16 years.

The source of infections of the orbit is usually the ethmoid sinuses but may also be the frontal and maxillary sinuses. The routes of spread are direct, hematogenous by arterial or venous thrombophlebitis, and lymphatic.[71] The medial orbital wall is an ineffective barrier against the spread of infection because it has natural dehiscences, suture lines, and thin bone. The orbital septum, the periosteal lining of the orbit, provides an effective barrier against the spread of infection into the orbit.[1] A CT scan with contrast confirms the diagnosis of periorbital complications. With any orbital complications, an ophthalmologic consultation is essential.

Chandler et al[72] divided orbital complications into five categories: (1) periorbital cellulitis, (2) orbital cellulitis, (3) subperiosteal abscess, (4) orbital abscess, and (5) cavernous sinus thrombosis (CST). Periorbital cellulitis is an inflammatory process limited to tissue anterior to the periorbita. Patients present with lid edema and erythema without any compromise of extraocular motion (EOM) or visual acuity. Orbital cellulitis is a diffuse inflammation of the orbital contents without

abscess formation. Associated symptoms consist of diplopia, EOM impairment, eyelid edema and erythema, and chemosis. A subperiosteal abscess (SPA) is a collection of purulent material between the periorbita and the orbital wall. It may cause lateral and/or inferior displacement of the globe. The symptoms are similar to those seen with orbital cellulitis but are more severe. An orbital abscess is a collection of purulent material within the orbital contents and presents with severe symptoms such as a fixed globe and diminishing visual acuity. CST is a life-threatening complication in which the infection has spread to the cavernous sinus via the ophthalmic vessels. There is rapid progression of bilateral orbital involvement with chemosis, ophthalmoplegia, severe retinal engorgement with poor visual acuity, high fevers to 40.5°C, and prostration.

The pathogens associated with orbital infections are the same as acute pediatric rhinosinusitis. In older children and those with chronic rhinosinusitis, *S. aureus* also becomes prevalent.[70]

Periorbital infections in younger children may be treated with aggressive medical management, whereas older children are more likely to require surgery.[73] Initial therapy should consist of a broad-spectrum IV antibiotic effective against the aerobic and anaerobic organisms. Nafcillin, metronidazole, ceftriaxone, and clindamycin are excellent choices.[6] Careful ophthalmologic management and monitoring are essential during treatment. Drainage of the abscess and involved sinuses is required if orbital or periorbital cellulitis progresses or fails to resolve or if there is an abscess or loss of visual acuity.

For a SPA, the traditional drainage procedure had been the external ethmoidectomy, which provides excellent exposure and a direct route to the ethmoids. ESS is a surgical modality that is becoming more common.[74] A total ethmoidectomy can be performed endoscopically, with the lamina papyracea skeletonized and removed, and the purulent collection can drain into the nasal cavity. If there is a localized orbital abscess, the periorbita can be incised and the abscess drained into the nasal cavity.[75] With frontal sinus disease, an external ethmoidectomy approach, frontal sinus trephination, or ESS can be utilized.[76]

Intracranial Complications

Intracranial complications include epidural abscess, subdural empyema, cerebral abscess, meningitis, and CST. Clayman et al[77] reported a 3.7% complication rate in children. Lerner et al[78] found 3% incidence. These complications have a 10 to 20% mortality rate.[79]

Pediatric intracranial abscesses are infrequent, with two-thirds of these abscesses having a sinogenic origin.[80] Cerebral abscesses and subdural empyemas are most common.[69,77,81] The symptoms in children are not readily apparent, and a high index of suspicion is necessary.[78] Fever, altered mental status, headaches, nausea, and vomiting are common presenting symptoms.[69] More ominous symptoms include signs of meningeal irritation, behavior changes, seizures, and neurologic deficits and are associated with greater morbidity, length of hospitalization, and mortality.[77] Diagnosis is confirmed by CT with contrast or MRI with gadolinium. The most common pathogenic microorganisms found in intracranial abscesses are anaerobes, including *Bacteroides* and *Peptostreptococcus* species. Aerobic microorganisms that are also recovered include *H. influenza, S. aureus,* and *Streptococcus* species.[78]

The frontal sinus is the most common source of intracranial complications, followed by the ethmoid, sphenoid, and maxillary sinuses.[77] Extension of infection from the paranasal sinuses occurs from hematogenous retrograde thrombophlebitis via the diploic veins of the skull, the veins of Breschet. Adolescence is associated with a peak in the vascularity of the diploic system and growth of the frontal sinus, predisposing this age group to the development of intracranial complications.[78] Other routes of spread include direct extension through normal anatomical pathways and erosion through bone.[6]

Rhinosinusitis is rarely reported in children with meningitis. Meningeal irritation and inflammation can result from the spread of infection from the nasal cavity and paranasal sinuses into the cranial vault. Meningitis symptoms include pain in the head and neck region, lethargy or altered mental status, fever, nausea and vomiting, and nuchal rigidity. The headaches are intense and diffuse. The usual pathogen is *S. pneumoniae*. The diagnosis is confirmed by lumbar puncture with culture.[69]

Management of these intracranial complications requires CT to evaluate the paranasal sinuses and the cranial vault. When an intracranial complication is suspected, immediate empiric treatment with systemic IV antibiotics should be instituted. The antimicrobial coverage should include high-dose, broad-spectrum, β-lactamase-resistant antibiotics with good CNS penetration and anaerobic coverage. A neurosurgic consultation should also be obtained. Anticonvulsant therapy is instituted, and intracranial pressure management is required.[69] Surgical drainage is the treatment of choice for intracranial abscesses.[77] The abscess and sinuses should be drained at the same time to prevent reseeding from the infected sinuses.[78]

Lower Respiratory Tract Complications

There has been a correlation between asthma and rhinosinusitis. Rhinosinusitis may act to trigger or exacerbate the asthma. If asthma is unresponsive to usual medical therapy, rhinosinusitis should be considered as an exacerbating factor. Children may benefit from treatment of both conditions.[82] Rosenfeld[83] reported that 67% of children with asthma and rhinosinusitis showed improvement following ESS.

The spread of infectious material from the upper to the lower respiratory tract has been a controversial subject. There are reports of children with rhinosinusitis having increased incidences of cough and recurrent pneumonitis.[84] Sinobronchial syndrome has been used to describe those patients without other metabolic or immunologic deficit that have malaise, low-grade fevers, rhinosinusitis, and recurrent tracheobronchitis or pneumonitis. The route of the infectious material is either direct extension via the pharynx with laryngeal aspiration or lymphatic spread. Sasaki and Kirchner[85] demonstrated the presence of a lymphatic path from the upper respiratory tract to the mediastinum and tracheobronchial tree.

■ Conclusion

Pediatric rhinosinusitis is a common entity. It is necessary to distinguish rhinosinusitis from other conditions. CT is the imaging study of choice to confirm the diagnosis. There is a high rate of spontaneous resolution; therefore, treatment should be conservative. Antibiotics are essential and are chosen to reflect the resistance profiles of microorganisms endemic to the region. Additional medical therapy includes topical nasal steroid sprays and nasal saline. Maximal medical therapy should be exhausted prior to considering surgery. Adenoidectomy may be considered as the initial surgical procedure. ESS is an important therapeutic option but should be reserved for children who have failed medical therapy. Communication between the patient, family, and physician is imperative to ensure realistic expectations for management of pediatric rhinosinusitis.

REFERENCES

1. Manning SC. Surgical management of sinus disease in children. *Ann Otol Rhinol Laryngol.* 1992;101:42–45.
2. Weinberg EA, Brodsky L, Brody A, et al. Clinical classification as a guide to treatment of sinusitis in children. *Laryngoscope.* 1997; 107:241–246.
3. Aitken M, Taylor JA. Prevalence of clinical sinusitis in young children followed up by primary care pediatricians. *Arch Pediatr Adolesc Med.* 1998;152(3):244–248.
4. Faust RA, Rimell FL. Chronic RS in children. *Curr Opin Otolaryngol Head Neck Surg.* 1996;4:373–377.
5. Szilagyi PG. What can we do about the common cold? *Contemp Pediatr.* 1990;7:215.
6. Gungor A, Corey JP. Pediatric sinusitis: a literature review with emphasis on the role of allergy. *Otolaryngol Head Neck Surg.* 1997; 116(1):4–15.
7. Parsons DS, Phillips SE. Functional endoscopic surgery in children: a retrospective analysis of results. *Laryngoscope.* 1993; 103:899–903.

8. Wald ER. Chronic sinusitis in children. *J Pediatr.* 1995; 127(3): 339–347.

9. Lanza DC, Kennedy DW. Adult RS defined. *Otolaryngol Head Neck Surg.* 1997;117(3):S1–S7.

10. Myer CM III, Cotton RT. Nasal obstruction in the pediatric patient. *Pediatrics.* 1983;72(6):766–777

11. Lucente FE. Rhinitis and nasal obstruction. *Otolaryngol Clin North Am* 1989;22:307–318.

12. Brown OE. Current management of pediatric nasal airway obstruction. *Curr Opin Otolaryngol Head Neck Surg.* 1995;3:396–401.

13. Anon JB, Rontal M, Zinreich SJ. *Anatomy of the Paranasal Sinuses.* New York:Thieme Medical Publishers; 1996:3–10.

14. Wolf G, Anderhuber W, Kuhn F. Development of the paranasal sinuses in children: implications for paranasal sinus surgery. *Ann Otol Rhinol Laryngol.* 1993;102:705–711.

15. Willner A, Lazar RH, Younis RT, et al. Sinusitis in children: current management. *Ear Nose Throat J.* 1994;73(7):485–491.

16. Wald ER. Sinusitis in infants and children. *Ann Otol Rhinol Laryngol.* 1992;101:37–41.

17. Gross CW, Gurucharri MJ, Lazar RH, et al. Functional endonasal sinus surgery in the pediatric age group. *Laryngoscope.* 1989;99:272–276.

18. Stankiewicz JA, ed. *Advanced Endoscopic Sinus Surgery.* Philadelphia: Mosby; 1995:33–39.

19. Stankiewicz JA. Pediatric endoscopic sinus surgery. *Otolaryngol Head Neck Surg.* 1995;113:204–210.

20. Shapiro GG, Virant SS, Furukawa CT, et al. Immunologic defects in patients with refractory sinusitis. *Pediatrics.* 1991;87:311–316.

21. Stanley P, MacWilliam L, Greenstone M, et al. Efficacy of a saccharine test for screening to detect abnormal mucociliary clearance. *Br J Dis Chest.* 1984;78:62–65.

22. Rossman CM, Newhouse MT. Primary ciliary dyskinesis: evaluation and management. *Pediatr Pulmonol.* 1988;5:36–50.

23. Davidson TM, Murphy C, Mitchell M, et al. Management of chronic sinusitis in cystic fibrosis. *Laryngoscope.* 1995;105:354–358.

24. Triglia JM, Nicollas R. Nasal and sinus polyposis in children. *Laryngoscope.* 1997;107:963–966.

25. Duplechain JK, White JA, Miller RH. Pediatric sinusitis: the role of endoscopic sinus surgery in cystic fibrosis and other forms of sinonasal disease. *Arch Otolaryngol Head Neck Surg.* 1991;117:422–426.

26. Arjmand EM, Lusk RP. Management of recurrent and chronic sinusitis in children. *Am J Otolaryngol.* 1995;16(6):367–382.

27. Lee D, Rosenfeld RM. Adenoid bacteriology and sinonasal symptoms in children. *Otolaryngol Head Neck Surg.* 1997;116(3):301–307.

28. Rosenfeld RM, Kenna MA, Reilly JS. To FESS or not to FESS: decisions in pediatric sinusitis. In: *Instructional Course Program.* Vol. 7. San Diego: Mosby; 1994.

29. Muntz HR, Lusk RP. Bacteriology of the ethmoid bullae in children with chronic sinusitis. *Arch Otolaryngol Head Neck Surg.* 1991;117:179–181.

30. Ros SP, Herman BE, Azar-Kia B. Acute sinusitis in children: is the Water's view sufficient? *Pediatr Radiol.* 1995;25:306–307.

31. McAlister WH, Lusk RP, Muntz HR. Comparison of plain radiographs and coronal CT scans in infants and children with recurrent sinusitis. *Am J Reontgenol.* 1989;153:1259–1264.

32. Lazar RH, Younis RT, Parvey LS. Comparison of plain radiographs, coronal CT, and intraoperative findings in children with chronic sinusitis. *Otolaryngol Head Neck Surg.* 1992;107:29–34.

33. Diament MJ, Senac MO, Gilsanz V, et al. Prevalence of incidental paranasal sinus opacification in pediatric patients: a CT study. *J Comput Assist Tomogr.* 1987;11:426–431.

34. Zinreich SJM, Kennedy DW, Kumar AL. MR imaging of normal nasal cycle: comparison with sinus pathology. *J Comput Assist Tomogr.* 1988;12:1014–1019.

35. Wald ER, Reilly JS, Casselbrant M, et al. Treatment of acute maxillary sinusitis in children: a comparative study of amoxicillin and cefaclor. *J Pediatr.* 1984;104:297–302.

36. Wald ER, Byers C, Guerra N, et al. Subacute sinusitis in children. *J Pediatr.* 1989;115:28–32.

37. Giebink GS. Childhood sinusitis: pathophysiology, diagnosis, and treatment. *Pediatr Infect Dis J.* 1994;13:S55–S58.

38. Stankiewicz J, Osguthorpe JD. Medical treatment of sinusitis. *Otolaryngol Head Neck Surg.* 1994;110(4):361–362.

39. Brook I. Bacteriologic features of chronic sinusitis in children. *JAMA.* 1981;246:967–969.

40. Davidson TM, Murphy C, Mitchell M, et al. Management of chronic sinusitis in cystic fibrosis. *Laryngoscope.* 1995;105:354–358.

41. Wald ER, Chiponis D, Ledesma-Medina J. Comparative effectiveness of amoxicillin and amoxicillin-clavulanate-potassium in acute paranasal sinus infections in children: a double blind placebo controlled trial. *Pediatrics.* 1986;77:795–800.

42. Lanza DC, Kennedy DW. Nose and sinus mucosal inflammation and infection, including medical therapy. *Curr Opin Otolaryngol Head Neck Surg.* 1994;2:27–32.

43. Lusk RP, Stankiewicz JA. Pediatric rhinosinutis. *Otolaryngol Head Neck Surg.* 1997;117(suppl 3):S53–S57

44. Benninger MS, Anon J, Mabry RL. The medical management of rhinosinusitis. *Otolaryngol Head Neck Surg.* 1997;117(suppl 3): S41–S49.

45. Wald ER. Rhinitis and acute and chronic sinusitis. In: Bluestone CD, ed. *Pediatric Otolaryngology.* 1996:843–873.

46. Siegel SC. Topical intranasal corticosteroid therapy in rhinitis. *L Allergy Clin Immunol.* 1988:934–991.

47. *Physicians' Desk Reference.* 52nd ed. Montvale, NJ: 1998.

48. Kravitz R, Scalin T, Pawlowski N. Internal review at Children's Hospital of Philadelphia, Divisions of Allergy Immunology/Infectious Diseases and Division of Pulmonary Medicine. 1998.

49. Hilding AC. Experimental sinus surgery: effects of operative windows on normal sinuses. *Ann Otol Rhinol Laryngol.* 1941; 50: 379–392.

50. Hempsted BE. End results of internasal operation for maxillary sinusitis. *Arch Otolaryngol Head Neck Surg.* 1939;30:711–715.

51. Muntz HR, Lusk RP. Nasal antral windows in children: a retrospective study. *Laryngoscope.* 1990;100:643–646.

52. Lund VJ. Fundamental considerations of the design and function of intranasal antrostomies. *Rhinology.* 1985;23:231–236.

53. Manning SC. Endoscopic management of medial subperiosteal orbital abscess. *Arch Otolaryngol Head Neck Surg.* 1993;119:789–791.

54. Lusk RP, Mair EA, Poole MD. Chronic sinusitis in a child. *Head Neck.* 1995;17:252–257.

55. Takahashi H, Fujita A, Honjo I. Effect of adenoidectomy on otitis media with effusion, tubal function and sinusitis. *Am J Otolaryngol.* 1989;10:208–213.

56. Brodsky L, Koch RJ. Bacteriology and immunology of normal and diseased adenoids in children. *Arch Otolaryngol Head Neck Surg.* 1993;119:821–829.

57. Kennedy DW, Zinreich SJ, Rosenbaum AE, et al. Functional endoscopic sinus surgery: theory and diagnostic evaluation. *Arch Otolaryngol Head Neck Surg.* 1985;111:576–582.

58. Messerklinger W. On the drainage of the normal frontal sinus of man. *Acta Otolaryngol.* 1967;63:178–181.

59. Lusk RP, Muntz HR. Endoscopic sinus surgery in children with sinusitis: a pilot study. *Laryngoscope.* 1990;100:654–658.

60. Lusk RP. Endoscopic approach to sinus disease. *J Allergy Clin Immunol.* 1992;90(3):496–504.

61. Lusk RP. Revision endoscopic sinus surgery in the pediatric patient. In: Stankiewicz JA, ed. *Advanced Endoscopic Sinus Surgery.* St. Louis: Mosby; 1995:41–49.

62. Lazar RH, Younis RT, Long TE, et al. Revision functional endonasal sinus surgery. *Ear Nose Throat J.* 1992;71:131–133.

63. Lazar RH, Younis RT, Gross CW, et al. Pediatric functional endonasal sinus surgery. review of 210 patients. *Head Neck.* 1992; 14:92–98.

64. Gurucharri MJ, Lazar RH, Younis RT. Current management and treatment of complications of sinusitis in children. *Ear Nose Throat J.* 1991;70:107–112.

65. Harrington PC. Complications of sinusitis. *Ear Nose Throat J.* 1984;63:163–171.

66. Wurster C, Levine T, Sisson G. Mucocele of the sphenoid sinus causing sudden onset of blindness. *Otolaryngol Head Neck Surg.* 1986;94:257–259.

67. Close LG, Oconner WE. Sphenoethmoidal mucocele with intracranial extension. *Otolaryngol Head Neck Surg.* 1983;91:350–357.

68. Small M, Dale BA. Intracranial suppuration 1968–1982: a 15 year review. *Clin Otolaryngol.* 1984;9:315–319.

69. Giannoni C, Sulek M, Friedman EM. Intracranial complications of sinusitis: a pediatric series. *Am J Rhinol.* 1998;12(3):173–178.

70. Schramm VL, Myers EN, Kennerdell JS. Orbital complications of acute sinusitis: evaluation, management and outcome. *Otolaryngology.* 1978;86(2):221–230.

71. Younis RT, Lazar RH. Endoscopic drainage of subperiosteal abscesses in children. *Am J Rhinol.* 1991;119:11–15.

72. Chandler JR, Langenbrunner DJ, Stevens ER. The pathogenesis of orbital complications in acute sinusitis. *Laryngoscope.* 1970;9:1414–1428.

73. Hawkins DB, Clark RW. Orbital involvement in acute sinusitis: lessons from 24 childhood patient. *Clin Pediatr (Phila).* 1977;16(5):464–471.

74. Mannings SC. Endoscopic management of medial subperiosteal orbital abscesses *Arch Otolaryngol Head Neck Surg.* 1993;119(7):789–791.

75. Burson JG, Gussack GS, Hudgins PS. Endoscopic approach to the pediatric orbit. *Laryngoscope.* 1995;105:771–773.

76. Clary RA, Cunningham MJ, Eavey RD. Orbital complications of acute sinusitis: a comparison of CT scan and surgical findings. *Ann Otol Rhinol Laryngol.* 1992;101:598–600.

77. Clayman GL, Adams GL, Paugh DR, et al. Intracranial complications of paranasal sinusitis: a combined institutional review. *Laryngoscope.* 1991;101:234–239.

78. Lerner DN, Choi SS, Zalzal GH, et al. Intracranial complications of sinusitis in childhood. *Ann Otol Rhinol Laryngol.* 1995;104:288–293.

79. Maniglia AJ, Goodwin WJ, Arnold JE, et al. Intracranial abscesses secondary to nasal, sinus, and orbital infections in adults and children. *Arch Otolaryngol Head Neck Surg.* 1989;115:1424–1429.

80. Nielsen H. Cerebral abscess in children. *Neuropediatrics.* 1983;14:76–80.

81. Wenig BL, Goldstein MN. Abramson AL. Frontal sinusitis and its intracranial complications. *Int J Pediatr Otorhinolaryngol.* 1983;5:285–302.

82. Rachelefsky GS, Katz RM, Siegel SC. Chronic sinus disease with associative reactive airway disease in children. *Pediatrics.* 1984;73:526–529.

83. Rosenfeld RM. Pilot study of outcomes in pediatric rhinosinusitis. *Arch Otolaryngol Head Neck Surg.* 1995;121:729–736.

84. Hengerer AS, Yanofsky SD. Complications of nasal and sinus infections. In: Bluestone CD, ed. *Pediatric Otolaryngology.* 3rd ed.. Philadelphia: WB Saunders; 1996:866–873.

85. Sasaki CT, Kirchner JA. A lymphatic pathway from the sinuses to the mediastinum. *Arch Otolaryngol Head Neck Surg.* 1967;85(4):432–444.

8

Headache and Rhinosinusitis

HOWARD L. LEVINE

Otolaryngologists frequently see patients with the symptom of headache, and the patient often believes the headache is sinus related. Yet, for the majority of patients who believe they have sinus headaches, it is not. Therefore, it behooves the otolaryngologist to have a thorough understanding of headache and how the symptomatology may or may not relate to the sinuses. Patients want the headache to be sinus related because it is far more socially acceptable if a patient is suffering from a "sinus headache" than from the most frequently seen headache, a "tension headache." The media have made sinus headaches appear quite common when in fact other types of headache are more common. Various over-the-counter cold and sinus medications relieve the headache, not because of the nasal and/or sinus medication they contain, but rather because of the analgesics or sedative effect of the antihistamines that are part of the medication.

Pain from nasal and/or sinus disease can be present in many areas of the face and be referred to a distant area of the head or neck. Physicians are taught that percussion of sinuses will reveal the site of sinusitis if pain is elicited, yet this is quite inexact and often provides misleading information. Because tension headaches can cause tenderness of the facial muscles and scalp, percussion of the forehead may elicit pain, causing the physician to suspect erroneously frontal sinusitis. The understanding and diagnosis of facial pain are far more complicated than this

Pain in the forehead may be a frontal or ethmoid sinus problem or a muscle contraction tension headache (Fig. 8–1). Pain in the maxillary sinus may be located over the maxillary sinus or radiate to the canine teeth and into the temporal region (Fig. 8–2). Ethmoid sinusitis can produce pain most often in the medial canthal area, but also the pain can extend into the parietal and temporal areas and into the upper cervical area (Fig. 8–3). Sphenoid sinusitis will generally produce a retro-orbital headache, but it can extend to the temporal area, vertex, occiput, and even into the shoulder and canine teeth (Fig. 8–4).

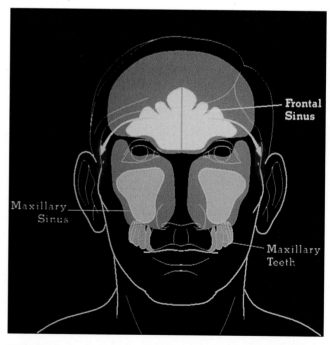

FIGURE 8–1 Pain in the forehead may be frontal or ethmoid sinus disease or muscle contraction tension headache.

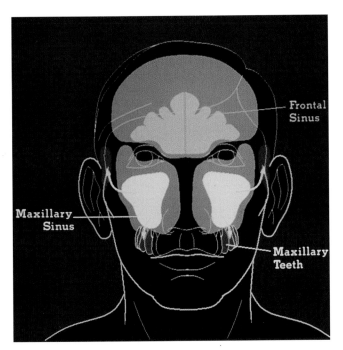

FIGURE 8–2 Pain in the maxillary sinus may be located over the maxillary sinus or radiate to the canine teeth and into the temporal region.

Although this breakdown of areas of pain is important and valuable, it is unusual for a patient to come to the physician with sinusitis in a single sinus. Involvement of multiple sinuses makes the pain and symptoms complicated. Multiple sinus involvement causes the pain to be

in several locations, and for the patient with other causes of facial pain, the etiology may be confusing for the practitioner (Fig. 8–5). Therefore, it often takes some understanding of symptomatology to be certain about the diagnosis. This is especially true as it relates to the symptom of facial pain and pressure.

The headache history is important in trying to sort out the etiology of facial pain and pressure. It is important to know the location of the pain, the nature of the pain (steady, pulsating, squeezing, vicelike, stabbing, sharp, dull, mild, severe, etc.), and the duration and frequency of the headache. Many patients have more than one kind of headache. It is important to know how many kinds of headaches are present, what makes the headache better or worse, and whether there are associated symptoms such as aura, nausea, vomiting, photophobia, and phonophobia. It is important to know about associated nasal and/or sinus symptoms such as nasal obstruction, nasal drainage, and alteration in taste and/or smell.

Many years ago a physician, H. G. Wolfe, wrote a textbook on headaches.[1] What Wolfe did was fascinating. He stimulated certain areas within the nasal cavity and showed to which head and neck locations pain was referred. If there is disease in the anterior nasal septum, such as ulceration, the pain was referred not only to the medial canthal area but also to the lateral part of the orbit (Fig. 8–6). Ulcerations like this can occur with atrophy of the nasal septum. This is seen in individuals with a severe nasal septal deviation and in some elderly individuals. Small polyps or edema putting pressure in

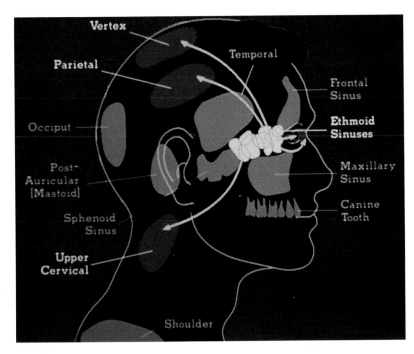

FIGURE 8–3 Ethmoid sinusitis can produce pain, most often in the medial canthal area. The pain also can extend into the parietal and temporal areas and into the upper cervical area.

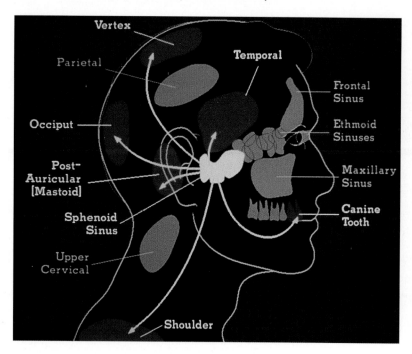

FIGURE 8–4 Sphenoid sinusitis will generally produce a retro-orbital headache, but it can extend to the temporal area, vertex, occiput, and even into the shoulder and canine teeth.

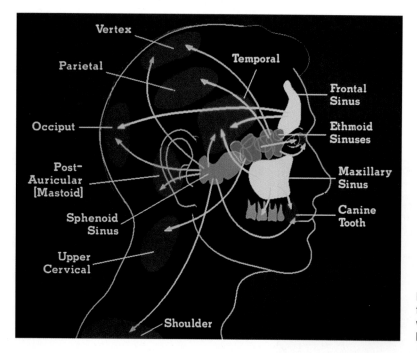

FIGURE 8–5 Multiple sinus involvement causes the pain to be in several locations. For the patient with other causes of facial pain, the etiology may be confusing.

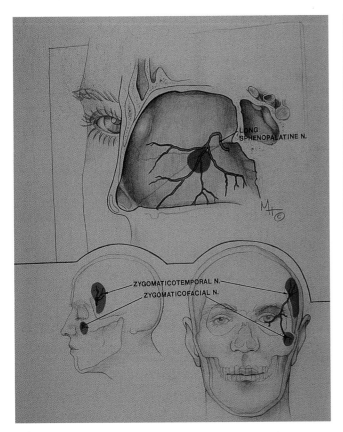

FIGURE 8–6 If there is disease in the anterior nasal septum, such as ulceration on the anterior septum, the pain was referred not only to the medial canthal area but also to the lateral part of the orbit.

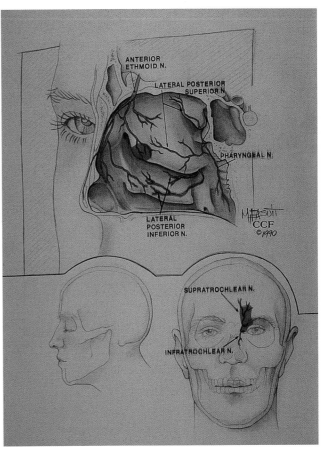

FIGURE 8–7 Small polyps or edema creating pressure in the anterior ostiomeatal complex may cause disease isolated to the anterior aspect of the middle turbinate.

the anterior ostiomeatal complex may cause disease isolated to the anterior aspect of the middle turbinate. Pain also may occur along the supratrochlear area (Fig. 8–7).

Patients may have disease and/or pathology in the ostiomeatal complex, perhaps from polyposis, an abnormality of the middle turbinate, which with a small amount of edema puts pressure on this area. A paradoxically bent middle turbinate may be asymptomatic, but it can cause pressure in the middle meatus that at times can cause pain in these various areas (Fig. 8–8). Minimal pathology may cause edema in the anterior osiomeatal complex, resulting from air pollutants, nasal congestion, or allergies. Abnormalities of the uncinate process may also cause intermittent obstruction in the anterior ostiomeatal complex. The pain from pathology in this region is along the zygomaticotemporal nerve laterally into the temporal region (Fig. 8–9).

Disease may occur in the posterior ostiomeatal complex (sphenoethmoid recess) caused by abnormalities of the superior turbinate such as a concha bullosa, edema, or polyposis.

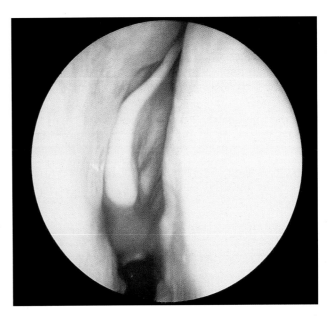

FIGURE 8–8 A paradoxically bent middle turbinate may be asymptomatic, but it can cause pressure in the middle meatus that at times can cause pain in these various areas.

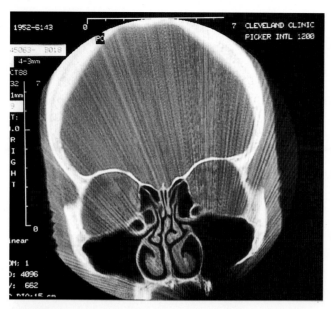

FIGURE 8–9 Abnormalities of the uncinate process may cause intermittent obstruction in the anterior osteomeatal complex. The pain from pathology in this region is along the zygomaticotemporal nerve laterally into the temporal region. The uncinate process may have several shapes, such as elongated (as seen on the right side) or short, thickened, and bent (as seen on the left side).

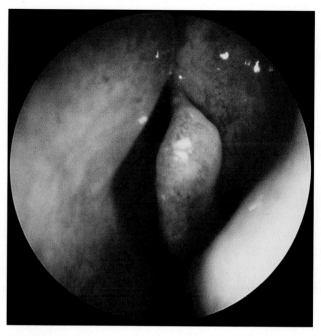

FIGURE 8–10 Agger nasi air cells obstructing the frontal sinus outflow.

Pain has a biochemical basis that is not totally understood. There are irritants, infection, thermal changes that cause the release of substance P, and probably many other mediators yet to be discovered. Substance P causes an orthodromic impulse that travels to the cerebral cortex and causes the sensation of both primary and referred pain. There is also an antidromic impulse that travels from the cerebral cortex to the nasal mucosa. This causes nasal dilatation and hypersecretion. The vasodilatation causes an increase in the mechanical pressure and mucosal contact. If there is already some degree of a compromised sinus outflow because of an anatomical abnormality, the problem is compounded and the pain worsened. This causes a greater release of substance P and subsequent increase in nasal congestion and hypersecretion, resulting in a vicious cycle. An attempt is made to break this cycle with decongestants, mucolytics, antibiotics, steroids, or surgery (Fig. 8–11).

PEARL

It has become common for rhinologists and radiologists to refer to the middle meatus as the ostiomeatal complex. This region comprises the uncinate process, infundibulum, hiatus semilunaris, and the adjacent associated structures. It is reasonable to call this the "anterior" ostiomeatal complex because there is a similar region posteriorly. The superior turbinate, the front face of the sphenoid, and the nasal septum form the sphenoid ethmoid recess. This should be referred to as the "posterior" ostiomeatal complex.

Enlarged agger nasi cells in the frontal recess region can become infected or obstructed and cause pain in this region.

PEARL

The anterosuperior attachment of the middle turbinate often has a rounded bulging region. It is important to recognize this endoscopically because agger nasi air cells that may or may not be causing pathology often form this bulge (Fig. 8–10).

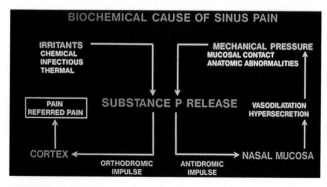

FIGURE 8–11 The vicious cycle created by the production of substance P.

From 1986 to 1991, the author examined 1165 patients, looking at their nasal and sinus symptoms. Some patients had more than one symptom. The most common symptoms were facial pressure (367), postnasal drainage (350), nasal obstruction (317), nasal congestion (243), change in sense of taste or smell (191), and ocular pain or pressure (189). There were less common symptoms such as headache (126), cough (114), itchy nose (99), watery eyes (95), bad breath (81), ear pressure (80), scratchy throat (80), runny nose (78), and fatigue (71).

It is important to understand the different symptoms of "discomfort." Facial pressure is a different sensation from facial or head pain. It is a feeling of fullness. Headache alone, as a single symptom, was not as common as the other symptoms of nasal and sinus disease. (The American Academy of Otolaryngology-Head and Neck Surgery Rhinology and Paranasal Sinus Committee has defined the major and minor symptoms that are needed for the diagnosis of rhinosinusitis. Headache is a minor symptom. See Chapter 4.) If a patient's main or only symptom is headache, he or she probably does not have sinus disease, but rather has another kind of headache. Far down the list are symptoms that are more allergic in origin: itchy eyes, cough, watery eyes, scratchy throat, and "runny" nose.

All of these patients with nasal and sinus symptoms had surgery. Facial pressure was relieved in 83.7% of the patients, and eye pain and pressure were relieved in 81.0%. Headache, when it was associated with other nasal sinus symptoms, was relieved in 74.6%. When headache was the only symptom present, only 32 of the 1165 patients (18.8%) were relieved of their headache. They had another cause for their headache other than sinus disease. Thus, patients with headache alone are rarely operative candidates.

From 1993 to 1994, the author looked at 126 patients, all of whom had headache as their major symptom but came to the author suspecting they had a nasal sinus problem. The patients had other symptoms of nasal sinus disease, such as nasal congestion, obstruction, drainage, and anosmia. Of those 126 patients, 71 did not have nasal sinus problems. Those who had nasal sinus pathology had deviated septum, vasomotor rhinitis, allergic rhinitis, and chronic sinusitis or nasal/sinus polyps. These findings support the concept that when headache is the major symptom, it is uncommon for the problem to be sinus related unless there are other nasal and/or sinus symptoms. The kinds of headaches that these patients had were mixed migraine and tension headache, tension headache or migraine alone, atypical facial pain, or cluster headaches.

In a similar study, of 184 patients who had CT scan–proven sinusitis, 66 (36%) had headaches.[2] The breakout of location of the headaches was frontal (39 patients), temporal (21), occipital (15), and parietal (5).

The characteristics of the headache were mainly dull (66 patients) and sharp pain (2). There was no special time of day for the occurrence of the headache. The headaches were muscle contraction.

Another suspected cause of facial pain is related to the middle turbinate. The primary innervation of the middle turbinate is the anterior ethmoid nerve. Compression can occur between the nasal septum and the middle turbinate, causing irritation of the anterior ethmoid nerve and pain. Most of the pain is in the medial canthus. It is unilateral and intermittent. It is worse when supine and less when upright, most likely because of the increased nasal congestion when supine. There is no aura. There is also no sympathetic hyperactivity, such as eye tearing or eye closure, that is seen with other headache problems. There are no sinusitis symptoms except those of obstruction from the contact between the middle turbinate and the nasal septum. One test to evaluate patients with suspected middle turbinate syndrome or nasal septal spur impaction is the use of a nasal spray, containing 4% lidocaine with an equal amount of 1% phenylephrine. Patients use this spray and keep a headache diary, noting the effectiveness of the spray. If the headache resolves most of the time with the decongestant and topical anesthetic, it is presumed that there is some nasal sinus pathology causing the symptomatology and that surgical management should be considered.

The physician caring for nasal and sinus problems seeing patients with nasal or sinus causes of headaches must be aware of the other common causes of headache, such as migraine, muscle contraction tension, cluster, and drug rebound. Although the physician specialist in nasal sinus disorders must have the ability to diagnose headaches of various causes, the specialist does not need to understand the complexities and subtleties of treatment.

Migraine headaches are recurring with periods free of pain. There are two types of migraine: migraine with aura (classical) and migraine without aura (common). Migraine headaches are typically moderate to severe in intensity, unilateral, pulsatile, and lasting for several hours. The headaches are usually associated with nausea, vomiting, photophobia, phonophobia, and irritability. During an attack, the migraine sufferer will usually have pale facies. During an attack, most sufferers will seek a dark, quiet room and find that sleep for several hours will help.

There are numerous triggers to bring on migraine headache. These include stress, fatigue, oversleeping, fasting or missing a meal, vasoactive substances in food (e.g., nitrates in processed meats), caffeine, alcohol, menses, change in barometric pressure, and changes in altitude. Such headaches often occur on weekends, when there is a change in typical sleep, eating, and activity schedules.

Most migraine sufferers are young adults, and women have migraine headaches three times more often than men. Many women have migraine headaches beginning a few days before the onset of their menstrual cycle. There is a positive family history for migraine in over 70% of patients. The onset is generally during adolescence, and migraine headaches tend to diminish by the fifth or sixth decade of life.

The aura associated with migraine usually begins about 1 or 2 hours before the actual headache. The aura may take any one of several forms: There may be visual disturbance, altered sensation, or altered speech, to name only a few.

Although nasal sinus symptoms are rarely part of the migraine symptom complex, many migraine sufferers have nasal sinus problems. Most likely this is because of the frequency of both entities. When nasal sinus disease is present, a migraine headache is occasionally stimulated. Therefore, a patient who has rhinosinusitis and also migraine may describe two kinds of headaches, one with related nasal sinus symptoms, and another with migraine-like symptoms occurring after the onset of the nasal/sinus problem. This can create confusion for the headache sufferer as to the exact cause of the headache. A careful history delineating the symptoms is needed. Often by caring for the nasal sinus problem the migraine headaches become less frequent and/or less severe.

Tension-type headache (muscle contraction headache) is the most common form. It is a combination of neurogenic, vascular, and muscular headache. The headache is usually a bandlike pain with pressure in the forehead, temples, over the top of the head, or down the neck and into the shoulders. It is described as a "pressing" or "tightness." It is most often of moderate intensity, but not disabling. Tension-type headaches are usually present more than half of the month. The discomfort worsens as the day progresses and rarely worsens with activity. Tension-type headaches are more of a "workweek" headache versus migraine, or "weekend-type," headaches. Tension-type headaches occur in ~3% of the population and in women more than men. They are triggered by stress, anxiety, drug habituation, cervical spine disorders, temporomandibular joint disorders, and some occupational situations. Because of the location of the pain in the forehead, patients come to the nasal-sinus physician frequently believing that they have a sinus headache when in fact they have a tension-type headache.

Cluster headaches are not as common as migraine or tension-type headaches. The pain of cluster headache is severe, beginning abruptly and lasting on average ~45 minutes. The episodes may occur many times in a 24-hour period and over several days. They will appear anywhere from 3 to 16 weeks at a time. Whereas migraine patients will go to a darkened room, seeking quiet, avoiding stimulation, and wanting to sleep, cluster headache patients become quite agitated. They often pace the floor, cannot sit still, and may even bang their head against a wall because of the excruciating pain. Unilateral periorbital pain, drooping eyelid, and conjunctival injection are often present. Cluster headache sufferers often have associated sweating, facial flushing, and nasal congestion. Alcohol, cold temperatures, or excitement can trigger the headache. Whereas migraine headaches occur most often at any time of the day, and tension headaches worsen as the day goes on, cluster headaches frequently awaken patients. The majority of cluster headache sufferers are men, and many are smokers. They often have a characteristic "lionlike" look to the face, with deep wrinkles in the forehead, deep nasolabial creases, and a ruddy face. Cluster headache is an important headache for the nasal-sinus physician because some of the symptoms are nasal in origin. Patients will often surmise that they have a sinus infection rather than cluster headache because of the associated nasal stuffiness and periorbital pain. Like other headaches, the history points to cluster rather than sinus headache.

Because there are now so many over-the-counter analgesics, many patients find it easy to self-medicate their headaches. The widespread use of acetaminophen and ibuprofen especially in combination with decongestants and/or antihistamines gives relief for many types of headache. This frequently occurs because of the analgesic property of the acetaminophen and ibuprofen and the sedative property of the antihistamine. Patients mistakenly believe that they have "sinus" headache because their headache goes away with these preparations. These analgesics are often taken alone or in combination every day or several times a day. Much like we see rebound with the decongestants, there may be rebound and withdrawal symptoms with the analgesics, leading to drug rebound headache.

A drug rebound headache usually occurs daily and often lasts the entire day. It is usually a bilateral frontal headache that is mild or moderate in severity. It is frequently present upon awakening, because there has been no analgesia throughout the night. Realizing that a headache is present, the drug rebound headache sufferer takes an analgesic medication that makes the symptoms resolve but perpetuates the problem. Many caffeine users have similar headaches and know that their "morning coffee" is what is needed to get them going. Treatment for drug rebound headaches is withdrawal from the offending drug and search for the etiology for the need for the drug.

When dealing with pain caused by a nasal sinus disorder, the site of obstruction is frequently much more important than the extent of the disease, and minor

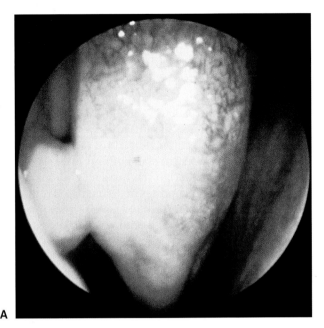

A

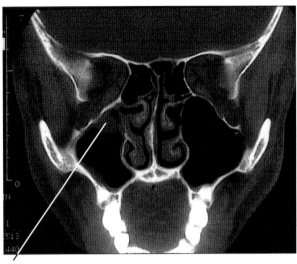

Polyp obstructing
B   left ostiomeatal complex

FIGURE 8–12   (A) Small lesions in the middle meatus may cause severe pain and pathology in the osteomeatal complex. (B) Plain sinus x-ray showing a small polyp obstructing the osteomeatal complex and causing recurrent acute rhinosinusitis.

obstruction can cause a great deal of pain. There may be a concentration of sensory nerve fibers around the ostia of the sinuses. This would result in small lesions and obstruction in the anterior or posterior ostiomeatal complex to produce a great deal of pain, pressure, and pansinusitis. Polyps may fill the nose and sinuses and cause little or no pain or pressure. There may be some accommodation of the nerves in and around the ostia, which adapt to the pathology, lessening the sensitivity and reducing the pain and pressure. This is substantiated when sinus surgery is performed under local anesthesia. There is much greater sensitivity around any of the ostia possibly because of greater concentration of sensory nerve fibers in this area (Fig. 8–12).

Barosinusitis is another type of nasal- sinus-related facial pain. This is not an infection and is therefore a misnomer. Barosinusitis is related to pressure changes in weather and/or altitude. Individuals initially have sharp pain, which then reduces fairly quickly, leaving a dull ache or pressure. There is no fever or purulent drainage because there is no true infection. Barosinusitis is the "eustachian tube dysfunction" of the sinus, with obstruction at the outflow from the sinus and subsequent buildup of negative pressure within the sinus. The etiology of most cases of barosinusitis is anatomical obstruction in the outflow from the sinus into the nose, such as a concha bullosa, rotated or enlarged uncinate process, a small polyp, or paradoxical middle turbinate (Fig. 8–13). (There is an important consideration concerning weather change and headache. There are many patients who believe that they have

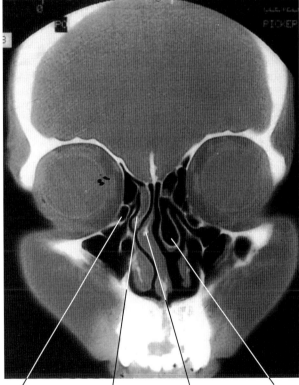

| Waller ethmoid air cells | Paradoxical right middle turbinate | Deviated nasal septum | Concha bullosa |

FIGURE 8–13   The etiology of most cases of barosinusitis is anatomical obstruction in the outflow from the sinus into the nose such as a concha bullosa, rotated or enlarged uncinate process, small polyp, or paradoxical middle turbinate.

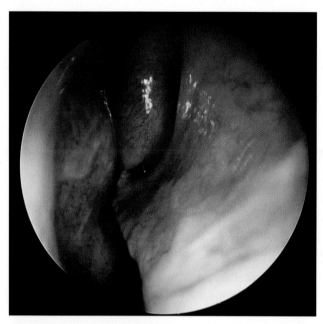

FIGURE 8–14   Nasal septal spurs may impact upon the lateral nasal wall and cause pain.

sinus disease because their symptoms worsen with weather changes or especially a low-pressure front. Though they may, often they have migraine headache that also can worsen with weather change and altered barometric pressure.)

Another entity that may cause facial pressure and headache is impaction of a nasal septal spur against the inferior or middle turbinate (Fig. 8–14). Wolfe's text-book on headaches mentions this. Many patients with septal spur impacting against the lateral nasal wall will have a sharp, severe, lancinating pain. It may also be dull and/or throbbing pain associated with eye tearing, eye closure, and nasal obstruction. This history can be confusing because it is similar to patients with cluster headaches or sphenopalatine ganglion neuralgia. To help differentiate these, patients are given a mixture of 4% Xylocaine and 1% phenylephrine, which is used at the time of the facial pain. The patients are instructed to keep a diary of how often the headache appears and how effective the medication is in resolving or reducing the facial pain. If the pain resolves most of the time, the cause is presumed to be nasal etiology.

■ Conclusion

Sinus headaches can be confused with headaches of other kinds, such as migraine, tension, and cluster. When headache is the only symptom, it is probably not sinus in origin. Subtle changes in the sinuses and ostiomeatal complex can cause pain that can be referred some distance from the sinuses.

REFERENCES

1. Wolfe HG. The nasal, paranasal, and aural structures as sources of headache and other pain. In: *Headache and Other Head Pain.* New York: Oxford University Press; 1948:532–560.
2. Tarabichi M. Characteristics of sinus-related pain. *Otolaryngol Head Neck Surg* 2000;122:842–847.

9

The Medical and Surgical Management of Allergic Fungal Rhinosinusitis

BERRYLIN J. FERGUSON

The medical and surgical treatment of fungal sinusitis is dependent on the manifestation of the fungal sinusitis along the immunologic spectrum.[1] This chapter will review in depth the management of allergic fungal sinusitis (AFS). This management is both surgical and medical. Recurrence rates of AFS following surgery alone are high.[2] Medical adjuncts that definitely or possibly reduce this recurrence rate include steroid therapy, antifungal therapy, and immunotherapy.[3] The evidence and recommended protocols will be reviewed.

The medical and surgical management of the other manifestations of fungal sinusitis, invasive (acute and chronic), granulomatous invasive, and fungus ball differ from AFS and will be briefly detailed to differentiate their management from AFS.

■ Management of the Various Manifestations of Fungal Sinusitis

Invasive fungal sinusitis, which occurs primarily in immunocompromised individuals, requires immediate surgical intervention to confirm the diagnosis and exenterate nonviable tissue.[4,5] Equally important is reversal of the source of the immunocompromise, if possible, with systemic and topical antifungal agents. *Aspergillus* species are the most common infecting agents; however, rare nonpathogenic fungi can also on occasion become invasive. Fungal cultures are necessary to determine sensitivity to the antifungal agents. Table 9–1 lists some common invasive fungal pathogens and the recommended systemic antifungal therapy.

Prognosis in invasive fungal sinusitis is linked directly to the ability to reverse the underlying source of immunocompromise. *Mucormycosis*, a term applied to infections from any of several species within the class of Zygomycetes, including *Mucor* and *Rhizopus,* should be considered a possible diagnosis in any poorly controlled diabetic with sinusitis.[5] The likelihood of recovery in diabetics with mucormycosis is 80%, and leukemics in relapse survive less than 20% of the time.[6] This difference in prognosis reflects the ability to reverse poorly controlled diabetes more easily than leukemia. Every attempt to provide the severely immunocompromised with a fungal free environment until recovery of their immune function should be made.[7]

Endoscopic sinus techniques can be utilized in invasive fungal sinusitis,[8] except in situations where thrombocytopenia or other coagulopathies exist. Although difficult-to-control bleeding makes any surgery difficult, it makes endoscopic techniques impossible. If surgery must be done, then correction of the coagulopathy for the time of surgery is imperative.

Occasionally invasive fungal infections of the paranasal sinuses occur in immunocompetent or mildly immunocompromised individuals. This is termed *chronic fungal sinusitis* or *granulomatous invasive sinusitis*, depending on the histopathology.[4] These infections may progress slowly yet relentlessly, and in some cases will be refractory to surgery and prolonged antifungal therapy.

Fungus balls, matted clumps of hyphae lying within the dark confines of a sinus cavity, occur in the immunocompetent and may be asymptomatic and discovered incidentally or the cause of pain, drainage, or congestion.[9]

TABLE 9–1   Recommended Systemic Antifungals for Invasive Fungal Sinusitis

Fungal Organism	Recommended Antifungal	Alternate
Aspergillus species	Voriconazole 4mg/kg IV q 12H, followed by 200 mg po q 12 H if >40 kg Amphotericin B 0.5–0.6 mg/kg IV; for rapidly progressive infections 1–1.5 mg/kg IV qid. Up to total dose of 3 g; a lipid formulation of amphotericin B (Abelcet) is dosed at 5 mg/kg IV qid (decreased renal toxicity)[1]	In serious invasive aspergillosis, voriconazole is superior to Amphotericin B; Some *Aspergillus* sp. are resistant to amphotericin and may respond to itraconazole (Sporonox) dosed at 200 mg po bid[2]
Fusarium, Mucorales	Amphotericin as above; Voriconazole has some activity against dematiaceous fungi, but none against those in the order Mucorales and limited against Fusarium	
Psuedoallescheria Alternaria, Curvularia, Bipolaris	Ketoconazole 400–800 mg po daily or miconazole IV Itraconazole (Sporonox) 200 mg bid; begin with a loading dose of 200 mg tid for 3 days; Voriconazole has some activity against dematiaceous fungi,	Itraconazole if less immunocompromised

[1] Fungi susceptible to amphotericin B have also been treated with topical ampthotericin B. A 0.5% nasal spray is produced when a 50 mg vial of IV amphotericin B is mixed with 10 mL of sterile water. A nasal spray can be dosed as two sprays two to six times per day. The solution is stable for 7 days but must be refrigerated and kept from light. There are no studies confirming the efficacy of nasal amphotericin; however, it has been used to prevent fungal infections in susceptible patients.[2] Liver function tests should be performed in patients taking itraconazole for more than 4 weeks.

The mean age is in the mid 60s, and the most frequent sinus involved is the maxillary sinus, followed by the sphenoid. Ethmoid sinus involvement is usually associated with maxillary sinus involvement, and frontal sinus involvement is rare. There is one case report in which a fungus ball became invasive following immunosuppresion of the patient for a kidney transplant. In the immunocompetent patient, no antifungal therapy is needed, and the disorder is resolved with surgical removal.[10] Endoscopic techniques lend themselves readily to removal of fungus balls. Endoscopic irrigation can be helpful in washing out the fungus. Occasionally, a Caldwell-Luc approach is required in maxillary infestations. Recurrence is uncommon. Frontal sinus fungus balls can be approached endoscopically endonasally, with a frontal sinus trephination, to provide a port to irrigate the fungus. Alternatively, a frontoethmoidectomy via a Lynch incision may be used.

Saprophytic fungal growth refers to the spores that grow on small crusts of mucus within the nasal cavity. This is more common after endoscopic sinus surgery, when mucociliary clearance pathways may be disrupted, leading to small mucous crusts residing on the middle turbinate or within the ethmoid cavity. These small growths of hyphae can be the early form of a fungus ball, but generally they are easily blown out by the patient or aspirated away at the time of nasal endoscopic evaluation. No further treatment is required. If the problem is recurrent, then the patient can be instructed in weekly saline irrigation of the nose with a baby bulb syringe or a powered water irrigation system.

The remaining sections of this chapter will deal with the management of AFS, which differs dramatically from the treatment of other manifestations of fungal sinusitis.

Table 9–2 summarizes the diagnostic criteria and management of the various forms of fungal sinusitis.

■ Management of AFS

Preoperatively, one suspects the existence of AFS because of the clinical characteristics outlined in Chapter 4. Ultimately, diagnosis requires surgery with histopathologic confirmation.[11] Nevertheless, recurrence is common. In treating the patient with AFS, conservative and nonmutilating surgical debridement of the affected sinuses is the primary modality of therapy. AFS is by and large a non-life-threatening disease, and one should not inflict potentially life-threatening procedures onto the disease process. The "cure" should not be worse than the disease. Removal of all the fungal-laden allergic mucin is important. If the fungal-laden mucin is not removed, then the disease persists. It may be quiescent during systemic steroid therapy, but it will almost always recur.[2] If removal of all fungal-laden allergic mucin is accomplished, the patient may be temporarily cured, but he or she faces the prospect of recurrent exposure to the ubiquitous fungal spores and recurrence of AFS because the underlying allergic predisposition persists. Thus, medical adjuncts are important in reducing recurrence of disease following surgery. These will be discussed following the section on special considerations in the surgery of AFS.

■ Surgery in AFS

Endoscopic surgical techniques were developed in the mid-1970s and introduced in the United States in the

TABLE 9–2   Diagnosis and Management of Fungal Sinusitis Manifestations

	Invasive Fungal Sinusitis	Chronic Indolent Invasive Fungal Sinusitis	Fungus Balls	Saprophytic Fungal Growth in the Nose	Allergic Fungal Rhinosinusitis
Incidence relative to all sinus surgeries	0.003%	Less than 0.003%	4%	Unknown	7%, but may be lower in certain areas
Immunologic status of the host	Immunocompromised; transplant, leukemia, neutropenia, poorly controlled diabetes	Immunocompetent or mildly immuno-compromised	Immunocompetent	Immunocompetent; may have had prior sinus surgery and disruption of mucociliary transport pathways	Allergic
Common fungal agents	*Mucormycosis* is found disproportionately in diabetics; *Aspergillus fumigatus, Candida* species, *Fusarium,* and multiple uncommon pathogens	*Aspergillus flavus, A. fumigatus*	*Aspergillus* species; *Pseudallescheria boydii*	Usually *Aspergillus* species, occasionally dematiaceous species such as *Alternaria*	Primarily dematiaceous species: *Bipolaris, Alternaria, Curvularia*; also *Aspergillus* species and multiple other molds such as *penicillium* usually growing concomitantly with other fungi
Clinical manifestations	Anesthesia of the face or nose is common as an early sign of mucormycosis; later the mucosa becomes necrotic and blackened. This is less usual in other fungal infections. There may be no purulence because of neutropenia; mild to severe nasal congestion; facial pain is variable; extension to surrounding structures—palate, orbit, brain, skin—is a late finding	Crusting, persistent granulomatous mucosal reaction, pain, bony erosion, orbital findings; may be nongranulomatous in mildly immuno-compromised	Frequently asymptomatic; may have complaints of nasal congestion, postnasal discharge, facial pain, headache, or seizure	Usually asymptomatic	Nasal obstruction, production of tenacious greenish to brown mucin casts, nasal polyps, anosmia, thick postnasal discharge; proptosis, nasal widening, headache or facial pain
Radiographic findings	Mild to extensive signs of sinusitis; bony erosion present only in advanced disease	Sinusitis and ultimately bony erosion	Hyperdense material on CT, usually with total or subtotal opacification; sclerosis of the bony walls common; bone destruction uncommon; air-fluid level rare	Not seen on imaging	Almost half have only unilateral disease, although involvement of multiple sinuses is common; bony erosion, mucoceles, orbital or intracranial extension along with hyperattenuated densities in the center of the sinuses or nasal cavity, surrounded by lower density mucosal hypertrophy; nasal cavity densities representing polyposis
Therapy	Reversal of underlying immunocompromise; systemic and topical appropriate antifungals; surgical debridement	Systemic and topical appropriate antifungals; surgical debridement	Surgical removal (usually endoscopic) of matted hyphae	Cleansing endoscopically in office or by patient with nasal irrigations	Conservative endoscopic removal of all fungal mucin, perioperative steroids and nasal steroid spray, postoperative fungal-containing immunotherapy; role of antifungals remains unproven
Prognosis	Dependent on source of immunosuppression 80–100% survival for diabetics; 20–40% for leukemics	Poor, but prolonged	Excellent; rare cases of fungus balls progressing to invasion, usually if patient is immuno-compromised	Excellent	Excellent; however, disease is frequently recurrent over 50% of the time

mid-1980s. Up until then, the surgical approach in AFS usually required external approaches, such as Caldwell-Lucs, external ethmoidectomies, and frontal sinus obliterative procedures. By and large, these procedures have all been replaced with endoscopic sinus surgery.[12–14] Occasionally, the allergic fungal mucin is so difficult to remove from the frontal sinuses or so recalcitrant in its recurrence that obliterative frontal sinus procedures are required. Frontal sinus trephination with irrigation may also be helpful in removing allergic fungal mucin from the frontal sinus. The other sinuses can usually be successfully exenterated endoscopically. Case reports of cranial facial resections for AFS exist. It is not clear that this surgery could not also have been accomplished with endoscopic techniques. Schubert and Goetz[15] have speculated that the mucosal sparing aspects of endoscopic sinus surgery may leave significant amounts of hypertrophic sinus mucosa with small rests of fungal infested mucin, which may predispose the patient to recurrence. It was their impression, without any statistical analysis, that prior sinus mucosal stripping procedures performed before the advent of endoscopic techniques were associated with less recurrence.

The most important recent technological advance in endoscopic sinus surgery is the microdebrider.[16] A variety of companies produce these instruments. Efficiency of aspiration varies with the microshaver and the size of the blade. The microdebrider is particularly efficient in the management of AFS. The microdebrider is able to suction and amputate the tenacious mucin. The attachment of a trap to the microdebrider suction allows collection of the mucin for histopathologic examination. Alternatively, one can harvest the eosinophilic mucin with a small forcep and send it to the laboratory. Mucin should also be sent for fungal cultures.

Although the microdebrider brings enhanced and more rapid debridement of the tenacious mucin and polyps of AFS, it also brings special dangers. AFS frequently erodes the lamina papyracea or the cranial vault. Dura may be all that separates the brain from polyps or allergic fungal mucin. Thus, the microdebrider can easily access dura or periorbita without the intervening protective bony layer.[17] For these reasons, very careful preoperative analysis of the sinus CT scan is required. The CT scan should be obtained within a few weeks of the surgery so one is aware of all bony dehiscences. In areas close to bony dehiscence, orbit, or skull base, a suction without a microdebrider is a safer instrument. Altough it is tedious to slowly aspirate the sticky, thick mucin with a large Fraser tip suction, it is far safer than the microdebrider in these areas.

Navigational instrumentation can be helpful. Frequently, the AFS has obscured all landmarks with its polyposis. Any of a variety of navigational systems that correlate the patient's anatomy to a CT image provided in sagittal, coronal, and axial sections may allow a more complete exeneration of the allergic fungal mucin by aiding the surgeon in pursuing persistent disease while avoiding intracranial or orbital complications. Nevertheless, no system is infallible, and the endoscopic rhinologic surgeon must know the anatomy and not rely completely on any technology. The margin of error in the most popular systems available for endoscopic sinus surgery is within 2 mm. However, in some cases, the margin of error may be greater.[18]

■ Steroid Therapy

Systemic steroids are important in the treatment of the pulmonary form of AFS, allergic bronchopulmonary aspergillosis (ABPA), and early on the use of steroids was extended to AFS, using similar dosages. Waxman and colleagues[19] started at a dosage of 60 mg a day and tapered it down over the course of several weeks to months. Kupferberg and colleagues[2] proved that objective evidence of recurrence of AFS is significantly reduced with the use of systemic steroids. Their steroid dosage schedule in the postoperative period, in a 70 kg (154 lb) patient, is as follows: prednisone 40 mg a day for 4 days, then 30 mg a day for 4 days, followed by 20 mg a day for 3 weeks. Kupferberg et al reported that dosages of less than 15 mg every other day led to recurrence. Schubert and Goetz,[15] in the largest series of consecutively reviewed patients, 67 patients with AFS, found that oral corticosteroid therapy significantly delayed the need for revision of surgery; however, at 2 years following the initial surgery, the need for revision surgery was very similar in patients regardless of steroid use. In fact, 70% of the 23 patients with revision surgery were still receiving oral steroid therapy at the time of the recurrence. Their oral corticosteroid dosage regimen was similar to Kupferberg et al's. Prednisone was begun perioperatively at a dose of 0.5 mg/kg each morning for 14 days, then decreased to 0.5 mg/kg every other day and gradually tapered to 5.0 to 7.5 mg every other day within 3 months, then maintained on 5 mg every other day for the duration of treatment. Intercurrent upper respiratory infections were treated with 20 to 30 mg of prednisone a day for 4 to 7 days, with a rapid taper back to 5 mg on alternate days within a week. Patients undergoing subsequent surgery for recurrent AFS were restarted on the original protocol.

Lower dosages of steroids, 0.5 to 1.0 mg/kg per day, are advocated in children, because of the concern of permanent growth retardation secondary to the steroids.[20] Steroids in both groups, but especially children, should be weaned as quickly as possible. Revision endoscopic sinus surgery is advocated in preference to continued steroid use in the pediatric population, because of the potential of irreversible loss of bone growth.[20]

Besides bone growth issues, the side effects of systemic steroids include accelerated osteoporosis, avascular necrosis of the hip, cataracts, and glaucoma. Because of increased osteoporosis risk, 1200 to 1800 mg of vitamin D–supplemented calcium should be considered in all adults on prolonged steroid therapy. In predisposed individuals, systemic steroids may unmask diabetes or make diabetes management quite difficult, exacerbate hypertension, or aggravate peptic ulcer disease. Acutely, systemic steroids may provoke personality changes, including depression, mania, hyperactivity, euphoria, and psychosis. If the patient has an adverse steroid reaction and has not been on steroids for over 2 weeks throughout the year, then the patient can probably safely stop the steroid without completing the taper.

■ Antifungal Therapy

Both topical and systemic antifungal therapies have been proposed for AFS. There are no published studies in clearly diagnosed AFS supporting either treatment.[3] The risks associated with topical therapy are minimal; however, systemic therapy is expensive and can be harmful. Ponikau and colleagues[21,22] reported a 70% symptomatic improvement in patients with chronic rhinosinusitis treated with 20 ml of Amphotericin B each nostril twice a day; however, this was an uncontrolled study, and saline washes alone are also therapeutic. No one currently advocates systemic amphotericin B therapy for AFS, although it is certainly clear that amphotericin has been administered in the past to patients with unrecognized AFS.

The most common pathogens in AFS are the dematiaceous species (*Curvularia, Bipolaris, Alternaria*). Bent and Kuhn[23] found that these species were sensitive to itraconazole, amphotericin B, nystatin, and ketoconazole, but rarely sensitive to fluconazole (Diflucan). They advocated the topical application of ketoconazole dissolved in an acetic acid solution (0.125% or 1 mg/mL) postoperatively. Alternatively, suspensions of amphotericin B at a dosage of 50 mg in 10 mL of sterile water (not saline or dextrose) irrigated into the nostrils two to four times a day have been used. Topical amphotericin B is not absorbed by the oral route. It does have a displeasing taste. There are no published randomized controlled studies regarding the efficacy of any topical antifungals.

Systemic antifungal therapy for AFS has not been studied in a systematic manner. Many of the fungi responsible for AFS are more sensitive to itraconazole (Sporanox) than to amphotericin B. Any study reporting efficacy or inefficacy of antifungal therapy must ascertain that the antifungal therapy utilized was effective, at least in vitro, with the fungal agent. In addition, we have no information as to whether even appropriate systemic antifungal agents achieve mucin levels sufficient to be effective. In the pulmonary manifestation of the disease, Denning et al[24] reported on six patients treated with itraconazole (200 mg twice daily for 1 to 6 months). After 2 months of itraconazole, prednisone requirements were halved, and total IgE fell from a pretreatment mean of 2500 U/mL to a posttreatment mean of 500 U/mL. Two of three patients had resolution of positive *Aspergillus* sputum cultures. Itraconazole must be taken by mouth. It is far less toxic than amphotericin B, but it is expensive.

Kupferberg et al[2] reported that three of five patients who received systemic antifungal therapy improved, but all showed objective evidence of recurrence. They did not detail the antifungal agent used. I treated one patient with prior endoscopic sinus surgery who developed a small accumulation of AFS (diagnosed by biopsy in the office). She was intolerant of oral corticosteroid therapy. Her disease resolved without surgery after 6 weeks of itraconazole 200 mg twice daily.

Rains[25] reported on 68 patients treated with endoscopic sinus surgery. Despite postoperative systemic steroids and itraconazole, he noted a 50% recurrence rate. These recurrences resolved with a repeated course of itraconazole combined with steroid sprays. The dosage he used was itraconazole 200 mg twice a day for 1 month, followed by 300 mg daily for 1 month, followed by 200 mg daily for 1 month after clinically clear. Unfortunately, his study lacked a control. Rains noted a 4% incidence of adverse reaction in his population with AFS treated with oral itraconazole. Liver functions should be monitored monthly with patients receiving itraconazole. The cost of the itraconazole regimen, as detailed by Rains, is in excess of $1500.

The bottom line is, to date, even the fairly benign use of itraconazole in this entity remains unproven. Voriconazole is an oral or systemic antibiotic which became available in 2003 and appears to have superior efficacy to amphotericin B for invasive aspergillosis.[26] Its role in AFS is unstudied.

■ Immunotherapy

For many years, immunotherapy was discouraged in patients with AFS. This is extrapolated from warnings regarding the use of immunotherapy in ABPA. These objections were theoretical and based on the fact that immunotherapy frequently results in a transient rise of IgE followed by a rise in IgG4, to the specific fungus. Because these diseases are associated with elevated specific IgE and IgG to the fungus, there was a concern that immunotherapy would exacerbate a condition already characterized by elevated levels of IgG and IgE. The role of immunotherapy in AFS patients was unstudied until recently.[3] In 1994, Goldstein et al[27] reviewed four cases of AFS and suggested that immunotherapy may have a role in preventing recurrences. In 1993, a report on five patients who failed to improve on immunotherapy prior to the recognition and surgical exeneration of AFS[28] stimulated Mabry and colleagues[29] to study the role of immunotherapy following endoscopic removal of AFS. They initiated immunotherapy for 1 month following surgery and initially used only fungal antigens. Immunotherapy was based on dilutional intradermal testing and advanced weekly to the highest tolerated dosage that did not promote a systemic reaction or local reaction larger than 3 cm in diameter. Their average maintenance antigen dosage was equal to 0.05 mL of a 1:100 weight/volume concentration. After 6 months of treatment, nonfungal antigens were added based on RAST testing. After a follow-up of 4 to 12 months, they reported no worsening of their patients' symptoms on immunotherapy. Mabry et al used this evidence to show that there were no adverse reactions to immunotherapy in this population. In an interim report they noted that one recurrence in a patient on immunotherapy actually reflected incompletely removed AFS.[30] In a subsequent cross-sectional analysis of these patients at 3 years compared with patients who elected not to receive immunotherapy,[31] they reported that the 11 patients receiving immunotherapy showed a statistical reduction in recurrence by endoscopic staging as well as symptomatic improvement. Immunotherapy also significantly reduced the reliance on the systemic corticosteroids. This single institution study suggests that controlling this recalcitrant disease may be possible with a relatively benign medical adjunct. The results need to be expanded to a multicenter study and ideally a randomized placebo-controlled trial. The duration of immunotherapy required is unknown, although Mabry[32] is currently studying patients whose immunotherapy was stopped after a 3-year period. In a more recent study, the same investigators reported that regardless of whether patients received immunotherapy or not, if followed for at least 4 years, most experienced disease remission.

■ Conclusion

The proper therapy of fungal sinusitis depends on the manifestation of the fungal sinusitis relative to the immunologic status of the host. In the immunosuppressed host, one finds invasive fungal sinusitis. Prognosis is often guarded and dependent on reversal of immunosuppression, combined with systemic antifungal therapy and surgical debridement. In rare situations, one has apparently normal individuals who suffer from a relentless, slow-growing invasive fungal infection, frequently only partially responsive to surgery and systemic antifungal therapy. Fungus balls occur in normal hosts and are readily resolved with the surgical removal of the matted hyphae from the sinus cavity. Recurrence is rare. The most recalcitrant and frequently seen of the fungal manifestations of rhinosinusitis is AFS.

The primary modality for therapy of AFS is surgery both for diagnosis and symptom relief. AFS is almost never life threatening, and the surgical procedure used should invoke as little morbidity as possible. The frontal sinus remains the most difficult sinus in which to extricate the AFS, and if the disease does not resolve with endoscopic techniques, oral corticosteroid therapy, and possibly oral antifungal therapy, then the patient may require frontal sinus obliteration.

Oral corticosteroid therapy is certainly effective in reducing nasal polyposis, patient symptoms, and disease recurrence; however, ultimately even on oral corticosteroids, the disease does recur. The long-term side effect profile of oral corticosteroids, including accelerated osteoporosis, potential for glaucoma, and increased cataract formation, makes its use unacceptable for prolonged periods. In children, potentially irreversible delays in bone growth may occur.[20] Nevertheless, it remains helpful in the perioperative period and should be used to minimize hyperplastic polypoid regrowth in the immediate postoperative period.

Systemic and topical antifungal therapies have been advocated but lack controlled trials to support their use.[31]

Immunotherapy is the most promising adjunctive modality in reducing recurrence of AFS. It appears to be most effective if the patient's AFS is exenterated completely prior to initiating immunotherapy.[31]

REFERENCES

1. Ence BK, Gourley DS, Jorgensen NL, Shagets FW, Parsons DS. Allergic fungal sinusitis. *Am J Rhinol.* 1990;4:169–178.
2. Kupferberg SB, Bent JP, Kuhn FA. Prognosis for allergic fungal sinusitis. *Otolaryngol Head Neck Surg.* 1997;117:35–41.
3. Ferguson BJ. What role do systemic corticosteroids, immunotherapy, and antifungal drugs play in the therapy of allergic fungal rhinosinusitis? *Arch Otolaryngol Head Neck Surg.* 1998;124:1174–1178.
4. DeShazo RD, O'Brien M, Chapin K, Soto-Aguilar M, Gardner L, Swain R. A new classification and diagnostic criteria for invasive fungal sinusitis. *Arch Otolaryngol Head Neck Surg.* 1997;123:1181–1188.
5. Blitzer A, Lawson W. Fungal infections of the nose and paranasal sinuses. *Otolaryngol Clin North Am.* 1993;26:1007–1035.
6. Sugar AM. Mucormycosis. *Clin Infect Dis.* 1992;14(suppl 1):S126–S129.
7. Trigg ME, Morgan D, Burns TL, et al. Successful program to prevent *Aspergillus* infections in children undergoing marrow transplantation: use of nasal amphotericin. *Bone Marrow Transplant.* 1997;19:43–47.

8. Avet PP, Kline LB, Sillers MJ. Endoscopic sinus surgery in the management of mucromycosis. *J Neuro-ophth.* 1999;19:56–61.

9. Klossek JM, Serrano E. Peloquin Ll, Pucodani J, Fontanel JP, Pessey JJ. Functional endoscopic sinus surgery and 109 mycetomas of paranasal sinuses. *Laryngoscope.* 1997;107:112–117.

10. Gungor A, Adusumilli V, Corey JP. Fungal sinusitis: progression of disease in immunosuppression—a case report. *Ear Nose Throat J.* 1998;77(3):207–215.

11. Katzenstein ALA, Sale SR, Greenberger PA. Allergic *Aspergillus* sinusitis: a newly recognized form of sinusitis. *J Allergy Clin Immunol.* 1983;72:89–93.

12. Kinsella JB, Rassekh CH, Bradfield JL, et al. Allergic fungal sinusitis with cranial base erosion. *Head Neck.* 1996;18:211–217.

13. Kinsella JB, Bradfield JJ, Gourley WK, Calhoun KH, Rasssekh CH. Allergic fungal sinusitis. *Clin Otolaryngol.* 1996;21:389–392.

14. Quraishi HA, Ramadon HH. Endoscopic treatment of allergic fungal sinusitis. *Otolaryngol Head Neck Surg.* 1997;117:29–34.

15. Schubert MS, Goetz DW. Evaluation and treatment of allergic fungal sinusitis: II. Treatment and follow up. *J Allergy Clin Immunol.* 1998;102:395–402.

16. Mirante JP, Krouse JH, Munier MA, Christmas DA. The role of powered instrumentation in the surgical treatment of allergic fungal sinusitis. *ENT.* 1998;678–682.

17. Ferguson BJ, DiBiase PA, D'Amico F. Quantitative analysis of microdebriders used in endoscopic sinus surgery. *Am J Otolaryngol.* 1999;20:1–5.

18. Gliklich R, Cosenza MA, Metson R. Comparison of image guidance systems for sinus surgery. *Laryngoscope.* 1998;108:164–170.

19. Waxman JE, Spector JG, Sale SR, Katzenstein ALA. Allergic *Aspergillus* sinusitis: concepts in diagnosis and treatment of a clinical entity. *Laryngoscope.* 1987;97:261–266.

20. Kupferberg SB, Bent JP. Allergic fungal sinusitis in the pediatric population. *Arch Otolaryngol Head Neck Surg.* 1996;122: 1381–1384.

21. Ponikau J, Sherris D, Kita H, Kern E. Intranasal antifungal treatment in 51 patients with chronic rhinosinusitis *J Allergy Clin Immunol.* 2002;110:862–866.

22. Ferguson BJ. Antifungal nasal washes for chronic rhinosinusitis: what's therapeutic—the wash or the antifungal? [Comment. Letter] *J Allergy Clin Immunol.* 2003;111:1137–1138.

23. Bent JP, Kuhn FA. Antifungal activity against allergic fungal sinusitis organisms. *Laryngoscope.* 1996;106:1331–1334.

24. Denning DW. Van Wye JE. Lewiston NJ, Stevens DA. Adjunctive therapy of allergic bronchopulmonary aspergillosis with itraconazole. *Chest.* 1991;100:813–819.

25. Rains M. Medical and surgical treatment of allergic fungal sinusitis. Paper presented at: International Sinus Symposium, Loyola University; October 17, 1997; Chicago.

26. Herbrecht R, Denning DW, Patterson TF, et al. Voriconazole versus amphotericin B for primary therapy of invasive aspergillosis. *New Eng J Med.* 2002;347:408–415.

27. Goldstein MF, Dunsky EH, Dvorin DJ, Lesser RW. Allergic fungal sinusitis: a review with four illustrated cases. *Am J Rhinol.* 1994;8:13–18.

28. Ferguson BJ. Immunotherapy and antifungal therapy in allergic fungal sinusitis. Paper presented at: Annual Meeting of the American Academy of Otolaryngic Allergy; September 1993; Minneapolis.

29. Mabry RL, Manning SC, Mabry CS. Immunotherapy in the treatment of allergic fungal sinusitis. *Otolaryngol Head Neck Surg.* 1997; 116:31–35.

30. Mabry RL, Mabry CS. Immunotherapy for allergic fungal sinusitis: the second year. *Otolaryngol Head Neck Surg.* 1997;117:367–371.

31. Folker RI, Marple BF, Mabry RL, Mabry CS. Treatment of allergic fungal sinusitis: a comparison trial of postoperative immunotherapy with specific fungal antigens. FL. *Laryngoscope.* 1998;108:1623–1627.

32. Marple B, Newcomer M, Schwade N, Mabry R. Natural history of allergic fungal rhinosinusitis: a 4- to 10-year follow-up. *Otolaryngol Head Neck Surg.* 2002;127:361–366.

10

Surgical Approaches: Endonasal Endoscopic

HOWARD L. LEVINE

Stammberger,[1] Messerklinger,[2] Wigand,[3] and Kennedy and colleagues[4,5] created a revolution in the thinking and surgical management of nasal sinus disease. The ability to use nasal endoscopy for the diagnosis, identification of sinus and nasal pathology within the narrow spaces and recesses of the nose, and delicate management of the disease has benefited the patient by more accurate surgery, preservation of function, and faster healing. From its introduction, the concepts of endoscopic sinus surgery continue to evolve because of increased understanding of the anatomy, improved endoscopes and video equipment, newer instrumentation, and improved technology.

The author's previous surgical concepts were described in a prior textbook, but they have since evolved as the concepts have changed and the technology has improved.[6] Although some of the principles and concepts remain the same, many others are different.

Although sinus surgery with endoscopes was initially called functional endoscopic sinus surgery (FESS), many would agree that this nomenclature is often misused because not all of the surgery is truly "functional." Because all of the surgery is endoscopic, it is appropriate to use the more general term *endoscopic sinus surgery* and realize that there are several types of procedures done in this manner. For all sinus surgeons there is a spectrum of procedures performed. At times the surgery is certainly "functional," and FESS is an appropriate term. There may be minimal disease, disease confined to the anterior or posterior ostiomeatal complex or nasal cavity. During FESS, the nasal and sinus mucous membrane lining, nasal turbinates, and sinus ostia mostly are preserved or nearly totally preserved. In other patients, there is extensive disease involving all of the sinuses, nasal turbinates, or nasal sinus mucous membranes. There may have been previous surgery or disease that has destroyed normal anatomy and/or sinus lining, leaving a scarred and distorted nasal sinus cavity. In these instances, the goal cannot be to re-create sinus function. Rather, the goal is to eradicate disease by creating a single large cavity that permits adequate aeration into the sinuses and adequate egress of mucus. Here, a marsupialized cavity is created. The author has called this marsupialization endoscopic sinus surgery (MESS). In between FESS and MESS there is a spectrum of operations depending on the pathology found.

■ Preparation for Surgery

Surgery is indicated for those patients who have medically unresponsive sinus disease, a complication of sinus disease such as orbital abscess, or an intracranial complication such as meningitis or abscess. Prior to surgery, all patients have had a nasal endoscopic evaluation and CT scan of the sinuses. The nasal endoscopic exam not only helps to identify the pathology, but also helps determine the areas of technical difficulty in performing an endoscopic sinus procedure. The CT scan used is a coronal CT visualizing the sinuses from the anterior wall of the frontal sinus through the posterior wall of the sphenoid sinus. Axial scans are occasionally obtained when frontal or sphenoid sinus pathology is seen. These axial CT scans aid in the endoscopic surgical management by determining the anterior to posterior dimensions of the sphenoid or frontal sinuses.

Patients with massive nasal and/or sinus polyps are placed on prednisone 40 mg each day beginning 1 week before surgery. If active infection is present, an appropriate antibiotic is used to lessen the inflammation and subsequent bleeding that may occur with this.

Patients avoid the use of any medications that may alter blood coagulation (e.g., aspirin, nonsteroidal anti-inflammatory drugs, or vitamin E) for at least 1 week prior to surgery.

■ The Operating Room

Patients are positioned on the operating table with a pillow placed under the knees to reduce strain on the lower back. In an effort to reduce bleeding and keep the blood pressure lowered, the head is slightly elevated, a soft roll or pillow is placed under the base of the neck, and the head rests upon a soft "doughnut" to bring the head and neck into a head forward sniffing position (Fig. 10–1).

The surgeon stands at the patient's side and operates from the monitor (the author is left-handed and therefore stands on the patient's left side) (Fig. 10–2). A Mayo stand with the most frequently used surgical instruments is at the head of the table. The scrub assistant stands opposite the surgeon, with the remainder of the instruments on the back table just behind the scrub technician. The video system cart with monitor, digital camera, recording, and still photographic capability is just above the Mayo stand. Image-guided triplanar localization surgical technological systems are just to the side of the video cart (Fig. 10–3).

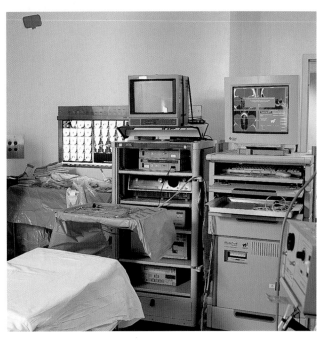

FIGURE 10–2   Organization of the operating room for endoscopic sinus surgery with the surgeon to the side, the anesthesiologist and operating room nurse opposite the surgeon and instruments at the head of the patient.

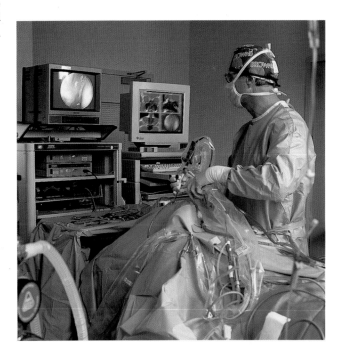

FIGURE 10–3   The CT scan is in view of the surgeon. The monitor off of which the surgery is done is at the head of the patient, and the computer-assisted navigational monitor (Visualization Technology Inc. [VTI], Wilmington, MA) is next to it. The surgeon in this case is left-handed and therefore stands at the left side of the patient.

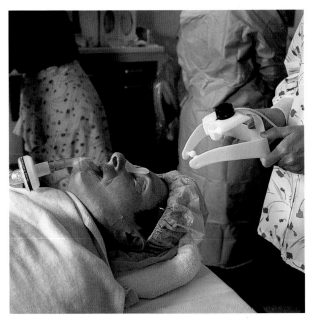

FIGURE 10–1   Positioning of the patient at the time of endoscopic sinus surgery, with the head slightly elevated and on a soft "doughnut" pillow. A pillow is placed beneath the knees.

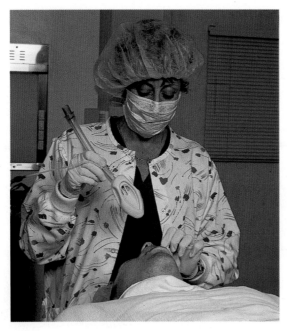

FIGURE 10–4   The laryngeal mask airway is inserted from the head of the patient.

The anesthesia team sits with their equipment at the patient's side. The CT scan is on an x-ray view box in full view of the surgeon for reference during the surgical procedure. The intravenous fluids and ports are located on the side closer to the anesthesia team for easy access. The blood pressure cuff is on the opposite side on the arm by the surgeon.

Nearly all cases are done under general anesthesia, which is chosen for several reasons. This is easiest especially for revision cases where there may be a great deal of scar tissue, making a regional block difficult. Intubation or laryngeal mask airway (LMA) protects the airway, especially in the patient with reactive airway disease, in which a small amount of blood in the trachea may cause

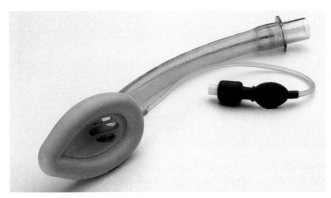

FIGURE 10–5   The laryngeal mask airway fits over the larynx and the hypopharynx and can be inflated appropriately to seal the laryngohypopharynx.

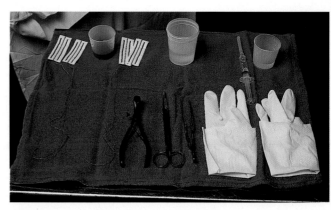

FIGURE 10–6   A separate table is set up with topical decongestants and injectable local anesthesia (if needed) so that the nose may be prepared prior to the surgeon scrubbing.

bronchospasm (Figs. 10–4, 10–5). (LMA is presently used in nearly all patients. It minimizes bronchospasm in the patient with reactive airway disease and seems to allow blood pressure to remain lower and more controlled with minimal use of medications. After several hundred patients undergoing ESS with LMA, no patient has had aspiration.) General anesthesia is valuable for those patients undergoing image-guided surgery, during which a headpiece is worn; it is imperative that there be minimal head movement during such surgery.

Once the patient is asleep, the endotracheal or LMA tube is secured to the lower lip and jaw, taking care to keep tape away from the nose, which might hamper visualization of the nasal/sinus cavity. The eyelids are taped closed to prevent corneal injury, and the eyes are left undraped in the field of surgery as a reference.

Prior to scrubbing, the surgeon uses a headlight and nasal speculum to decongest the nose using oxymetazoline (Fig. 10–6). The oxymetazoline is colored with gentian violet to prevent its being confused with another solution on the operating table. Neurosurgical cottonoids are soaked in the oxymetazoline and placed medial to the middle turbinate, in the region of the anterior ostiomeatal complex and along the inferior turbinate. These are left in place with their strings extending out from the nares until after the surgeon has scrubbed and the patient has been draped. The patient's face and nose are not prepped because the inside of the nose is laden with bacteria and cannot be adequately sterilized. (In several thousand cases, the author has not seen any postoperative infection caused by lack of facial preparation.)

Once the oxymetazoline has produced adequate vasoconstriction, the patient has been draped, and the blood pressure is in the range of less than 100 mm Hg systolic, the procedure is begun. The nasal cavity is initially examined with a 0-degree, 4 mm endoscope. Xylocaine 1% with 1:100,000 epinephrine is injected into the

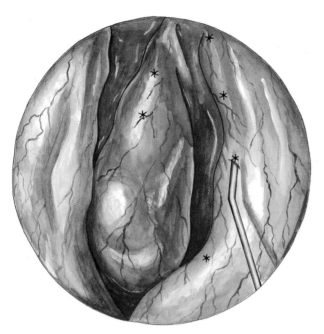

FIGURE 10–7 Injection of local anesthesia for vasoconstriction into the anterior ostiomeatal complex.

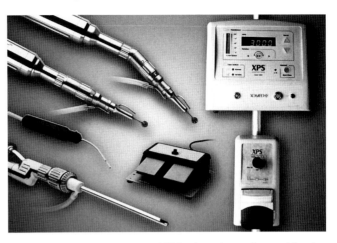

FIGURE 10–8 The Xomed XPS microshaver is used for the majority of endoscopic sinus surgeries.

region of the uncinate process and attachment of the middle turbinate. The anesthetic is injected slowly and allowed to flow posteriorly into the ostiomeatal complex (Fig. 10–7). The injection is used not because of the anesthetic but rather because of the vasoconstriction the epinephrine produces. Preoperative photographs are taken of the anterior ostiomeatal complex and any pertinent pathology. These intraoperative photographs are kept as part of the patient's office record and referred to during subsequent follow-up visits. These photographs (combined with a photograph taken at the end of the procedure) provide a valuable reminder to the surgeon of what was found and what was accomplished at surgery.

■ Nasal Septal Surgery

If a deviated nasal septum is present, obstructing the nasal cavity and limiting the nasal airway or access to the sinus cavities, a septoplasty is performed prior to beginning the sinus surgery. The septoplasty is performed in a traditional manner or with a microshaver, removing bony spurs as needed. Following the septoplasty, cottonoids with oxymetazoline are placed in the nose while the instruments are changed over from the septoplasty to the sinus surgery. These cottonoids provide additional vasoconstriction and minimize the edema along the nasal septal flap that occurred from the septal surgery.

■ General Principles of Endoscopic Sinus Surgery

Most endoscopic sinus surgery is done using the Xomed XPS microshaver (Medtronic Xomed, Jacksonville, FL) (Fig. 10–8). The microshaver is delicate and provides accurate and atraumatic tissue removal. Bleeding is minimal. Normal mucosa is better preserved while pathologic tissue is removed. The irrigating system that is an integral part of the Xomed microshaver minimizes the blockage in the system and permits ease and efficiency of use. The attached suction draws bone and soft tissue into the blade. An additional irrigating system (Clear-ESS) (SLT Laser, Mongomeryville, PA) is added to the microshaver (Fig. 10–9). Saline is used either continuously or intermittently, as determined by the surgeon, through trumpet-type control valves on the endoscope, to irrigate away secretions or blood. Several blades and burs are available and used, depending on the pathology and its location. A 4.2 mm Tricot blade is used for most of the procedure. When disease is present in the frontal recess, frontal sinus, or maxillary sinus, a 40- or 60-degree angulated Tricut blade is used. These blades are used in an oscillating mode at 1500 rpm. This is slow enough to permit the suction to draw tissue into the blade opening. It is generally used for polyps, soft tissue, and thin bone. When a moderate amount of thin bone is present, the microshaver is used at 3000 rpm to enhance the bone-cutting capacity. The mode can be shifted into a continuous mode to cut through thin to medium bone.

Straight burs with one side protected or 55-degree burs permit access into the heavier bony areas of the frontal or sphenoid sinus. The burs are used in a continuous mode generally at 5000 rpm.

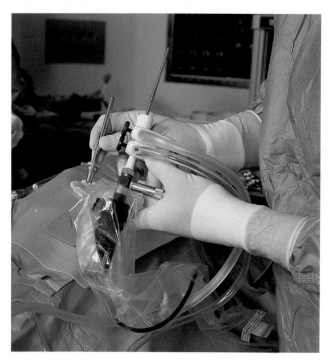

FIGURE 10–9 The Clear ESS system can be attached to the microshaver, permitting intermittent or continuous irrigation of blood and/or debris from the sinus cavity.

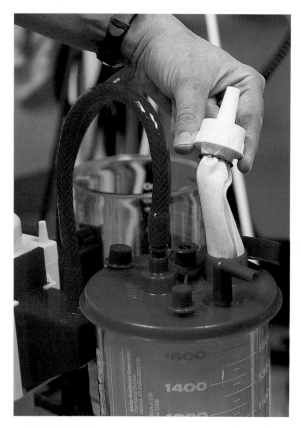

FIGURE 10–10 Collection of the specimen in the "sock" within the operating room suction apparatus.

Specimens from the microshaver are collected in a "sock" (Fig. 10–10) in the suction. This is sent to pathology for histological examination. A recent report (personal communication) demonstrated that pathologists could accurately identify various tumors sent for histological examination, which were sampled with a microshaver.

Throughout the procedure, the sinus cavity is periodically irrigated with warmed saline to wash away both blood and bony debris. The saline is instilled with a soft angiocatheter and 20 cc syringe or the ClearESS system.

If intraoperative bleeding occurs and is bothersome, the nose is packed with cottonoids moistened with oxymetazoline and the surgery continued on the opposite side. Hydrogen peroxide–moistened cottonoids also help in reducing bleeding, clearing the soft tissues of blood staining to allow better visualization of the operative field and to clear purulent secretions from the mucous membrane.

If purulence is seen, intraoperative cultures, typically, aerobic, anaerobic, fungal, and tuberculous, are obtained. Swab, tissue, and mucous trap collections are obtained.

■ Operative Techniques

The "Traditional" Endoscopic Sinus Surgical Approach

Since the introduction of endoscopic sinus surgery over a decade ago, some aspects of the surgical technique have become standard. For the patient with generalized pansinusitis or diffuse sinus disease, a "traditional" endoscopic sinus surgical procedure is performed.

After waiting for ~10 minutes after the injection of Xylocaine with epinephrine to be certain maximal vasoconstriction is achieved, the procedure is begun. A complete endoscopic examination is performed, which is generally easier to do under anesthesia than as an outpatient procedure. This ensures that there is no pathology or anatomical abnormality present that may have been overlooked in the outpatient nasal endoscopic evaluation. It also orients the surgeon to the normal and previously identified pathologic anatomy.

The Uncinate Process

For the patient who has not had previous sinus surgery, the procedure is usually begun anteriorly. Initially, the uncinate process is removed. Care must always be taken when working around the uncinate process to avoid penetration of the lamina papyracea, resulting in exposed orbital fat or intraorbital bleeding (Fig. 10–11). A ball-tipped probe is used to enter the hiatus semilunaris and slightly reflect the uncinate process medially. A microbackbiter is used to remove a small portion of

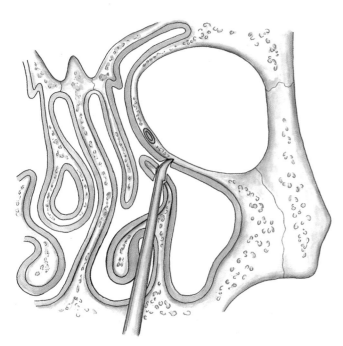

FIGURE 10–11   When removing the uncinate process, care must be taken to avoid injury to the lamina papyracea.

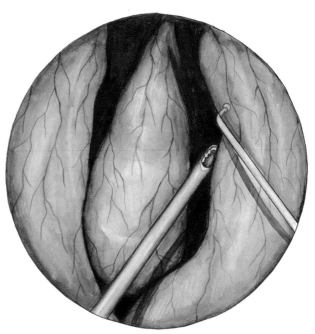

FIGURE 10–13   An incision may be made in the uncinate process to medialize it and allow the microshaver to remove it.

the uncinate process and create a "raw" edge for engagement of the microshaver. This minimizes the risk to the underlying lamina papyracea (Fig. 10–12). The microshaver is used to remove the raw edge of the uncinate process. If the uncinate process is tightly adherent to the

underlying ethmoid bulla, an incision is made with a sickle knife, and the uncinate is displaced medially (Fig. 10–13). This then allows removal with the microshaver. At times a microbackbiting forceps is used to remove the uncinate process in a retrograde manner. If disease is present only in the maxillary sinus and a deformed uncinate process or ethmoid bulla is present, only the inferior portion of the uncinate process is removed.

Anterior Ethmoid Sinus

Once the uncinate process is removed, the microshaver is used to open the ethmoid bulla. It is safest to open the ethmoid bulla anteriorly, medially, and inferiorly away from the orbit and the roof of the sinus (Fig. 10–14). The anterior and medial wall is initially removed gradually, working superiorly and laterally looking for the thin, vertically positioned plate of bone that identifies the lamina papyracea. It typically has a yellow appearance because of the underlying orbital fat. Once the uncinate process and ethmoid bulla are removed, the frontal recess, maxillary sinus ostium, and basal lamella are usually visible.

Posterior Ethmoid Sinus

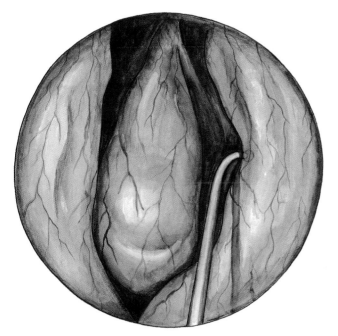

FIGURE 10–12   A ball-tipped probe is inserted into the hiatus semilunaris and used to reflect the uncinate process medially. This helps avoid injury to the underlying lamina papyracea when removing the uncinate process.

If there is disease in the posterior ethmoid or sphenoid sinus, the basal lamella is perforated and the posterior ethmoid sinuses entered. The basal lamella is entered with the microshaver on the medial and inferior aspect to prevent any injury to the fovea ethmoidalis or lamina

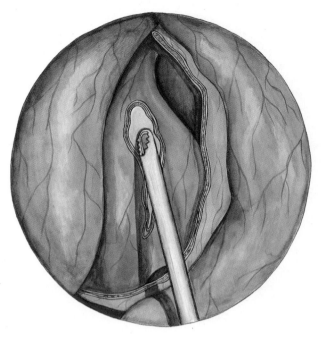

FIGURE 10–14   Drawing showing entrance into the medial and inferior aspect of the ethmoid bulla, where it is safe to avoid injury to the lamina papyracea and/or fovea ethmoidalis.

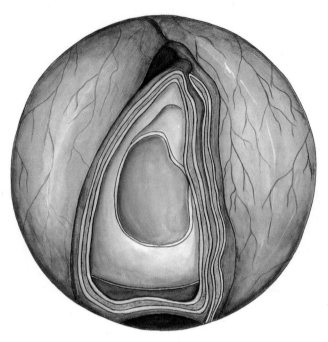

FIGURE 10–16   Drawing showing entrance into the posterior ethmoid sinus air cells, leaving the basal lamina as a support for the middle turbinate.

papyracea (Fig. 10–15). The anterior portion of the basal lamella is removed to gain access to the posterior ethmoid sinus. Every attempt is made to keep the inferior basal lamella intact because this may help to support the middle turbinate and keep it in its medial position

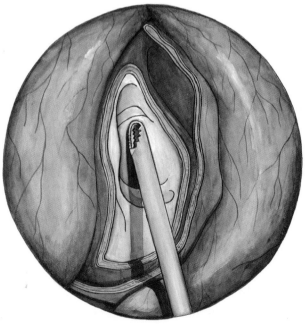

FIGURE 10–15   The basal lamella separating the anterior from the posterior ethmoid sinus air cells is perforated inferiorly and medially to avoid injury to the lamina papyracea and the fovea ethmoidalis.

(Fig. 10–16). Throughout the entire ethmoid sinus dissection, care is taken to identify the fovea ethmoidalis and lamina papyracea. The fovea ethmoidalis appears as a flat, white plate of bone. When working medially, great care must be taken superiorly near the junction of the fovea ethmoidalis and middle turbinate attachment because of the thin bone and potential for its injury, causing a cerebrospinal fluid leak. Posteriorly and superiorly in the ethmoid, care is taken because of the possibility of optic nerve exposure.

Sphenoid Sinus

If there is disease in the sphenoid sinus, it is opened. This is typically done once the posterior ethmoid sinus is opened and the fovea ethmoidalis, lamina papyracea, and lateral aspect of the middle turbinate are exposed.

There are several landmarks that permit safe and accurate entry into the sphenoid sinus. No matter which method is used, the mucosa over the front face is gently dissected inferiorly to expose the underlying bone. This minimizes any injury and bleeding from the sphenopalatine artery that has a branch crossing the inferior border of the sinus.

In opening the sphenoid sinus, instruments are always used in an inferior and medial direction to avoid injury to the internal carotid artery optic nerves, which are lateral and superior in the sinus walls.

The natural ostium of the sphenoid sinus can be identified in the posterior ostiomeatal complex medial to

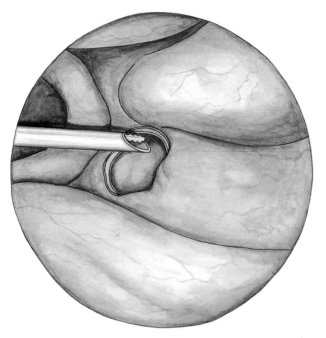

FIGURE 10–17 Entering into the sphenoid sinus medially and inferiorly minimizes the chances of injury to the sphenoid sinus roof, internal carotid artery, or optic nerve. This is done by medializing the middle turbinate.

the superior turbinate. This may be difficult if there is extensive pathology in the sphenoethmoid recess or the region is narrow because of the superior or supreme turbinate or a deviated nasal septum.

Another method of entering the sphenoid sinus is through the posterior ethmoid air cells (Fig. 10–17). The posteroinferior attachment of the middle turbinate is identified where it joins the front face of the sphenoid sinus. The middle turbinate is medialized in this area, and the front face of the sphenoid sinus is palpated. This is over the soft fontanel of the sinus inferior to the ostium and medial and inferior to the carotid artery and optic nerve. The front face can be opened safely and joined to the natural ostium. Soft tissue is elevated off the front face to protect the sphenopalatine artery.

If there is any question about where the front face of the sphenoid sinus is located, the choana of the nose is another useful landmark. The front face of the sphenoid sinus is on the same plane as the choana. By merely following the choana superiorly, the front of the sphenoid sinus can be identified.

On occasion, an inconsistent posterosuperior ethmoid sinus air cell (Onodi cell) may be mistaken for the sphenoid sinus. The Onodi cell, if present, is generally superior, whereas the sphenoid sinus is inferior. Here also, the choana and posterior middle turbinate attachment is helpful in differentiating these two.

Maxillary Sinus

The ostium to the maxillary sinus is identified in the infundibulum. It is generally anterior and inferior in the infundibulum. Once the uncinate process is removed, the ostium is seen. If an opening is seen going into the maxillary sinus when the uncinate process is intact, this opening is nearly never the natural but rather an accessory ostium. If the middle turbinate is intact, it may be a reasonable landmark to identify the ostium that generally lies on the same plane as the inferior edge of the middle turbinate.

If an accessory ostium is present, it is connected to the natural ostium to minimize the chances of ciliary flow of mucus through the natural ostium reentering the maxillary sinus through the accessory ostium.

If the natural ostium is small, it is enlarged using back-biting forceps, removing tissue toward the nasal lacrimal duct. The bone surrounding the nasolacrimal duct is thick. The dissection is stopped if the bone feels thick because the nasolacrimal duct will be in this region. The natural ostium may also be opened posteriorly using sharp through-cutting forceps. Caution is used proceeding posteriorly to avoid injury to the sphenopalatine artery. Also, the ostium may be opened inferiorly using a downbiting forceps. Working too far inferiorly may result in trauma to the inferior turbinate and excessive bleeding.

Once the maxillary sinus ostium is opened, it is inspected with a 0-, 30-, or 70-degree endoscope if pathology is present. Mucus is suctioned. Polyps are removed with the 40- or 60-degree microshaver blades (Fig. 10–18).

Frontal Sinus

The frontal sinus is the most challenging sinus to manage because of the small recess through which the sinus empties and because of its location anteriorly and superiorly in the nasal cavity close to the orbit, cribriform plate, fovea ethmoidalis, and anterior ethmoid artery. Even opening it and removing pathology does not always guarantee success. Pathology may recur and the recess becomes stenotic unless care, caution, and expertise are used in managing the frontal sinus. (Because the frontal sinus disease is unique and challenging, Chapter 14 is devoted to the topic.)

Posterior Wigand Approach to Sinuses

One of the early descriptions of ESS was that of Wigand[3] in which a posterior to anterior approach was used. This is especially helpful when there has been previous sinus surgery or there are few landmarks, and a consistent landmark needs to be identified to begin the sinus surgery. This is similar to traditional techniques of

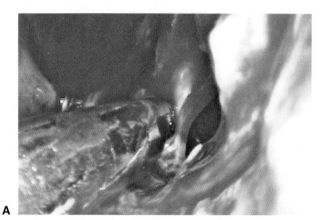
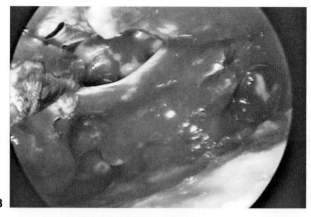

FIGURE 10–18   Removing disease from the maxillary sinus with a 40- (A) or 60-degree (B) microshaver.

intranasal ethmoidectomy and sphenoidotomy accomplished by first identifying the front face of the sphenoid sinus. This is done because the one consistent point is the entrance to the sphenoid sinus.

The choana and the front face of the sphenoid sinus superior to it are identified. The sphenoid sinus can be opened and the roof of the sinus identified. The roof is then followed anteriorly along the fovea ethmoidalis into the posterior and then anterior ethmoid sinuses. Working laterally, the lamina papyracea is identified, then the natural ostium to the maxillary sinus. Wigand[3] described this posterior-to-anterior approach, and it is effective in situations where the anatomy is uncertain. However, when any sinus procedure is performed, especially when there are few landmarks, the identification of any landmark permits the dissection to extend from the known region to other easily recognized areas.

■ Marsupialization Endoscopic Sinus Surgery

For some patients, there has been previous surgery or there is extensive pathology that has a high chance of recurrence or extensive scar tissue. In these instances, many of the normal landmarks are missing either because of previous surgery or because of destruction from disease. Thus, a functional procedure cannot be performed. For these patients, an attempt is made to create a single ethmoid sinus cavity in which the frontal, maxillary, and sphenoid sinuses can adequately drain. In the majority of these cases most of the middle turbinate is missing. This procedure is similar to the older intranasal ethmoidectomy, maxillary antrostomy with sphenoidotomy done with headlight and nasal speculum, but in this instance it is done with nasal endoscopes. The nasal endoscopic approach provides excellent visualization to manage pathology in the previously operated, scarred,

and/or diseased sinus cavity. It leaves a marsupialized cavity that can be irrigated and has the best chance for drainage. The author calls this marsupialization endoscopic sinus surgery (MESS). This is not a functional procedure; however, it is needed to eradicate disease and promote the best possible drainage.

■ Minimally Invasive Functional Endoscopic Sinus Surgery

Many patients present with minimal CT-proven sinus disease and minimal changes on nasal endoscopy but with recurrent acute and subacute rhinosinusitis. Most of these patients have anatomical abnormalities in the anterior or posterior ostiomeatal complex. These may be such abnormalities as a paradoxically bent middle turbinate, concha bullosa, enlarged ethmoid bulla, deformed uncinate process, accessory sinus ostium, or narrowed outflow from the frontal or sphenoid sinus (Fig. 10–19). When medical management has failed, these deformities can be corrected with a minimally invasive functional endoscopic sinus procedure. Micro-endoscopic sinus instruments are used along with miniature powered instruments to remove small bits of tissue, correct the abnormality, preserve normal mucosa, and restore function. Healing is rapid because surgical trauma is limited to the areas of pathology (see Chapter 12).

■ Nasal Turbinates and Sinus Surgery

The nasal turbinates play an important role in the pathophysiology of sinus disease. Although they may obstruct the nose, causing nasal congestion, they may also obstruct the outflow from the sinuses into the nose, causing rhinosinusitis.

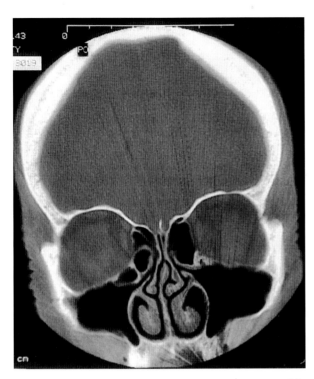

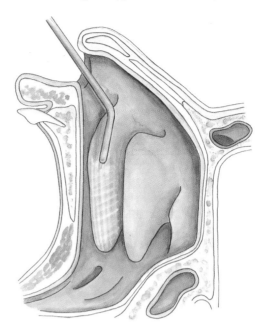

FIGURE 10–20 Cross-hatching of the inferior turbinates to create scar in the submucosa and reduce the size of the turbinate.

FIGURE 10–19 Examples of anatomical abnormalities obstructing the outflow from the infundibulum into the nasal cavity and placing the patient at risk for subacute or recurrent acute rhinosinusitis.

Inferior Turbinate

The inferior turbinate may become congested or polypoid from allergic or vasomotor rhinitis. Also, rhinosinusitis may affect the sinuses by causing inflammation and edema of the inferior turbinate from drainage from the middle meatus. Initial management of inferior turbinate dysfunction is medical using decongestants and/or topical nasal steroid sprays: beclomethasone (Beconase, Vancenase), flunisolide (Flonase), fluticasone propionate (Nasarel), mometasone furoate monohydrate (Nasonex), and triamcinolone acetonide (Nasacort).

If medical management fails, then a laser or radiofrequency reduction of the turbinate is performed.

Laser turbinate reduction is performed using the KTP/532 laser (Laserscope, San Jose, CA). The inferior turbinate is crosshatched using the laser at 8 W in a continuous mode and with the laser tip in contact (Fig. 10–20). (A complete discussion of laser techniques for sinus and nasal pathology is included in Chapters 15a and 15b.)

Radiofrequency (RF) turbinate reduction uses the Somnus radiofrequency generator (Somnus, Sunnyvale, CA) (Fig. 10–21). The radiofrequency creates a controlled destructive lesion within the turbinate, causing it to shrink and contract over a 4- to 6-week period. The radiofrequency energy dispels through the tissue most easily when the turbinate is congested. Therefore, efforts are made to avoid decongestion of the turbinate prior to the procedure.

RF reduction of the inferior turbinate can be performed under local or general anesthesia. When using local anesthesia, the nose is sprayed with topical lidocaine. Lidocaine (with epinephrine) is injected into the anterior aspect of the inferior turbinate. After adequate anesthesia is achieved, the RF turbinate needle probe is inserted into the anterior aspect of the inferior turbinate (Fig. 10–22). Usually 550 J of RF energy is delivered into the turbinate. If the turbinate is large, a second site is treated either superiorly or inferiorly to the

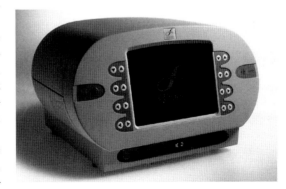

FIGURE 10–21 The Somnus radiofrequency generating unit (Somnus, Sunnyvale, CA).

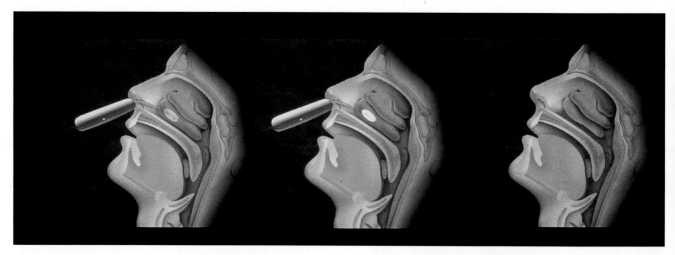

FIGURE 10–22   Somnoplasty (radiofrequency) reduction of the inferior turbinate.

first. When two sites are treated, 500 J of energy are delivered to each.

If the RF reduction is combined with a septoplasty and the procedure is done under general anesthesia, it is usually done after the septoplasty. Because the nose had been decongested for the septoplasty, the inferior turbinate is "recongested" using approximated 5 to 8 cc of normal saline injected into the turbinate. The same technique is then used as if the procedure is performed under local anesthesia.

RF reduction is described in a pilot study of 22 patients used by Somnus for gaining U.S. FDA approval.[7] There were no adverse effects. Mild edema was noted in the first 24 to 48 hours. There was minimal crusting and moderate edema for a few weeks. Posttreatment analgesia was maintained with acetaminophen. Eight weeks after treatment nasal breathing was improved in 21 of 22 patients, with a 58.5% reduction in the severity and a 56.5% decrease in the frequency of nasal obstruction. Postoperative care merely involves the use of topical saline spray as a nasal moisturizer.

Middle Turbinate

The middle turbinate can obstruct the nose because of the presence of a choncha bullosa, paradoxically bent middle turbinate, or polypoid change on the turbinate.

A concha bullosa is frequently associated with a deviated nasal septum, and the concha bullosa sits in the concavity of the septum. The septal deviation occurs to the opposite side, and the middle turbinate is frequently deformed, causing a paradoxically bent middle turbinate. The paradoxical middle turbinate has its concavity medial instead of lateral (Fig. 10–23). Although this may not cause any difficulty for most patients, for some it causes obstruction in the outflow from the

anterior ostiomeatal complex. A small amount of edema of the inferior turbinate from any cause can incite sinusitis.

If a concha bullosa is obstructing either the anterior ostiomeatal complex or the nasal cavity, the lateral

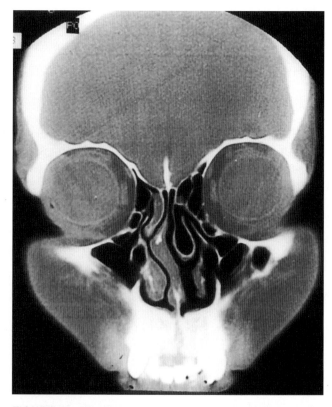

FIGURE 10–23   Paradoxically bent middle turbinate causing potential obstruction of the outflow from the osteomeatal complex into the nasal cavity.

lamella of the concha is removed, leaving the mucosal lined medial lamella. This preserves and re creates the middle turbinate.

The paradoxically bent middle turbinate is more difficult to correct. On occasion, merely fracturing and displacing it medially will suffice to open the anterior ostiomeatal complex. At other times, it is fractured longitudinally in several places to straighten it. At still other times, it is necessary to resect a portion of the inferior anterior edge as the only method of opening the anterior ostiomeatal complex. Stents are rarely used in keeping the turbinate medial; however, if a septoplasty is performed, a Silastic nasal septal splint is placed into the middle meatus to keep the turbinate from scarring and lateralizing. Gelfilm is sometimes used and rolled into an inverted U to keep the turbinate from lateralizing. The Gelfilm dissolves after several weeks in the nasal cavity.

Superior Turbinate

If the superior turbinate obstructs the posterior ostiomeatal complex, posterior ethmoid and/or sphenoid sinusitis may occur. If the superior turbinate obstructs the cribriform plate region, anosmia may occur. The obstruction may occur because the superior turbinate is bulbous, has a concha bullosa within it, or is merely in a narrow region, with crowding from the nasal septum. In all of these instances, it may be necessary to reconstruct or resect portions of the superior turbinate.

■ Image-guided Triplanar Localization Sinus Surgery

Traditionally, surgeons have used a coronal and occasionally axial CT scan obtained preoperatively and viewed on an x-ray view box in the operating room as their reference. The newer technology of image-guided surgery allows more rapid and accurate intraoperative anatomical localization during endoscopic sinus surgery (see Chapter 13 for a complete discussion). Prior to surgery, a helical CT scan is obtained, during which time a special headset with seven electromagnetic sensors is placed on the patient's head and rests in the external ear canal and the bridge of the nose (Figs. 10–24, 10–25). (Some systems use optical sensors.) The helical scan data are either transmitted electronically to a workstation used in the operating room or sent by computer floppy disk to the operating room. In the operating room, the same headset is placed on the patient after he or she is asleep, and the headset is linked to a CT workstation. The headset is registered via the computer workstation software so that the computer is aware of the anatomical structures. Straight and angulated suction aspirators are also linked to the computer workstation. When these are placed within the nasal or sinus cavity, the tip of the aspirator can be located on the screen of the workstation with 3 mm accuracy and seen on axial, coronal, and sagittal views (Figs. 10–26, 10–27).

Image-guided surgery typically is used for revision sinus surgery and complicated cases such as mucoceles, neoplasm, CSF leaks, and meningoencephaloceles.

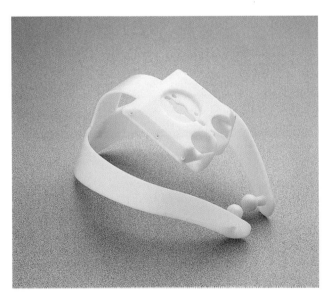

FIGURE 10–24   The VTI headset fits over the head, into the ears, and on the nose.

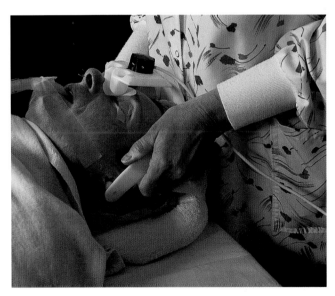

FIGURE 10–25   The VTI headset in place on the patient and linked to the computer workstation.

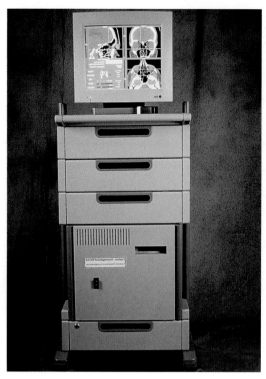

FIGURE 10–26 VTI workstation and monitor.

■ Dressing and Packing

The ideal postoperative dressing for endoscopic sinus surgery would be hemostatic and bactericidal or bacteriostatic and would promote wound healing and ciliary regeneration. This dressing does not yet exist.

With care during surgery, most patients have minimal or little bleeding. For these patients a small strip of telfa covered in Bactroban ointment is inserted in the middle meatus and left in place for about 1 hour. The Bactroban ointment is used to help lubricate the telfa dressing, making it easier to remove. The ointment is also water-soluble and helps avoid the problems of myospherulosis.

Revision sinus surgery and asthmatic patients often have moderate postnasal drainage following surgery. This drainage may cause bronchospasm in patients with reactive airway disease and therefore needs to be kept to a minimum. For these patients, Oxycel cotton

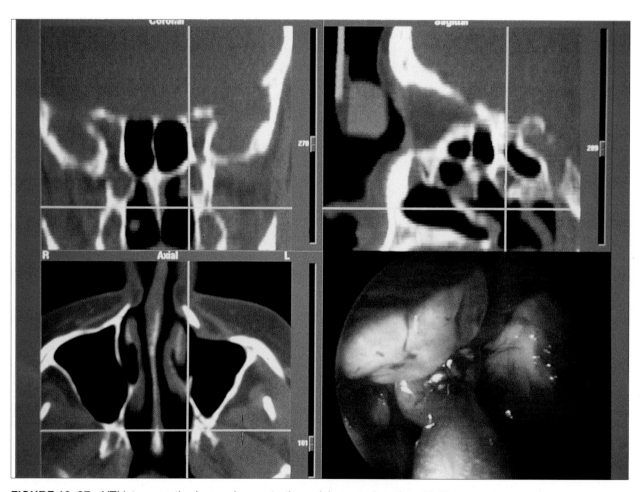

FIGURE 10–27 VTI intraoperative image demonstrating axial, coronal, and sagittal images.

(oxidized cellulose) is inserted into the sinus cavity. The Oxycel cotton is divided into small strips, loosely rolled, and coated with Bactroban ointment. These are placed into the sinus cavity. Over several days following surgery mucous and saline nasal sprays instilled into the nose cause the Oxycel cotton to become a mushlike substance easily suctioned from the nose endoscopically. The Oxycel cotton dressing is hemostatic.

For the rare patient who has severe bleeding, a Merocel tampon is placed in the middle meatus and left there for at least 24 hours.

Newer dressings of hyaluronic acid, a naturally occurring constituent of extracellular matrix, are being developed (Merogel, Xomed Surgical Products, Jacksonville, FL). These dressings seem to control bleeding, minimize adhesion formation, and change into a viscous fluid over several days.

REFERENCES

1. Stammberger H. Endoscopic endonasal surgery-new concepts and treatment of recurring rhinosinusitis: I. Anatomic and pathophysiologic considerations, II: Surgical considerations. *Otolaryngol Head Neck Surg.* 1986;94:143–156.
2. Messerklinger W. *Endoscopy of the Nose.* Baltimore: Urban & Schwartzenberg; 1978.
3. Wigand ME. *Transnasal Endoscopic Surgery of the Anterior Skull Base: Proceedings of the Twelfth ORL World Congress, Budapest, 1981.* Publ. House Hungary. Acad. Sci.; 1981.
4. Kennedy DW, Zinreich SJ, Rosenbaum AE, et al. Functional endoscopic sinus surgery: theory and diagnostic evaluation. *Arch Otolaryngol.* 1985;111:576–582.
5. Kennedy DW. Functional endoscopic sinus surgery, technique. *Arch Otolaryngol.* 1985;111:643–649.
6. Levine HL, May M. *Endoscopic Sinus Surgery.* New York: Thieme Medical Publishers; 1993.
7. Kasey KL, Powell NB, Riley RW, Troell RJ, Guilleminault C. Radiofrequency volumetric tissue reduction for the treatment of turbinate hypertrophy: a pilot study. *Otolaryngol Head Neck Surg.* 1998;119:569–573.

11

Combined Microscopic and Endoscopic Technique (COMET Surgery)

M. PAIS CLEMENTE

Over the past three decades there has been great evolution in nose and paranasal sinus surgery compared with classical approach techniques that have been used. Interest in nasal anatomy dates to practitioners in ancient Egyptian (c. 1500 B.C.) who used the nose as a route for removing the contents of the cranial vault as part of the mummification process to avoid any facial disfiguration.[1] From those times until the last century, the progress of medical science, technological developments, and the contribution of excellent physicians throughout the years havemade the techniques performed today possible. By reviewing the medical literature related with the history of paranasal sinus, diagnosis, and treatment, it is possible to conclude that there are five important reasons for the present state of the field of nose and paranasal sinus surgery.

The first reason is the introduction of the binocular Zeiss operating microscope with coaxial illumination for endonasal surgery invented by Hans Heermann (1958).[2] At about the same time, Harold Hopkins (1956) applied a new concept of lens systems and proximal illumination to the rigid telescope and used glass fibers for transmission of cold light.[3] Nowadays, endoscopes use a light source connected by fiberglass cable that is fitted with a halogen lamp and is available with assorted angles of vision. With its improved illumination and wider field of vision, this newly designed endoscope was immediately used for diagnostic endoscopy. However, the use of telescopes for intranasal surgical procedures is a more recent development because it was necessary to improve the endoscopes and manufacture finer microinstruments that would be suitable for endoscopic sinus surgery.

The second reason is the concept pioneered by Messerklinger (1972),[4] who showed that most of the sinus pathology occurs in the anterior ethmoid sinus at the level of the ostiomeatal unit. He used endoscopy in fresh cadaver specimens to demonstrate a disruption of mucociliary clearance in areas obstructed by the contact of two mucosal-covered surfaces in the middle meatus. Stasis of secretions follows this obstruction, which, in turn, leads to infection. According to Messerklinger, such areas of obstruction are most likely to develop in the middle meatus and to involve the anterior and middle ethmoids, with possible involvement of the maxillary, frontal, and posterior ethmoid sinuses and eventually the sphenoid sinus. If these obstructive areas can be removed with an endoscopic approach with restoration of drainage and ventilation through the natural ostia can be established, then resolution of limited or extensive disease in the dependent sinus can be achieved and its mucosa preserved. This represents a revolutionary concept compared with the classical surgical techniques of paranasal sinus surgery, which preferred creation of radical cavities, sometimes with removal of the mucosal coverage, or even intranasal total ethmoidectomy when there was only limited disease. The development of functional endoscopic sinus surgery contributed tremendously by providing a means to remove localized disease obstructing the narrow ethmoid clefts and thereby restoring normal mucociliary drainage and ventilation. Spontaneous resolution of mucosal disease in the maxillary and frontal sinuses could occur without the need for radical mucosal removal. Unfortunately, Messerklinger's surgical approach for treatment of paranasal sinus disease was not published in the English literature until 1978.[5]

The third reason is the development of the CT scan, which is considered an essential examination for the diagnosis of paranasal sinus disease. A CT scan can show the different anatomical structures of the paranasal sinuses (including the delicate bony leaflets), identify the anatomical variants that may compromise the ventilation of the sinus, and demonstrate extensive pathologic areas or discrete points of diseased mucosa that are responsible for recurrent disease.

The fourth reason is the general improvement of medical care, particularly anesthesia, and the administration of antibiotics to prevent local and intracranial complications.

The fifth reason is related to the contribution of many excellent specialists throughout the world practicing rhinology in different locations and teaching these new surgical techniques to the younger generation of doctors. In this regard, the contributions of (in historical order) Prades,[6] Dixon,[7–9] and Park[10] in microsurgery of the paranasal sinus are very valuable. The concept of functional endoscopic sinus surgery was popularized and disseminated throughout the world by Stammberger (1985)[11–15] and Kennedy (1985).[16–21] Wigand,[22–27] Rice,[28–33] and Levine[34–39] also shared their experience to achieve widespread circulation of this procedure with numerous publications.

Today the concept of functional surgery can be applied to three basic surgical procedures: microscopic sinus surgery, endoscopic sinus surgery, or a combination of both techniques, which has been the author's preference since 1986.[40–42] Other surgeons, including Draf,[43–44] Rudert,[45] and Stamm,[46] are using the same combined technique.

■ Surgical Principles

General Overview

Contemporary sinus surgery has made tremendous progress over the last three decades. This is the natural consequence of a clear understanding of the pathogenesis of sinus diseases, the improvement of imaging studies, and the development of new optical technologies for better diagnosis and surgical treatment. Also the concept of the ostiomeatal complex, pioneered by Messerklinger,[4] has gained wide acceptance. A set of general surgical principles that are applicable to virtually any surgical procedure has been established (Table 11–1).

1. Sinus surgery should be performed after an accurate sinus diagnosis based on clinical history, endoscopic nasal findings, and imaging studies (the basic principle for surgical management of sinus patients). The pathology of the sinus should be clearly established by CT scan prior to any scheduled sinus procedure.

TABLE 11–1   General Principles for Sinus Surgery

1. Accurate sinus diagnosis
2. Sinus surgery should be performed after failure of appropriate medical management
3. Proper surgical planning
4. One-stage integrated treatment of the nose and paranasal sinus
5. Combined management of sinus disease
6. A thorough knowledge of the nose and paranasal sinus anatomy
7. Excellent visualization and minimal bleeding in the surgical field
8. Removal of diseased tissue from the sinuses
9. Restoration of normal drainage and ventilation in the affected sinuses
10. Adequate postoperative follow-up

2. Surgical treatment of sinus disease should be performed after failure of appropriate medical management. This should be the general rule of contemporary sinus surgery, and conservative medical treatment should be the first choice for treating sinus problems. Even with massive nasal polyposis a significant decrease of the polyp mass is achieved after systemic administration of steroids. In this situation, preceding medical management will render the surgical procedure easier and less hazardous by decreasing the polyp mass.

3. Proper surgical planning should be the guideline for a comprehensive and accurate surgical plan supported by the clinical history, the nasal findings by endoscopy, and the preoperative CT scan, although it is possible to find unexpected pathology that should be taken care of during surgery.

4. The concept of one-stage integrated treatment of the nose and paranasal sinus is an adequate approach to treat combined nasal problems and sinus diseases during the same surgical procedure (Table 11–2). The importance of correcting local morphological alterations of the nasal cavity, such as septal deviations, septal perforations, concha bullosa, and hypertrophy of the inferior turbinates, during the same operative procedure should be emphasized. These alterations may decrease the nasal airflow and may affect their mucosal drainage and the ventilation of the sinus and, consequently, may cause sinus problems. On the contrary, an infected sinus may drain purulent material to the nasal cavity, adversely affecting the nasal mucosa, which aggravates sinusitis, particularly when there are

TABLE 11–2   Concept of One-Stage Integrated Treatment of the Nose and Paranasal Sinuses

1. Septoplasty and/or rhinoplasty
2. Reduction of hyperthrophic inferior turbinates
3. General surgical principles for endoscopic sinus surgery

nasal abnormalities. In this situation, a vicious circle is generated between the affected sinus and the pathologic mucosa of the nasal cavity.

This concept of integrated treatment of the nose and paranasal sinuses represents a great advantage for the patient and avoids a second-stage procedure with an acceptable operating time at no increased morbidity and with reduced costs.

5. Combined management of sinus diseases including pre- and/or postoperative medical treatment should be programmed before any surgical intervention and explained to the patient. The pathogenesis and natural course of chronic hypertrophic inflammatory sinusitis are incompletely understood, and many patients with diffuse nasal polyposis, aspirin sensitivity, and asthma require continued medical therapy such as topical nasal steroids and immunotherapy following surgery to maintain control of their symptoms and to decrease the risk of recurrent disease.

It must be recognized that sinus surgery techniques do not provide a cure for all of the inflammatory sinus diseases because the underlying factors are multiple. Allergies, systemic diseases, genetic influences, and environmental pollution are associated with reactive airway disease. Surgical treatment may correct anatomical abnormalities of the nose and sinus, remove the diseased tissues, restore drainage and ventilation, and possibly control the nature of the disease. However, there are other factors including those mentioned before that should also be taken into consideration and may influence the final outcome of the treatment. Tobacco smoking and exposure to environmental tobacco smoke are also important factors implicated in chronic nasal irritation and other respiratory symptoms in children and adults.[47–49] Children exposed to the parental smoking are also at higher risk to develop chronic middle ear effusions and allergic disorders, including allergic rhinitis. It might be expected that after chronic nasal irritation caused by active and passive smoking, such exposure may result in an increased incidence of respiratory disorders of the nose and paranasal sinus, and/or may potentiate the effects of allergies on nasal and sinus functions, and/or may induce the recurrence of sinus disorders after medical/surgical treatment.

6. A thorough knowledge of the nose and paranasal sinus anatomy is of paramount importance. Recognition of the anatomical landmarks that provide surgical guidance is crucial for an effective and safe surgery. The great variability of anatomical structures is a constant feature, and even in the same individual variability occurs from one side to another. Because of these anatomical variations, previous surgical dissections in cadaveric specimens of paranasal sinus should be mandatory before starting surgical treatment of patients with paranasal sinus pathology.

7. Excellent visualization and minimal bleeding are basic surgical requirements for a safe surgery. The use of optical instruments such as the microscope and endoscope allows the surgeon to have an excellent view of the surgical field, including clefts, recesses, niches, and even the inside of the sinus cavities. The contribution of local vasoconstriction to keep bleeding to a minimum is very important.

8. Removal of diseased tissue from the sinus with minimal surgical trauma is another principle of contemporary sinus surgery. One of the priorities of this surgical procedure is the complete and accurate resection of the diseased tissue with maximum preservation of normal-looking mucosa. This concept of functional surgery directed only to a limited removal of irreversibly damaged mucosa and the obstructing anatomy has gained wide acceptance. Even massive inflammatory changes in the sinus mucosa have the capacity to undergo spontaneous healing after restoration of drainage and ventilation. This concept of "reversibility" of mucosal disease has been debated in our specialty for many years, and the merits of aeration versus radical procedures have been discussed. At what point does mucosal disease become irreversible? It is probably better to remove questionable mucosa than to leave it behind and hope that it undergoes transition back to normal tissue, providing that such removal can be safely accomplished.

In severe cases of chronic sinusitis, it is important to remove osteitic bony partitions as thoroughly as possible from the areas of severe mucosal disease. It is possible that these sites have a low-grade chronic osteomyelitis that may be responsible for the recurrent focus of chronic sinusitis.[50] Although the concept of minimally invasive surgical therapy to remove obstructive areas to improve mucociliary clearance and restore normal sinus drainage and ventilation should be applied particularly in early and mild diseases, a more aggressive surgery should be performed with removal of bony partitions where there is more extensive pathology, while at the same time preserving the normal-looking mucosa. However, complete removal of mucosa from the bony surfaces should be avoided because this will increase the possibility of postoperative osteitis and scar formation (Fig. 11–1A and B).

9. Restoration of normal drainage and ventilation from the affected sinus is the concept introduced by Messerklinger.[5] In the past it was believed that chronic inflammatory disorder of the paranasal

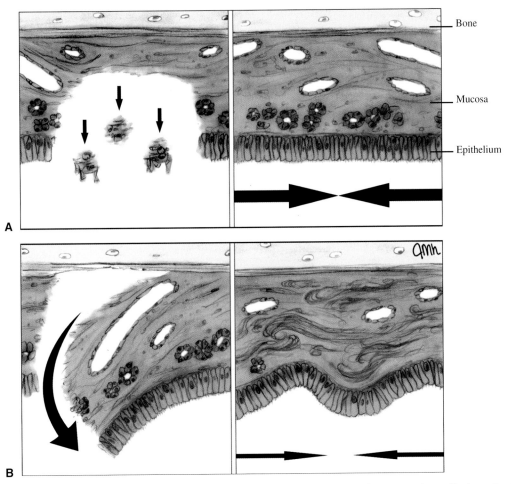

Bone

Mucosa

Epithelium

FIGURE 11–1 Surgical dissection of the sinus mucosa should be very gentle, leaving normal-looking mucosa behind and avoiding exposure of the bony surface as much as possible. (A) The reepithelization with ciliated epithelium is more rapid, with less scarring effect and with a more uniform aspect. (B) Same dissection with denuded bone, more scarring and a less uniform appearance result.

sinuses was an infectious process arising primarily from the affected sinus itself. However, based on studies of mucociliary clearance, Messerklinger was able to demonstrate that the etiology in most patients with chronic or recurrent sinusitis in the ethmoid, maxillary, and frontal sinuses is related to anatomical abnormalities and/or mucosal pathology obstructing the drainage system of these sinuses. Classical surgical procedures for treatment of chronic infections of the sinuses and other disorders, such as nasal polyposis, direct the surgeon to remove diseased tissues in the nose and/or paranasal sinuses. The new surgical openings in the sinus caused by those conventional surgical techniques are in locations distant from the natural ostium, and so treatment of the disease interferes with the mechanism of drainage of secretions of the sinus already disturbed by the infection.

The mucus produced in the anterior ethmoid sinus, maxillary sinus, and frontal sinus drains into an anatomically complex region of the lateral nasal wall called the ostiomeatal complex. The ostiomeatal complex is a narrow anatomical region consisting of multiple bony structures (middle turbinate, uncinate process, ethmoid bulla), air spaces (frontal recess, ethmoid infundibulum, middle meatus), and the ostia of the anterior ethmoid, maxillary, and frontal sinuses. In this area the mucosal surfaces are very close or even in contact with each other, and mucous secretions can be removed easily from the sinus because of the ciliary sweeping motion, which keeps the drainage system functioning. If, however, the opposing mucosal surfaces in this cleft become inflamed and swollen, drainage and ventilation of the sinus may be seriously impaired because the ciliary sweeping motion decreases and eventually ceases. When edema develops, the ostium quickly becomes blocked because of its small diameter, and consequently mucus can no longer be excreted. Also, ventilation that ensures gaseous exchange can be affected, and any alteration of this mechanism can have deleterious consequences. Hypoxia, increasing edema, decreased ciliary motion, and transudate form a vicious circle that facilitates possible infection. Supuration then develops either as a result of aerobic bacterial infection that consumes large amounts of oxygen or by a gradual decrease in pO_2 pressure that makes phagocytosis less effective and permits colonization by anaerobic organisms.

The concept that restoration of the drainage and ventilation systems through the natural ostia using endoscopic sinus surgery can reestablish normal function of the sinus and treat pathological changes in the dependent sinus has radically revolutionized the surgical treatment of sinus diseases.

10. Adequate postoperative follow-up after sinus surgery is mandatory at regular intervals until healing is complete. Endoscopic examination of the nose is advised to clean the crusts, clotted blood, and thick mucus from the nose, ostiomeatal complex area, and accessible regions of the sinus cavities. Synechiae must be removed at an early stage, and lateralization of the middle turbinate should be avoided.

All patients who have undergone endonasal sinus surgery will benefit postoperatively from a prolonged course of nasal irrigations using a saline nasal spray and an aerosol nasal corticosteroid for a shorter period of time following initial healing and diminution of crusting. Patients with allergic rhinitis should be maintained on topical corticosteroids and appropriate pharmacotherapy and immunotherapy.

Surgical Indications

The current indications for surgical treatment of paranasal sinus disease are defined by our knowledge of its pathogenesis, its natural evolution, and how that course can be changed by different treatment modalities. Certainly surgery is one option, and the ultimate goal is to eradicate the disease. However, we should keep in mind that we cannot cure all patients even with the most up-to-date equipment and the best surgical techniques available and properly executed.

The main and most frequent indications for paranasal sinus surgery are summarized in Table 11–3, but their range will continue to increase and expand with new sophisticated equipment and more refined surgical procedures. The surgeon must tailor the operation to the disease and its characteristics, location, and extent. However, the patient's clinical condition, ability to withstand general anesthesia, prolonged postoperative care, and expectations must be considered.

TABLE 11–3   Indications for Paranasal Sinus Surgery

– Inflammatory diseases
  • Chronic sinusitis
  • Complicated acute sinusitis
  • Recurrent acute sinusitis
  • Hyperplastic sinusitis (sinonasal polyposis)
  • Sinus mucoceles
  • Allergic fungal sinusitis
– Neurorhinologic disorders
  • Rhinopathic headaches resistant to medical therapy
– Orbital indications
  • Severe exophthalmos
  • Nasolacrimal duct obstruction
– Restorative indications
  • Cerebrospinal fluid rhinorrhea
  • Severe posterior epistaxis
  • Choanal atresia/stenosis
– Neoplastic diseases
  • Benign tumors (osteoma, hemangiopercytioma, juvenile angiofibroma, and pituitary tumors)
  • Malignant tumors (biopsy for diagnosis and assistance in craniofacial resection)

The most common indication for performing paranasal sinus surgery is chronic sinusitis. However, if adequate medical therapy can control the patient's symptoms and the evolution of the disease, then the benefit of surgery is difficult to justify, and it should be avoided. Most patients with acute sinusitis can be treated with appropriate medical management without the need for surgical intervention. In certain cases with threatening or established complications (e.g., abscess formation), surgery should be performed to achieve drainage of the involved sinuses. In cases of acute sinusitis with periorbital or intraorbital complications, sinus surgery can provide access to the medial orbital wall (lamina papyracea), and resecting the lamina will expose the periorbital fascia to drain the periorbital abscess or to incise the fascia to decompress orbital cellulitis.

Recurrent acute sinusitis is an uncommon indication, and the patient should be evaluated very carefully before the decision to undergo surgery is made. This condition is defined by the absence of significant mucosal disease during the intervals of acute sinusitis episodes. A variety of anatomical abnormalities may be visualized on CT scan in this type of sinusitis, including the concha bullosa and the paradoxical middle turbinate (Fig. 11–2).

Variations of the uncinate process (with either pneumatization or lateralization), excessive aeration of anterior ethmoid cells, enlarged Haller's cells, and agger nasi cells may also be found. These alterations may decrease sinus drainage and ventilation and predispose the patient to recurrent acute sinusitis. An excessively deviated nasal septum may have the same effect by impinging upon the middle turbinate and narrowing the infundibulum. In these cases, medical management may help control the frequency and severity of the infections, but

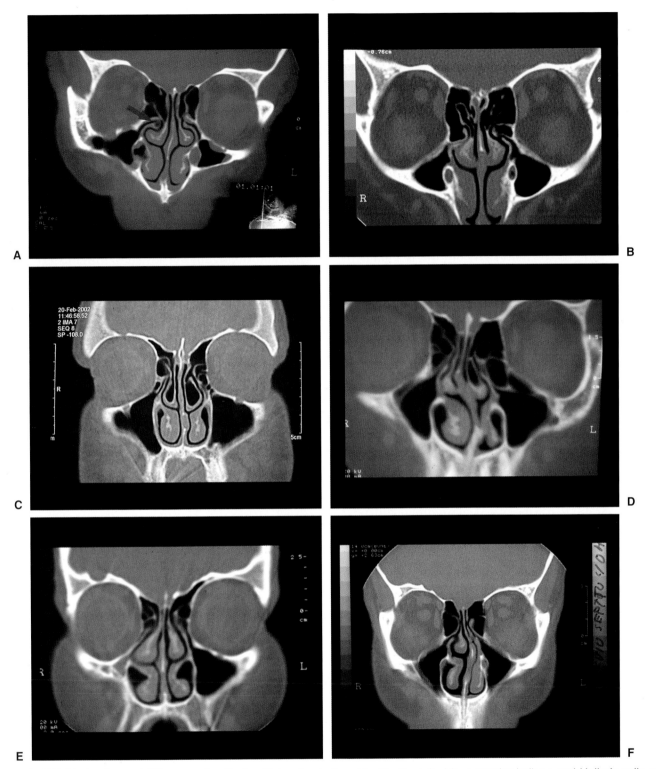

FIGURE 11–2   Coronal CT scans of patients with anatomical abnormalities of the nose and paranasal sinus. (A) Pneumatized right uncinate process. (B) Hypertrophy of the ethmoid bulla obstructing, the right ostiomeatal complex. (C). Bilateral concha bullosa. (D) Deviated nasal septum toward the right side. On the left side a concha bullosa and Haller's cells are obstructing the ostiomeatal complex. (E). Hypoplasia of the right maxillary sinus. (F) Deviated nasal septum pushing the middle turbinate laterally, causing obstruction of the left ostiomeatal complex. (Images courtesy of J. Almeida Pinto.)

only surgery can solve the problem. Usually the maxillary sinus is the affected sinus, and a very limited approach to enlarge the natural ostium is the treatment of choice. The other abnormalities should be surgically treated also using techniques like septoplasty, resection of the lateral lamella of the concha bullosa and partial resection of the middle turbinate to remove the lateralized segment.

Sinonasal polyposis frequently requires both medical and surgical treatment to achieve clinical improvement. The goal of sinus surgery in these patients is to remove the polyps and restore sinus drainage and ventilation. In the presence of extensive polyposis, a complete surgical cure of this disease is unlikely. This situation is related to an underlying mucosal hyperreactivity and general tendency to form polyps. Sinonasal polyposis is a multifactorial disorder, and it should be looked at as a nonspecific local reaction of the mucosa to a great variety of inflammatory, allergic, thermal, toxic, and mechanical stimuli. Consequently, other treatment options should be considered for management of this entity such as adjuvant therapy.

Another indication for sinus surgery is the endoscopic drainage of the sinus mucoceles. The frontal sinus is most commonly involved, followed, in order of frequency, by the ethmoid, sphenoid, and maxillary sinuses.

Allergic fungal sinusitis is an absolute indication for endonasal sinus surgery, and surgery should be considered in patients who do not respond to conventional medical therapy. The goal of this surgical treatment is the complete removal of diseased mucosa, bony partitions, and inspissated material containing fungus that should be sent for staining and culture tests for positive identification. Postoperatively, all patients require adjunctive medical treatment with antibiotics, topical and oral steroids, and oral antifungal agents.

Endoscopic surgery for management of rhinopathic headaches refractory to medical therapy is one of the most controversial indications of sinus surgery. It is possible that, in the absence of sinus inflammation, structural abnormalities may create an intermittent obstruction of the sinus that may induce chronic facial pain syndrome. This phenomenon can be compared with others related to the ear and eustachian tube dysfunction. The sinus CT scan may only reveal bony anatomical variations or abnormalities. In the author's experience, this condition may be misdiagnosed despite a very careful evaluation and screening. During surgical treatment of a limited number of cases, a lateralized uncinate process, a small concha bullosa, or a paradoxical middle turbinate was found. In all cases the mucosa of the infundibulum was edematous, and the maxillary sinus ostium was closed. The procedure itself consisted only of removal of the anatomical abnormalities and the enlargement of the maxillary sinus ostium. In all patients the symptoms

disappeared. Definitive proof of this association, though, depends on resolution of the syndrome after surgical correction. However, in patients complaining of headaches with limited sinus symptomatology, negative neurological work-up, and prolonged medical therapy with nasal steroid spray and decongestant, surgery should be considered the treatment of last resort when other methods have not controlled the complaints.

Endoscopic orbital decompression may be used for surgical treatment of severe exophthalmos (thyroid orbitopathy or Graves' disease), and the results are similar to the conventional techniques with the added advantages of an endoscopic approach.

Nasolacrimal duct obstruction and chronic dacryocystitis requiring surgical intervention can also be managed endoscopically with significant advantages over external intervention.

Cerebrospinal fluid rhinorrhea can be treated with an endoscopic nasal approach with higher success rates using mucosal grafts and, for lesions greater than 5 mm, free bone or cartilage grafts along with a local pedicled mucosal flap. Certainly craniotomy may be required for larger defects, but the endoscopic management of skull base defects avoids the significant morbidity associated with a craniotomy.

Even posterior epistaxis can be treated endoscopically through cauterization or clipping of the sphenopalatine artery. Choanal atresia/stenosis may be managed by removing the stenotic area using this technique.

The role of endoscopic sinus surgery in neoplastic diseases is primarily to treat selected cases of benign tumors, such as osteomas, hemangiopericytomas, juvenile angiofibromas, and pituitary tumors. Vascular lesions should have preoperative embolization to decrease intraoperative bleeding to a minimum. In the author's experience this is an excellent approach, with decreased morbidity and a better postoperative period.

The contribution of endoscopic techniques in relation to malignant tumors is to assist in craniofacial resection. During the tumor resection an endonasal approach provides excellent illumination of the roof of the nasal cavity and guides anterior fossa osteotomies from the cranial side under microscopic visualization of the vertical cuts on both the medial orbital walls after the brain has been retracted posteriorly. The extensive skull base defect following the resection of both ethmoid bones (en bloc resection of anterior cranial floor) is then closed with a bone graft from the internal table of the cranium. Additional resection of adjacent structures can be performed depending on the extent of disease. This is the perfect example of the benefit of combined microscopic and endoscopic sinus surgery (COMET surgery).

Other indications for paranasal sinus surgery and special procedures will be covered in other chapters of this book.

TABLE 11–4   Preoperative Evaluation of Patients with Sinus Diseases

Absolute	Relative
• Clinical history • Complete ORL examination • Nasal endoscopy • Computed tomography (coronal and axial scans)	• Rhinomanometry and acoustic rhinometry • Allergy testing • Olfactometry • Mucociliary testing • Nasal citology • Sweat test (children) • Immunoglobulin studies • Nasal mucosal biopsy

Preoperative Evaluation

The outcome of paranasal sinus surgery depends on a very careful preoperative evaluation, including a complete otorhinolaryngologic examination with special emphasis on the nose and paranasal sinuses, and a collection of general medical information about the clinical condition of the patient. The routine examination comprehends a clinical history, physical examination, and complementary testing considered necessary for an accurate diagnosis (Table 11–4).

The clinical history related with the nose and paranasal sinuses is directed to the most common symptoms: nasal obstruction, nasal stuffiness, anterior nasal discharge, postnasal drip, mucopurulent rhinorrhea, itchy nose, sneezing, disorders of smell, facial pain, pressure, and headaches. Questioning should be systematic and should also cover the symptoms of ear diseases (e.g., hearing loss, popping and itching in the ears, and sensations of pressure). Chronic throat symptoms, such as slight discomfort, pain, dry sensation, scratchy throat, and frequent throat clearing, are often due to discharge from an infected nasal region and/or chronic sinusitis flowing down the pharynx. Also, pulmonary symptoms (coughing, spitting, wheezing, etc.), diseases of the teeth and jaws, allergic symptoms, eye complaints (eye pressure, pain, watery eyes, etc.), dizziness, chronic fatigue, weight loss, inflammatory diseases of the joints, autonomic disorders, and skin and systemic diseases, such as diabetes and hypertension, should be inquired about. The clinical history should establish the timing of the symptoms, duration of the disease (acute, chronic, or recurrent), tobacco smoking, current medications, previous surgeries, and complications.

The nasal examination should be performed in a routine fashion looking for morphologic abnormalities and characteristics of the nasal mucosa and its secretions. Particular attention should be paid to the lateral nasal wall and the middle turbinate area, although often this cannot be accomplished until a nasal spray decongestant is applied. This nasal inspection can also be accomplished using the microscope as the light source instead of a headlight (Fig. 11–3). The author has used the microscope for routine otorhinolaryngologic examination for the past 20 years because it provides better illumination and amplification.

If the nasal abnormalities are detected by anterior or posterior microrhinoscopy, no further examination is necessary. However, if the nasal examination under the microscope needs further evaluation or is otherwise incomplete, it should be combined with nasal endoscopy.

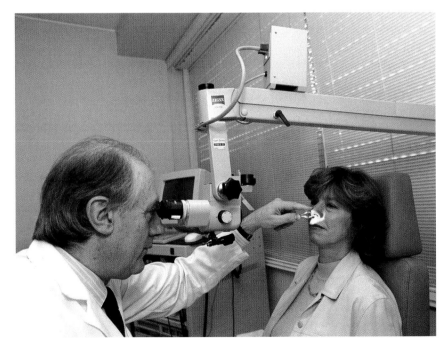

FIGURE 11–3   Routine otorhinolaryngologic examination using the microscope.

This diagnostic technique is best performed by spraying the nose with a vasoconstrictor (0.5% phenilephrine hydrochloride) and an anesthetic agent (10% lidocaine) and allowing them to work for a few minutes. Then the entire nasal cavity should be systematically examined (including the nasopharynx) with a rigid 0-degree, 4 mm endoscope, or, if it is difficult to pass between the middle turbinate and the lateral nasal wall, a 30-degree, 2.7 mm endoscope. The flexible 3.2 mm endoscope is preferable with children. Again, particular attention should be paid to the middle meatus, where it is likely that the main changes will be found. Using videoendoscopy, these findings can be stored on a digital videotape, and with a laser printer the resulting images can be printed for the patient's chart.

Computed tomography has become the main radiological investigation for sinonasal pathology and is absolutely mandatory for sinus surgery. By presenting bone and soft tissue details, it defines structural abnormalities, as well as the location and extension of disease, and often indicates the diagnosis when certain characteristic features are present. A coronal CT scan and axial CT projections provide comprehensive and detailed information about the nose and the paranasal sinus anatomy, its variations, relationships of important surrounding structures, and pathologic findings.

The rhinologist must develop a special expertise in this imaging technique that will allow him or her to read the images, follow them carefully in the operating room, and compare them with the intraoperative findings. The clinical examination is mandatory, but the correlation with the imaging studies is absolutely necessary to make an accurate diagnosis and to manage the patient correctly according to his or her problem.

Other tests, such as the rhinomanometry and acoustic rhinometry,[51–60] are performed on patients complaining of nasal obstruction in the routine preoperative evaluation. The rhinomanometry is an objective nasal test that measures nasal airway resistance by making a quantitative measurement of nasal flow and pressure. Acoustic rhinometry is another nasal test based on sound reflection that provides an estimate of the cross-sectional area as a function of distance from the nostril. Both are indicated mainly for quantification of pre- and posttherapy (medical and/or surgical) for nasal obstruction, for exclusion of functional disorders, and for medicolegal purposes. Nasal respiration and paranasal sinus aeration are not always correlated. However, improvement of the nasal air passages will contribute to the recovery of the sinus from sinusitis. In this situation, surgical treatment of the deviated nasal septum and/or the hyperthrophic inferior turbinates together with paranasal sinus surgery is essential to correct the nose and paranasal sinus unit. All of these procedures can be performed during the same operation, which the author calls one-stage integrated surgical treatment.

If there are systemic allergic disorders such as asthma, dermatitis, conjunctivitis, or gastrointestinal disturbances, or an underlying allergy coupled with nasal symptoms, then allergy testing is requested. The skin prick test, IgE antibodies (RAST) test, and serum IgE (PRIST) test are very useful for identification of the allergens responsible for the symptoms.[61–66]

Preoperative olfactometry is very valuable for assessing disturbances of the olfaction and the results of ethmoid procedures in diffuse polyposis. Dysosmia is often caused by inflammation of the olfactory mucosa, and it improves after careful endoscopic management of the polypoid mucosa of the olfactory cleft. Other tests, such as mucociliary testing and nasal cytology, may be useful for additional information, but they should not be considered routine tests for preoperative evaluation.[67–74]

In children with chronic recurrent sinusitis, the sweat test should be used to rule out cystic fibrosis, and determination of immunoglobulins and immunoglobulin classes, along with nasal mucosa biopsy to establish the diagnosis of ciliary diskinesia.[75–78]

After reviewing these tests for preoperative evaluation, it should be concluded that clinical examination of the patient together with the imaging studies is essential for an accurate diagnosis. Other tests should be performed according to the clinical judgment. Correct diagnosis and the establishment of a surgical plan can be achieved in most situations by combining clinical examination, endoscopic results, and imaging studies.

The author strongly advises having a protocol for sinus surgery to evaluate sinus symptoms and to describe the nasal endoscopic and CT scan findings, surgical planning, and the results of surgery. It is a great effort toward data standardization that can be stored in a computer for a better update and follow-up, analysis of long-term results, and interchange of medical information.

Surgical Planning

After a careful preoperative evaluation, an accurate diagnosis can be established, and a treatment plan must be developed and introduced to the patient. The surgical procedure should be defined by the clinical examination, and the objective findings encountered during the preoperative evaluation must follow the surgical principles already described and must be performed according to the surgeon's experience. The age of the patient and his or her medical conditions, expectations should also be considered before a final decision is made and the patient is scheduled for surgery.

Preoperative medication should be recommended before surgery in patients who have suppurative sinusitis. They should receive an appropriate oral antibiotic for

10 to 12 days before the surgical procedure. Patients with massive polyposis should take a short treatment of oral corticosteroids immediately before surgical treatment with a "booster" dose intraoperatively. Hypertension and diabetes must be controlled before surgical intervention with the cooperation of an internist. Medications, such as aspirin and nonsteroidal anti-inflammatory drugs that prolong bleeding should be discontinued before the operation.

The different phases of the treatment plan, including preoperative remarks, type and extent of surgery, and the postoperative follow-up, should be discussed with the patient. The final outcome of the treatment, including possible risks and complications of surgery, should also be stressed. Certainly the surgeon's experience and his or her trust in the results are very important factors in convincing the patient to accept the proposed treatment plan and sign the informed consent.

■ Instrumentation

Surgical Equipment

Two optical systems are used to surgically treat the nose and paranasal sinuses: the microscope and the endoscope. The combination of both systems during the same surgical procedure is called combined microscopic and endoscopic technique (COMET surgery).

The majority of the surgical operation is performed with the Zeiss operating microscope OPMI ORL (Fig. 11–4) equipped with coaxial fiberoptic, cold-light illumination with a 12 V, 100 W halogen reflector lamp (cold light), spot illumination, 0-degree central illumination, 1:6 zoom magnification, 180-degree wide field tiltable tubes with eyepieces, and motorized internal fine focusing. A stereo co-observation tube with excellent ergonomic conditions is used for the assistant, and another

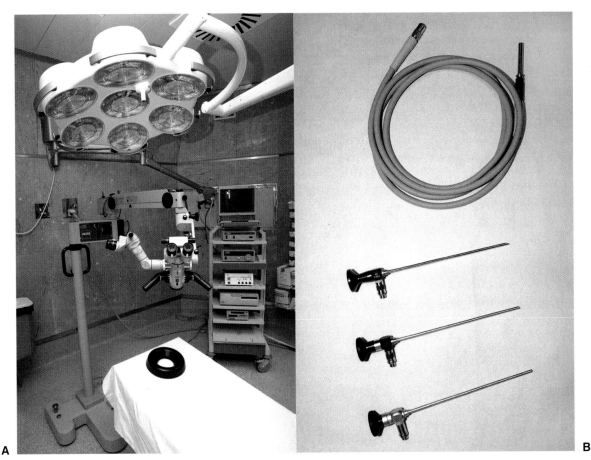

A   B

FIGURE 11–4 The two optical systems used in COMET surgery. (A) Zeiss operating microscope OPM1 with 300 mm lens. Next to the microscope is the Karl Storz Mobile Videocart (Karl Storz, Tuttlingen, Germany) containing the video endoscopic system (color monitor, cold-light fountain, endo-camera, video recorder, and video printer). (B) Standard 4 mm Hopkins rod telescopes with 0-, 30-, and 70-degree angled lenses.

arm with a video camera system is adapted to the microscope and fitted with a lens with a focal length of 300 mm.

Another optical aid is the endoscope. Several endoscopes are available for performing endoscopic procedures. A rigid telescope with a brighter illumination source provides an excellent clear field of vision. The improved telescopes incorporate wide views of the peripheral field along with magnified images of the anatomical structures. The built-in mechanism of angled vision in the rigid telescopes provides the further advantage of viewing deeper areas located in narrow clefts. Angled telescopes are therefore useful to see inside the sinuses, around corners, and into niches, recesses, or ducts.

The viewing angles of telescopes range from 0 to 120 degrees. They are all available in standard or wide angles. The standard diameter is 4 mm for surgical procedures in adults. The smaller diameter 30-degree, 2.7 mm telescopes are used to view through the trocar sleeve and are also used for pediatric patients. The 0- and 30-degree, 4 mm diameter telescopes are the most useful. The 70-degree telescope is often required to visualize hidden pathology or deep lateral wall structures inside the sinuses. The telescopes have a length of 18 cm, and they have a connection for a fiberoptic light cable. The relationship between the diameter and the length of an endoscope requires a complex optical rod system. The intermediate image produced by the lens is transposed through a series of rod-lens inversion systems over the length of the endoscope sheath. The term *inversion system* means that each one of these systems inverts the image. The image is always returned to its correct position if there is an even number of rod lenses in the system. The intermediate image from the last (proximal) inversion system is displayed and enlarged through the eyepiece of the telescope. Cold-light illumination, provided by a powerful xenon light source and conducted by film optic light cables, is always used.

Video recording of the images obtained with a small change-coupled device (CCD-type) video camera attached to both the microscope and the telescope is extremely important for surgical demonstration of endonasal surgery and, therefore, for teaching purposes and for medical documentation. The high light sensitivity of modern video systems permits their use with moderate-intensity light sources. For video recording, the most widely used and best for compatibility are VHS and $_S$VHS 8 mm formats. The 8 mm formats have the convenience of small tape size, which facilitates storage. For most purposes, the $_S$VHS is a good compromise between convenient size and image quality. The recording techniques of still photography and video imaging permit retention of images for later retrieval and also offer the ability to compare images before and after treatment. Recently, with the introduction of a digital still recorder with superior image quality, images can be obtained as still pictures of video recording. Because of their superior quality, these images are recommended for publication and teaching.

In a teaching hospital, an endoscopic camera is a necessity and can be linked to an endoscope or to the sidearm on the operating microscope, permitting all the staff or those outside the operating room to follow the surgery. Although cameras are available using couplings with or without beam splitters (which provide the surgeon with visualization through the endoscope), the former is recommended.

A wide range of microsurgical instruments is available for endoscopic nasal surgery, including sickle knives, rasps, probes, elevators, suction tubes, curettes, and microscissors. The basic set also contains punches and forceps. The backbiting forceps have a through-cutting mechanism that prevents tearing and stripping of the mucosa and leaves a smoother cut than the standard grasping/biting jaws. The cutting punches allow removal of tissue with preservation of neighboring viable mucosa. These instruments have been modified since the beginning of endoscopic sinus surgery to have a more narrow profile and a longer jaw. Other modifications include downbiting forceps, sidebiting forceps, and a forceps with a rotating head that allows any orientation of the jaws. The set also contains giraffe forceps with a long, thin shaft capable of changing angles (hence the name giraffe forceps). The standard set should also have a drill with an angulated hand piece and extra-long diamond burs (used in sphenoid sinus and transnasal surgery of the hypohysis). Other instruments, such as forceps with offset handles for intranasal bipolar coagulation and semi-rigid coagulation probes, complete the set of surgical equipment to perform sinus surgery.

■ Optical Principles

Microscopes have been well-established magnifying equipment in practical use in otorhinolaryngology, and their sophistication has reached powerful limits with the current technologies. In 1923, Holmgren introduced the binocular operative microscope without coaxial light for ear surgery.[79]

Endonasal surgery and laryngeal microsurgery accompany the historical developments of ear surgery. In 1958, Heermann pioneered the use of the binocular Zeiss operating microscope with coaxial illumination in endonasal surgery.[2] Kleinsasser was the founder of modern laryngeal microsurgery in 1962, using a Zeiss operating microscope.[80]

Since the beginning, the application of the operating microscope has been the standard method of optical aid in otorhinolaryngology. In 1972, Messerklinger developed the concept of endoscopic sinus surgery using

TABLE 11–5   Main Parameters of Any Optical System

- Focal distance (working distance)
- Depth of field (focus)
- Numerical aperture
- Field of view
- Resolution limit
- Luminance (brightness)
- Distortion
- Cleanliness and protection

nasal endoscopes. This has revolutionized, improved, and radically changed the techniques used for the diagnosis and treatment of patients with sinus disease.

Other surgeons, including this author, are continuing to use both instruments, combining microscopic and endoscopic techniques (COMET surgery).

Optical Performances

The two basic optical instruments used for sinus surgery are the microscope and the endoscope. It is absolutely necessary for technical knowledge and teaching purposes to describe the main parameters of any optical system[81] and to compare the characteristics of these optical aids based on optical performance and ergonomic capabilities. Although there are several relationships between the main characteristic parameters of any optical system, for practical reasons, the most important and currently used ones are described here (Tables 11–5 and 11–6).

The focal distance (working distance) defines the clearance or distance between the object and the first surface of a lens system. It affects the user's ability to image and manipulate the sample at the same time. The working distance increases with the objective focal length. For the microscope, the focal distance is variable and finely adjustable. The range is in the order of 300 mm, giving very ample volume for all surgical work. The head of the surgeon, once working on a region, remains steady behind the ocular, and the adjustment of the focus is simple by rotating the focusing knob.

For the endoscope, the focal distance is fixed, not adjustable. The range is in the order of a few millimeters. The working volume is very small. The head and one of the hands of the surgeon have to move to focus. The surgeon has to bow his or her head over the patient and remain at a close distance to see through the endoscope.

The depth of field (focus) is the distance by which the image (or object) may be shifted longitudinally with respect to a reference plane (retina of optical system) without introducing unacceptable blur. In practice, this represents the visible depth of the object.

The microscope presents a much larger depth of field, providing a deeper volume of visibility. Also, the depth of focus is much greater, and the surgeon can comfortably move his or her eyes behind the ocular lens. With the endoscope, the depth of field is shorter; therefore, the endoscope must be finely moved by hand to examine in depth. The depth of focus is short, and consequently the eyes of the surgeon have to move together with the endoscope to keep the image in focus.

The numerical aperture is related to the depth of field (focus), the luminance, and the resolution of the system. The illumination of an image is proportional to the square of the numerical aperture. The numerical

TABLE 11–6   Microscopic versus Endoscopic Optical Characteristics

Optical characteristics	Microscope	Endoscope
Focal distance	• Variable and finely adjustable • Larger working volume	Fixed, not adjustable Small working volume
Depth of field (Focus)	Larger, with a deeper volume of visibility	Shorter; the surgeon's eyes move in sync with the endoscope
Numerical aperture	More light is required; when illuminating a larger area, resolution is smaller	Image looks brighter, better fine details, although field extension is much smaller
Field of view	More extended (as is the volume); surgeon observes the full movement of the total body of surgical	Smaller; surgeon sees only the tip of the surgical instruments and cannot follow the movement
except		
	Instruments	within a short range
Resolution limit	Smaller but very adequate; can be varied and adjusted	Higher, giving finer details; resolution is fixed, and the endoscope must be changed whenever resolution has to be adjusted
Luminance (brightness of image)	Smaller, can be adjusted by using a stronger light source; uniform without bright spots	Higher, with strong reflections; bright spots occur with frequency, which may cause temporary discomfort to the surgeon
Distortion	**Smaller**	**Higher**
Cleanliness and protection	The entire optical system is away from the surgical field, so the system is clean and protected	Part of the optical system is placed within the working surgical volume and constantly affected by fogging, staining, and accidental scratching

aperture in the microscope is smaller, more light is required (illuminating a larger area), and resolution limit is smaller than in the endoscope. However, it can be varied and adjusted. In the endoscope, the numerical aperture is higher and the image looks brighter and has better fine details, although the image field extension is much smaller. The numerical aperture is fixed, and the endoscope must be moved.

The field of view is the volume within which there is image formation. In the microscope, the field of view is much more extended, as is the volume. The surgeon is able to follow the movement of almost the entire body of the surgical instruments. With the endoscope, the field of view is much smaller. The surgeon can see only the tip of the surgical tools and therefore follow the movement only within a short range (Fig. 11–5).

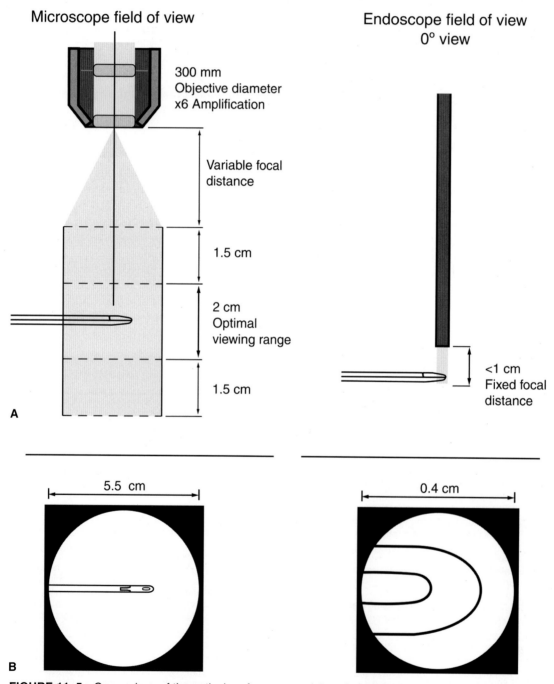

FIGURE 11–5 Comparison of the optical performances of the microscope versus the endoscope. (A) Field of view of the microscope. (B) Field of view of the endoscope.

The resolution limit expresses the distance between two points that can be still separated at the image plane. With the microscope, the resolution limit is smaller, but only by less then an order of magnitude, which is very adequate. Resolution can be varied and adjusted.

With the endoscope, the resolution, in principle, is higher, giving finer details in a clear form. However, the resolution is fixed, and the endoscope must be changed whenever the numerical aperture and the resolution have to be adjusted.

The luminance (brightness of the image) is the quantity of light flux passing through a point on a specific surface, in a specified direction per unit of projected area, and per unit solid angle in the given direction. For the microscope, the luminance is smaller, but it can be adjusted, either by using a stronger light source or by increasing the numerical aperture. In practice, it does not represent a disadvantage. The luminance is uniform without bright spots. The endoscope intrinsically presents a higher luminance. However, due to the mechanism, if illumination is by fiber optics and the image forming process is fiber optics, the used light source has to be more intense. In practice, the problem is solved, and the luminance of the image is good. Nevertheless, as the tip of the endoscope acts as a light source very close to the surgical instruments with highly reflective surfaces, strong reflections occur during the procedure that saturate the image, and bright spots occur with frequency. This may cause temporary discomfort to the surgeon, but slight adjustments of light intensity during surgery can be performed.

The distortion is related to technical performance of the optical system, which has imperfections and does not handle perfect spherical waves. Distortion is one of the so-called primary aberrations Efforts are being made to design an optical system that minimizes aberrations and optimizes its performance for this application.

The design of the optical microscope leads to smaller distortion. In the endoscope, the number of optical elements for aberration correction generally causes a higher distortion.

Cleanliness and protection are relevant for preservation and operation purposes. Because the microscope

TABLE 11–7 Microscopic and Endoscopic Main Optical Performances

Optical characteristics	Microscope	Endoscope
Objective focal length	0.5–100 mm	0.2–5 mm
Magnification	5X–5000X	2X–26X
Numerical aperture	0.10–0.96	0.25–0.7
Resolution power	<430 l p/mm	250–400 l p/mm
Depth of field	Few μm	Mm to ∞
Field of view	6–20 mm	30°–120°
Distortion	Smaller	Larger

has all optical systems far away from the surgical field, it presents as an ideal solution. The endoscope is placed within the area to be treated, and so is constantly affected by fogging, staining, and accidental scratching.

Table 11–7 summarizes the main optical performances of the microscope and endoscope.

Ergonomic Performances

The main ergonomic differences between the microscope and endoscope are presented in Table 11–8.

The microscope is ideal, as the instrument itself is far away, there is a large field of view and large volume depth, and both hands of the surgeon remain free for the surgical work. A unique optical instrument is used during the full intervention. The instrument is rigid and self-supported, permitting a point of view for the surgeon that is easily adjustable. The main advantages are total freedom of both hands combined with binocular view and large working volume under global visual monitoring. The endoscope requires the use of one of the surgeon's hands. The surgeon eye is closed to the endoscopic viewer and one hand has to follow all of the fine movements of the instrument. This is a monocular system that intrinsically causes fatigue (CCD cameras can be used to release freedom). The surgical instruments are only seen clearly when close to the tip of the endoscope. A set of various endoscopes are used during surgery. They have the advantage of an angled view, but the surgeon must keep the plane of reference in mind once the field of view is small. The resolution is intrinsically higher, and the images give crisp details.

TABLE 11–8 Microscopic versus Endoscopic Ergonomic Capabilities

Microscope	Endoscope
One instrument during surgery, rigid and self-supported, easy adjustments	Various sets of endoscopes during surgery
Binocular vision, large working volume under global visual monitoring at all times (CCD cameras can be incorporated)	Monocular system producing tiredness (CCD cameras can be incorporated)
Instrument is far away from the surgical field, and both hands of surgeon remain free	Generally requires the use of one of the surgeon's hands
The optical system is away from the surgical field ⇒ cleanliness and protection	Part of the optical system is placed within the working surgical volume, affected by bleeding, fogging, staining, and accidental scratching
Easier manipulation, less training is needed	More difficult, requires more training

TABLE 11–9 Advantages of the Combined Microscopic and Endoscopic Techniques (COMET Surgery)

Main characteristics	Microscopic	Endoscopic	Combined
Binocular vision	Yes	No	Yes
Permanent exposure of operative field	Yes	No	Yes
Magnification	Yes	No	Yes
Three-dimensional view	Yes	No	Yes
Angled view	No	Yes	Yes
Two hands for surgery	Yes	Generally No	Yes

Combined Microscopic and Endoscopic Optical and Ergonomic Performances

The advantages and disadvantages of both surgical instruments have been demonstrated. Thus, an adequate combination and integration of both systems with new imaging technologies (namely, with CCD cameras) may offer an optimization of available optical capabilities and ergonomic advantages (Table 11–9).

Positioning

Patients of COMET surgery are always under general anesthesia and placed in the supine position, with the head slightly elevated and gently rotated toward the direction opposite the surgeon (Fig. 11–6). This position

is very comfortable for the standing posture of the surgeon because the patient's nose is right in front of the surgeon's eyes.

The surgical team is positioned as shown in Figure 11–7, with the surgeon and the assistant at the right side of the patient for surgery on the nose and left sinuses. The surgeon will move to the left side (the assistant stays on the right side) for surgery of the right sinus. The anesthesiologist stands at the left side monitoring the anesthesia, and the scrub nurse remains at the right side of the surgeon and patient.

The assistant is always following the surgery through the co-observation tube of the microscope or viewing the monitor while the surgeon is doing the endoscopy. When a self-retaining speculum is not used, the assistant can also hold the nasal speculum, which gives the surgeon two free hands to proceed with the different steps of the planned sinus surgery with the help of a third hand from the assistant.

There are two tables: one in front of the nurse across the patient's legs containing surgical instruments for nasal surgery, and the other behind the nurse with microinstruments for paranasal surgery and endoscopes (Fig. 11–8). The Zeiss operating microscope is placed behind the patient and moved into position whenever necessary. The mobile video cart (containing a cold-light fountain, a color monitor, and a complete video system) stays on the left side of the patient, close to the Zeiss operating microscope.

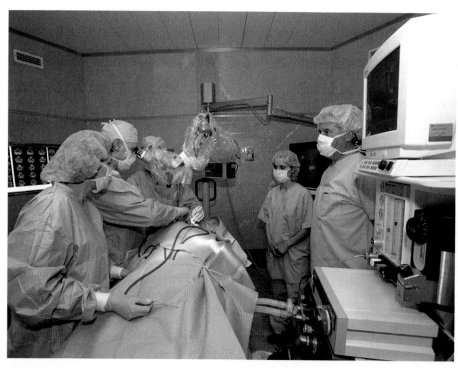

FIGURE 11–6 Position of the patient for COMET surgery. Patient is under general anesthesia, with his head slightly elevated and gently rotated toward the direction opposite the surgeon.

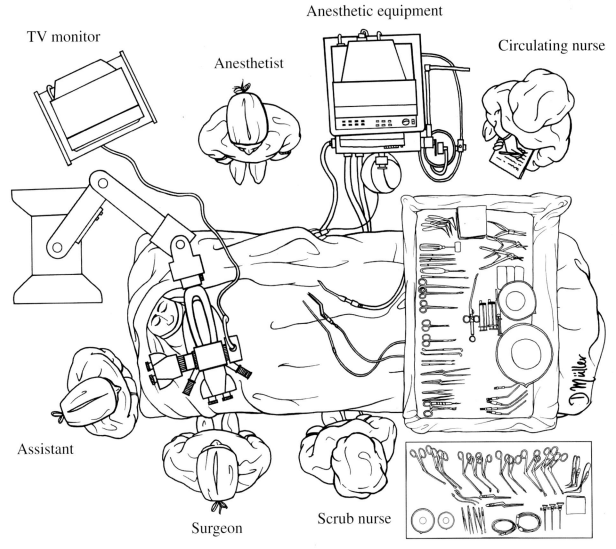

FIGURE 11–7 Operating room setup and position of the surgical team.

The CT scans are displayed in the operating room and should be visible for immediate reading if necessary.

Anesthesia Considerations

The choice of anesthesia depends on former training, and personal experience of the surgeon. The author prefers general endotracheal anesthesia (with controlled hypotension, if possible), combined with local vasoconstriction. For more extensive procedures involving one-stage integrated treatment with correction of nasal problems and sinus pathology, general anesthesia should always be recommended to spare the patient anxiety. To prevent the swallowing of blood, nasal secretions, and fluid from irrigation of the nasal tissues, pharyngeal packing is used.

The primary reasons for the choice of general anesthesia are efficiency, immobilization of the patient, thesia are efficiency, immobilization of the patient, freedom of instrument use due to lack of intraoperative pain and anxiety, controlled ventilation (especially important for asthmatics), and avoidance of aspiration. No increased bleeding is observed, and even suction irrigation is not a problem for the intubated patient (Table 11–10).

The patient receives a premedication with diazepam 2 hours prior to surgery. Also, there is a protocol for general anesthesia covering various intravenous medications before intubation: a hypnotic (propofol), an analgesic (fentanyl), and a muscular relaxant (vecuronium). Then the patient is intubated, and a gas mixture of O_2, N_2O, and sevoflurane is used for anesthesia. An endotracheal tube must be fixed to the chin with nonallergic tape, and a modern silicone tube with a special wire and a high-volume, low-pressure cuff should be used to prevent narrowing due to kinking. The oropharynx is packed with a moist gauze roll.

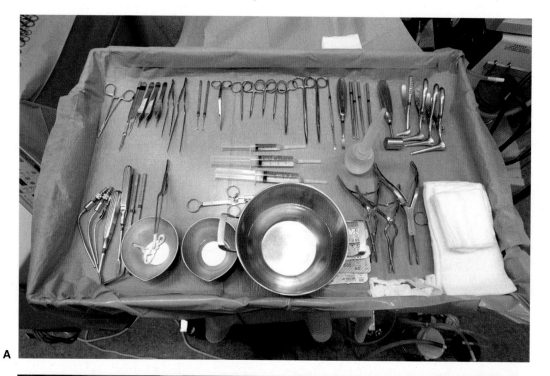

A

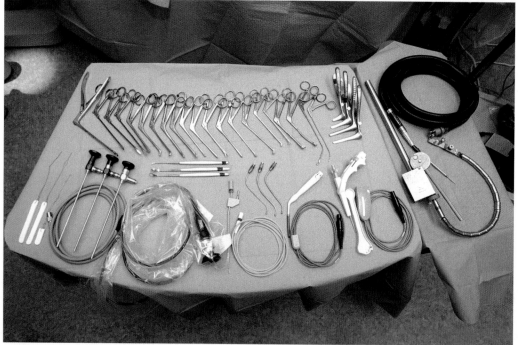

B

FIGURE 11–8 Surgical instruments used for (A) nasal surgery and (B) endoscopic sinus surgery, including different instrumentation for treatment of the hypertrophic inferior turbinates.

Next, the intubated patient is draped and prepared, leaving the nasal area and the internal corners of the eyes uncovered. Topical anesthesia of the nasal cavity is started with small gauze sponges soaked with 1% lidocaine and 1:100,000 epinephrine prepared in a small metal cup. The sponges are introduced with a bayonet forceps into the nasal cavity and left in place for 3 minutes. Following topical anesthesia, a local infiltration with a three-ring syringe and a special septal needle containing 5 to 10 mL of a mixture of 1% lidocaine and

TABLE 11–10   Features of General Anesthesia with Controlled Hypotension Combined with Local Vasconstriction

1. Very safe procedure
2. Excellent efficiency
3. Controlled ventilation, especially important for asthmatics
4. No increased risk of cardiopulmonary complications with monitoring
5. Avoidance of aspiration of postnasal drainage of blood, secretions, and saline from irrigation
6. Excellent hemostasis
7. Great visibility
8. Easier instrumentation
9. Possibility of suction-irrigation
10. More comfortable for the patient

1:200,000 epinephrine is used for vasoconstriction of the septum and the tip of the nose under microscopic guidance. Finally, cocaine paste is applied topically with moist cotton pledgets. The formula contains 18% cocaine hydrochloride and 0.03% epinephrine. The dose must be limited to a small amount, 100 to 150 mg of cocaine paste for each side of the nose for at least 5 minutes. Table 11–11 indicates the protocol for controlled local vasoconstriction under monitored vital signs after general anesthesia.

It is usually recommended to maintain the blood pressure stable with mean values between 7.5 and 8 mm Hg. Care should be taken to avoid low hypotension because of the arterial compromise of cerebral vascularization. To do so, the concentration of sevoflurane can be increased or decreased but should never exceed 2%. If hypotension cannot be reached with this measure, a solution of labetalol should be administered in small and fractionated doses.

General anesthesia with controlled hypotension and local vasconstriction reduces the intraoperative bleeding to a minimum and provides a bloodless field as if working with local anesthesia. In over 1000 combined sinus procedures performed with the patient under general anesthesia, the author has never had any intraoperative anesthetic complication or even any complication immediately following surgery.

TABLE 11–11   Protocol for Mucosal Vasoconstriction

1. Topical application of small gauze strips soaked in 1% lidocaine with 1:100,000 epinephrine
2. Local infiltration of 1% lidocaine with 1:200,000 epinephrine from 5 to 10 mL
3. Minimal topical application of 18% cocaine paste containing 0.03% epinephrine

Surgical Technique

Endonasal sinus surgery can be performed following different surgical steps that are dependent on the nature, location, and extent of the disease. For a better understanding of the surgical plan, a systematic step-by-step scenario is described, according to the concept of one-stage integrated treatment (Table 11–12).

Septoplasty and/or Rhinoplasty

Surgery should follow the initial treatment plan. If this plan involves surgical treatment of the deviated nasal septum for improvement of nasal ventilation, the septoplasty will be performed under controlled vision of the microscope at all times. This technique is thus named microseptoplasty. If this situation is associated with a cosmetic problem, a rhinoplasty is added to the initial procedure. The use of the microscope offers great advantages for this procedure by providing excellent illumination all along the nasal cavity with amplification (particularly important in revision cases). For almost 20 years the author has used the microscope for nasal procedures, and his degree of personal satisfaction with

TABLE 11–12   Strategic Approach to Endonasal Sinus Surgery (COMET Surgery)

Step 1: Patient under general anesthesia
Step 2: Local vasoconstriction of the nasal cavity
Step 3: Septoplasty and/or rhinoplasty, if necessary (microscopic)
Step 4: Management of the middle turbinate (removal of concha bullosa, if necessary)
Step 5: Uncinectomy (microscopic)
Step 6: Maxillary antrostomy (COMET)
- Removal of sinus disease
- Irrigation with warm normal saline
- Endoscopy of the maxillary sinus with 30-, 70-degree, 4 mm telescopes
- Removal of residual diseased tissue with angled forceps (if necessary)
Step 7: Ethmoidectomy (partial and/or total) (microscopic)
- Removal of sinus disease
- Irrigation with warm normal saline
Step 8: Frontal sinusotomy (COMET)
- Endoscopy of the frontal recess with 30-degree, 4 mm telescope
- Removal of polypoid tissue with curved forceps (if necessary)
- Irrigation with warm normal saline
Step 9: Sphenoidotomy (COMET)
- Removal of sinus disease
- Endoscopy of the sphenoid sinus with 30-, 70-degree, 4 mm telescopes
- Removal of residual diseased tissue with angled forceps (if necessary)
- Irrigation with warm normal saline
Step 10: Removal of the posterior third and radiofrequency thermal ablation of the anterior and middle thirds of the hypertrophic inferior turbinates (microscopic)

its application in the nasal area is enormous. The surgical technique used for septoplasty under microscopic vision is the classical technique, modified by the author, and adapted to each individual case.

The surgical procedure continues with the approach to the paranasal sinuses after septal correction. However, in a nose crowded with nasal polyps, a microscopic polypectomy is performed prior to sinus surgery to open the nasal airway and allow for identification of landmarks.

Management of the Middle Turbinate

The anatomical variants of the middle turbinate may cause middle meatal obstruction. This problem should be handled under microscopic control before sinus surgery. A small concha bullosa that does not interfere with sinus drainage or that does not cause obstruction generally is not resected unless diseased. However, in the presence of a large concha bullosa where the head of the middle turbinate is enlarged, round, and smooth, resection of the concha bullosa should take place. After local vasoconstriction using the protocol decribed in Table 11–11, the turbinoplasty is performed by incising the inferior free border of the middle turbinate along its length and carrying the incision up to the neck. The incision is then carried forward to the anterior end. The mucosa of the neck and the upper part of the head of the turbinate facing the lateral nasal wall should be preserved to prevent adhesions (Table 11–13).

The incision is further enlarged using the microscissors, and the lateral half of the concha is removed after elevating the mucosal flap from the lateral bony wall (Fig. 11–9). There is sometimes polypoid mucosa inside

the concha bullosa with a plug of mucus that can be infected also. It should be removed. Then, a mucosal flap on the medial side is elevated to expose the bony lamella of the middle turbinate. The redundant inferior portion of the middle turbinate is then trimmed with turbinate scissors. The elevated medial mucosal flap is rolled up and laterally to cover the inferior border and

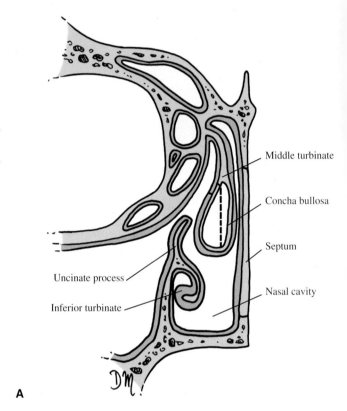

Middle turbinate

Concha bullosa

Septum

Nasal cavity

Uncinate process

Inferior turbinate

A

TABLE 11–13   Surgical Remarks about the Middle Turbinate

Landmarks	Lateral nasal wall
	Skull base
Anatomical variants	Concha bullosa
	Paradoxical middle turbinate
	Lateralized middle turbinate
Surgical technique	Exposure of conchal bullosa
	Partial conchal resection using the local mucosa flap
	Resection of the portion of the paradoxical turbinate that compresses the lateral nasal wall
Recommendations	Preserve the medial portion of the middle turbinate to protect the lamina cribriform unless there is a concha bullosa
	Surgical dissection only lateral to the middle turbinate, never medial to it
	Avoid twisting or fracture the middle turbinate CSF fistula
Goals	Removal of secretions, mucus, and polypoid material from inside the conchal bullosa
	Enlargement of the middle meatus air space for improved drainage and ventilation

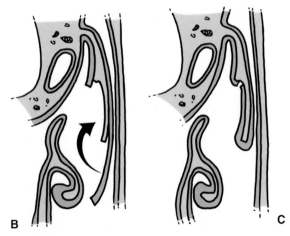

B   **C**

FIGURE 11–9 Surgical management of a concha bullosa. (A) Resection of the lateral half of a concha bullosa. The resection line is shown by a dotted line. (B–C) Plastic reconstruction of the remaining middle turbinate.

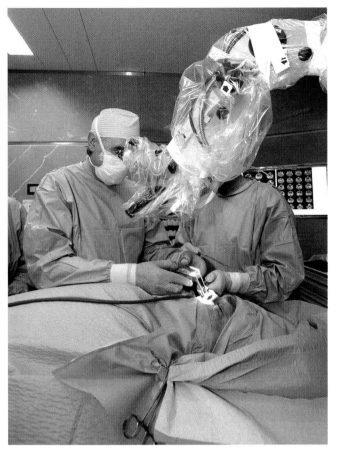

FIGURE 11–10 COMET surgery in progress. Removal of the concha bullosa and formation of a mucosal flap on the medial side of the middle turbinate using the microscissors in the right hand and the straight Blakesley ethmoid forceps in the left hand. The assistant holds the nasal speculum, which opens the middle meatus, and his second hand is ready for suction if necessary.

the excised raw lateral surface of the bone. The lateral mucosal flap is relaid on the raw lateral surface of the middle turbinate (Fig. 11–10).

If, at the end of surgery, a floppy middle turbinate is identified, the mucosa of a small area of the medial surface of the middle turbinate and the opposing mucosa of the nasal septum should be scarified to form an adhesion. As a consequence, the adhesion between the nasal septum and the middle turbinate mucosa displaces the middle turbinate medially and holds it in place, avoiding lateralization during the healing period.[82]

Uncinectomy

The middle turbinate is medialized using a Freer elevator by applying firm pressure against the lateral aspect of the upper part of the turbinate, and a nasal speculum is inserted into the middle meatus under microscopic guidance, which gives an excellent view of its

structures (Fig. 11–11). Cocaine paste containing 18% cocaine hydrochloride and 0.03% epinephrine is applied topically over the mucosa of the middle meatus for at least 5 minutes. Initially, the self-holding nasal speculum was used, which was fixed to the operating table by a flexible arm, and the surgeon was in a sitting position with the microscope in front of him or her, like a routine otological procedure. However, during the last few years the technique has changed, and now the assistant holds the nasal speculum with one hand to speed up the surgery. Then the standing position was adopted.

After mucosal vasoconstriction of the middle meatus, the next procedure is to expose the ethmoid infundibulum by removing the uncinate process. This is the first step of all the techniques for paranasal sinus surgery working in the anterior-to-posterior direction (Fig. 11–12). The removal of the uncinate process is termed uncinectomy.

This procedure begins with an incision of the uncinate process at its anterior attachment. The incision is extended with a sawing motion posteriorly and inferiorly, parallel to the upper edge of the hiatus semilunaris and toward the natural ostium of the maxillary sinus. The knife blade should always be oriented parallel to the lamina papyracea to avoid orbital penetration. The incised uncinate process is then grasped and, using microscissors, the superior and inferior attachments are gently cut and the uncinate process is removed (Fig. 11–13).

The uncinectomy exposes the base of the infundibulum and the anterior wall of the ethmoid bulla. The infundibulum is now open, and diseased mucosa or polyps should be removed (Table 11–14). The procedure may be terminated at this time, but if there is more sinus pathology, it is necessary to continue with a maxillary antrostomy.

Maxillary Antrostomy

The uncinectomy has been performed, and the infundibulum and the ethmoid bulla are identified. Therefore, it is important to expose the lower part of the ethmoid infundibulum to visualize the natural ostium of the maxillary sinus. Attention to the maxillary sinus opening within the middle meatus is a basic part of almost every endonasal surgical procedure.

If an uncinectomy is performed without enlargement of the maxillary ostium, the patient will be at risk for stenosis, leading to subsequent problems. It is necessary to incorporate the natural ostium into the middle meatus antrostomy. If the surgical antrostomy does not include the natural ostium, a recirculation problem may occur. In those cases, mucus flows out of the natural ostium, reentering the maxillary sinus through the surgical antrostomy. This recirculation of mucus can lead to chronic inflammation.

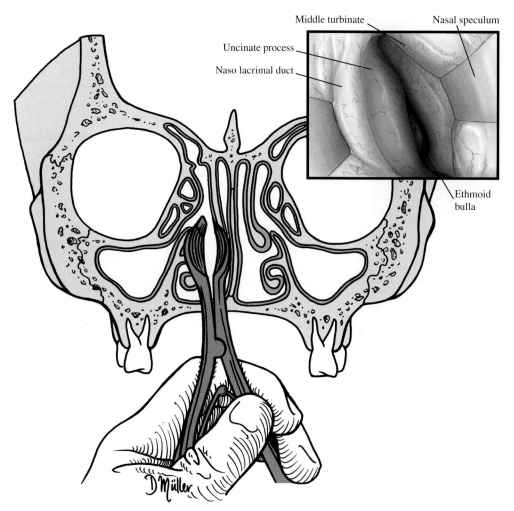

FIGURE 11–11 (A) Medial retraction of the right middle turbinate with a nasal speculum, which opens up the right middle meatus. (B) Microscopic view of the right nasal wall, with the right middle turbinate retracted with the nasal speculum toward the septum to bring the uncinate process and ethmoid bulla into view.

The key to performing a middle meatus antrostomy lies in the initial identification of the natural ostium. The natural ostium is very consistent, always being anterior and inferior within the middle meatus. The ostium may sometimes be difficult to identify because it can be obstructed by inflamed mucosa, polyps, or scar tissue. Landmarks for locating the natural ostium are of crucial importance. The ostium usually is at the same level as the inferior margin of the middle turbinate, anterior to the ethmoid bulla. Theoretically, the ostium is located at the midportion of the middle turbinate. The ostium is almost always in the same sagittal plane as the lamina papyracea. If the ostium is not immediately apparent, it can be located with a probe.

After identifying the natural ostium of the maxillary sinus, this opening is then further enlarged posteriorly into the posterior fontanelle with the backward-biting punch forceps and anteriorly with the upturned Blakesley-Wilde ethmoid forceps (Fig. 11–14). Small pieces of bone and fragments of mucosa around the opening should be removed. The edges of the antrostomy should be smooth, and, if possible, the mucosa of the maxillary sinus should be rolled out from the sinus to cover the edges of the antrostomy.

The maxillary sinus ostium is immediately posterior to the nasolacrimal duct. This relationship is important because it means that an agressive enlargement in the anterior direction will open the nasolacrimal duct into the maxillary sinus and middle meatus. It is best to avoid this complication because stenosis of the duct can result causing epiphora or pooling of tears into the sinus, with subsequent intermittent drainage of tears. Patients with this problem will complain of sudden drainage of clear fluid from the nose upon

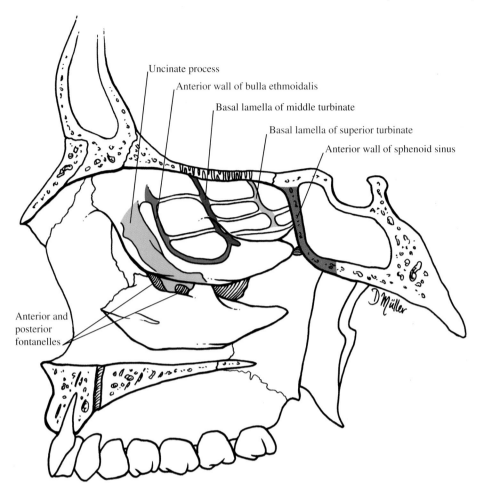

Uncinate process
Anterior wall of bulla ethmoidalis
Basal lamella of middle turbinate
Basal lamella of superior turbinate
Anterior wall of sphenoid sinus

Anterior and posterior fontanelles

D Müller

FIGURE 11–12   Progressive bony landmarks of paranasal sinus surgery encountered as the surgeon works from the uncinate process to the sphenoid sinus.

positional change from supine to upright or when leaning over.

It is sometimes extremely difficult to find the natural ostium, especially when disease is present (polyposis) or when there is long-standing sinusitis. Also, the anatomical landmarks around the infundibulum and anterior fontanelle are often difficult to recognize. In this case, we have to identify the area of the posterior fontanelle. The area of the posterior fontanelle is palpated with the tip of the angled forceps or suction tube. This area is posterior to the inferior limit of the ethmoid bulla and courses close to the superior border of the inferior turbinate. An accessory ostium in the posterior fontanelle should be identified. Gentle removal of the nasal mucosa over the posterior fontanelle will facilitate its opening into the sinus. The area anterior and inferior to the lower border of the ethmoid bulla and close to the upper border of the inferior turbinates is the site for middle meatal antrostomy. This area can be punched with the upturned Blakesley-Wilde ethmoid forceps used for making the antrostomy opening. The tip of the surgical instrument should always be pointing toward the floor of

TABLE 11–14   Surgical Remarks for Uncinectomy

Landmarks	• Middle turbinate
	• Uncinate process
	• Lamina papyracea
	• Basal lamella
	• Skull base
Surgical technique	• Incision runs medially and inferiorly toward the natural ostium of the maxillary sinus
Recommendations	• Displace the uncinate process away from the orbit
	• Avoid deep penetration of the tip of the sickle knife during uncinectomy because it may injure the lamina papyracea
	• Dissection should be parallel to the orbit
	• When necessary, palpate the eye while working near the lamina papyracea, looking for possible herniation of orbital fat
Goals	• Removal of diseased mucosa of the sinus ethmoid infundibulum
	• Open the access to the maxillary, ethmoid, and frontal sinuses
Problems after incomplete removal	• Upper portion
	• Obstruction and/or adhesions to the drainage region of the frontal sinus
	• Lower portion
	• Difficulty finding the maxillary ostium
	• Obstruction and/or adhesions to the infundibulum

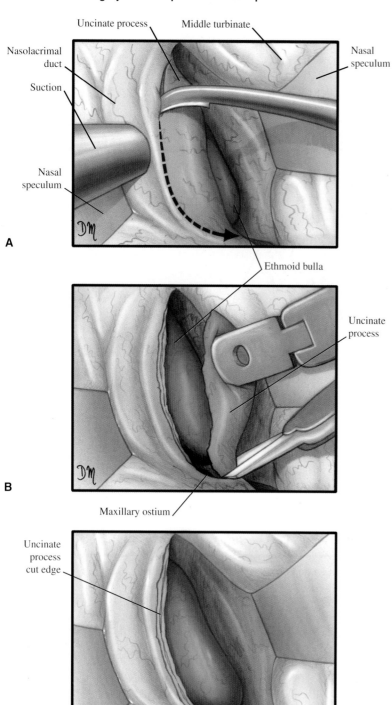

FIGURE 11–13 Uncinectomy process under microscopic view. (A) The right middle turbinate is retracted toward the septum with a nasal speculum held by an assistant to bring the uncinate process and ethmoid bulla into view. The incision of the uncinate process is then carried out with a sickle knife. (B) The uncinate process is grasped by the Blakesley forceps, and the superior and inferior attachments are gently cut and the uncinate process removed. (C) Microscopic view of the uncinate process remnant.

the maxillary sinus and never medially. Once the fontanelle is perforated (under microscopic guidance), it is enlarged with backward-biting punch forceps.

The antrostomy should be carried far enough forward to include the natural ostium of the maxillary sinus in the infundibulum. Inferior and anterior removal of tissue is usually all that is necessary. Hard bone anteriorly in-dicates the nasolacrimal duct. As a general rule, the antrostomy should not be made more anterior than the anterior end of the middle turbinate.

Polypoid tissue, diseased mucosa, mucous plugs, and secretions should be removed using this technique under microscopic view, with two hands free to manipu-late the microsurgical instruments. In one hand, is the

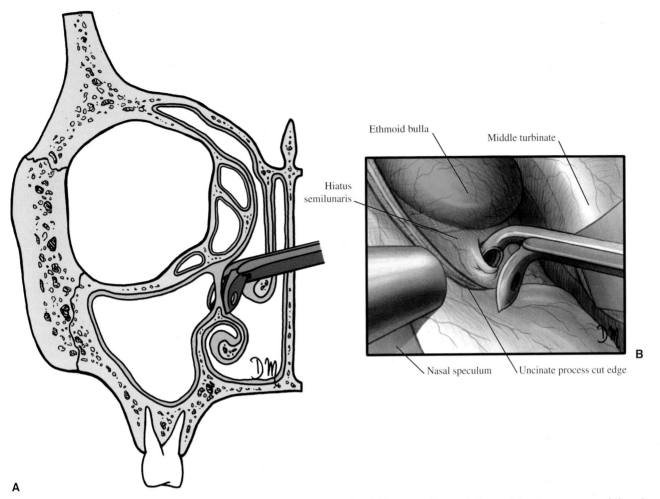

FIGURE 11–14 (A) Middle meatal antrostomy under microscopic view. (B) Enlargement of the maxillary sinus ostium with the backward-biting forceps. The edges of the neo-ostium should be smooth, and, if possible, the mucosa of the sinus should be rolled out to cover the edges of the antrostomy.

suction tube; in the other hand, adequate nasal forceps. Sometimes the assistant gives an extra hand with a suction tube or another nasal forceps to aid in the removal of the material. This is another great advantage to microscopic sinus surgery, particularly in benign tumor surgery, when an extra hand is always welcome. There is still some room available for this help with the microscopic technique.

Next, irrigation with warm normal saline is performed, which facilitates the extrusion of some mucous plugs, hard secretions, and/or fragments of diseased tissue that behave as foreign bodies and possible sources of reinfection. Also, it will improve the view of the surgical field by removing blood clots and/or small bony particles in preparation for the endoscopic examination (Fig. 11–15).

Endoscopy with a 30-degree, 4 mm telescope should be performed through the 8 to 10 mm opening of the maxillary sinus (Fig. 11–16), and a curved grasping forceps can be introduced along with the telescope for removal of residual diseased mucosa from the maxillary sinus cavity (Table 11–15).

Ethmoidectomy

If there is evidence of ethmoid disease, the surgery will proceed with ethmoidectomy. The technique described in this section is the complete ethmoidectomy, including removal of the cells of the ethmoid labyrinth, performed with the microscope and with the standard surgical instruments for endoscopic sinus surgery. However, it is important to tailor the operative procedure to the endoscopic findings and to the amount of disease observed on CT scans. Following these guidelines, an anterior ethmoidectomy may be sufficient, but if the posterior ethmoid is also involved, a total ethmoidectomy should be performed. Unlike the maxillary sinus, which is a single cavity with a distinct ostium,

TABLE 11–15 Surgical Remarks for Antrostomy

Identification	– Natural ostium • Located in lower part of the infundibulum bounded anteriorly by the uncinate process and posteriorly by the ethmoid bulla • Located in anterior fontanelle • Lies more obliquely • Oval-shaped – Accessory ostium • Located in posterior fontanelle • Lies in sagittal plane • Circular-shaped • Sometimes multiple
Surgical technique	• Complete uncinectomy • Identification of natural ostium • If not possible, identification of accessory ostium • Puncture the area of posterior fontanelle to enter the sinus if the identification of natural ostium fails • Enlargement of natural ostium or creation of a large window (8–10 mm) connecting both ostia points • Irrigation with warm normal saline and aspiration of mucus, secretions, and inspissated material • Removal of polypoid tissue and/or diseased mucosa
Recommendations	• First, locate the maxillary sinus ostium before entering the sinus. If it is not possible, palpate the posterior fontanelle area with the tip of a suction tube • Penetration of the sinus should be performed with the tip of a surgical instrument pointing down, toward the floor of the sinus cavity and on the top of the inferior turbinate • Antrostomy should be placed just above the inferior turbinate and not more anteriorly than the anterior end of the middle turbinate
Goals	• Enlargement of natural ostium and/or performance of a large neo-ostium • Treatment of the sinus pathology

the ethmoid sinus consists of multiple cavities of interconnected cells. The basal lamella of the middle turbinate plays a key role in separating the ethmoid labyrinth into two distinct anatomical and physiologic compartments.

The anterior group of cells drains its secretions into the infundibulum together with the maxillary and frontal sinuses. The ethmoid cells lying posterior to the attachment of the middle turbinate drain their mucus into the superior meatus. These cells belonging to the posterior compartment are more independent, and the mucus flows normally. The anterior group of cells, however, depends on anatomical variations in the structure of the ethmoid, maxillary, and frontal sinuses, and such variations may impede the flow. Mucociliary drainage can be restored by correcting the obstructive structure and treating the disease.

The main anatomical landmark for performing an ethmoidectomy is the identification of the ethmoid bulla (Fig. 11–17). This structure is easily visualized and

approached. The mucosa is dissected away very carefully over the bony surface of the ethmoid bulla with the tip of a straight Blakesley through-cutting, tissue-sparing forceps, which is particularly important when there are swollen mucosa or polypoid tissue. After identification of the bony anatomical area, the ethmoid cells are opened cell by cell and removed with gentle movements until the anterior compartment is reduced to one common cavity covered by mucosa (Fig. 11–18). It is possible to use warm normal saline irrigation with the help of the assistant to wash the surgical field with all the recognized advantages of this cleaning effect. This surgical technique is easily performed under microscopic view, and the principle is very simple: dissection instead of tearing to save healthy mucosa and reduce stripping and unwanted tearing of the mucosa as it is removed.

After the bulla is removed, the lamina papyracea can usually be identified, and the basal lamella can generally be visualized. The other borders, such as the skull base and the boundary with the frontal sinus, are reached relatively safely in this way. The goal of an anterior ethmoidectomy is the complete exposure of the anterior ethmoid cells. This technique can be properly executed with two hands under microscope view, one handling the suction tube to aspirate small tissue fragments and the other operating the nasal forceps. The assistant is holding the nasal speculum, and sometimes a third hand is quite welcome for suction. This allows the surgeon to operate with both hands when using the microscope, as is commonly done with microsurgery of the ear and/or larynx.

The anterior ethmoidectomy as it is described has proven to be a particularly safe procedure. It is performed after the initial meatal antrostomy (Table 11–16). The antrostomy exposes the antral roof; thus, the orbital wall can be constantly monitored, and removal of the neighboring ethmoid cells is safe. Also, the antrostomy is often indicated because the maxillary sinus is frequently involved.

Sometimes it is necessary to open the agger nasi cells (because they may be inflamed) depending on the extent of the ethmoid disease as determined by CT scan and the microscopic appearance of the bulla. Dissection should never be performed in front of the small prominence of bone where the anterior end of the middle turbinate meets the agger nasi because the base of the skull and the olfactory cleft begin in front of or above this point.

A posterior ethmoidectomy may be indicated if there is involvement of the posterior compartment of the ethmoid bone, although inflammatory diseases mainly affect the anterior ethmoid. After dissecting the anterior ethmoid cells, the basal lamella of the middle turbinate is usually encountered. It divides the anterior from the posterior ethmoid compartments. The basal lamella is

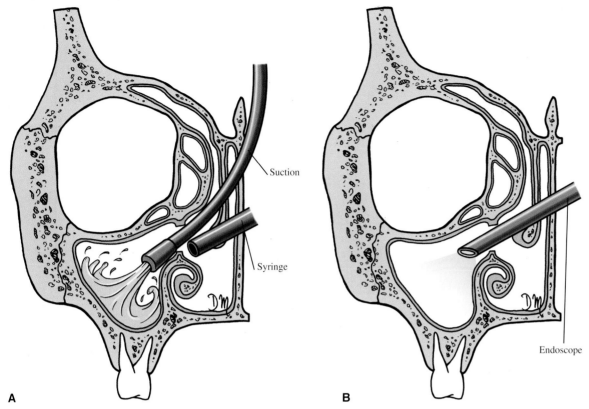

A

B

FIGURE 11–15 Middle meatal antrostomy. (A). Irrigation with warm normal saline to remove mucus, hard secretions, and/or fragments of diseased tissue under microscopic view.

(B) Endoscopic view of the inferior portion of the sinus cavity with a 30-degree, 4 mm telescope while looking for morphologic abnormalities.

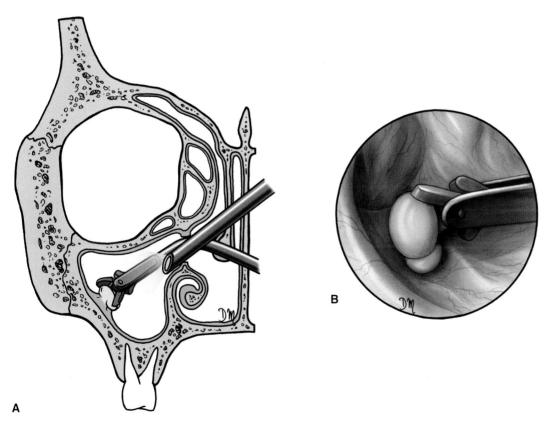

A

B

FIGURE 11–16 (A) Middle meatal antrostomy. (B) Removal of residual diseased mucosa using a 30-degree, 4 mm telescope and antrum grasping forceps.

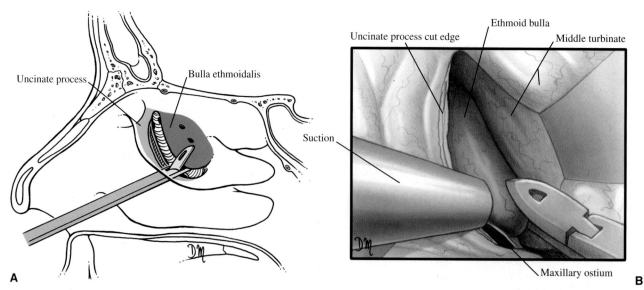

FIGURE 11–17   Anterior ethmoidectomy under microscopic view. (A) The initial step is to identify and palpate the ethmoid bulla. Then the mucosa is dissected away with Blakesley forceps, and the ethmoid cells are opened. (B) Microscopic view with the surgeon's left hand holding the suction tube and the right hand controlling the nasal forceps, which is ready to open.

perforated medially and inferiorly, and the posterior ethmoid cells are removed stepwise until the anterior wall of the sphenoid sinus is exposed (Fig. 11–19).

Once the posterior ethmoid is open, the upturned through-cutting tissue-sparing forceps are used to work toward the skull base. The forceps are placed behind each partition to ensure that the partition is below the skull base. The vertically oriented bony partitions are removed until the roof of the ethmoid bone is visualized. This roof is identified by the relatively smooth contour of its surface, the slightly white color of the bone, and its typical, more solid feel when palpated with the tip of the angled forceps. The posterior ethmoid artery can frequently be seen at this point, and this landmark defines the anterior edge of the most posterior ethmoid cell in most patients.

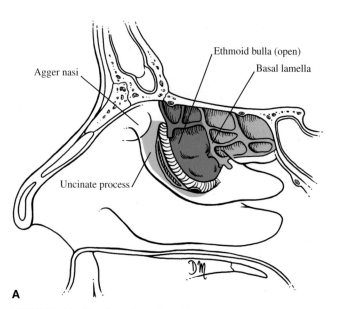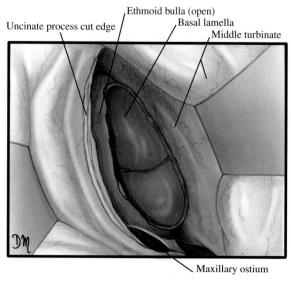

FIGURE 11–18   Anterior ethmoidectomy under microscopic view. (A) Completion of an anterior ethmoidectomy with removal of the anterior ethmoid cells until the anterior compartment is reduced to one common cavity. (B) Microscopic view presenting the anterior ethmoid cavity with the basal lamella of the middle turbinate clearly illustrated.

TABLE 11–16   Surgical Remarks for Ethmoidectomy

Landmarks	• Ethmoid bulla • Lamina papyracea • Skull base • Basal lamella • Anterior wall of sphenoid sinus
Surgical technique	• Anterior ethmoidectomy (removal of anterior ethmoid cells up to the basal lamella) • Posterior ethmoidectomy (removal of posterior ethmoid cells up to the anterior wall of the sphenoid sinus) • Total ethmoidectomy (anterior + posterior ethmoidectomies)
Recommendations	• It is important to open the cells of the anterior and posterior ethmoid region at their lowest portion parallel to the floor of the nasal cavity and, therefore, parallel to the skull base. • The dissection along the roof of the ethmoid bone is most safely executed in a posterior-anterior direction after the ethmoid sinus has been opened carefully in an anterior-posterior course. • The removal of the cells along the skull base must be performed with a punch or through-cutting forceps to avoid stripping of the mucosa of the ethmoid roof and injury to the dura, which may induce CSF fistula. • The skull base slants downward as the surgeon moves posteriorly, putting the posterior ethmoid and sphenoid areas at risk. • Be aware of several dehiscences of the ethmoid sinus mainly along the anterolateral roof of the ethmoid cells, the medial wall of the ethmoid sinus, the origin of the middle turbinate, and the anterior and posterior ethmoid vessels and nerves.
Goals	• Removal of polypoid tissue and/or diseased mucosa

Once the skull base is clearly identified in the posterior ethmoid region, this plane can be followed anteriorly to skeletonize the more anterior skull base. It is then followed anteriorly up to the anterior ethmoid artery. Removal of the bony partitions should be as close as possible to the level of the skull base, but without unnecessary removal of the skull base mucosa. Preservation of the skull base mucosa is a basic principle of endoscopic sinus surgery, and it should be done as much as possible.

At this point, any residual bony ridges with loose mucosa are removed from the lamina papyracea, preserving its mucosa. Again, the dissection should be completed leaving a smooth surface contour of the medial orbital wall and without removing unnecessary mucosa along this plane.

Frontal Sinusotomy

The surgical steps that follow ethmoidectomy include inspection of the frontal recess using a 30- and 70-

degree, 4 mm telescopes. The CT scan is very helpful in identifying the anatomical variations of this area and the pathologic abnormalities. In most cases the frontal sinus does not show any evidence of disease; consequently, this sinus does not need to be entered nor its ostium routinely enlarged. The aperatura of the frontal sinus should be manipulated as little as possible. When frontal sinusitis is caused by infundibular inflammatory disease, the uncinate process is displaced medially. The frontal recess accompanies this displacement further medially and, in some cases, may result in mucosal fusion between the uncinate process and the anterior attachment of the middle turbinate. Less common is frontal sinus obstruction secondary to agger nasi inflammatory disease. In this case, the frontal recess may be displaced posteriorly and superiorly close to the skull base, and it becomes very difficult to find. Also, severe and longstanding sinus disease may cause stenosis of the frontal recess and bony destruction (osteitis), which make endoscopic enlargement very difficult.

Intranasal frontal sinusotomy is the most challenging and potentially dangerous procedure performed in endonasal sinus surgery (Table 11–17). The important landmark for this procedure is the anterior ethmoid artery, which is posterior to the frontal recess. Sometimes it may be necessary to remove a superior remnant of the uncinate process to localize the frontal recess. The anterior ethmoid artery usually lies posteroinferior to the dome of the ethmoid bone or slightly behind the point where the skull base becomes horizontal. Its position is variable, and it can be absent intranasally in some patients, but it is typically posterior to the supraorbital ethmoid cells. Occasionally this vessel can lie more anteriorly (between a supraorbital cell and the frontal sinus), and in other patients it may lie up to 4 mm below the skull base. Therefore, care is needed when dissecting in this area because of the vessel anatomy and the thin skull base medially. One must be particularly careful medially because the skull base is very thin and easily perforated at this point.

The agger nasi cells are extremely common, and, depending on their size, the approach to the frontal recess may become difficult. Also, the frontal sinus drainage system may be restricted. The frontal sinus infundibulum, frontal sinus ostium, and frontal recess comprise a functional unit for drainage that has been named the frontal sinus outflow tract.[83] The frontal sinus drainage can be posterior and medial to the agger nasi cells, but never anterior to these cells.

To visualize the frontal recess area adequately, it is most often necessary to remove the agger nasi cells widely (Fig. 11–20) under microscopic view. Then, the frontal recess is enlarged using the sharp curette to break down the anterior ethmoid cells, the spina nasalis frontalis (nasofrontal "beak"), and any remaining anterior wall of the bulla under endoscopic control (Fig. 11–21).

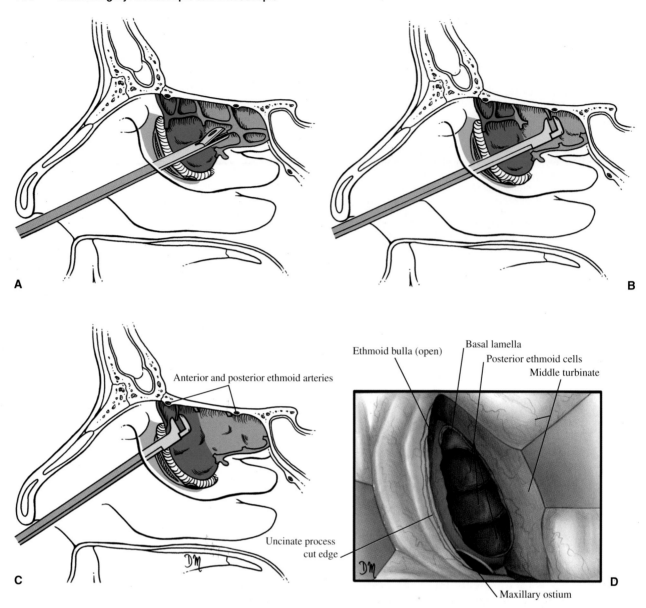

Anterior and posterior ethmoid arteries

Ethmoid bulla (open) **Basal lamella** **Posterior ethmoid cells** **Middle turbinate**

Uncinate process cut edge

Maxillary ostium

FIGURE 11–19 Total ethmoidectomy under microscopic view. (A) Posterior ethmoidectomy with removal of posterior ethmoid cells with straight Blakesley forceps. (B–C) Total ethmoidectomy is completed with resection of residual bony partitions at skull base with through-cutting forceps (not by blunt ethmoid forceps) working in a posterior-anterior direction. Note the relationship with the anterior and posterior ethmoid arteries. (D) Microscopic view of total ethmoidectomy. Observe the remnants of the ethmoid bulla and some bony partitions.

However, removal of the inferior cells of the agger nasi may be insufficient when the residual dome of these cells is still compromising the frontal recess, constricting the outflow tract of the frontal sinus, and remaining the cause of persistent frontal sinusitis. It may appear that the sinus has already been opened when viewed from below, and in this case it is important to identify the communication to the frontal sinus posteriorly or medially. If there is any difficulty in identifying the ostium, a curved probe or frontal sinus seeker can be used to palpate along the skull base, above and anterior to the ethmoid artery. If there is a supraorbital ethmoid air cell, then the frontal ostium will be more medial. In this case the best approach is to follow the lateral surface of the middle turbinate superiorly. Then, it is possible to remove the dome of these cells with a special slim, curved curette introduced between the skull base and the dome of the agger nasi cells. This bony roof is then fractured anteriorly or laterally, depending on whether the opening is posterior or medial. Directly perforating

TABLE 11–17   Surgical Remarks for Frontal Sinusotomy

Landmarks	• Skull base • Anterior ethmoid artery • Agger nasi cells • Ethmoid infundibulum
Surgical technique	• Difficult visualization • Dangerous area, as it is close to the orbit and to the skull base • Keep the cribriform plate and anterior attachment of the middle turbinate in view during the procedure • Always work in an anterior to posterior direction • Gentle probing of the ostium • Meticulous atraumatic technique
Recommendations	• Only remove the agger nasi cells or enlarge the frontal recess if the patient has long-standing chronic sinusitis. • Be aware of the anatomical variations of the frontal sinus area, namely, duplication of the drainage channels, which may lead to false judgments in frontal sinusotomy. • This is a technically challenging area that can be managed by the combined technique (COMET surgery).
Goals	• Removal of enlarged agger nasi cells • Removal of stenotic areas and polypoid tissue obstructing the ostium • Mucosa preservation at the ostium when possible

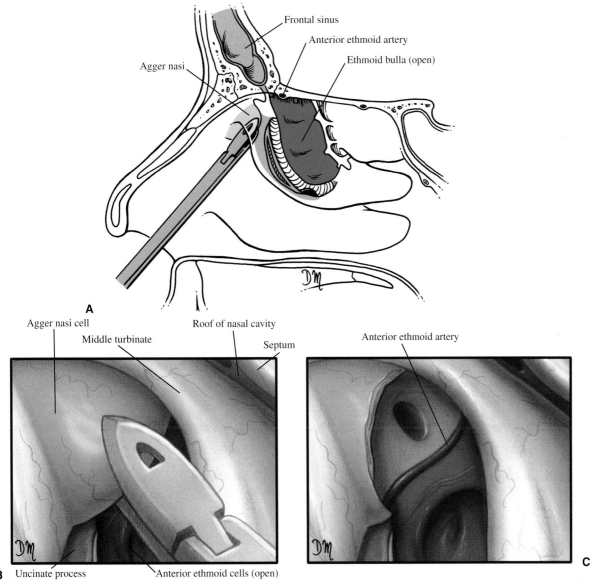

FIGURE 11–20 Frontal sinusotomy under microscopic view. (A) Beginning of a frontal sinusotomy. The agger nasi cells are removed to improve the access to the frontal recess. (B) Microscopic view of the agger nasi area, with the tip of the ethmoid forceps starting the procedure. (C) Removal of the agger nasi cells.

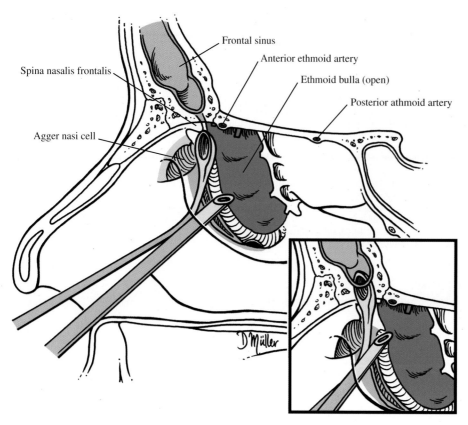

FIGURE 11–21   Frontal sinusotomy under endoscopic view. The frontal recess is enlarged using a sharp curette. The surgeon works with a surgical curette guided by an angled endoscope.

this cell remnant for frontal sinusotomy endangers the local frontobasal mucosa. Bony fragments are removed under endoscopic vision using Kuhn giraffe forceps with cupped jaws. This procedure has been popularized as "uncapping the egg."[84]

Great care should be taken to avoid stripping the mucosa, particularly in the area of the ostium of the frontal sinus, to avoid stenosis postoperatively. However, if there are osteitic bony partitions, they need to be removed with forward or side-to-side through-cutting forceps. The size of the frontal opening to be formed depends on the degree of bony thickening and mucosal inflammation present. However, it is necessary that the opening communicates with the natural ostium if a good mucociliary clearance is to be achieved and secondary closure is to be avoided. In general, an opening of at least 4 to 5 mm is sufficient (Fig. 11–22).

In revision cases undertaken for treatment of stenosis of the ostium, or in cases in which a very narrow opening is present due to the natural bony anatomy, more aggressive bone removal is necessary. Various techniques and instruments are available for removal of the bone in this area, including curettes, rasps, and drills.

Sphenoidotomy

The decision to open the sphenoid sinus should be planned ahead and included in the treatment surgical plan. The decision is based on generalized mucosal disease of all of the paranasal sinuses or on localized disease. In all cases, the author uses the transnasal approach under microscopic guidance, which is considered very safe. With the sphenoid sinus, this approach is very easy because the sinus has an anatomical structure quite visible due to its anterior contour over the posterior choana and is straight in front of the surgeon's view. The most reliable landmark in the posterior section of the nasal cavity is the posterior choana nasopharynx (Fig. 11–23). If a previous septoplasty and/or rhinoplasty for correction of nasal septum and/or nasal deformity has been performed before this procedure, an excellent and improved visibility of this area will be noted.

The sphenoid sinus can be opened safely 10 mm above the choana just lateral to the midline septum at the rostrum of the sphenoid. If an instrument is placed at an angle of 30 degrees to the anterior floor of the nose, the anterior wall of the sphenoid sinus should lie at a depth of 7 cm.

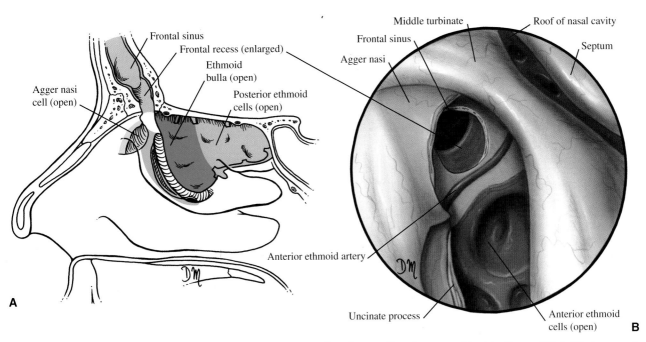

FIGURE 11–22   Frontal sinusotomy. (A). Sagittal section of the right frontal sinus after the agger nasi cells have been removed, the frontal recess enlarged, and the diameter of the sinus ostium increased to 4 to 5 mm. (B) A 30-degree, 4 mm endoscopic view.

If the ostium cannot be seen, it may be located by palpation with the tip of a suction tube. Sometimes the ostium is closed with fibrous tissue or new bone formation. A small mucosal flap is performed with an elevator at the ostium level for a better visualization. If identi-fied, the opening is enlarged in a lateral and inferior direction. The initial opening can be made with the straight Blakesley forceps. With the opening enlarged a micro-Kerrison punch can be introduced into the sinus and the remainder of the anterior wall removed

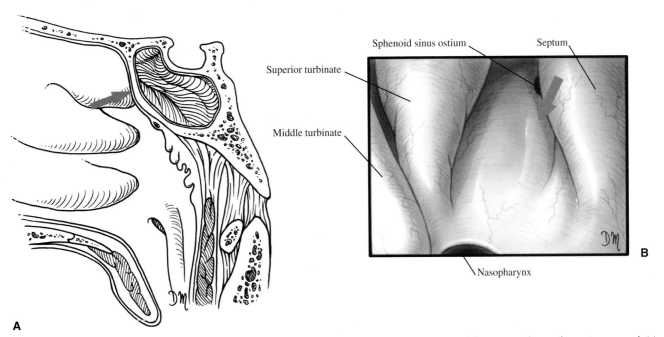

FIGURE 11–23   Sphenoidotomy under microscopic view. (A) Sagittal section showing the anterior wall of the sphenoid sinus. (B) Microscopic view presenting the anatomical landmarks of the sinus. The arrow shows the entrance point to the sinus during sphenoidotomy.

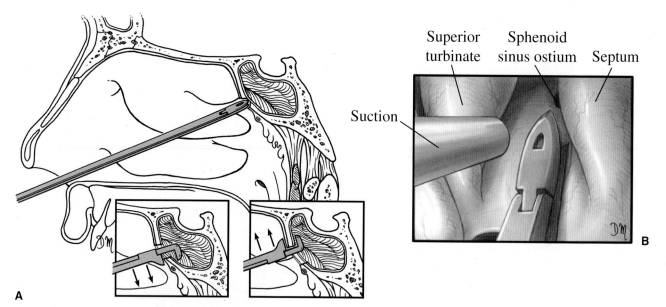

A

B

Superior
turbinate   Sphenoid
sinus ostium   Septum

Suction

FIGURE 11–24 Sphenoidotomy under microscopic view. (A) Sagittal section showing the opening of the sphenoid sinus using straight Blakesley forceps through a transnasal, direct approach, and the opening enlarged with a micro-Kerrison punch forceps. (B) Microscopic view of the opening of the anterior wall of the sphenoid sinus after the middle turbinate has been slightly retracted laterally.

(Fig. 11–24). If the entire anterior wall of the sinus is thick and the ostium cannot be visualized, an angulated hand piece with an extra-long diamond bur (12.5 cm) should be used to make an opening in the ostium area (Fig. 11–25). The enlargement of the opening may continue with the use of the diamond bur and suction irrigation as a routine otologic procedure. However, as the opening is enlarged, care must be taken with branches of the sphenopalatine artery (the medial posterior nasal artery and the nasal septal artery), which

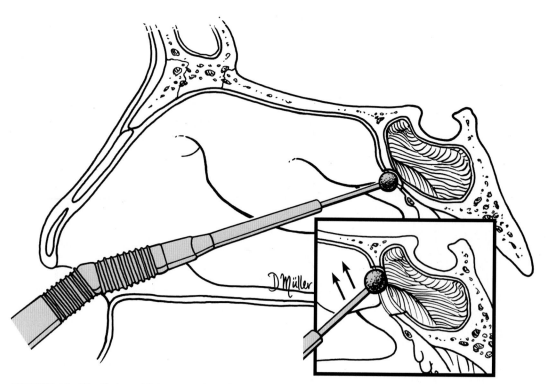

FIGURE 11–25 Sphenoidotomy under microscopic view. Microsurgical technique for sphenoidotomy using the angulated hand piece with an extra-long diamond bur.

run across the face of the sphenoid sinus at a level slightly superior to the sinus floor as they pass toward the nasal septum. They can be damaged, and bleeding may occur. In this situation, it may be safest to cauterize with monopolar suction cautery.

With the anterior wall opened, the mucus, secretions, inspissated material, and pathologic tissue can be gently suctioned and removed. After irrigation with warm normal saline, the 30-degree, 4 mm endoscope is introduced into the sinus and the entire cavity visualized for further clearance of the sinus. However, extreme caution should be used whenever operating in the sphenoid sinus. Both the optic nerve and the carotid artery are located along the lateral and posterior wall, and the bone over these structures can be incomplete. Also, the sella turcica (which contains the pituitary gland) is situated medial and superior to the sinus, and the cavernous sinus is located laterally. With these vital structures surrounding the walls of the sphenoid sinus, the surgeon should be aware that extreme care should be taken in biting away tissue laterally close to the carotid artery and the optic nerve. The optic nerve travels in a lateral to medial direction, crossing the superolateral wall of the sphenoid sinus. Also, the sphenoid sinus roof is extremely thin, presenting the potential risk of a CSF leak if the dissection is too vigorous superiorly. Nevertheless, if the techniques described are properly followed, the surgical goals can be achieved, and the potential risks can be avoided (Table 11–18).

Management of the Inferior Turbinate

There are many factors (anatomical, physiological, and pathological) that may lead to hypertrophy of the inferior turbinates and cause nasal obstruction. It is important

TABLE 11–18 Surgical Remarks for Sphenoidotomy

Landmarks	• Skull base • Middle and superior turbinates • Posterior nasal septum • Posterior choana
Surgical technique	• Identification of the ostium • Perforation of the sinus wall at this level and enlargement of the opening • Always work medially. • Extreme care should be taken during lateral dissection inside the sinus (risk of damaging carotid artery and optic nerve). • Preservation of normal middle and superior turbinates
Recommendations	• Identify and cannulate the sphenoid ostium if possible, and start the sphenoidotomy from there. • To open the sphenoid sinus safely, use the transnasal approach, and follow the landmarks: relative to the arch of the posterior choana, above the posterior attachment of the middle turbinate and close to the septum. • Be careful with the dissection close to the lateral wall of the sphenoid sinus because of its rich anatomical relationship with vital structures such as the internal carotid artery and the optic nerve, which can be dehiscents.
Goals	• Removal of mucous secretions and pathologic tissue • Closure of CSF fistulas • Biopsy and excision of benign tumors

to evaluate this condition preoperatively to treat this problem during the same surgical procedure: one-stage integrated treatment.

After taking care of septal deviation and paranasal sinus disease, the last step is to treat the hypertrophy of the inferior turbinates (Fig. 11–26).

A long nasal speculum is introduced along the inferior turbinate, and with microscopic view, the posterior

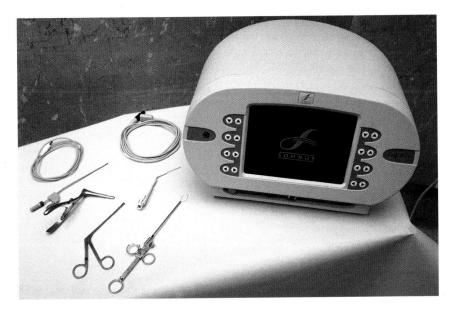

FIGURE 11–26 Surgical instruments and equipment used for treatment of the hypertrophic inferior turbinates.

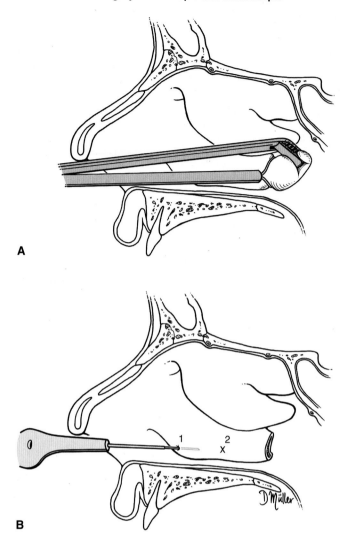

FIGURE 11–27 Management of the inferior turbinate. (A) Resection of the tail of the inferior turbinate with a nasal polyp snare. (B) Radiofrequency thermal ablation of the anterior and middle thirds of the inferior turbinate (1x and 2x indicate the site of the introduction of the needle electrode).

third of the inferior turbinate is then visualized. Sometimes the tail of the turbinate is so enlarged that it almost completely obstructs the posterior choana, even extending to the nasopharynx. A nasal snare is introduced along the floor of the nasal cavity, and the soft tissues of the posterior portion of the inferior turbinate are removed after being retracted medially with a straight Blakesley forceps (Fig. 11–27). Minimal bleeding from the stump is cauterized with monopolar cautery. The same technique is applied to the contralateral side. It is obvious that this feature is one more factor causing nasal obstruction, and if not removed, even after septoplasty and treatment of paranasal sinus disease, the patient will probably continue to complain of nasal obstruction.

The anterior and middle thirds of the hypertrophic inferior turbinates are treated with radiofrequency thermal ablation (RFTA) for tissue volume reduction.[85–87] With the patient still under general anesthesia, a short nasal speculum is used to identify the anterior portion of the inferior turbinate. A special needle electrode is then introduced in the anterior part and along the body of the inferior turbinate. The needle has a 40 mm total length, of which the distal 15 mm is an exposed active electrode. The proximal 25 mm is insulated. A thermocouple at the needle tip and at the junction of the exposed and insulated portions of the needle provides temperature feedback to control power delivery. The radiofrequency selected is 200 J with 10 W at a temperature of 80°C on the Somnus model S_2 radiofrequency generator (Somnus Medical Technologies, Inc.).

The needle electrode is reinserted into the middle portion of the inferior turbinate from an inferomedial approach, and 200 J is delivered one more time. The depth of insertion is 5 mm or greater, so that the exposed needle is not in contact with mucosa. The procedure is then performed on the contralateral side. Over a period of 3 to 6 weeks the resulting heated turbinate tissue is reabsorbed, with a secondary decrease of volume of the hypertrophic inferior turbinate and improvement of the nasal airway.

Before ending the one-stage integrated surgical procedure, it is necessary to close the anterior septal incision with 3–0 Monocryl stitches. A bilateral silicone sheet 1 mm thick is introduced along the nasal cavity to keep the mucoperichondrial flaps together and to stabilize the septum in the midline, and it is sutured with two stitches of 2–0 Mersilk (Fig. 11–28). A small Merocel sinus pack (3.5 cm) is inserted to stent the middle turbinate laterally, and a long Merocel nasal packing (10 cm) is placed along the floor of both nasal cavities to provide pressure, to absorb blood, and to provide a gentle tamponade. All Merocel sponges are coated with antibiotic ointment (bacitracin) to minimize mucosal trauma. The strings of the sponges are tied loosely across the columella, and an external nasal dressing is applied over the nose and secured in place with nonallergic adhesive tape. If the patient underwent a rhinoplasty, an external nasal splint is placed over the nasal dorsum.

The total operating time for the entire procedure (one-stage integrated treatment) is close to 2½ hours, which is acceptable if we take into consideration that the goals of the surgical planning were accomplished and that the patient needs no further treatment. Medications are prescribed for pain and to control infection. This surgical procedure is not very painful, and acetaminophen is sufficient. The antibiotics are continued for a minimum of 12 days after surgery. The nasal packs are left in place for 2 days after surgery, and the patient is discharged on the third postoperative day after removing the nasal packing. On the night of sur-

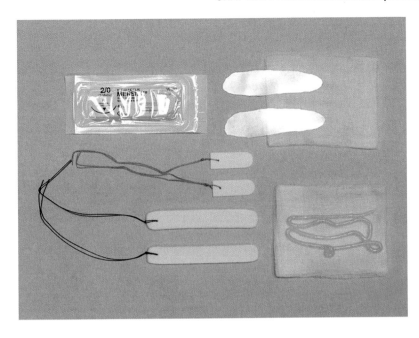

FIGURE 11–28 Supplies needed for nasal packing.

gery the patient is advised to remain at rest, with the head elevated. On the following day, the patient is up and moving around his or her room.

Postoperative Care

The successful outcome for patients undergoing endonasal and/or sinus surgery relies on very careful postoperative care and management. The standard postoperative regimen includes repeated office visits for meticulous follow-up associated with medical therapy. The first postoperative visit is scheduled 1 week after surgery to clean the nasal cavity and sinus area under microscopic view, removing clots and crusts and suctioning mucus and inspissated secretions. During the second visit 2 weeks after surgery, the internal nasal silicone splint is removed, and cleaning of the nasal cavities is repeated. If necessary, nasal endoscopy with topical anesthesia and decongestion should be performed to remove areas of granulation tissue, regenerative mucosal cysts, and any synechiae using suction and Blakesley forceps. Additional follow-up visits may be scheduled, depending on the needs of the individual patient, but normally return visits are planned 1, 3, and 6 months after surgery, then every 6 months for the period of time considered necessary. The patient is informed that it will take 4 to 8 weeks for mucosal healing, but in most cases this regenerative process will be complete in 4 weeks. Synechiae between the lateral wall and the middle turbinate and between this structure and the nasal septum can develop postoperatively. The best way to avoid this development is to perform minimally traumatic surgery and to avoid damaging the mucosa of the nasal septum and the turbinates as much as possible. The medical therapy consists of an-

tibiotic coverage, topical saline sprays, topical steroid sprays, and oral steroids.

Antibiotics are administered for a minimum of 12 days, and cephalosporin is used routinely. However, if during the healing phase the nose and the sinus cavity demonstrate an active infection, then cultures are taken, and as soon as the results are available, the antibiotic is selected to cover the cultured bacteria. Patients are advised to use topical saline sprays frequently after removal of the nasal packing to minimize crusting and to continue spraying the nose twice daily for at least 6 months. Also, patients are instructed to use topical steroids once daily for long term to prevent recurrent mucosal disease. A tapering dose of oral steroids is prescribed before surgery and for 2 or more weeks for patients with extensive nasal polyposis, depending on the endoscopic appearance of the mucosa and if not medically contraindicated. Other adjunctive medical therapy, including allergy desensitization for patients with allergic rhinitis, should be considered.

Patients who do smoke are always advised to stop smoking, and if they cannot do so by themselves, a smoking cessation clinic is recommended. It is believed that tobacco smoking is one of the leading causes of recurrent paranasal mucosal disease.

Tobacco smoke is a heterogeneous mixture of several hundred compounds, and some of them have the ability to damage almost all of the cells and tissues in the body. Over 4200 chemical components have been identified in the form of gases, uncondensed vapors, and liquid particulate matter. Other products in tobacco include nicotine and related substances that produce dependence; benzopyrene and its derivatives with well-known carcinogenic effects; and some gases, such as formaldehyde, acrolein,

TABLE 11–19   Recommended Postoperative Care

Postoperative visits	• 1 and 2 weeks • 1, 3, and 6 months, then every 6 months for a limited period of time according to the clinical evolution
Medical therapy	• Antibiotic coverage • Topical saline sprays • Topical steroid sprays • Oral steroids (if necessary)
Adjunctive medical therapy	• Allergy desensitization
Stop smoking	• Self-motivation • Smoking cessation clinic

methanol, ammonia, and nitrogen dioxide, which are potent irritants for the respiratory mucosa. Inhibition of ciliary mobility following exposure to tobacco smoke constituents has been demonstrated frequently in animal studies, and similar results have been obtained with ciliated human respiratory epithelium.[88–92] Also, there is enough clinical evidence that tobacco smoking and environmental tobacco smoke are irritating agents for nasal mucosa, and exposure may contribute to the aggravation and prolongation of chronic sinusitis.[93–94]

For the above reasons, the cessation of smoking must always be in the first line of priorities of postoperative care. The author has much experience in this field over the past 10 years and recognizes that it is not enough to say "stop smoking." The surgeon must monitor this problem very carefully and advise the smokers who are unable to stop by themselves to attend a smoking cessation clinic for nicotine replacement therapy, associated pharmacotherapy, and a complete change of health lifestyle[95–98] (Table 11–19).

Clinical symptoms usually respond quite well to the surgical procedure, particularly nasal obstruction and pain and pressure, unless there is persistent or recurrent mucosal disease. Olfaction is also a symptom that monitors the improvement or failure of the surgical treatment and may predict late recurrence. A postoperative CT is indicated only if there is clinical evidence of recurrent sinus disease.

The final outcome of this treatment depends not only on the competence of the surgeon and his or her surgical expertise, but also on the quality of postoperative care. Meticulous cleaning and debridement of the nasal cavity will almost always contribute to normal healing and good results.

■ Results

The Concept of Major and Minor Nasal Units

Before discussing the results of COMET surgery of the nose and paranasal sinuses, it is important to understand the philosophy behind the treatment of patients complaining of sinonasal symptoms.

What are we treating? Just the patient's problems related with that small part of the nasal lateral wall, called the ostiomeatal unit? Are we absolutely convinced that the patient's complaints, even after a careful preoperative evaluation, are related only to that small area of the lateral wall? How about the anatomical structures composing the nose and the paranasal sinus, which we call the major unit, and their influence on the ostiomeatal unit, which we name the minor unit? Do we have a clear understanding of the role of the major unit over the minor unit? What is the real impact of other medical conditions (allergic diseases, genetic influences, immunologic disorders, etc.) and environmental pollution (tobacco smoking) and lifestyle on the final outcome of the medical/surgical treatment of those patients? Should endoscopic sinus surgery be performed for treatment of sinus diseases and, sometimes, septoplasty to improve the surgeon's surgical field? Or should we approach the nose and paranasal sinuses as a total functional major unit, treating the diseased sinus and performing septoplasty because of nasal obstruction due to anatomical abnormalities and their impact on sinus function?

Certainly, if the results of the surgical treatment of patients with disease mainly located at the level of the minor unit alone are compared with the data of patients treated for clinical problems in the major unit, the results must be completely different. There is no contradiction about the impact of the major unit over the minor unit if there is a general consensus on the influence of the total unit, the human body (genetic problems, allergic diseases, and immunologic disorders, etc.) over the nose and paranasal sinus. This conclusion may justify the concept of the major unit (nose and paranasal sinus) and its effect on the minor unit (paranasal sinuses), and consequently, the treatment of the nose and the paranasal sinuses together and the presentation of their results combined. Surgically speaking, should we pay more attention to the sinuses than the nasal structures, even performing surgical procedures in different stages? If so, what is the logical approach behind that? Conversely, should the nasal problems be treated together with the sinus diseases during the same operative procedure to reinforce the concept of the major unit and its impact on the minor unit and the concept of one-stage integrated treatment as we recommend? It does make sense to treat both clinical problems during the same intervention, if it is surgically justified. However, there are still questions without answers related to the progress of science in this fascinating field of rhinology. Future research, adoption of universal criteria for classification of the involved sinonasal diseases, consensual staging systems, standardization of surgical techniques, and technological development of surgical instrumentation will eventually lead to better treatment and prevention of these disorders. Progress is made by individual steps, and the contribution of well-known surgeons throughout the last century has had an enormous impact on where we stand now. The Messerklinger concept is a historical contribution, but there is still a long way to go, and the next step is expectation. The future should be regarded with hope for solving some of the raised questions.

Problems of Classification, Standardization, and Documentation of Results

Classification and standardization of results present a difficult task because of the large number of parameters involved that may influence the results, such as referral patterns, time of evaluation, indications for surgery, surgical techniques, variations in surgical skills, and postoperative care. Furthermore, the overall results may improve over the course of time, even for the same surgeon. On the contrary, the patient's final outcome may deteriorate with time, and what is a success today may become a failure in the next 5 or 10 years.[99–104] Observations of this kind have led some authors to call attention to the need for longer follow-up periods of about 3 or more years. There is no point in evaluating results sooner than 6 months after surgery, but rather at least 3 years, as in ear surgery.[105–108]

It is well recognized that there are difficulties in reporting the final outcome of paranasal diseases: Methods to report the final results are variable, as are follow-up studies. A great number of patients participating in follow-up studies give up, and even after several years the number of participants is often reduced to half or less. Other pertinent information is not included in studies, such as septal deviation, hypertrophic inferior turbinates, or the condition of mucosa and bony pathologies after previous surgery. Other questions not included pertain to the effect of preoperative conditions such as allergic rhinitis, asthma or other allergic disorders, and aspirin sensitivity on the final outcome of sinus surgery. These issues do not yet have definite answers. What are the factors that determine success or failure? Certainly, nasal deformity, the type of sinus pathology, and particularly the presence of polyps can affect the results.[109–112] Another problem is to develop a stage system to classify and grade the results of a surgical treatment and to monitor the follow-up. What "very good," "good," and "moderate" signify in the assessment of treatment of chronic sinusitis may differ from one author to another. Despite the fact that patients often report a subjective improvement in their general condition, postoperative CT scans frequently demonstrate some persistent opacification in the sinuses. Thus, postoperative radiological findings must be assessed individually for each patient in conjunction with the clinical and endoscopic findings.[113–115]

However, as a rule, repeated CT scans should be performed only in symptomatic patients. Various sinus surgery reports also refer to successful results after one procedure, and others evaluate results after several revisions or procedures. Recurrences are usually observed after 1 year, but they may be seen up to several years after the operation. If mucosal normalization does occur, the majority of patients remain stable over the years. In this situation, should every recurrent polypoid mucosa require revisional surgery, because symptomatology correlates weakly with objective findings (nasal endoscopy and/or CT scan)?

All of these parameters can have a marked effect on the results, so the choice of homogeneous groups for comparison is difficult and validation of the results is not always possible, even with a large series of patients. This kind of information is normally important for a surgeon who wants to start a new operative technique, by allowing him or her to judge whether it is worthwhile to perform a technique after comparing his or her own results with those of other authors. Also, standard values must be available for a better interchange of medical information among colleagues, for detailed explanation to patients, and for medicolegal purposes. It is difficult to compare results published from different authors because no consensual rhinosinusitis staging system and reporting criteria for success and failure exist.

Kennedy[116] has proposed a classification system based on the extent of the disease (CT and endoscopic surgical findings). May and Levine[117] have introduced a classification system for reporting results of sinus surgery that takes several factors into account: anatomical variations, inflammatory diseases, severity of the disease, outcome of the surgery, and the time frame for follow-up evaluations and care. Lund and Mackay[118] have presented a simple staging system based on subjective (visual analogue score) and objective data (CT scan assessment and endoscopic findings). However, without a generally accepted method of classifying clinical and objective findings, surgical procedures and outcomes, as well as the comparison of the different surgical techniques, will continue to be difficult in the future. In the absence of a standardized staging system and grading method for the results of surgical treatment for chronic rhinosinusitis, the success rate is reported as >80% in adult patients.[119]

In view of these problems with the analysis of reported results, the development of a consensual system for classification of sinonasal diseases, surgical techniques, and results is essentially needed. Because of the related problems of classification, standardization, and presentation of results, it is most important to rely on personal statistical data and the credibility of several surgeons who, often after many years of specialization in the field of sinus surgery, have demonstrated the efficacy of their surgical skills, techniques, and results.

COMET Surgery Results

Over the past 18 years, over 1000 surgical procedures were performed by this author combining the microscope and endoscope to treat sinonasal diseases. If 10 more years of using the microscope alone for surgical management of sinus diseases before the combining procedure (COMET surgery) is added, significant surgical experience has been gained in this field since 1977.

Of the series of 1000 patients treated, a group of 200 were studied retrospectively, with a minimum follow-up of 3 years. A clinical history and a complete head and neck physical examination were performed. All patients had CT scans (coronal and axial plans) preoperatively. When there was a nasal obstruction and a suspicious allergic disease, rhinomanometry, acoustic rhinometry and allergy testing were also performed. Olfactometry testing was indicated when there was a smell dysfunction.

Surgical planning was conducted according to the clinical history, objectives, objective radiological findings, and patient's general condition. Patients with diabetes mellitus, oral steroid use, immunologic problems, and genetic disorders, as well as those with revision surgery, were excluded from this study. The approach was planned according to the type, location, and extent of the disease in the nose and paranasal sinuses (one-stage integrated treatment). With the combined technique, the postoperative care was the one recommended (Table 11–19). The overall results of 200 patients with chronic sinusitis after a 3-year follow-up period is 82% with improvement of their symptoms after surgery. However, preoperative nasal obstruction is improved in ~87% of cases. This high percentage is based on concomitant surgery in

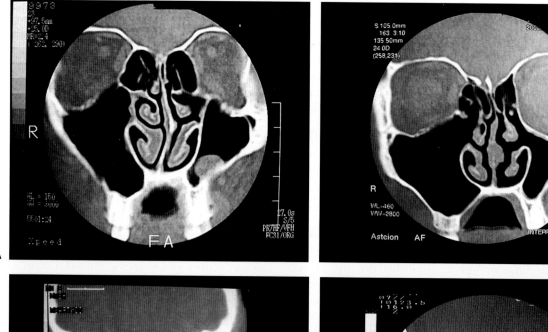

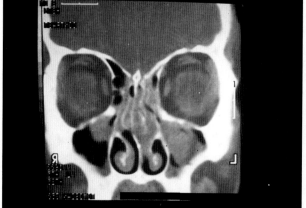

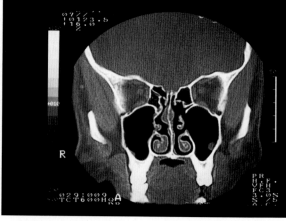

FIGURE 11–29 Preoperative (A) and postoperative (B) coronal CT scans of a patient with a deviated nasal septum and a mucous retention cyst of the left maxillary sinus. The patient underwent a rhinoseptoplasty, a middle meatal antros-tomy, and an anterior ethmoidectomy on both sides. Preoperative (C) and postoperative (D) coronal CT scans of a patient with bilateral nasal polyposis who underwent a middle meatal antrostomy and an anterior ethmoidectomy, bilaterally.

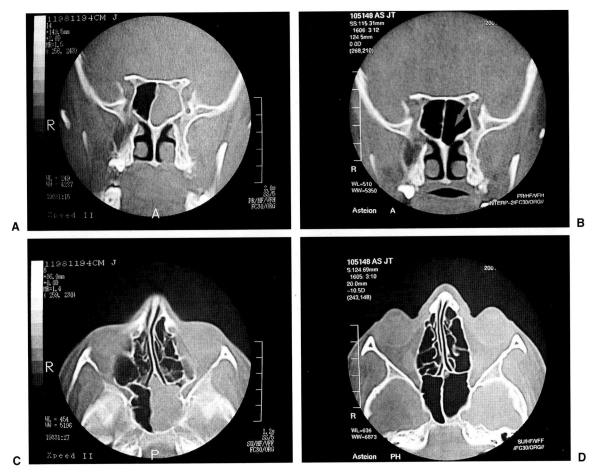

FIGURE 11–30 Preoperative (A) and postoperative (B) coronal CT scans of a patient with chronic sphenoiditis. The patient underwent a left sphenoidotomy. Note the neo-ostium of the left sphenoid sinus indicated by the arrow. Preoperative (C) and postoperative (D) axial CT scans of the same patient.

the nasal septum, tip of the nose, and nasal dorsum if necessary, together with the treatment of the inferior turbinates.[120]

Patients with headaches and facial pain respond quite well to surgery, with an improvement of 86%, although headaches often take 4 to 8 weeks to disappear after sinus surgery. Individuals with impaired sense of smell have a significant improvement of 72%. Most of the symptoms usually resolve early following the surgical procedure, with the exception of posterior rhinorrea, which remains longer. Some of the CT scan results are indicated in Figures 11–28, 11–29, 11–30, and 11–31. The overall results, including the subjective and objective data, are in accordance with results presented in the literature. However, we prefer not to mention "cure" or "success," but only "improvement," because it is difficult to be sure that the "converted" normal mucosa is going to stabilize or if there is any focus of possible recurrent disease. In any case, caution is the correct attitude to have because the long-term results of this surgical technique are still not known.

Despite the fact that patients often report a gratifying subjective improvement in their condition, postoperative radiological examination in some patients demonstrates some persistent mucosal swelling in the maxillary sinus and sometimes the frontal sinus. However, even if this fact indicates residual disease or a new focus of disease, revision surgery is not advised if the patient continues to feel well, and repeated CT scans should be requested only in symptomatic patients to rule out recurrent disease. In this situation, revision surgery should be decided according to the clinical judgment and should be based on intensity of symptoms, physical examination, endoscopic and radiological findings.

Always keep in mind that surgery, even performed by the most skilled surgeon with proper and meticulous surgical technique, does not cure all patients. We are dealing only with a small part of the body, and sinus

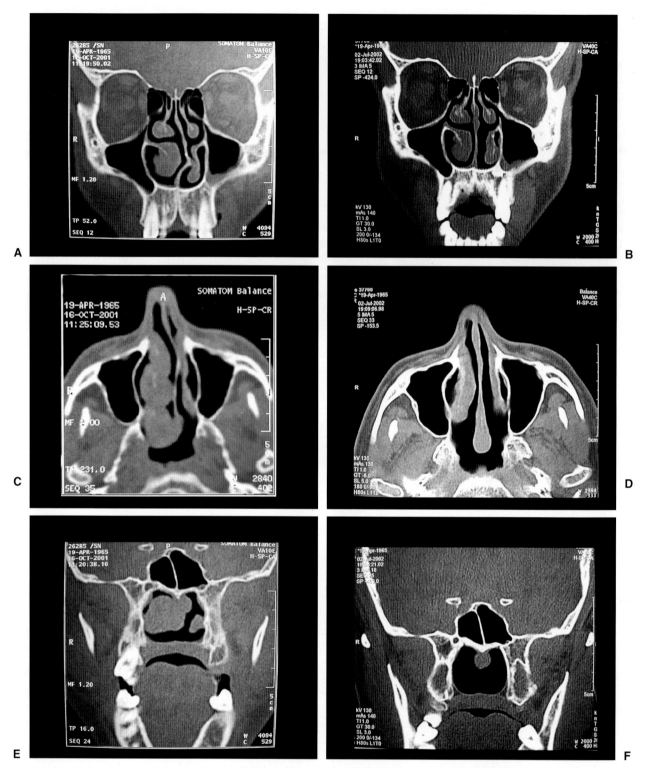

FIGURE 11–31 Preoperative (A) and postoperative (B) coronal CT scans at the level of the crista galli of a patient with nasal septum deviation, left chronic sinusitis, and a hypertrophic right inferior turbinate. Preoperative (C) and postoperative (D) axial CT scans of the same patient. Preoperative (E) and postoperative (F) coronal CT scans at the level of the posterior choana showing the hypertrophic right inferior turbinate obstructing the right nasal cavity and protruding into the nasopharynx.

disease is a multifactorial disorder. It is our opinion that the key for successful results (besides technical knowledge and surgical expertise) is clinical judgment.

■ Complications

Potential complications associated with surgery of the nose and paranasal sinuses range in severity from minimal to catastrophic. The surgeon must be aware of each of these, and the best approach to handle these surgical problems is to prevent, rather than to treat. Most complications of sinus surgery are associated with ethmoidectomy, frontal sinusotomy, and sphenoidotomy. The rate of complications depends on several factors, including the specific anatomy of the patient, location and severity of the disease, previous procedures, the surgeon's skills, and the techniques used.[121-127]

Complications of endonasal sinus surgery are listed in Table 11–20. A discussion of these complications is presented in Chapter 18.

One of the major advantages of COMET surgery is the almost complete lack of complications. As a matter of fact, the excellent visualization obtained with the microscope; the possibility of having two hands, one for dissection and the other for suction; the cleaning of the surgical field; and the ability to view the anatomical structures and the tip of the surgical instruments at all times are responsible for a very low rate of complications. In our patient population of over 1000 cases over the past 18 years using COMET surgery, we never had a major complication. In the study group of 200 patients, only two cases of minor complications (1%), one orbital emphysema and one case of orbital ecchymosis, were observed. The incidence of complications in endoscopic sinus surgery in a large series of patients is 0.85% (major) and 6.9% (minor) for a total population of 2108 patients.[128]

TABLE 11–20 Intraoperative Complications of Endonasal Sinus Surgery

Minor	• Orbital
	• Orbital emphysema
	• Orbital echymosis
	• Nasolacrimal duct injury (epiphora)
	• Disturbance of olfaction
	• Dental or lip pain and/or numbness
Major	• Orbital
	• Orbital hematoma
	• Optic nerve injury
	• Dural
	• CSF fistula
	• Brain
	• Laceration
	• Hemorrhage
	• Ethmoid arteries
	• Anterior communicating artery (or its branches)
	• Internal carotid artery
	• Internal carotid artery and cavernous sinus fistula

■ Conclusion

The combined microscopic and endoscopic techique (COMET surgery) is an excellent technique for surgical treatment of nose and paranasal sinus diseases. Today optical aids are very important for assisting the surgeon in performing accurate surgery with excellent results and fewer complications, and by combining the optical advantages of the microscope with the optical features of the endoscope, theoretically, this is the ideal surgical technique to achieve these goals.

The results obtained with COMET surgery are identical to those reported in the literature about endoscopic sinus surgery. The complication rate is minimal due to the optical characteristics and ergonomic performances of both optical instruments, which contribute to safe surgery when properly used. Also, the operating time of the described one-stage integrated treatment is acceptable, considering that the treatment of the nasal problems and the sinus diseases was accomplished during the same surgical procedure. Besides the importance of this concept of one-stage integrated treatment for patient care, avoiding a second operation and the relation cost/benefit is another valuable factor that should be applied in hospital practice.[129,130] This is an excellent surgical technique for the beginner who is trained to use the microscope in routine ear and laryngeal surgeries and with some more additional training can learn to handle the endoscopes. Later, when the surgeon feels more confident with nose and sinus surgery, he or she should consider the options and find the technique he or she chooses to follow in the future: microscopic, endoscopic or combined sinus surgery.

REFERENCES

1. Willemot J, et al. Anatomie et traumatismes du nez. Septo-rhinoplastie—nez et esthétique: la médicine antique au temps des pharaons. In: Willemot J., coordenateur. Naissance et développment de l'oto-rhino-laryngologie dans l'histoire de la médecine. Brussel, Belgium: *Acta Medica Belgica.* 1981:201–210. *Acta Oto-Rhino-Laryngol.* 1981:201–210.

2. Heermann H. Über endonasale Chirurgie unter Verwendung des binocularen Mikroskopes. *Arch Ohren Nase Kehlk Heilk.* 1958; 171:295–297.

3. Mehta D. Historical attraisal. In: Mehta D, ed. *Atlas of Endoscopic Sinonasal Surgery.* Philadelphia: Lea & Febiger; 1993:1–4.

4. Messerklinger W. Technik und möglichkeiten der nasenendoskopie. *HNO.* 1972;20:133–135.

5. Messerklinger W. *Endoscopy of the Nose.* Baltimore: Urban & Schwarzenberg; 1978.

6. Prades J. *Microcirurgia endonasal de la fosa pterigomaxilar y del meato medio.* Barcelona: Salvat; 1980.

7. Dixon HS. Microscopic antrostomies in children: a review of the literature in chronic sinusitis and a plan of medical and surgical treatment. *Laryngoscope.* 1976;86:1796–1814.

8. Dixon HS. Microscopic sinus surgery, transnasal ethmoidectomy and sphenoidectomy. *Laryngoscope.* 1983;93:440–444.

9. Dixon HS. The use of the operating microscope in ethmoid surgery. *Otolaryngol Clin North Am.* 1985;18:75–86.

10. Park IY. Improved endonasal sinus surgery by use of an operating microscope and a self-retaining retractor speculum. *Acta Otolaryngol.* 1988;458(suppl):27–33.

11. Stammberger H. Endoscopic surgery for mycotic and chronic recurring sinusitis. *Ann Otol Rhinol Laryngol.* 1985;119(suppl):1–11.

12. Stammberger H. Endoscopic endonasal surgery—concepts in treatment of recurring rhinosinusitis: 1. Anatomic and pathophysiological considerations. *Otolaryngol Head Neck Surg.* 1986; 94:143–147.

13. Stammberger H. Endoscopic endonasal surgery—concepts in treatment of recurring rhinosinusitis: 2. Surgical technique. *Otolaryngol Head Neck Surg.* 1986;94:147–156.

14. Stammberger H. *Functional Endoscopic Sinus Surgery: The Messerklinger Technique.* Philadelphia: BC Decker; 1991.

15. Stammberger H, Hawke M. *Essentials of Functional Endoscopic Sinus Surgery.* St. Louis: Mosby; 1993.

16. Kennedy DW. Functional endoscopic sinus surgery: technique. *Arch Otolaryngol.* 1985;111:643–649.

17. Kennedy DW, Zinreich SJ, Rosenbaum AE, Johns ME. Functional endoscopic sinus surgery: theory and diagnostic evaluation. *Arch Otolaryngol.* 1985;111:576–582.

18. Kennedy DW, Zinreich SJ. The functional endoscopic approach to inflammatory sinus disease: current perspectives and technique modifications. *Am J Rhinol.* 1988;2:89–96.

19. Kennedy DW. Prognostic factors, outcomes and staging in ethmoid sinus surgery. *Laryngoscope.* 1992;101:1–18.

20. Kennedy DW, Shaman P, Han W, Selman H, Deems DA, Lanza DC. Complications of ethmoidectomy: a survey of fellows of the American Academy of Otolaryngology—Head and Neck Surgery. *Arch Otolaryngol Head Neck Surg.* 1994;111:589–599.

21. Kennedy DW, Borger WE, Zinreich SJ. *Diseases of the Sinuses.* Hamilton, BC: Decker; 2001.

22. Wigand ME, Steiner W, Jaumann MP. Endonasal sinus surgery with endoscopical control: from radical operation to rehabilitation of the mucosa. *Endoscopy.* 1978;10:255–260.

23. Wigand ME. Transnasal ehtmoidectomy under endoscopical control. *Rhinology.* 1981;19:7–15.

24. Wigand ME. Renaissance des opérations transnasales des sinus par l'endoscopie chirurgicale. *J Franc Oto-Rhino-Laryngol.* 1982; 5:319–322.

25. Wigand ME, Buiter CT, Griffits MV, Perko D. Treatment of antral pathology—which surgical route? *Rhinology.* 1988;26:253–255.

26. Wigand ME. *Endoscopic Sinus Surgery of the Paranasal Sinuses and Anterior Skull Base.* New York: Thieme Medical Publishers; 1990.

27. Wigand ME, Hosemann W. Endoscopic surgery for frontal sinusitis and its complications. *Am J Rhinol.* 1991;5:85–89.

28. Rice DH. Endoscopic sinus surgery: results at 2-year follow up. *Arch Otolaryngol Head Neck Surg.* 1989;101:476–479.

29. Rice DH. Basic surgical techniques and variations of endoscopic sinus surgery. *Otolaryngol Clin North Am.* 1989;22(4):713–726.

30. Rice DH. Endoscopic sinus surgery. *Otolaryngol Clin North Am.* 1993;26:613–618.

31. Rice DH. Chronic frontal sinus disease. *Otolaryngol Clin North Am.* 1993;26:619–622.

32. Rice DH, Kennedy DW, Schaefer SD, Weymuller EA. Difficult decisions in endoscopic sinus surgery. *Otolaryngol Clin North Am.* 1993;26:695–700.

33. Rice DH, Schaefer SD. *Endoscopic Paranasal Sinus Surgery.* 2nd ed. New York: Raven Press; 1993.

34. Levine HL. Endoscopy and the KTP 532 laser for nasal sinus disease. *Ann Otorhinolaryngol.* 1989;98:46–51.

35. Levine HL. Functional endoscopic sinus surgery: evaluation surgery, and follow-up of 250 patients. *Laryngoscope.* 1990;100:79–84.

36. Levine HL. The office diagnosis of nasal and sinus disorders using rigid nasal endoscopy. *Otolaryngol Head Neck Surg.* 1990; 102:370–373.

37. Levine HL. The potassium-titanyl phosphate laser for treatment of turbinate dysfunction. *Otolaryngol Head Neck Surg.* 1991; 104:247–251.

38. Levine HL, May M. *Endoscopic Sinus Surgery.* New York: Thieme Medical Publishers; 1993.

39. Levine HL. Lasers in endonasal surgery. *Otolaryngol Clin North Am.* 1997;30:451–455.

40. Ochoa C, Silva HF, Pais Clemente M, et al. Mucocelo do seio esfenoidasl com resposta pseudo-sarcomatosa dos tecidos envolventes. A propósito de um caso clínico. *Rev Port ORL.* 1992; 30(4):227–232.

41. Antunes A, Santos M, Pais Clemente et al. Complicações orbitárias da etmoidite aguda—Estudo retrospectivo de 39 doentes. *Rev Port ORL.* 1995;33(6):305–315.

42. Pereira C, Pais Clemente L, Pais Clemente M, et al. Complicações da sinusite aguda na criança. Estudo retrospectivo de 76 casos. *Rev Port ORL.* 2002;40(2):133.

43. Draf W. Endonasal micro-endoscopic frontal sinus surgery: the Fulda concept. *Op Tech Otolaryngol Head Neck Surg.* 1991; 2:234–240.

44. Draf W, Weber R. Endonasal micro-endoscopic pansinus operation in chronic sinusitis: 1. Indications and operation technique. *Am J Otolaryngol.* 1993;14:394–398.

45. Rudert H. Mikroskop und endoskopgestützte chirurgie der entzündlichen nasennebhöhle nerkrankungen. *HNO.* 1988; 36:475–482.

46. Stamm AC, Draf W. *Micro-endoscopic Surgery of the Paranasal Sinuses and the Skull Base.* Heidelberg: Springer; 2000.

47. Benninger MS. The impact of cigarette smoking and environmental tobacco smoke on nasal and sinus disease: a review of the literature. *Am J Rhinol.* 1999;13:435–438.

48. Brook I, Gober AE. Resistance to antimicrobials used for therapy of otitis media and sinusitis: effect of previous antimicrobial therapy and smoking. *Ann Otol Rhinol Laryngol.* 1999;108:645–647.

49. Lieu JEC, Feinstein AR. Confirmation and suprises in the association of tobacco use with sinusitis. *Arch Otolaryngol Head Neck Surg.* 2000;126:940–946.

50. Kennedy DW, Senior BA, Gannon FH, et al. Histology and histomorphometry of ethmoid bone in chronic rhinosinusitis. *Laryngoscope.* 1998;108:502–507.

51. Clement PAR. Committe report on standardization of rhinomanometry. *Rhinology.* 1984;22:151–155.

52. Pais-Clemente M, Ribeiro M, Barros GC. Rinomanometria computorizada. *Rev Port ORL.* 1989;27(3):161–172.

53. Maran AGD, Lund VJ. Rhinomanometry. In: Maran AGD, Lund VJ, eds. *Clinical Rhinology.* New York: Thieme Medical Publishers; 1990:51–53.

54. Cole P, Roithmann R. Rhinomanometry. In: Gershwin ME, Incaudo GA, ed. *Diseases of the Sinuses: A Comprehensive Textbook of Diagnosis and Treatment.* Totowa, NJ: Humana Press; 1996:451–468.

55. Santos M, Vales F, Silva HF, Pais-Clemente M. Rinometria acústica: princípios e aplicações clínicas. *Rev Port ORL.* 1999;37(2):127–131.

56. Quine SM, Eccles R. Nasal resistance from the laboratory to the clinic. *Curr Op Otolaryngol Head Neck Surg.* 1999;7:20–25.

57. Parvez L, Erasala G, Noronha A. Novel techniques standardization tools to enhance reliability of acoustic rhinometry measurements. *Rhinol.* 2000;16(suppl):18–28.

58. Cole P. Acoustic rhinometry and rhinomanometry. *Rhinol.* 2000;16(suppl):29–34.

59. Grymer LF. Clinical applications of acoustic rhinometry. *Rhinol.* 2000;16(suppl):35–43.

60. Corey JP, Patel A, Mamikoglu B. Clinical applications of acoustic rhinometry. *Curr Opin Otolaryngol Head Neck Surg.* 2002;10:22–25.

61. Calvario F, Nunes R, Pais-Clemente M. Imuno-alergologia em patologia sinusal. *Rev Port ORL.* 1989;27(3):175–186.

62. Ward WA Jr. Diagnostic skin testing: skin end point titration. In: Krause HF, ed. *Otolaryngic Allergy and Immunology.* Philadelphia: WB Saunders; 1989:133–140.

63. Weeke B, Poulsen LK. Diagnostic tests for allergy. In: Holgate ST, Church MK, eds. *Allergy*. London: Gower Medical Publishing; 1993:11.1–11.14.

64. Donald PJ. Basic allergy and immunology. In: Donald PJ, Gluckman JL, Rice DH, eds. *The Sinuses*. New York: Raven Press; 1995:101–144.

65. Marks SC. Allergy diagnosis and management. In: Marks SC, ed. *Nasal and Sinus Surgery*. Philadelphia: WB Saunders; 2000: 83–104.

66. Krouse HJ, Davis JE, Krouse JH. Immune mediators in allergic rhinitis and sleep. *Otolaryngol Head Neck Surg*. 2002;126(6): 607–613.

67. Deitmer Th. Methods of investigation of mucociliary transport. In: Pfaltz CR, ed. *Physiology and Pathology of the Mucociliary System*. Basel: Karger; 1989:26–34.

68. Passàli D. Mucociliary clearance: our experience. In: Passàli D, ed. XIV Congress of the European Rhinologic Society (ERS) and XI International Symposium on Infection and Allergy of the Nose (ISIAN). Rome, Italy, October 6–10, 1992. *Rhinol Up-to-Date: Proceedings of the Fourteenth ERS Congress and Eleventh ISIAN*. 1992:105–107.

69. Passàli D, Bellussi L, Paganelli II, Rossi S. Surfactant in upper airways. In: Passàli D, ed. XIV Congress of the European Rhinologic Society (ERS) and XI International Symposium on Infection and Allergy of the Nose (ISIAN). Rome, Italy, October 6–10, 1992. *Rhinol Up-to-Date: Proceedings of the Fourteenth ERS Congress and Eleventh ISIAN*. 1992:150–155.

70. Baroody FM. Mucosal cytology. In: McCaffrey TV, ed. *Rhinologic Diagnosis and Treatment*. New York: Thieme Medical Publishers; 1997:175–192.

71. Jankowski R, Persoons M, Foliguet B, Coffinet L, Thomas C, Verient-Montaut B. Eosinophil count in nasal secretions of subjects with and without nasal symptoms. *Rhinology*. 2000;38:23–32.

72. Iguchi Y, Yao K, Okamoto M. A characteristic protein in nasal discharge differentiating non-allergic chronic rhinosinusitis from allergic rhinitis. *Rhinology*. 2002;40:13–17.

73. Besançon-Watelet C, Béné MC, Montagne P, Faure GC, Jankowski R. Eosinophilia and cell activation mediators in nasal secretions. *Laryngoscope*. 2002;112:43–46.

74. Boek WE, Graamans K, Natzijl H, Van Rijk PP, Huizing EH. Nasal mucociliary transport: new evidence for a key role of ciliary beat frequency. *Laryngoscope*. 2002;112:570–573.

75. Fernandes F, Duarte D, Castedo S, Simões MS, Gomes AM, Pais-Clemente M. Síndrome de Kartagener: a propósito de um caso clínico. *Bol Soc Port ORL*. 1986;24(2):31–42.

76. Duarte D, Pais Clemente M. Um caso de situs inversus com alterações morfológicas ciliares. *Acta ORL Gallega*. 1987:151–163.

77. Slavit DH, Kasperbauer JL. Ciliary dysfunction syndrome and cystic fibrosis. In: McCaffrey TV, ed. *Systemic Disease and the Nasal Airway*. New York: Thieme Medical Publishers; 1993:131–149.

78. Loft LM. Sinus surgery in cystic fibrosis. *Op Techni Otolaryngol Head Neck Surg*. 1999;7(3):242–247.

79. Shambaugh GE Jr. Stapes operations for otosclerosis. In: Shambaugh GE Jr, ed. *Surgery of the Ear*. 2nd ed. Philadelphia: WB Saunders; 1967:503–504.

80. Kleinsasser D. Microlaryngoscopy. In: Kleinsasser O, ed. *Tumors of the Larynx and Hypopharynx*. New York: Thieme Medical Publishers; 1988:128–130.

81. Hech E. *Optics*. New York: Addison-Wesley; 1997:148–246.

82. Bolger WE, Kuhn FA, Kennedy DW. Middle turbinate stabilization after functional endoscopic sinus surgery: the controlled synechiae technique. *Laryngoscope* 1999;109:1859–1853.

83. Zeifer B. Update on sinonasal imaging anatomy and inflammatory disease. *Neuro Imaging Clin Nor Am*. 1998;8:607–614.

84. Stammberger H. *FESS—"uncapping the Egg": The Endoscopic Approach to Frontal Recess and Sinuses. A Surgical technique of the Graz University Medical School*. Tuttlingen, Germany: Endo-Press; 1999:7–30.

85. Utley DS, Goode RL, Hakim S. Radiofrequency energy tissue ablation for the treatment of nasal obstruction secondary to turbinate hypertrophy. *Laryngoscope*. 1999;109:683–686.

86. Myrthe KS, Huizing H, Huizing E. Treatment of inferior turbinate pathology: a review and critical evaluation of the different techniques. *Rhinology*. 2000;38:157–166.

87. Lee KC, Hwang PH, Kingdom TT. Surgical management of inferior turbinate hypertrophy in the office: three mucosal sparing techniques. *Op Tech Otorryngol Head Neck Surg*. 2001;12:107–111.

88. Hilding AC. On cigarette smoking, bronchial carcinoma and ciliary action: experimental study on the filtering action of cow's lungs, the deposition of tar in the bronchial tree and removal by ciliary action. *N Engl J Med*. 1956;254:1155–1160.

89. Ide G, Suntzeff U, Cowdry EV. A comparison of the histopathology of the tracheal and bronchial epithelium of smokers and non-smokers. *Cancer*. 1959;12:473–484.

90. Ballenger JJ. Experimental effect of cigarette smoke on human respiratory cilia. *N Engl J Med*. 1960;263:832–835.

91. Kensler CJ, Battista SP. Components of cigarette smoke with ciliary-depressant activity. *N Engl J Med*. 1963;269:1161–1166.

92. Gross CW. Animal studies of the effects of inhaled air toxins on nasal mucosa. *Cur Opin Otolaryngol Head Neck Surg*. 1996;4:50–51.

93. Willes SR, Fitzgerald TK, Bascom R. Nasal inhalation: challenge studies with sidestream tobacco smoke. *Arch Environ Health*. 1992;47:223–230.

94. Keles N, Ilicali C. The impact of outdoor pollution on upper respiratory diseases. *Rhinology*. 1998;36:24–27.

95. Kunze M. Epidemiology of nicotine dependence and general aspects of smoking cessation. *Cardiovasc Risk Factors*. 1996; 6:130–134.

96. Raw M, McNeil A, West R. Smoking cessation guidelines for health professionals: a guide to effective smoking cessation interventions for the health care system. *Thorax BMJ London*. 1998; 53(5):3–38.

97. Pou A, Snyderman CH. Strategies for curing tobacco addiction. *Curr Opin Otolaryngol Head Neck Surg*. 1999;7:79–83.

98. Peto R, Darby S, Deo H, Silcock SP, Whitley E, Doll R. Smoking, smoking cessation and lung cancer in the UK since 1950: combination of national statistics with two case-control studies. *BMJ*. 2000;321:323–329.

99. Stankiewicz JA, Donzelli JJ, Chow JM. Failures of functional endoscopic sinus surgery and their surgical correction. *Op Technic Otolaryngol Head Neck Surg*. 1996;7(3):297–304.

100. Kerrebijn JDF, Drost HE, Spoelstra HAA, Knegh PP. If functional sinus surgery fails: a radical approach to sinus surgery. *Otolaryngol Head Neck Surg*. 1996;114(6):745–747.

101. Ramadan HH. Surgical causes of failure in endoscopic sinus surgery. *Laryngoscope*. 1999;109:27–29.

102. Stankiewicz JA. Management of endoscopic sinus surgery failures. *Curr Opin Otolaryngol Head Neck Surg*. 2001;9:48–52.

103. Richtsmeier WJ. Top 10 reasons for endoscopic maxillary sinus surgery failure. *Laryngoscope*. 2001;111:1952–1956.

104. Chow JM. Technical reasons for endoscopic sinus surgery failures. *Curr Opin Otolaryngol Head Neck Surg*. 2002;10:33–35.

105. Danielsen A, Olofsson J. Endoscopic endonasal sinus surgery: a long-term follow-up study. *Acta Otolaryngol*. 1996;116(4): 611–619.

106. Klossek JM, Peloquin L, Friedman WH, Ferrier JC, Fontanel JP. Diffuse nasal polyposis: postoperative long-term results after endoscopic sinus surgery and frontal irrigation. *Otolaryngol Head Neck Surg*. 1997;117(4):355–361.

107. Rosenstiel DB, Sillers MJ. The long-term results of functional endoscopic sinus surgery. *Curr Opin Otolaryngol Head Neck Surg*. 2000;8:27–31.

108. Senior BA, Kennedy DW, Tanabodee J, Kroger H, Hassab M, Lanza D. Long-term results of functional endoscopic sinus surgery. *Laryngoscope*. 1998;108(2):151–157.

109. Drake-Lee AB. Medical treatments of nasal polyps. *Rhinology.* 1994;32:1–4.

110. Van Camp C, Clement PAR. Results of oral steroid treatment in nasal polyposis. *Rhinology.* 1994;32:5–9.

111. Passàli D, Ferri R, Becchini G, Passàli GC, Bellussi L. Alterations of nasal mucociliary transport in patients with hypertrophy of the inferior turbinates, deviations of the nasal septum and chronic sinusitis. *Eur Arch Otorhinolaryngol.* 1999;256:335–337.

112. Assanasen P, Naclerio RM. Medical and surgical management of nasal polyps. *Curr Opin Otolaryngol Head Neck Surg.* 2001;9:27–36.

113. Shankar L, Evans K, Hawke M, Stammberger H. The postoperative appearances of the paranasal sinuses. In: Sankar L, Evans K, Hawker M, Stammberger H, eds. *An Atlas of Imaging of the Paranasal Sinuses.* Philadelphia: JP Lippincott; 1994:122–139.

114. Smith MM, Smith TL. The role of CT imaging in rhinosinusitis and the need for a standardized CT reading system. *Curr Opin Otolaryngol Head Neck Surg.* 2001;9:17–22.

115. Kenny TJ, Duncavage J, Bracikowski J, Yildirim A, Murray JJ, Tanner SB. Prospective analysis of sinus symptoms and correlation with paranasal computed tomography scan. *Otolaryngol Head Neck Surg.* 2001;125:40–43.

116. Kennedy DW. Prognostic factors, outcomes and staging in ethmoid sinus surgery. *Laryngoscope.* 1992;102:1–18.

117. May M, Levine H. Sinus surgery results reporting system of May and Levine. In: Levine HL, May M, eds. *Endoscopic Sinus Surgery.* New York: Thieme Medical Publishers; 1993:182–184.

118. Lund VJ, Mackay IS. Staging in rhinosinusitis. *Rhinology.* 1993; 31:183–184.

119. Hoseman WG, Weber RK, Keerl RE, Lund VJ. Results of endonasal sinus surgery for chronic rhinosinusitis. In: Hoseman WG, Weber RK, Keerl RE, Lund VJ, eds. *Minimally Invasive Endonasal Sinus Surgery: Principles, Techniques, Results, Complications, Revision Surgery.* New York: Thieme Medical Publishers; 2000:32–50.

120. Silva HF. Conceitos actuais do tratamento cirúrgico das sinusites crónicas. Estudo experimental e clínico. Ph. D. Thesis Porto, 1972;137–153.

121. Anand VK, Panje WR. Avoidance and successful management of complications of endoscopic sinus surgery. In: Anand VK, Panje WR, eds. *Practical Endoscopic Sinus Surgery.* New York: McGraw-Hill; 1993:87–98.

122. King HC, Mabry RL. Complications of sinus surgery. In: King HC, Mabry RL, eds. *A Practical Guide to the Management of Nasal and Sinus Disorders.* New York: Thieme Medical Publishers; 1993:161–181.

123. Stankiewicz JA. Complications of endoscopic sinus surgery and malpractice. In: Stankiewicz JA, ed. *Advanced Endoscopic Sinus Surgery.* St. Louis: Mosby; 1995:151–160.

124. Klossek JM, Fontanel JP, Dessi P, Serrano E. Complications et soins postopératoires. In: Klossek JM, Fontanel JP, Dessi P, Serrano E, eds. *Chirurgie endonasale sous guidage endoscopique.* Paris: Masson; 1995: 118–128.

125. Castillo L, Verschuur HP, Poissonnet G, Vaille G, Santini J. Complications of endoscopically guided sinus surgery. *Rhinology.* 1996;34:215–218.

126. Kaluskor SK. Complications in FESS. In: Kaluskar SK, ed. *Endoscopic Sinus Surgery: A Practical Approach.* London: Springer; 1997:79–90.

127. Stankiewicz JA. Complications of microdebriders in endoscopic nasal and sinus surgery. *Curr Opin Otolaryngol Head Neck Surg.* 2002;10:26–28.

128. May M, Levine HL, Schaitkin B, Mester SJ. Complications of endoscopic sinus surgery. In: Levine HL, May M, eds. *Endoscopic Sinus Surgery.* New York: Thieme Medical Publishers; 1993:193–243.

129. Kezirian EJ, Yueh B. Accuracy of terminology and methodology in economic analysis in otolaryngology. *Otolaryngol Head Neck Surg.* 2001;124(5):496–502.

130. Gross CW, Schlosser RJ. Prevalence and economic impact of rhinosinusitis. *Curr Opin Otolaryngol Head Neck Surg.* 2001;9:8–10.

12

Minimally Invasive Endoscopic Sinus Surgery with Powered Instrumentation

PETER DOBLE

■ History

Rueben Setliff was the first physician to successfully demonstrate that powered cutting tools could be used with precision, control, and safety in the nose and the paranasal sinuses in humans.[1] While seeking to improve the surgical approach and the outcomes of nasal sinus surgery, he recognized that the precision that controlled powered cutting could afford a surgeon was available to others but had not been examined and attempted in the field of otolaryngology. To that end, he began to use equipment that was available and had been designed for use in the small joint spaces of the hand and the temporomandibular joint (TMJ). In the late 1980s and early 1009s the first efforts offered a great deal of success and demonstrated that the equipment would work but that the requirements of the tissues in the paranasal sinuses would demand a more specifically designed tool. Setliff then began to engage medical instrument companies to improve and promote their instrument design. Through his pioneering vision and his tireless effort to seek the medical instrument establishment's acceptance of this procedure, we as physicians today have an entirely new tool to use in the field of nasal surgery.

The application of power to a surgical procedure is not new by any standard, but over time the advent of a series of new and more progressive technical improvements in specifically nasal surgery has occurred. The most obvious examples can be appreciated with a review of the application of power and optical improvement in the field of otologic surgery. The use of the dental engine and the advent of the use of the operating microscope appeared almost at the same time and were met at first with only lukewarm acceptance. However, within a short period it was obvious that surgical procedures were improving with the new tools, and surgeons began to understand that previously established limits were technical barriers only and that new limits could be explored.

The introductions of optical endoscopes and powered cutting tools in surgery on the nose and paranasal sinuses seem to be directly parallel. The ability today to proceed in a more defined, surgically clean field with ever increasing precision and delicacy allows surgeons great choice with respect to tissue preservation.

Type of Cutter and the Position of the Cutter

The important aspect of what Setliff accomplished was the choice of a cutter that had the blade face positioned so that the opening of the cutter was able to be seen by the operator through the endoscope at the same time he or she was operating. The previous choice had involved cutter designs that employed end-mounted cutters. These were not effective because of the viewpoint that the surgical field presented. The limits of the exposure do not allow the operator to see the end of the cutter during the actual time that tissue is being cut, and therefore the surgeon was cutting blindly.

The choice of using a cutter with a cutter face mounted in such a fashion so as to allow the working portion of the tool to be seen at all times was a bold and obvious move. This addressed all of the visualization problems that previous attempts in designing appropriate tools for nasal surgery had failed to see.

■ Development of the Micro-Debrider Tool

Micro-Debrider

The first Micro-Debrider (Stryker Leibinger, Kalamazoo, MI) was adapted from a tool produced for use in small joint arthroscopy in the wrist and the TMJ. It is our good fortune that the tool was so nearly ideally designed for the newly identified use. It required very little design change and was rapidly able to be approved for use in this new area by appropriate government agencies.

Suction

The real breakthrough that allowed the cutting tool to work and achieve early success and usefulness was the continuous suction at the working end of the tool. The suction allows the tool to remove tissue and blood from the field as the surgery proceeds. This allows the surgeon to work with two hands. One hand holds the working tool, while the other hand holds the endoscope and controls the surgical field of view. Although the two-handed approach had been promoted by others, it previously had been difficult to put into practice because of the technical demands the procedure requires of not only the surgeon but also the operating room team and staff.

The continuous suction at the distal tip of the cutting instrument meant that the surgeon could now operate and clear the field at the same time and remain in control and in full view of the procedure at all times.

Irrigation

The problem that this system had in its early development was its lack of effectiveness with respect to tissue removal. The instrument could clog with tissue that was being cut free and removed from the field. This presented many difficulties in the early days of the development of the Micro-Debrider tool. When the suction became blocked, it failed to present new tissue to the cutter and failed to remove cut tissue from the blade. The failure of the suction system was one problem that the surgeon needed to keep in mind because it appeared to be so subtle that it was often unrecognized.

This problem required an immediate fix and resulted in a field repair.

STOPCOCK SYSTEM

The first fix to this problem was the insertion of an in-line three-way stopcock that allowed the assistant to cut off the suction and direct a stream of hand-pressurized water to the clogged instrument. This system worked fairly well, but it required the assistant to fill and replace the syringes often and to divide his or her attention between the operating field and the stopcock system while the surgeon was operating. This system is still available. It fits the requirements of the individual surgeon.

PRESSURE SYSTEM

The importance of maintaining the Micro-Debrider tool in its best state of function led to the development of the pressurized irrigator and tissue trap system. This system places a large volume of irrigating solution under pressure via a pressurized infusion bag. The stopcock was replaced by a two-way lever valve and inline tissue trap. The tissue trap allowed the system to collect two separate specimens and submit them for pathological examination. The advantages are that the system remains closed and the nursing staff does not come in contact with tissue or fluids.

SELF-IRRIGATION SYSTEM

The self-irrigation system, which has evolved into its third generation, has addressed many, but not all, of the problems associated with clogging. The ideal system setup includes a self-irrigating handpiece as well as a pressure irrigator.

Tissue Trap

The advent of the tissue trap has allowed the surgeon to continue to send the entire resected specimen to the pathologist rather than representative samples. These traps are widely available and are always mounted in the suction line after the cutter. They may be placed in the suction canister as well as in the field. It is good medical practice to obtain tissue for study, whether using microshavers or cutters.

Cutters

The designs of today's cutters all feature a partly forward-facing cutter window and a revolving inner cutter blade with variously shaped cutting edges.

Basic blades come in different diameters. The appropriate size is determined not only by the age of the patient but also by the size of the nasal and sinus cavities. The different blades allow careful and thorough access to these areas. Basic blades are straight. They vary with respect to their shape and size, as well as the location and dimension of the cutter window. The choice depends on the specific application.

A recent change has been the availability of bent or angled blades. These blades represent a dynamic effort on the part of the medical instrument industry, as the development of these tools requires a large amount of research and development time and effort. Blades are available now in both fixed and adjustable shapes. Obviously, the marketplace will decide which is better or at least more supported.

Burs

Burs have great use in complex procedures such as intranasal removal of osteomas, removal of heavy bone around the front face of the sphenoid sinus and bone thickened from chronic infection, and the treatment of the frontal sinus duct. They also have great application for the plastic surgeon in bone remodeling.

Image-guided Triplanar Navigation

The availability of the multiplanar intraoperative tracking system (VTI, General Electric System, Lawrence, MA; Micro-Debrider, Stryker Leibinger, Kalamazoo, MI) has given surgeons new margins of safety. These systems are all based on the use of a high-speed computer and a system for reference to the patient intraoperatively. They require the patient to have had a super-high-resolution CT scan with a registration device in place prior to the operation. Surgical instruments are linked to the computer, and the computer displays a real-time image of the location of the cutting tool. This location is referenced in simultaneous axial, coronal, and sagittal images on the monitor screen. In the case of paranasal sinus surgery, this allows the surgeon to identify the location of surgical instruments. Accuracy is ~0.25 mm. This is important because of the proximity to the orbital contents, carotid siphon, and intracranial space.

■ Minimally Invasive Endoscopic Sinus Surgery

Most nasal and sinus surgical procedures in the United States are performed in an ambulatory surgery center. The procedure as outlined below can be modified depending on the needs of the particular surgical setup. However, the requirements that are noted are very important and if not respected will lead to results that differ from the experiences presented.

Anesthesia

The anesthesia of choice for this operation is a combination of regional nasal blocks, topical local anesthesia, and IV sedation or general inhalation techniques. The choice of IV or general inhalation techniques is personal and should be discussed with the patient before the operation. However, the use of regional nasal blocks and topical local anesthesia is required.

Oxymetazoline

The nasal membranes are vigorously decongested and vasoconstricted with oxymetazoline in the preoperative phase. This is needed to allow the operator better access to the nasal cavities and their structures. The use of oxymetazoline appears to allow a more aggressive application of cocaine. The nasal membranes are sprayed every 3 to 5 minutes for the duration of the preoperative period, or up to 45 minutes.

Cocaine

The application of oxymetazoline is followed by a solution of 10% cocaine. This is used for its severe vasoconstrictor effect as well as its excellent topical anesthetic properties. The cocaine is placed in the nose by aerosol spray delivered every 3 to 5 minutes up to the time of instrumentation and the start of the procedure. The remaining solution is reserved on the operating field and is applied as needed during the procedure. The amount of cocaine required varies from patient to patient, but 10 to 20cc of 10% solution is the normal amount.

A debate has raged over the concomitant use of multiple vasoconstricting agents, but the regimen given above has been used successfully in multiple centers over many years and many thousands of cases without complications. As with all endoscopic procedures, the ability to have an unimpeded surgical view is paramount to a successful outcome, and the above outlined regimen will routinely accomplish that very necessary goal.

Injection

The injections for the regional block of the anatomy of the nose have been documented elsewhere. The block we employ is used to complement the topical anesthesia and to enhance the vasoconstriction already in place following preoperative treatment. The blocks are placed at the superior root and along the inferior horizontal portion of the middle turbinate. The required amount of anesthetic varies but is usually 10 to 15cc of 1% xylocaine with 1:100,000 epinephrine. This is delivered by the use of a #27 1½-inch needle in a very superficial plane. The fewest injection sites that are employed, the better, as some small amount of bleeding from the injection sites will happen. This can cause some difficulty with the procedure because of the interference with the endoscope.

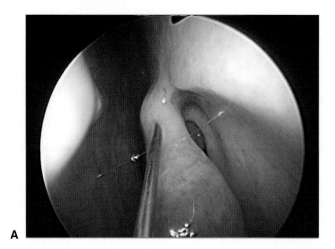
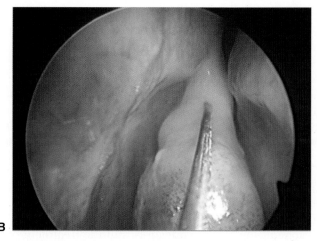

FIGURE 12–1   (A,B) Injection of the root of the middle turbinate, left and right.

The use of a transpalatine nerve block has not been shown to be critical to the technique described here. The block is accomplished transorally. The foramen of the palatine nerves is located in a standard fashion, and 5 to 10 cc of the local anesthetic is infiltrated into the canal.

Injection into the middle turbinate is shown in Figures 12–1 and 12–2.

Details of the Procedure

Once the injections have been completed and the patient's condition is stable, the operation is begun. The technique of using the hand Micro-Debrider tool demands attention to detail and requires that the surgeon make a commitment to the discipline of learning the subtle movement that makes the tool function properly.

The tool is held in the surgeon's dominant hand as if it were a pen or pencil.

The microshaver is used to remove tissue from the surface of the sinuses and the interior of the nasal cavity. The microshaver must be moved continuously and must not be held in one fixed position for a prolonged period of time. Although the risk of burning tissue is not present, the tool works most effectively if it is allowed to be in contact with the tissue in a rapid and intermittent fashion. This allows the suction to present new tissue to the cutter face each time the blade turns.

The cutter controls allow the cutter to rotate selectively left, right, and in an oscillating mode. The cutter blades generally are used in the oscillating mode when removing soft tissue and in the continuous mode when removing bone. This allows the cutter blade to bring new material to the working portion of the blade with each rotational change. This also allows for the irrigation system to function more effectively and to keep the blade set for clogging.

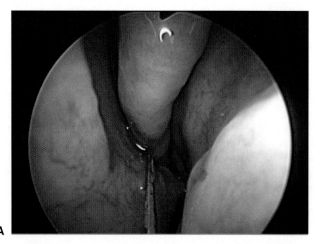
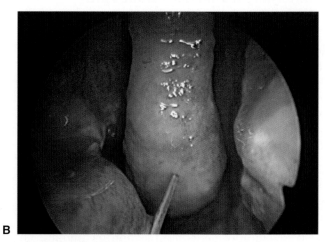

FIGURE 12–2   (A,B) Injection of the inferior portion of the middle turbinate, left and right.

HAND POSITION

The handpiece is held in the surgeon's dominant hand and is grasped as lightly as possible and as firmly as needed for the action desired and the control needed. As in otologic procedures where the drill is used and the action required is extremely delicate and close to important structures, the hand control required is identical and demands exceptional strength with delicate fine movements.

The tool should be held in a comfortable fashion, with the weight of the instrument carried slightly behind the balance point. The best grasp is one that mimics holding a pen or pencil. The tool will have some vibration, but the surgeon should quickly become comfortable with the tool's characteristics. The hand should rest as comfortably as possible on the operating field so that the wrist is supported and the hand can move as required to approach the unusual anatomical relationships that the nose presents.

Wrist and Arm Position

The wrist and arm must be supported as much as possible. The resting position of the wrist and arm must be worked out so that the operator places his or her arm in this position without restriction. The wrist should be supported by the fifth finger and advanced as needed by the wrist and forearm.

This position must allow the surgeon to hold and move the Micro-Debrider tool with as much or as little force as needed. This position is best if the arm and wrist are at rest and supported as if the tool were an otologic drill.

SURGEON'S POSITION

The surgeon's position during the operation is one of choice. The decision to sit or stand while operating is left to the surgeon.

POSITION OF THE VIDEO SYSTEM

The use of the video system appears to be the best method of visualization. The safety of the video system is twofold. First, it allows the surgeon to remove himself or herself from the immediate area of the operating field. This reduces the risk of bloodborne pathogens. Second, it reduces the risk of damage to the macula from the intense light of the optical systems. Significant damage to the retina from the use of direct-view fiberoptic scopes has led to the widespread use of videoscopes by our gastrointestinal colleagues.

The field of view that the endoscope provides is limited by the television camera itself, and the camera is less sensitive than the human eye. The perspective provided for the surgeon by the endoscope may be less than the eye, but it is controllable and gives the surgeon the opportunity to learn the limits of the endoscope. The limits of the camera and the endoscope can be learned and can be used as constant aids by the surgeon with placement and surgical location.

The comfort provided by a video system cannot be understated. The freedom that can be obtained by using a video system allows the surgeon choices in positions and operating styles.

FINE CONTROL

The fine control of the hand tool is based on the concept of two interrelated arcs or circles. The wrist describes a larger series of arcs. These arcs are made by the wrist rotating on the forearm and the wrist bones.

The smaller arcs are formed by the fingertips rotating the hand tool on the thumb. These arcs allow the surgeon to make very fine movements. When combined with the larger arcs from the wrists' movements, these two motions allow for fine, delicate control and placement of the tool.

Middle Turbinate

The middle turbinate is the first anatomical landmark encountered in an endoscopic surgical approach. In the normal position it will appear as an overhanging mass of tissue in the midcentral area of the nasal airway arising from the lateral nasal wall (Fig. 12–3).

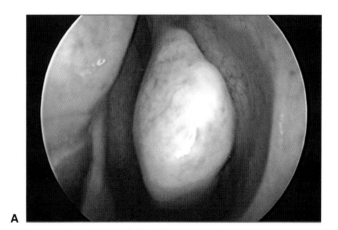

A

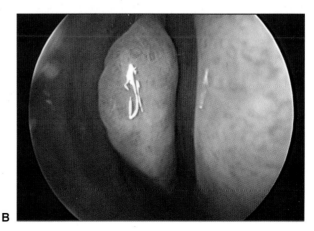

B

FIGURE 12–3   (A,B) Normal appearance of a middle turbinate.

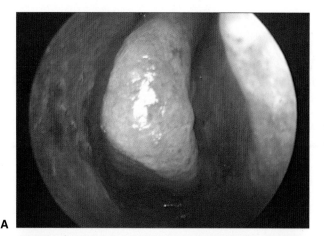

A

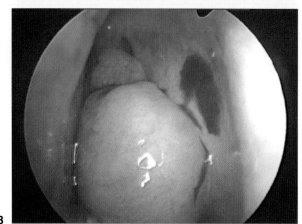

B

FIGURE 12–4 (A,B) Polypoid turbinates, left and right.

The middle turbinate arises from a thin, finely developed plate of bone from the ethmoid sinus and is the medial limit of the ethomid system. The middle turbinate is almost always identifiable in this location. In the event that polypoid material is present from the ethmoid or

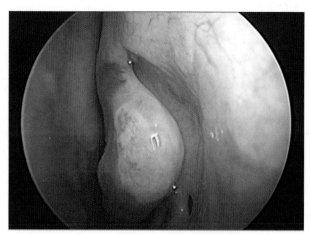

FIGURE 12–6 Paradoxical middle turbinate.

the superior ethmoid cavities, the view may obscure and may require diligent effort on the part of the operator to obtain a satisfactory block and vasoconstriction to define the anatomy.

The presence of polypoid changes, or polypoid degeneration of the middle turbinate, causes the clear delineation of the anatomy to be more difficult but more important. With a carefully considered and technically adequate local block and topical block, the middle turbinate can be defined (Figs. 12–4, 12–5).

The various shapes of the middle turbinate will determine the required approach to the structure and will define the reshaping needed to accomplish the desired form to accommodate the changed airflow and drainage pathways (Figs. 12–6, 12–7, 12–8).

Uncinate/Maxillary Ostium

The uncinate and the maxillary ostium are considered to be an interrelated anatomical and physiologic structure.

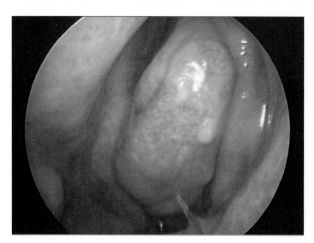

FIGURE 12–5 Thick middle turbinate.

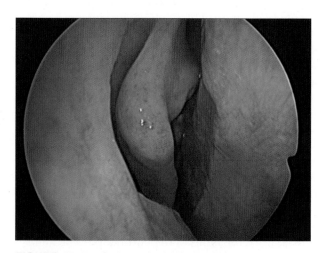

FIGURE 12–7 S-shaped middle turbinate.

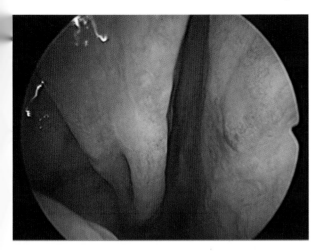

FIGURE 12–8   Bifid middle turbinate.

The shape defined by the medial surface of the nasal wall to the inner surface of the middle turbinate is considered the ostiomeatal complex. The highly vascular tissues in this area are subject to edema from all of the insults that the entire nasal membranes suffer. The normally tight environment that encompasses these structures does not allow them to expand to accommodate the swelling caused by these insults; therefore, the edema sets up causes contact between the tissues. This contact in turn causes the mucociliated transport to stop. The stoppage of flow results in the onset of stasis, which leads to infection.

The uncinate is located at the posterior edge of the lacrimal crest and is bordered superiorly by the attachment of the middle turbinate. The inferior border is the insertion into the lateral nasal wall at the level of the posterior membranous fontanelle. The posterior edge of the uncinate is free and is in close proximation with the anterior edge of the ethmoid bulla. The area where the free edge of the uncinate joins the ethmoid bulla is the ideal site to locate the incision into the uncinate.

The backbiter is placed into this area, and the retrograde dissection is performed until the tip of the instrument is gently felt to be in contact with the intact posterior border of the lacrimal crest, as this is the anterior limit of the dissection (Fig. 12–9).

Using the endoscopic power tool or microshaver, the free edge of the incised uncinate is sharply removed to the level of the joining of the uncinate to the lateral nasal wall. This is the final common pathway for the drainage of the maxillary sinus and the frontal sinus. The area just below and posterior to the location is the membranous fontanelle. A delicate set of dissecting instruments is employed to gently remove the uncinate bone from the cut surface of the dissection. This requires that the bone be dissected with a great deal of care to respect the interior mucous membrane. The

interior leaflets of this membrane's cilia are oriented in such a fashion that following the creation of the "final common" pathway the cilia will be positioned so as to assist in the removal of mucus from the natural ostium of the maxillary sinus (Figs. 12–10, 12–11).

Uncinate to Agger Nasi

Once the dissection of the natural ostium of the maxillary sinus has been accomplished, the approach to the frontal sinus can be started. The landmark that appears to be the most consistent and the most readily located is the anteriormost air cell in the ethmoid system, the agger nasi cell. This is seen on the CT scan in the coronal projection as the first cell encountered before the root attachment of the middle turbinate. In the case of a patient who is to have revision surgery, this landmark is still usually discernible.

The anterior attachment of the uncinate leaflet is the anterior bone wall of the agger nasi cell. The approach to this area is simply the application of the power tool in a gentle manner to remove tissue until the agger nasi cell is entered from below. Once the cell is opened inferiorly, the cell is opened to the nasal cavity working within the classic surgical precept of "known to unknown." The important structures in this area are well protected, and the exposure of the agger nasi cell allows the immediate approach to the frontal duct and the frontal system (Fig. 12–12).

Agger Nasi to Frontal Sinus

The agger nasi cell's posterior border is the anterior wall of the frontal "duct." The opening of the agger nasi cell allows the surgeon to instrument the duct with whatever technique he or she has chosen. This is usually not needed, as free drainage from the frontal system can be established by the manipulation of the agger nasi system. This allows drainage down the anterior portion of the uncinate fold and into the final common pathway (Fig. 12–13).

Frontal Sinus Location

The actual duct drains in the posterior and medial position to the location of the agger nasi cell. The location is fairly constant because of the embryology of the ethmoid cell system's development with respect to the frontal sinus system's development (Fig. 12–14).

Ethmoid Bulla

Immediately posterior to the free edge of the uncinate is the anterior border of the ethmoid bulla. The shape,

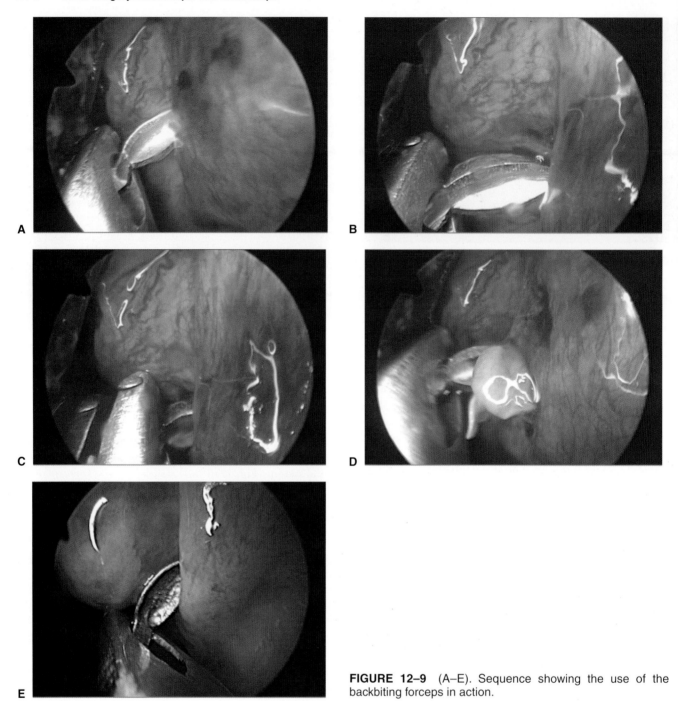

FIGURE 12–9 (A–E). Sequence showing the use of the backbiting forceps in action.

size, and pneumatization of the bulla are highly variable. The medial and internal margins are the inner surfaces of the middle turbinate. The posterior border is the anterior wall of the sphenoid sinus (Fig. 12–15).

Anterior Ethmoid Sinus

The surgical approach to the ethmoid bulla is begun by placing the power instrument on the surface of the bulla and dissecting toward the lateral nasal wall. Proceeding

from anterior to posterior and from inferior to superior while moving from medial to lateral, the dissection is accomplished under complete control and under direct vision at all times.

Hiatus Semilunaris Posterior

The entrance to the posterior ethmoid air cells is located immediately posterior to the lamella basalis and lies directly behind the attachment of the middle

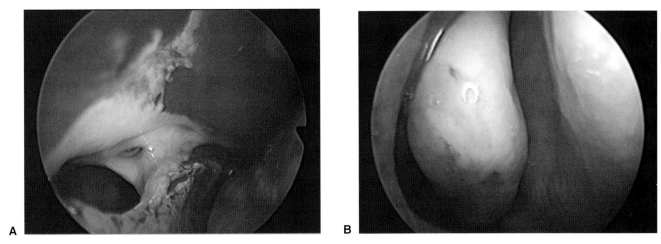

FIGURE 12–10   Final common pathway (A) and outflow track (B) of the natural ostium.

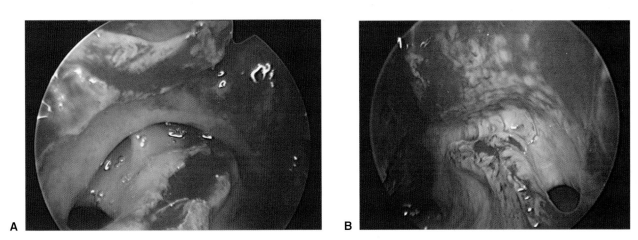

FIGURE 12–11   Outflow track (A) and pathway (B) of the natural ostium.

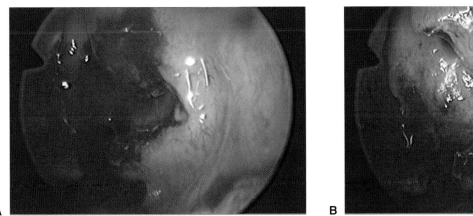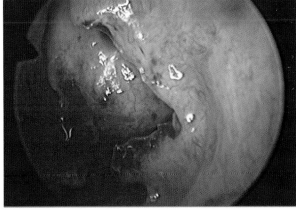

FIGURE 12–12   (A,B) Dissection of the uncinate process   superiorly to the agger nasi cell system.

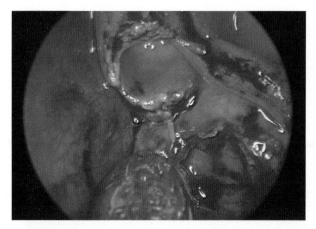

FIGURE 12–13   Dissection of the agger nasi cell to the frontal sinus.

turbinate to the lateral nasal wall (Fig. 12–16). This structure has been called the hiatus semilunaris posterior by Setliff[1] and others. This structure is formed by the air cells of the posterior cells, which cause a change in the conformation of the horizontal section of the

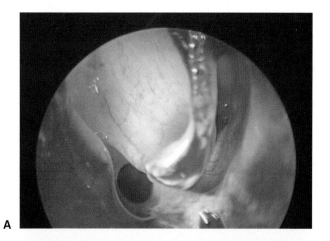

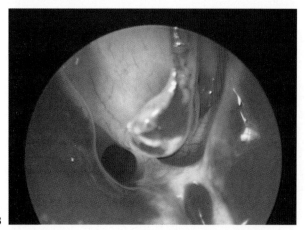

FIGURE 12–14   (A,B) Dissection of the frontal sinus duct as it drains medially and posteriorly to the agger nasi cell system.

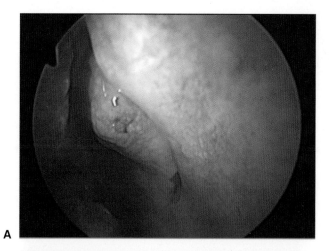

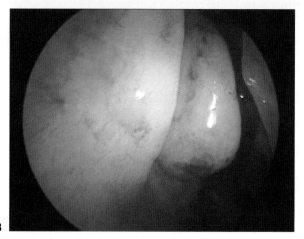

FIGURE 12–15   (A,B) Dissection of the ethmoid bulla.

middle turbinate's projection and attachment to the lateral nasal wall (Fig. 12–17).

Posterior Ethmoid Sinus

The anterior border of the posterior system is the posterior surface of the horizontal projection of the middle turbinate. The lateral border is the medial surface of the middle and superior turbinate. The medial border is the lateralmost surface of the orbit. The superior border is the inferior portion of the anterior cranial fossa and rarely a portion of the frontal sinus. The posterior border is the anterior wall of the sphenoid sinus.

Sphenoid Sinus

The sphenoid sinus develops at the most posterior and medial section of the nasal cavity and is located superior to the posterior oral nasal vault. Usually but not always this structure has a left and right side. The structure may

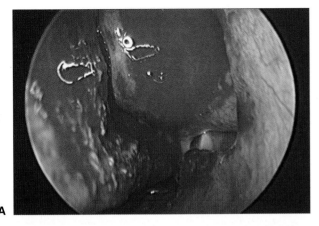

A

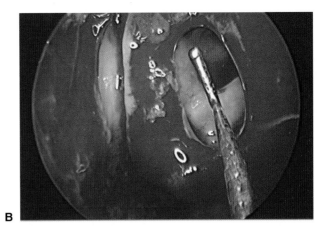

B

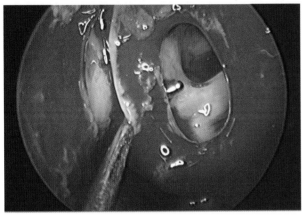

C

FIGURE 12–16 (A–C) Dissection of the posterior ethmoid viewed through the transition of the anterior ethmoid space, already dissected.

exist in a variable fashion and may have more than one cell per side.

■ Immediate Postoperative Care

After the procedure has been completed, the nasal cavity is dressed in the following fashion. The middle turbinates are injected with a depo-steroid product in the areas that have been addressed surgically or that have suffered superficial damage from the passage of the instruments. The steroid is one of the surgeon's choices, with multiple products on the market.

The ethmoid and ostiomeatal complex are filled with an ointment of choice. The surgeon is encouraged to choose one of the aqueous-soluble types for this application.

The use of nasal packs is a hotly debated issue. Should you choose to pack, there are many types to select. The choice and selection are up to the surgeon.

If a septoplasty has been performed, the next choice is stenting. Again, this is the surgeon's preference.

In any case, the removal of the packing or the stenting should be done as soon as possible and in a manner that causes the least secondary trauma to the nasal mucosa.

The patient is placed on a hypertonic saline nasal rinse as soon as possible postoperatively, usually that same day. The postoperative regimen includes antibiotics, analgesics, oral or injectable steroids, and nasal steroids. Oral steroids are administered in a decreasing dosage over a 10- to 12-day period and usually started at 20 mg bid. If injectable steroids are given, a single dose of 60 to 80 mg of a long-acting steroid is sufficient.

A light dressing under the nose to catch the small amount of drainage is usually all that is required and can normally be discontinued the following morning.

■ Postoperative Care

Postoperative care is simple and straightforward. Patients are seen in the office at whatever interval has been determined as the optimal time. In the author's office, patients are seen at 1-week intervals for the first month. They are seen as required following the first month.

During the first month, patients require very little debridement, and that debridement is reserved to as little as needed and only if absolutely indicated. The author does not debride at all until the third weekly visit.

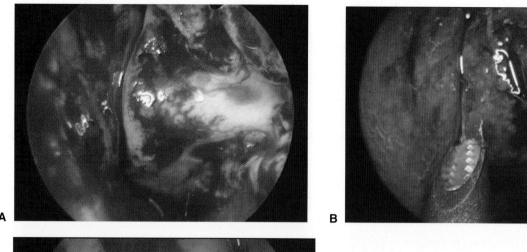

FIGURE 12–17 (A–C) Anatomical demonstration of the outflow system of the anterior ethmoid air cell system, also known as the hiatus semilunaris posterior.

Packing if placed is removed at the end of the first week. If septal stents are used, they are removed at that time as well.

As in all nasal surgery it is important to avoid synechiae. This has been demonstrated to be less of a problem with this minimally invasive approach, but it remains a cause for careful observation. Minimal postoperative debridement and judicious use of injectable steroids have proven to be most effective. Early irrigation with hypertonic saline solutions also appears to be helpful. Patients are started on saline solution rinses the evening of the procedure and are continued for 6 weeks at a twice-a-day regimen. The better the compliance, the quicker the healing and the lesser the appearance of scar tissue.

REFERENCES

1. Setliff RC. The hummer: a remedy for apprehension in functional endoscopic sinus surgery. *Otolaryngol Clin North Am.* 1996;29(1): 95–104.

13

Stereotactic Surgery

JACK B. ANON AND LUDGER KLIMEK

Endonasal sinus surgery is the procedure of choice for most patients with acute or chronic rhinosinusitis that fails to respond to appropriate medical therapy. The close proximity of the ethmoid, frontal, and sphenoid sinuses to the orbit and skull base provides for only a small margin of error. Though rare occurrences, violation into these important surrounding structures may lead to visual disturbances, CSF leak, and even death. Therefore, it is important for the surgeon to continually know the precise location of the surgical instruments. We have previously described the use of various computer-aided (aka image-guided and computer-assisted) devices that provide a precise two- and three-dimensional graphic interface between the operative site, a computer system, and a high-resolution monitor (Fig. 13–1). This interface may utilize an arm-based, infrared, electromagnetic, or sonic sensor system (no longer available) manufactured by several companies. This chapter will address four specific navigational devices: the VTI (Woburn, MA) electromagnetic InstaTrak, the Xomed (Jacksonville, FL) active/passive infrared LandmarX, the BrainLAB (Palo Alto, CA and Heimstetten, Germany) passive infrared VectorVision, and the Stryker (Kalamazoo, MI) active infrared Navigation System.

■ Historical Background

Neurosurgeons were the first to use surgical guidance systems. Framed stereotactic units using CT scans were developed in the mid-1970s, and although they provided for instrument trajectory, they did not show real-time instrument localization.[1,2] Roberts et al[3] were among the

first in the English literature to describe a frameless navigational system to "improve the integration of imaging data with the operative procedure." Radiopaque glass beads were taped to the patient's head, and a CT scan was performed. The intraoperative computer was linked to a microscope via an acoustical localizer and had an accuracy of ~2.0 mm. Over the ensuing years, other authors have described their own experiences of variations on the same theme.

In the mid-1980s, Schlöndorff et al,[4] and others at the University of Aachen, Germany, were some of the first to realize the potential for these same systems to be utilized in otolaryngology for skull base and sinus surgery. Over the course of several articles during the ensuing years, they described their laboratory and clinical experiences with a passive arm-based system, an optical arm-based digitizer, an infrared localizer, and an acoustical probe.

In the mid-1990's in the United States, Anon and colleagues[5,6] reported on the use of the mechanical arm and infrared freehand ISG (Mississauga, Ontario, Canada) Viewing Wand.

Recently, Anon et al[7] examined the evolution of computer-aided surgery, and reviewed the different types of localizers currently available.[7]

■ VTI InstaTrak

The InstaTrak system is an intraoperative computer-aided surgical system that utilizes electromagnetic tracking technology to provide real-time positional feedback of instrument location on prerecorded CT and MR images.

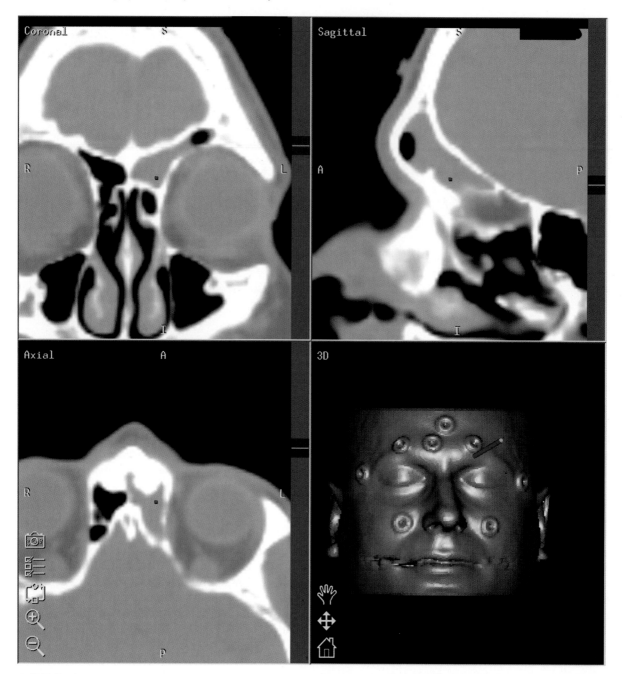

FIGURE 13–1 Medtronic Xomed LandmarX triplanar screen shot of a preoperative scan.

The system is composed of a Sun Sparc-5 computer workstation with 20-inch high-resolution monitor, an electromagnetic transmitter-receiver pair with associated electronics, and a plastic headset frame worn by the patient during both the preoperative CT scan and surgery.

Computer

The Sun Sparc-5 computer workstation uses a Solaris operating system that is capable of simultaneously displaying an original axial CT scan as well as reformatted coronal and sagittal two-dimensional views on a 20-inch high-resolution monitor. The workstation processes position and orientation information from the electromagnetic locating system and in real time displays the instrument tip with respect to the CT images of the patient as a "crosshair."

Headset

The headset allows for automatic registration of the preoperative CT images with the electromagnetic tracking

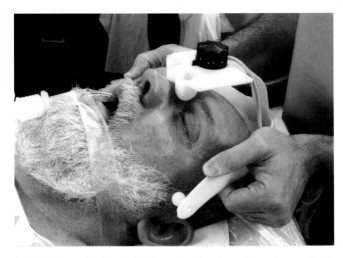

FIGURE 13–2 The VTI headset is placed on the patient. Note how the headset sits on the nose. The ear pieces are rounded and fit into the meatus of the external auditory canal. The black piece is the electromagnetic transmitter.

the electromagnetic transmitter, consisting of a geometric arrangement of coils, serves as a magnetic field source generator. The coils are driven through a series of excitation states to produce a continuously varying magnetic field in the target surgical area. When the receiver (attached to a variety of straight and curved suctions, powered dissectors, and forceps via a docking mechanism) is introduced into the magnetic field, voltages are induced in sensors inside the receiver assembly. The strength and polarity of these signals are determined by the position and orientation (x, y, and z axes, azimuth, elevation, and roll) of the receiver relative to the transmitter. A dedicated computer processor measures these received signals and calculates the appropriate position and orientation of the receiver based on a mathematical model of the magnetic fields and calibration data. The electromagnetic system has a positional accuracy of 0.5 mm and an angular (orientation) accuracy of 0.5 degree.

system and adjusts the computer's positioning system with head movement during the surgical procedure. The VTI headset is a molded disposable plastic reference frame with two rubberized earpieces that fit into each external auditory meatus and a double nasal piece that fits onto the nasal dorsum. The headset is placed on the patient prior to the preoperative CT scan and is placed back on the patient at the time of surgery (Fig. 13–2). The design of this headset allows for secure, reproducible positioning of the device each time it is applied on the patient. In a recent study, 25 subjects each had 4 different headsets placed in position by 2 different technicians 4 different times, for a total of 16 applications. These headsets were specially marked with a positional marking system, and each patient had an adhesive millimeter coordinate grid attached to strategic areas on his or her face. The exact position of the headset was able to be determined for each application, and the coordinates were compared. This study showed that the VTI headset can be placed on a patient each time with an accuracy of 0.6 mm (JB Anon, unpublished data).

The headset also contains seven 2.0 mm diameter metal balls affixed into the plastic structure of the headset. After acquiring the preoperative CT scan, the InstaTrak system software automatically searches for the densities of the metal balls, which all need to be within the same plane of scanning. If they are all in position, the computer is able to "autoregister."

The headset also serves as the attachment point of the electromagnetic transmitter.

Electromagnetic Transmitter and Receiver

All position measurements are made by an electromagnetic location-finding system. In this proprietary system,

Radiology

As noted above, the InstaTrak system employs axial, coronal, and sagittal views of the patient's CT scanned anatomy. The coronal and sagittal views are reformatted by the InstaTrak system from the patient's single helical scan data taken in the axial plane and transferred to the InstaTrak via a network or media connection.

In radiology, the headset is placed on the patient, and the patient is prepared for an axial plane sinus CT scan. A lateral scout view is taken, and the scan area is defined from the inferior aspect of the maxilla superior to a level ~1.5 cm above the uppermost CT bright metal markers in the headset. The display field of view (DFOV) is ~20 cm and centered about the sella turcica so that all nasal cavity and sinus anatomy is included in the scan.

With the CT scanner's gantry angle at 0 degree, the archive matrix set to 512, and an axial plane established, a helical 3×3 scan of the patient is made. The 3×3 scan refers to a 3 mm slice thickness by a 3 mm table movement. The CT data are reconstructed to a 1 mm table increment using a standard bone algorithm. The standard bone algorithm is used to visually enhance the bone tissue as opposed to soft tissue or edges. It is noted that this method of obtaining the required scan data subjects the patient to minimal doses of ionizing radiation compared with an axial scan, where 1 mm slices are individually obtained.

Most CT scanners configure their patient scan data in accordance with a NEMA standard entitled "Digital Imaging and Communication in Medicine," which is commonly referred to as DICOM 3. The InstaTrak system and its companion workstation, called ConneCTstat, are designed to communicate with and accept DICOM 3 scan data via network transfer. Therefore, the patient's

CT scan data are sent via network transfer to either the InstaTrak or the ConneCTstat systems. Typically, the ConneCTstat resides in radiology, where the scan data transfer takes place. The ConneCTstat reformats the patient's data to provide all three views (axial, coronal, and sagittal) and writes this data to an optical media cartridge. The media cartridge may then be physically taken to the InstaTrak instrument, typically residing in the operating room or surgical suite, where the patient's CT data are installed. If the OR is equipped with a network outlet, the patient's CT data may be pushed directly to the InstaTrak system over the network, making the ConneCTstat workstation unnecessary. It would also be unnecessary if the radiology department and surgical suite were close enough to allow the InstaTrak to be physically taken to radiology for network transfer of the patient's CT data.

Operating Room

The metal operating room table is shielded from the patient by securing a 6-inch foam pad along the length of the table. Once the patient is anesthetized and intubated (we do our procedures under general anesthesia), the headset with attached electromagnetic transmitter is placed in position, and sterile plastic drapes are applied. Any preparation, injections, and so on are performed, and prior to beginning the procedure, a calibration is performed. The calibration procedure allows the user to correlate the position of the instrument/receiver unit being used to the location of the receiver assembly. This procedure is performed by placing the tip of the instrument in a small dimpled center of the transmitter assembly and activating the "tip offset" button display on the computer screen. The system measures the distance of the receiver from the transmitter from several different orientations and calculates the instrument tip location relative to the receiver. Next, a "drift point" is established by touching the instrument to a set point on the patient's nose and activating the "drift set point" button on the computer screen. During the operation, an internal timer necessitates checking this "drift point." If the accuracy changes by more then 2.0 mm, then recalibration is required to maintain consistent accuracy. Calibration and "drift point" setting take approximately 2 minutes.

Surgery commences in the usual fashion, and the instrument/receiver unit is used intranasally to confirm the surgeon's precise location as shown on the computer screen

Instrumentation

The VTI InstaTrak has been adapted for use with a variety of suctions (straight and curved) and forceps, as well as shavers, such as the Xomed Magnum system. Smaller

electromagnetic receivers allow for flexibility and ease of use. A flat-screen touchpad monitor, which can be covered with a sterile drape, is now available. It gives the surgeon a clear view of the operating site as well as control of the computer functions.

■ Medtronic Xomed LandmarX System

The LandmarX ENT Image Guidance System is a dual-modality optical system that utilizes both infrared emitting diodes (IREDs) and reflective passive markers attached to an intraoperative headset and a variety of instrumentation. A camera array, attached on a movable boom to the LandmarX cart, tracks the light emissions from the IREDs or passive markers, then relays that positional information to the computer.

A high-resolution monitor is mounted on the cart on which the surgeon can select one, two, four, six, or nine views: orthogonal views (axial, sagittal, and coronal), various navigational views (based on the actual position of the instrumentation), the endoscopic view, and various three-dimensional models (skull, skin, sinuses, etc.).

Computer

A Silicon Graphics Model R12000 computer processes data at speeds upwards of 2.1 gigabytes per second and utilizes a Unix operating system. There is built-in modem and an uninterruptible power supply (UPS). The modem allows a technical support staff to "talk to" the LandmarX system, thus providing immediate diagnostics, maintenance, and software upgrades. The UPS protects the system in the event of power surges or outages, but more importantly, it facilitates moving the system from one OR suite to another without having to reboot.

Radiology

The patient is not required to wear any device during the scanning process, as anatomical fiducials may be used to register the dataset. Scanning protocol requires axial scans from 1 to 3 mm, contiguous and nonoverlapping. The LandmarX system can utilize scans from either helical (or spiral) or nonhelical CT scanners. MRI datasets may also be used.

The CT datasets may be transferred to the LandmarX system by two methods. First, the system will accept information transferred over a DICOM 3 network. Alternatively, the LandmarX system can be configured with a variety of media drives. So, if a scanner archives to a DAT tape or optical disk, the corresponding drive(s) can be built into the LandmarX system. The tape or disk is then loaded into the system just as a floppy disk is in a personal computer. These scanner interfaces allow for easy interface with off-site scanners and as a backup should you prefer a network interface. There is no need for an off-site workstation, as the LandmarX software performs the multiplanar reconstruction.

Operating Room Setup

The headset is placed onto the patient and secured using an elastic silicone band. The camera array is aimed at the surgical site and placed in its optimum position by using a visual aid on the software screen. The surgeon calibrates the surgical instruments by placing each one into a divot located in the headset. The calibration process is a safety feature that confirms the instrument has not been damaged and conforms to the specifications that have been programmed into the software.

Registration Process

The surgeon selects from 4 to 10 anatomical fiducials on the three-dimensional model that has been reconstructed from the dataset. These are selected via a simple "point and click" with the mouse. The point selected is also displayed on all three orthogonal views, giving the surgeon confidence in the point selected. The surgeon then touches those same points on the patient with the registration probe. The computer software matches those two sets of points (the three-dimensional model and the patient), thus correlating the patient to the dataset.

The LandmarX system registration process has several unique features. It utilizes a proprietary, multifactor equation that includes consideration of the mean fiducial error of the selected points, the spread of the points, the number of points, the slice spacing, and the scan field of view. The resulting value is a prediction of true intraoperative accuracy or how accurately the instrument tip will be displayed in the orthogonal views. Because the fiducials are selected from various planes and cover the volume of the sinuses, the instrument tip accuracy will be reflected throughout the sinus. The LandmarX system also offers a graphical representation of the intraoperative accuracy throughout the anatomy in addition to the numerical value resulting from that registration. The software also gives the surgeon the ability to improve the registration accuracy.

An advanced software algorithm, known as Surface-Merge, is also available to further refine the PointMerge registration process. In this process, the surgeon touches 40 random points with a probe on the surface anatomy, depressing the footswitch to enter each point. This process draws a map of the facial contours, tightly correlating the anatomy to the CT dataset. Although this process may add another 2 minutes to setup time, it improves localization accuracy.

A third registration process employs the FAZER Contour Laser Device to acquire surface registration points without physically touching the patient. This device utilizes a safe, low-intensity laser beam to easily map out the contours on the patient's face. An advanced software algorithm matches these contours to the patient's CT data, and an accurate registration is achieved in under a minute.

Operating with the LandmarX System

Once registered, the patient and/or the system may be moved without loss of registration through a patented process known as "dynamic referencing."

A "sustained accuracy checkpoint" may be selected to verify that the headset has not slipped in relationship to the anatomy. A point is selected (by touching with the registration probe) and stored. Then, anytime throughout the procedure, the surgeon may touch that point. A numeric message will inform him or her whether the headset has changed position relative to the anatomy.

Because the LandmarX system is an optical device, the IREDs and passive markers on the instrumentation must be visible to the camera array when the surgeon wishes to localize a point. This issue, commonly known as the "line of sight" issue, can be minimized by proper OR setup and becomes fairly transparent after the learning curve of just a few cases. In addition, the IREDs and passive markers display a great deal of flexibility in positioning in that the camera array can detect light emissions from obtuse angles. Medtronic Xomed has also developed IRED and passive marker attachments that are offset to face the camera to further minimize this issue.

The surgeon may choose to operate in continuous or freeze mode. In continuous mode, the system is tracking the instrument's location constantly, and the orthogonal views move in real time. In the freeze mode, the surgeon may, with the footswitch, freeze the picture so that the anatomy may be studied and/or on-screen images may be captured.

Surgeon Control Options

The LandmarX system offers two means by which the surgeon can control the system from the sterile field. The patented TouchPad comes with the system and attaches in multiple positions to the headframe. It is sterilizable and wireless. To activate, the surgeon touches all four corners of the TouchPad, thus drawing a grid in space that the computer recognizes. The surgeon can then use any navigational instrument to activate the functions on the TouchPad. The latest generation system, the LamdmarX Evolution System (Fig. 13–3), offers a high-resolution 21-inch, flat-panel touch screen that can be pulled up to the OR table. The surgeon can then

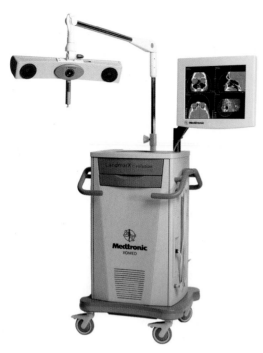

FIGURE 13–3   The Medtronic Xomed Evolution system.

operate all functions of the system using a set of sterile pointers from the surgical field.

Instrumentation

Any standard OR instrument may be used with the LandmarX system via one of three methods.

An instrument may be modified with a post that will accept the modular "tracker." With this methodology, each instrument is listed on a drop-down menu of instruments available. When an instrument is selected with the mouse or the TouchPad, the software knows exactly where the tip of the instrument is in relation to the IREDs in the tracker and displays the crosshairs accordingly. Medtronic Xomed currently has a microresector (Fig. 13–4), ostium seekers, a variety of suctions, forceps, and other instruments available in posted versions.

An optional software upgrade, known as the SureTrak Universal Instrument Adapter System, enables navigation

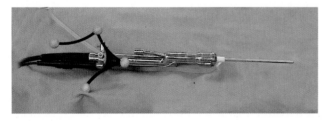

FIGURE 13–4   The Medtronic Xomed Magnum shaver with passive infrared array.

with any rigid instrument in the surgical field by securely clamping IRED and passive marker arrays. A simple calibration procedure enables this software to write the specifications "on the fly," precluding the need to have them entered into the software.

Archiving Information

The LandmarX contains a CD-ROM drive on which entire datasets (including three-dimensional models and surgical plans) or screen "snapshots" may be stored for patient files or publication. The snapshots are archived in a JPEG format that is easily viewed, printed, or saved on a PC.

■ BrainLAB's VectorVision and Kolibri ENT

The VectorVision system links a wireless freehand probe, tracked by a passive marker sensor system, to a virtual computer image space on a patient's preoperative CT or MR images. The system runs under Windows-XP, which enables the easy installation and maintenance of the entire software program. Upgrades to the existing software are easily applied. The proprietary infrared dual cameras from NDI are part of the integrated image-guided surgery system. The cameras are both infrared flash emitter and receiver. These infrared flashes are reflected by passive marker spheres mounted on a wide variety of instrument adapter arrays that can be attached to preexisting surgical instruments. The infrared reflection images from the markers of the instrument adapter array on the selected instrumentation are "seen" by the two cameras from different angles. The computer software geometrically analyzes the angles of reflectance to calculate the three-dimensional position of each marker sphere, and therefore the position of the entire instrument relative to the patient.

When designing the software, one of the major challenges was to determine the identity of the various marker images seen by each of the cameras. Which markers seen by one camera correspond to which markers seen by the other camera? In addition, it was necessary to deduce which markers correspond to which tool. This is a specific problem that occurs only in passive marker systems, making the software design much more complicated than that for active infrared optical systems. These problems were solved by tracking the sequential instrument positions as they move. Using known distances and other geometrical information available, the software is able to deduce the identity of the markers. This principle requires that the cameras have an unobstructed view of the tool markers at all times that navigation is desired during surgery.

Diagnostic Examination

FIDUCIAL MARKERS

To provide a link between patient anatomy and the diagnostic image data, it is necessary to establish a fixed reference between these two points; that is, the system needs to know the patient's orientation in three-dimensional space relative to the cameras. When the system was first shown in 1997, special low-profile fiducials were developed that are adhered to the patient's skin before the preoperative CT is obtained. These fiducials consist of two parts, an adhesive socket that is attached to the patient's scalp near the area of projected exposure and draping and an 8 mm spherical aluminum marker that is inserted into the sockets for preoperative CT. This design allows the scan to be performed at least several days before the procedure and also allows the patient to sleep with the attached sockets. For security, a circle can be drawn with a felt-tip marker around the sockets so they can be reattached in the same location in the event they are detached.

The marker sites are selected on minimally mobile scalp areas to provide proximity to the planned surgical site so they can be palpated under surgical draping and to provide as much distance as possible between individual sites. Although only three marker sites are essential, the attachment of two more is recommended to provide redundancy; the software can handle up to five markers. After the diagnostic examination, the spherical aluminum markers are replaced by indented patient fiducials and inserted into the sockets. The cone in the middle represents the center of gravity of the spherical markers and ensures precise referencing of the patient because a defined point is used for registration. Because all system components can be used in a sterile environment, the process of registration is truly straightforward.

As an alternative to using fiducial markers, mouthpieces have been applied to achieve dynamic referencing.[8,9] A similar mouthpiece has been used in the Vector Vision system. The central element is an individual dental cast, made from a rapidly hardening, nonirritant, and form-stable dental material (Impregum, ESPE, Seefeld, Germany). This is glued to carbon fiber plate with two rods. A vacuum pump is connected to the plate to create a pressure difference that squeezes the teeth cast to the upper jaw, thus repositioning the mouthpiece precisely. Two other rods are connected at right angles, and a reference clamp with three spherical reflective markers is connected. All components (except the markers) are made of carbon fiber with plastic screws, so that artifacts during radiologic imaging can be avoided. Additionally, this design gives maximum stability with minimum weight.

Z-Touch Laser Registration

In 2000 BrainLAB developed a new proprietary technology to provide a link between diagnostic data and patient in the OR. With the development of the z-touch laser registration, it was no longer necessary to apply fiducial markers, mouthpieces, or headsets for the diagnostic CT/MRI scan (Fig. 13–5). With this technology it

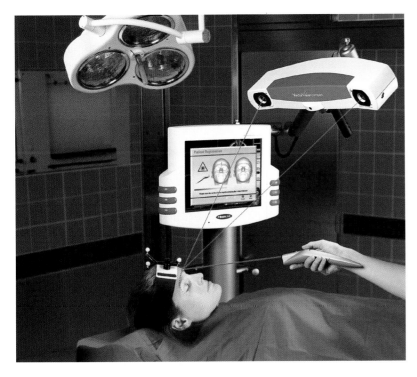

FIGURE 13–5 BrainLAB VectorVision with z-touch laser registration.

is now possible to scan the patient without having to worry about applying any kind of reference device for preoperative scanning. With recent additions to the data transfer module it is now also possible to use original diagnostic data as long as they have been acquired in a slice thickness that lies between 1 and 3 mm. The addition of z-touch has changed the approach for image-guided surgery procedures. Reducing effort for preoperative scanning and clinical setup time is crucial for the use of IGS technology.

Radiology

VectorVision employs axial, sagittal, or coronal views from CT or nuclear magnetic resonance (NMR). Additionally, digital subtraction angiography (DSA) data can be included. We use these data not in endonasal surgery for inflammatory diseases, but for example, in tumors invading the base of the skull, the orbit, or the fossa retromandibularis.

In paranasal sinus surgery, CT scans with the following properties are used (Table 13–1):

TABLE 13–1   Properties of CT Scans in Paranasal Sinus Surgery

Field of view scan range	Include all sinus cavities and all superficial facial anatomy. Do not include complete brain and skull if not necessary.
	Do not include the table or headrest in the field of view.
	Include all fiducial markers/landmarks (defined by responsible surgeon).
	z-touch: Include the face containing the forehead, eyes, and complete nose (tip of nose must not be cut off).
	No restraints across face or ears (across chin is OK).
Scan properties	• Axial only
	• Contrast chemicals allowed
	• Scan with kernel for soft tissue windowing.
	• Scan patient with eyes closed.
	• Pixel size, matrix size, and table height must remain the same during the scan.
	• Sequential scans
	• 1–3 mm, contiguous or overlapping slices
	• Do not scan with gap.
	• Slice distance can be changed during the scan.
	• Spiral/helical scans
	• Pitch (table-scan ratio) ≤2:1
	• Reconstruction scan slice increment ≤3 mm (recommend 2 mm)
Gantry tilt/ angulation	• Positive and negative values are allowed, but they must remain the same during scanning.
	Any kind of gantry angles can be used.
Patient orientation	Strict supine position
Image compression	If transferring via CD-ROM, save images in uncompressed format.
Matrix size	Any, recommend squared (e.g., 256 × 256 or 512 × 512)

1 to 2 mm slice thickness with 2 mm table movement
Continuously nonoverlapping
Axial helical scan slices taken for suppression of dental amalgam artifacts (these are reformatted by the system into a three-dimensional model including coronal and sagittal views)
~30–60 slices
Gantry angle at 0 degrees
Matrix set to 512 (or higher, depending on CT scanner)
DFOV centered to sphenoid or sella turcica
Standard bone algorithm
Data configuration according to DICOM 3

Data may be transmitted via a fiberoptic network or CD-ROM in DICOM 3 format. If data are obtained by NMR or DSA, special properties are used that will be individually adjusted.

If the z-touch laser registration is used for intraoperative registration, the patient is not required to wear a headset or fiducial markers during diagnostic imaging. The scan is taken with a standard CT/MR protocol that ensures the optimum accuracy and resolution required for image-guided surgery. In a typical case situation, the patient will be seen by the surgeon who schedules a CT scan without having to apply fiducial markers or headset. The scan procedure is performed according to the scan protocol mentioned above. The surgeon can even use original diagnostic imaging data in image-guided surgery. The surgeon can decide to use image guidance at any time and does not have to schedule an additional CT scan.

System Calibration

In contrast to the camera arrays of the very first optical tracking systems,[10] VectorVision uses NDI infrared cameras with high-resolution field matrix CCD chips. The cameras are built into a housing and can be flexibly adjusted to the operational approach.

The cameras are precalibrated, and therefore no calibration has to be performed.

Operating Room

The system is placed at the head of the patient. Our standard is to perform computer-aided surgery procedures under general anesthesia. The setup is very easy and straightforward because the system will be booted by a single switch. The assistant nurse can load the data from a zip disk or network and can then prepare the patient with the reference headband. The headband is applied by sticking the adhesive pad directly to the forehead of the patient and then tightening it with a Velcro band. After applying the headband and the reference array with reflective spheres, the patient's head will be randomly scanned with a special laser pointer that allows the system to utilize each patient's head and facial anatomy for registration. Once the surface is scanned, the advanced software algorithm calculates the alignment of the patient's anatomy to the CT or MR imaging data in the computer system.

The registration process is completely performed in a sterile environment. All components are autoclaved, as are the reference clamps or the various pointer tools.

After registration, accuracy checks are performed by making a visual check of landmarks such as the lateral canthi and by comparing the position of identifiable landmarks on the patient relative to the coordinates of the same landmark on the image reconstruction. Additionally, the root mean square can be determined (i.e., the overall deviation for the registration set).

Instrumentation

This system is easily adaptable to any already existing instrument in the OR. Although a special pointer is available for this system, this tool has no further function other than pointing to a target. Additionally, different lightweight passive marker arrays were designed that can simply be attached with adjustable brackets to any instrument, enabling its simultaneous use for surgical navigation (Fig. 13–6). After mounting one of the four arrays to the instrument, the tip only must be calibrated in an instrument calibration matrix (Fig. 13–7). This is done by touching the tip to the center of one of the pivot points of the instrument calibration matrix. The software then recognizes automatically the specific array

and calibrates the length of the instrument. In this manner, any surgical instruments or endoscopes are turned into pointing devices, and the surgeon does not have to change his or her tool during surgery. Furthermore, there are a variety of suctions and IGS-ready instruments that increase the ease of use of IGS systems.

Kolibri ENT

The Kolibri ENT system was designed with the goal of making image-guided surgery available to every patient. Kolibri is a small portable system that is easily integrated into the surgical setup. The procedure from CT scan to navigation is highly simplified, and the process is sped up. After the scan, the data are put on a CD-ROM or transferred via network. After the data are transferred to the Kolibri ENT, the data will be automatically loaded. After attaching the previously mentioned reference headband, the patient will be scanned with the z-touch laser registration. The software then calculates the alignment of the patient to the CT scan.

Optical Digitizers (Not Related to BrainLAB)

Replacement of the rigid arm by active optical digitizers for computer-assisted surgery was a big step toward more flexibility and ease of use. Active optical digitizers rely on IREDs placed on the operating probe or instruments in a known geometric pattern. A camera array near the operating table detects the position of the IREDs, and, using triangulation techniques, the position of the probe or instrument can be determined. If IREDs are placed on the patient, the motion of the patient can be

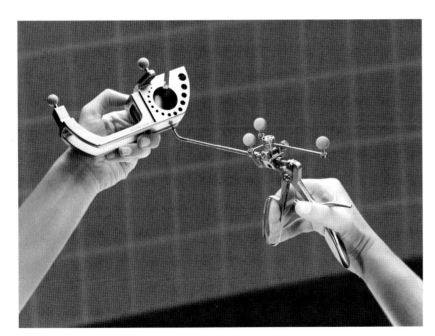

FIGURE 13–6 BrainLAB Instrument calibration with the ICM 4 instrument calibration matrix.

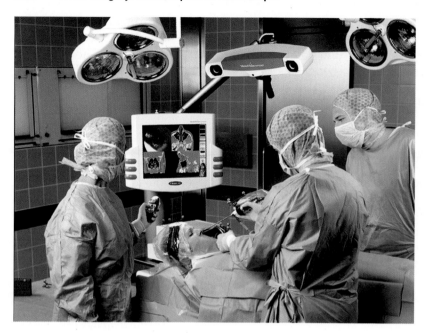

FIGURE 13–7 Operating with the BrainLAB VectorVision system.

detected by the computer. Surgery can then be performed under either local or general anesthesia.

The first optical digitizing system used for otolaryngologic surgery had a triangular camera array attached to an aluminum frame placed above the patient. The instrument handle had five IREDs strategically placed, and there was another set of five IREDs attached to the patient's head. This system has found widespread use in several fields of otolaryngologic surgery.[11–13]

We have performed a laboratory trial as well as clinical studies with this system.

■ Stryker Navigation System

The Stryker Navigation System guides the surgeon with an active tracking system and software written on a Windows 2000 platform. After the patient is imaged, the images are imported into the navigation system and reformatted so the surgeon can visualize the relative orientation of the diseased tissue and the surrounding healthy tissue. From these images, the system also creates a virtual model of the patient that is later linked with the real patient through a registration process. Once the patient is registered, the surgeon can track the surgery progress on the patient's virtual model. In this way the surgeon adds another dimension of visual feedback to his or her surgical tool kit.

Radiology

The Stryker Navigation System does not require any headsets or fiducial markers to be attached to the patient prior to imaging. CT and/or MR images can be used with the system, and an imaging protocol is provided to the technologist with the parameters that yield optimum results. The most important part of the protocol requires that the acquired images are thin (roughly 2 mm thick) compared with standard radiologic images (typically 5–7 mm thick). Thin images yield the best image quality when the image stack is reformatted and cut along planes other than the acquisition plane. The images can be downloaded to an optical disk, CD, or tape, or they can be transferred to the navigation system over a network transfer.

Platform

Stryker offers cart and laptop systems as well as a navigation suite where the monitor and camera are ceiling mounted. Each platform uses the Windows 2000 operating system and a Dell computer. The monitor has a high-resolution, flat-panel display that was designed specifically for Stryker Navigation and Stryker Endoscopy monitors. Even though it is a flat-panel display its characteristics (contrast, brightness, and lumens) more closely resemble those of a cathode ray tube (CRT) monitor (Fig. 13–8). The tracking camera is Stryker's own technology and has the ability to pinpoint a tracked light emitting diode (LED) to within 0.25 mm.

Instrumentation

Stryker's navigable instruments have embedded LEDs in predefined locations that are calibrated so that the LED locations can be translated to yield the instrument's need for a touch screen or a second person to run the navigation software. All of the Stryker Navigation System handpieces, including their electronics, are autoclavable.

Registration

Registration with the Stryker system is done in one of three ways: paired points, surface matching, or with Stryker's Mask autoregistration system.

Paired-points registration is done by selecting distinct anatomical points (e.g., the tragus, medial and lateral canthi, and nasion) on both the virtual patient and the real patient. The system then takes these points and merges the virtual world and the real world. Following registration, any moves made by the navigable instrument are shown in the virtual world against the backdrop of the patient's image data.

Surface matching is similar to paired points except the pointer is used to define the patient's surface anatomy instead of distinct points. The system merges the "real" surface with the virtual surface created from the image data.

Stryker's Mask autoregistration system is a unique device that enables a consistent and accurate registration (Fig. 13–10). The mask is composed of a form-fitting adhesive strip (with embedded LEDs) that is affixed to the patient's face, plus a communication unit (much like the communication unit of the handpieces). When the mask is turned on (with the push of a button), the system recognizes it and automatically registers the patient to the contour map (automatically calculated from the patient's images). After the registration process is complete, the LEDs on the forehead section of the mask serve as the patient tracker. This eliminates the need for a head strap or fixation device to mount the tracker to the patient's head, which, in turn, eliminates the possibility of head strap slippage. The mask can also be rearranged to accommodate frontal approaches (e.g., frontal sinus trephination).

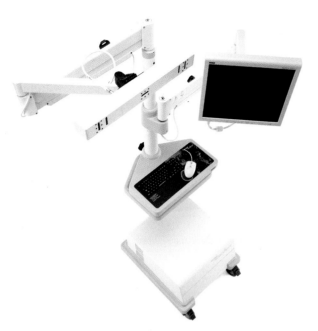

FIGURE 13–8 The Stryker Navigation System.

tip location when navigating (Fig. 13–9). There are several precalibrated instruments (pointers, frontal sinus seeker, frontal sinus suction, maxillary sinus seeker, and maxillary sinus suction) with angled offsets that eliminate line-of-sight issues. Adapters are also available that can be affixed to nonnavigable instruments (including microdebriders) to convert them for navigation. Handheld calibration tools are used to calibrate these instruments. In addition to the tracking LEDs on each navigable instrument, there are embedded communication electronics that turn the instrument into a two-way communication device. Each instrument has buttons much like a computer's mouse that the surgeon can push to control the software. The software interface was designed so that all of the software features can be accessed and controlled with the handpiece. This remote function was added to eliminate the

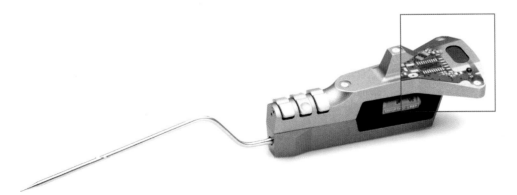

FIGURE 13–9 The Stryker active infrared handpiece.

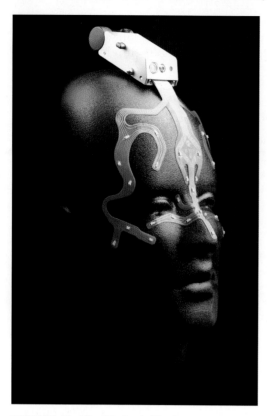

FIGURE 13–10   Stryker's Mask autoregistration system.

Navigation

After the patient is registered, computer operations that can be performed via the various handpieces include

- Zooming (in and out)
- Screen captures
- Image-view manipulations (there are five predefined viewing templates plus a tool for setting up user-defined templates)
- Virtual-tip extension
- Registration refinement and/or surface matching

At the end of the operation the patient's images can be archived onto a CD with the read/write CD drive that comes with both the cart and the laptop systems.

■ Conclusion

Computer-aided surgery is an important tool for the sinus surgeon. TheVTI InstaTrak, Xomed LandmarX, BrainLab VectorVision, and Stryker Navigation System provide for 1 to 3 mm accuracy in the clinical setting, which gives the operator real-time accurate knowledge regarding his or her location within the sinus complex. It is our assumption that this knowledge can only be beneficial for the patient, allowing for safer and more complete dissection within the operating field.

REFERENCES

1. Bergstrom M, Greitz T. Stereotactic computed tomography. *Am J Roentgenol.* 1976;127:167–170
2. Brown R. A computerized tomography–computer graphics approach to stereotaxic localization. *J Neurosurg.* 1979;50:715–720.
3. Roberts DW, Stronbehn JW, Hatch JF, et al. A frameless stereotaxic integration of computerized tomographic imaging and the operating microscope. *J Neurosurg.* 1986;65:545–549.
4. Schlöndorff G, Meyer-Ebrecht D, Mösges R, et al. CAS computer assisted surgery: final project report to the North-Rhine-Westfalian Ministry of Science and Technology. 400–09886. 1986.
5. Anon JB, Lipman SP, Oppenheim D, Halt RA. Computer-assisted endoscopic surgery. *Laryngoscope.* 1994;104:901–905.
6. Anon JB, Rontal M, Zinreich SJ. Computer assisted endoscopic sinus surgery—current experience and future developments. *OP Tech Otolaryngol Head Neck Surg.* 1995;6:163–170.
7. Anon JB, Klimek L, Mosges R, Zinreich SJ. Computer-assisted endoscopic sinus surgery: an international review. *Otol Clin North Am.* 1997;30:389–401.
8. Bale RJ, Vogele M, Freysinger W, et al. Minimally invasive head holder to improve the performance of frameless stereotactic surgery. *Laryngoscope.* 1997;107:373–377.
9. Nitsche N, Hilbert M, Strasser G, Tümmler HP, Arnold W. Einsatz eines berührungsfreien computergestützten Orientierungssystems bei Nasennebenhöhlenoperationen: II. Anatomische Studien und erste klinische Erfahrungen. *Otorhinolaryngol Nova.* 1993;3:173–179.
10. Krybus W, Knepper A, Adams L, Rüger R, Meyer-Ebrecht D. Navigation support for surgery by means of optical position detection. In:. Lemke HU, Rhodes ML, Jaffe CC, Felix J, eds. *Proceedings of the CAR '91.* Berlin: Springer Publishers; 1991:362–366.
11. Klimek L, Kainz J, Reul J. Advoidance of vascular complications in paranasal sinus surgery: 2. Pre- and intraoperative imaging. *HNO.* 1993;41:582–586.
12. Klimek L, Wenzel M, Mösges R. Computer-assisted orbital surgery. *Ophthalmic Surg.* 1993;24:411–417.
13. Mösges R, Klimek L. Computer-assisted surgery of the paranasal sinuses. *J Otolaryngol.* 1993;22:69–71.

14

The Frontal Sinus: The Endoscopic Approach

BARRY SCHAITKIN

This chapter is dedicated to the treatment of frontal sinusitis. Although separate chapters in this book have been devoted to embryology, radiology, and anatomy, some brief discussion of these with specific reference to the frontal sinus seems obligatory. The frontal sinus remains the most difficult of the dependent sinuses for the endoscopic surgeon. It is the most difficult sinus to treat in a functional way by clearing the natural outflow tract without causing iatrogenic stenosis of the ostium, and it is the sinus that requires the greatest surgical expertise and level of intervention once ostium stenosis has occurred. Within this chapter, I will stress my own philosophy of treating the frontal sinus while attempting to avoid this most unwanted complication.

■ Embryology

Kasper[1] described four frontal sinus pits or furrows. These are the ethmoidal pneumatization into the frontal bone, which will become the frontal sinus, and the outflow tract structures. The first pit generally becomes the agger nasi cell, the second, the frontal sinus, and the third and fourth, the anterior or supraorbital ethmoid cells (if these are present). At about age 2 years the pneumatization enters the vertical portion of the frontal bone and progressively enlarges over the next 15 to 18 years.

■ Anatomy

Understanding frontal sinus anatomy for an endoscopic surgeon requires a detailed understanding of the frontal

recess. The term *internal frontal ostium* will be used for the bony orifice leading into the frontal sinus, and the term *frontal recess* will be used for that anatomy comprising the outflow tract of the frontal sinus, between the internal frontal ostium and the middle meatus. Most authors have tried to get away from the older term *nasofrontal duct* that suggested a more tubular bony structure that rarely exists.

If one thinks of the level of the ostium as the central part of an hourglass, as suggested by Stammberger and Hawke,[2] it is visually helpful. From the central portion down we find the frontal recess, most notable for the agger nasi. The agger nasi cell, a highly reliable landmark present in over 90% of patients (Fig. 14–1), is the

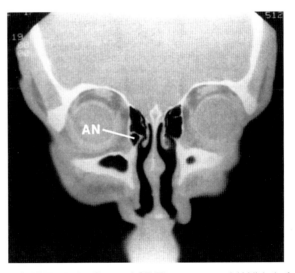

FIGURE 14–1 Coronal CT. The agger nasi (AN) is in front of the anterior attachment of the middle turbinate.

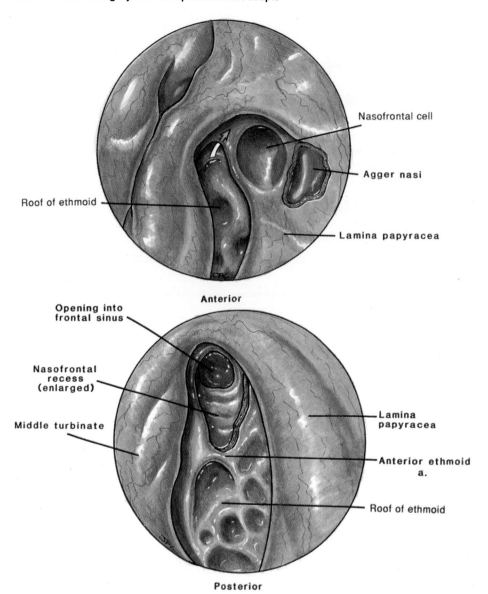

FIGURE 14–2   (A,B) Endoscopic views of the left nasofrontal recess after the agger nasi cell has been opened. In this case, the frontal sinus drains medial to the infundibulum.

key to the frontal recess. The agger nasi cell has as its boundaries laterally the lacrimal sac and orbit, medially the uncinate process, posteriorly the anterior ethmoid artery and skull base, and superiorly the frontal recess. The medial border of the frontal recess is almost always the lateral surface of the anterior portion of the middle turbinate. This, however, is dependent on the type of insertion that the uncinate process takes.

In the vast majority of cases (85%) the uncinate process will merge with the medial wall of the agger nasi cell; therefore, the frontal sinus will drain between the uncinate process and the middle turbinate (Fig. 14–2), thus using the middle turbinate lateral surface as the medial border of the frontal recess.[1] However, in a small number

of cases the uncinate process will attach either to the insertion site of the middle turbinate along the lateral lamella of the cribriform plate or to the skull base. In this small number of cases (less than 15%) the frontal recess will have a direct entry into the infundibulum (Fig. 14–3).

The upper part of the hourglass then starts at the internal frontal ostium. The lateral aspect of the upper hourglass is the curved upper portion of the orbital roof. Anteriorly, the ostium is made up of a thick plate of bone that is the confluence of the nasal bone and the frontal bone. The primary frontal sinus ostium is located within the medial aspect of the frontal sinus floor close to the inner sinus septum. The size of this ostium has been variably reported but is felt to average 3 to 4 mm.

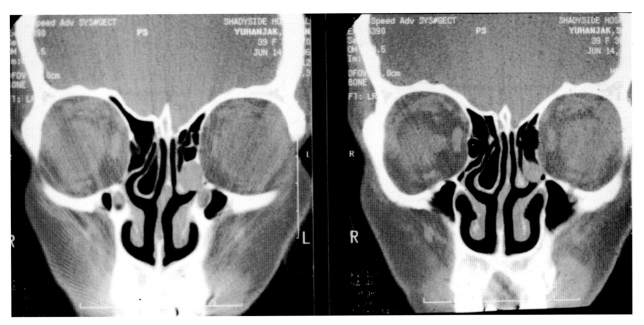

FIGURE 14–3   The uncinate attaches to the skull base. In this case, the frontal sinus drains into the infundibulum.

In most cases the frontal sinus consists of two large cells separated by an inner sinus septum. In 15% of patients there may be an absence of one of these cells, and in 5% of patients neither frontal sinus may become pneumatized (Fig. 14–4). The position of these cells in relation to the orbit and anterior cranial fossa is of paramount importance to the frontal sinus surgeon. Figure 14–5 shows the relationship of the frontal sinus to the anterior cranial fossa and orbit at six levels in the axial plane; the most inferior section shows how the frontal sinus narrows to the nasal frontal isthmus, which lies between the cribriform plate posteriorly and the lacrimal sac anteriorly and laterally. Figure 14–5C is a three-dimensional

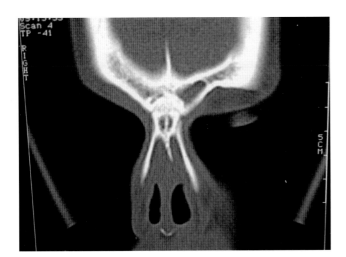

FIGURE 14–4   Unilateral frontal sinus.

representation of a right frontal sinus showing the frontal sinus in its relationship to the cribriform plate and anterior cranial fossa. Figure 14–5D shows the frontal sinus in a coronal plane in its relationship to the agger nasi cell and middle turbinate.

■ Pathophysiology

Like other paranasal sinuses discussed heretofore the frontal sinus relies on the mucociliary clearance. Any procedure done on the frontal sinus must respect this mucociliary clearance if it is to be successful. Any disease process that affects the ability of secretions to enter into the ethmoid from the frontal sinus will cause pathology in this location. Most commonly edema, polyps, and a variety of benign neoplasms are encountered. However, of a more worrisome nature is the increasing frequency with which scarring and adhesions in the nasofrontal region due to iatrogenic trauma are becoming the main indication for surgery. It is the combination of obstruction and infection that causes symptoms for the patient with frontal sinusitis and is the establishment of free drainage into the nose that relieves this condition. The surgeon must understand the pathophysiology of the individual patient's problem with a keen eye toward the anatomical abnormalities, a firm understanding of the particular pathophysiology at work in the patient, and a highly developed level of surgical expertise. The reader should review the original papers by Kasper,[1] Schaffer,[3] and Van Alyea,[4] as well as the more recent work by Kuhn et al[5] to master this anatomical region.

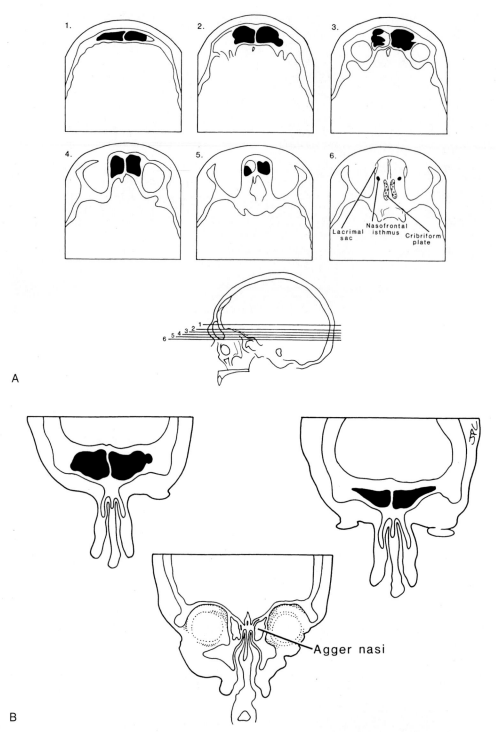

FIGURE 14–5 Survey CT of the frontal sinus used to determine dimensions of the sinus and anatomical relationships to nasofrontal recess. (A) Axial CT, cuts 1 through 6. Frontal sinus narrows to a small isthmus as it drains into the nasofrontal recess. (B) Coronal CT scan shows the relationship of the frontal sinus to the orbit and agger nasi cells (C,D) Demonstration of these relationships and the nasofrontal drillout approach to enlarge the frontal sinus outflow tract.

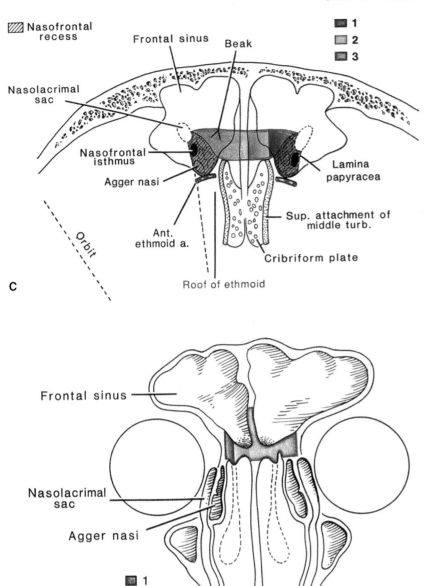

Nasofrontal recess

Frontal sinus Beak

Nasolacrimal sac

Nasofrontal isthmus

Agger nasi

Lamina papyracea

Ant. ethmoid a.

Sup. attachment of middle turb.

Cribriform plate

Roof of ethmoid

Orbit

1
2
3

C

Frontal sinus

Nasolacrimal sac

Agger nasi

1
2
3

D

FIGURE 14–5 *(Continued)*

Adding to the frontal sinus surgeon's difficulty is the healing burden of chronic inflamed tissue, the potential bone loss from the disease process or previous surgery, and the presence of scar from the previous surgeon's procedure. The following philosophy is drawn out of my own expertise in treating over 2000 patients surgically for sinusitis with an eye toward preventing iatrogenic frontal sinus problems (Table 14–1).

Surgical Treatment

The endoscopic approach has revolutionized the thinking in regard to diseases of the paranasal sinuses. The

TABLE 14–1 Factors Influencing Failure and Revision Surgery

1. Symptomatic patient
2. Nasal polyps
3. Asthma
4. Aspirin sensitivity
5. Extensive disease
6. Previous surgery
7. Underlying problems—allergy immunodeficiency:
   - Cystic fibrosis
   - Cilial dysfunction
8. Anatomy problems—septum
   - Concha bullosa
   - Others

9. Wrong diagnosis
10. Inadequate surgery
11. Inappropriate surgery
12. Poor technique
13. Synechia
14. Complications
15. Insufficient/inadequate postoperative surgical therapy
16. Inadequate postoperative medical therapy

TABLE 14–2 Most Common Causes of FESS Failure

1. Maxillary sinus ostia
   Maxillary sinus recirculation
   Maxillary natural ostia obstruction
   Ciliary dysfunction
2. Retained uncinate process
   Missed natural ostia
   Blocked agger nasi/infundibulum
3. Middle turbinate lateralization/destabilization
   Middle turbinate pushed/scarred laterally
   Blocked frontal
   Blocked maxillary
   Blocked ethmoid
   Middle turbinate pushed medially
   Blocked sphenoid recess
4. Overly aggressive surgical technique
   Stenotic maxillary antrostomy
   Closed maxillary antrostomy
   Closed sphenoid antrostomy

work of Messerklinger[6] and Stammberger and Hawke[2] and all of their disciples has strengthened the belief in the reestablishment of mucociliary clearance as the "gold standard." To this end, I offer the following treatment philosophy based on individual patient presentation to maximize surgical success and minimize iatrogenic trauma (Tables 14–2 and 14–3).

From 1989 to 1995, 699 adult patients were seen with CT-proven frontal sinus disease. Five hundred and thirty patients had more than 50% of the frontal sinus aerated. In this group only an anterior ethmoidectomy alone was performed. Of this group, 497 (93.8%) had reduction in their frontal sinus signs and symptoms. One hundred and fifty-six of the patients had either a complete or nearly complete opacification of the frontal sinus. These patients had a primary endoscopic osteoplasty by either (1) removal of polypoid tissue alone and the surrounding agger nasi air cells or (2) a drillout procedure as described in this chapter. There were 33 patients who failed either the anterior ethmoid surgery or the frontal sinus surgery. There were 21 osteoplastic frontal sinusotomies performed. Most of these were in the earlier years, demonstrating improved technology and improved ability

TABLE 14–3 Most Common Causes/Symptoms in ESS Failure

Recurrent infection
    Purulent drainage   5. Loss of smell
    Congestion—nose and ear   6. Obstruction (polyp patients)
    Cough   7. "Bad" smell
    Bad breath
Postnasal drainage only—esophageal reflux
Nasal obstruction (nonpolyp patient)
Turbinate swelling
Septal deformity
Nasal valve problem
Headache: factitious or nonnasal sinus etiology

to intervene and manage frontal sinus disease endoscopically. From this it appears as if the vast majority of patients with CT-proven frontal sinus disease can be managed with anterior ethmoid sinus surgery. Only a small number require frontal sinus surgery, and an even smaller number require osteoplastic frontal sinusotomy.

■ Normal Frontal Sinus Preoperatively

The patient who presents without frontal sinus symptoms, with a normal nasal endoscopy of the frontal recess and a normal CT scan of this area, should have the most minimal of intervention in the frontal recess area. This includes the patient with an enlarged agger nasi cell that previously some authors may have recommended to be taken down. In my own hands, the patient with ostiomeatal complex disease, maxillary sinus outflow obstruction, and posterior ethmoid disturbances can be treated without completely visualizing the frontal recess. These patients have a procedure very much in keeping with the philosophy suggested by Setliff.[7] An uncinate window is created in a retrograde fashion using an Instrumentarium (Quebec, Canada) pediatric side biter. The microdebrider allows for marsupialization of the maxillary sinus ostium and outflow tract without mucosal injury to the maxillary sinus ostium. The uncinate process is taken up high enough to establish good ethmoid visualization and assume patency of the outflow tract of the agger nasi cell. The ethmoid surgery is performed to the extent required by the pathophysiology. The nasal frontal recess, however, is not manipulated. The upper border of the uncinate is not touched. This eliminates any scar tissue formation between the uncinate process and the lateral surface of the middle turbinate, thus leaving the nasal frontal area untraumatized.

■ Patients with Frontal Sinus Symptoms and Objective Abnormalities

In patients who have frontal sinus symptoms or objective abnormalities, the frontal recess is assessed for patency. This is accomplished with a frontal sinus trephine technique that was first introduced to me by Jean-Michel Klossek. Figure 14–6 shows the anatomical reference points of the supraorbital foramina. In a patient with a well-pneumatized frontal sinus as appreciated on both axial and coronal scans of the paranasal sinuses, a line is drawn between these two supraorbital foramina. Local anesthesia can be employed, with the local injected into the medial aspect of the brow, and a small incision is made. The drill, in a forward mode, is then used to penetrate the anterior table of the frontal sinus. Direct measurements taken off the axial scans allow for the

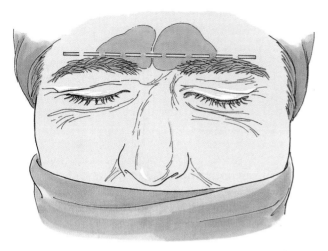

FIGURE 14–6 Anatomical reference points for frontal sinus trephine procedure are the supraorbital foramen. (Courtesy of Xomed Surgical Products, Inc., Jacksonville, FL.)

turbinate will be appreciated by the surgeon's hand on the barrel of the syringe. Likewise, the character of the secretions is immediately apparent to the endoscopic viewer as the irrigation is initiated. This technique works exceedingly well with a wide range of pathologies, including eosinophilic mucin sinusitis.

In patients with eosinophilic mucin sinusitis, all of the material must be cleaned out of all of the paranasal sinuses to establish the return of health. The most atraumatic way to do this in the frontal sinus has been to use this irrigation technique. The success of this has been documented with an endoscopic view and postoperative imaging. Removing this material through a completely endonasal technique does run the risk of scar in the nasal frontal recess as the suction cannula is generally inserted and reinserted a series of times to clear all of the viscous material.

elimination of penetration of the posterior wall. The cannula system is then hooked in place, as depicted in Figure 14–7. Negative pressure in the syringe confirms either mucopus or air before irrigation commences. If there is no return of either air or mucopus, the position is checked again prior to instilling water to eliminate the possibility of injecting into the wrong space.

At this point, with a 30-degree endoscope visualizing the nasal frontal recess, the surgeon can assess the patency of the entire hourglass as judged by the pressure required to deliver the water from the syringe into the ethmoid region. The amount of pressure required is a learned skill but correlates with the level of patency of the entire outflow tract. Anything obstructing within the frontal sinus, in the internal ostium or in the outflow tract involving the agger nasi, uncinate, and middle

■ Patients Who Fail to Irrigate Easily

A failure of the patient to irrigate in a freely flowing manner with the technique described above indicates outflow obstruction of the irrigation fluid. Most commonly this obstruction is at the level of the outflow tract. However, before resorting to enlarging the outflow tract, the surgeon should once again refresh his or her impression of the frontal sinus and outflow tract. Not infrequently a frontal cell as described by Bent et al[8] can be the cause of this. These frontal cells have been described as existing in four types. In the absence of such a frontal cell the main culprit is likely to be the frontal recess. The agger nasi cell is appreciated in a standardized fashion. By following the uncinate process to its superior limit, the floor of the agger nasi can always be appreciated. With the trephine in place, the water can generally

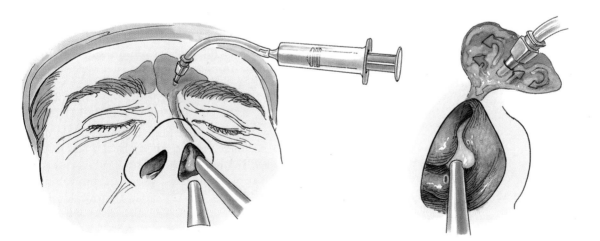

FIGURE 14–7 Frontal sinus trephine system assembled for use. (Courtesy of Xomed Surgical Products, Inc., Jacksonville, FL.)

be appreciated traveling through its most common location that is between the medial wall of the agger nasi cell and the lateral wall of the middle turbinate. To expose the internal frontal ostium at this point, the medial wall and dome of the agger nasi cell must be reflected using a through-biting or powered instrument. This avoids the previous grab-and-tear technique that caused stripping of the mucosa around the internal frontal ostium. The agger nasi cell is thus taken down until the frontal ostium is appreciated, and the water at this point should be freely flowing. Having ruled out a problem in the superior part of the hourglass and having cleared surgically the inferior part of the hourglass, if obstruction still exists, it is at the level of the internal frontal ostium. This is the most unusual of all of the sites of possible obstruction. If this is the case, however, then the next level of intervention is required.

■ Frontal Sinus Drillout

Patients who have failed all the above techniques require a more aggressive approach. Attention to the level of the internal frontal ostium and its enlargement must be at the anterior aspect of the ostium at the confluence of the nasal bone and the frontal bone. This is the only safe area to work within the frontal recess. Laterally, the surgeon will find himself or herself perforating the nasal bone, entering the lacrimal system, or entering the orbit. Posteriorly, the surgeon will find himself or herself in the anterior cranial fossa and violating the anterior ethmoid artery. Patients who are candidates for any of the following endonasal approaches to the frontal sinus are also candidates for an osteoplastic procedure. That is to say that one should not embark on an endoscopic approach to the frontal sinus lightly.

In my own series of 2000 sinus cases, only 78 frontal sinus drillout procedures have been done. The patient who is not a candidate for an endoscopic approach would not be a candidate for an external approach and vice versa. This should add to the surgeon's mind the gravity by which he or she embarks to enlarge the internal frontal ostium. In 1915 Lathrup and Jawma[9] described a median drainage approach to the frontal sinus. Lathrup started by removing the anterior end of the middle turbinate and breaking up the anterior ethmoid cells. He felt that this should be attempted first because it may effect a cure. In patients who failed this technique, the eyebrow was marked out, and an external incision was used to enter the frontal sinus. Rasps were passed from above and below through the enlarged ostium, cutting forward and laterally. The burs and rasps were used alternatively at the discretion of the operator. Gradually all of the dense bone and floor of the frontal sinus was removed. This bone included the nasal crest and spine

of the frontal bone and the thickened area of the nasal bones and the nasal process of the superior maxilla. The inner frontal sinus septum was perforated and burred away where the contralateral side was then addressed both from inside the nose and through the external approach. In all instances, even in the case of unilateral disease, Lathrop performed a bilateral midline drainage procedure.

The endonasal approach of this area was pioneered by Draf.[10] Draf described simple, extended, and median drainage involving both frontal sinuses. The endoscopic approach to the advanced frontal sinus case was pioneered by May and Schaitkin[11] and later discussed by multiple authors.[12–17]

■ Indications and Contraindications

Candidates for frontal sinus ostioplasty include (1) those with persistent symptoms of nasofrontal recess obstruction after intensive medical management and endoscopic sinus surgery, (2) those with extensively pneumatized frontal sinuses (because it is difficult with an external procedure to ensure that all mucosa has been removed), and (3) those who object strongly to an external incision.

Contraindications to endonasal ostioplasty include (1) the presence of a laterally based frontal sinus osteoma or tumor, (2) inflammatory disease that is limited to the lateralmost recesses of the frontal sinus and cannot be reached endonasally, (3) most cases of displaced fractures of the anterior or posterior table of the frontal sinus, (4) CSF leaks through the posterior table of the frontal sinus, and (5) osteomyelitis involving the anterior or posterior wall that requires extensive removal of bone. A relative contraindication is a small frontal sinus, as these are difficult to keep open postoperatively.

■ Technique

After identification of the natural ostium, the key landmarks for the nasofrontal recess approach are identified (Table 14–4). These landmarks are the anterior attachment of the middle turbinate and the arch formed by the frontal process of the maxilla where it meets the junction of the perpendicular plate of the ethmoid and quadrangular cartilage. This arch is also known as the nasofrontal beak. In the nasofrontal arch (NFA) 2 and 3, the nasofrontal beak is removed using a drill, upbiting Kerrison punch forceps, J curettes, and giraffe forceps. In this manner the floor of the frontal sinus is opened in continuity with the natural ostium. In the NFA 2, the sinus floor is opened from the lamina papyracea to the middle turbinate. In the NFA 3, the opening is extended

TABLE 14–4   Six Friendly Landmarks

1. Anterior arch	Defines the medial and lateral borders of the anterior ethmoid dissection; it protects inadvertent entry into the cribriform plate if one stays lateral to the middle turbinate remnant.
2. Maxillary sinus antrostomy	This is an absolute landmark for identifying the floor of the orbit if one moves medially along the floor, it becomes easy to identify the lamina papyracea. One must be careful not to miss the natural ostia, which might not have been included in the original antrostomy.
3. Lamina papyracea	This marks the lateral extent of the ethmoid dissection protecting inadvertent orbital injury; its continuity must be established radiographically before operative management.
4. The ridge	Defined as the bone that lies between the lamina papyracea and antrostomy site; when followed posteriorly, it isolates the posterior ethmoid cells superior to it and the sphenoid sinus inferiorly.
5. Posterior choanal arch	Leads the surgeon to the anterior face of the sphenoid sinus.
6. Sphenoid sinus roof	Dictates the most superior extent of the posterior ethmoid dissection; the sphenoids share the same level for their roof.

medially to the septum. Upon opening of the sinus floor, an olive-tipped suction is placed into the frontal sinus, and copious irrigation is undertaken. If the sinus does not easily irrigate, a wider osteoplasty is undertaken.

In the NFA 4, a window of the septum is removed superiorly at the junction of the quadrangular cartilage and the perpendicular plate of the ethmoid. Once this septum is removed, the nasofrontal beaks are followed medially to where they meet at a triangular wedge of bone in the midline. By drilling away this bone, keeping anterior to the beaks, the floor of the frontal sinus can be safely removed without injury to the posterior table or anterior ethmoid artery and without entry into the anterior cranial fossa. Care is taken to avoid drilling too far anteriorly to avoid injury to the nasal bones with resulting cosmetic deformity. When drilling anteriorly, the surgeon's finger is placed over the nasal bones to help avoid this untoward event. When drilling laterally, care is taken to spare the lacrimal sac. Frequent palpation of the globe while observing endoscopically for movement along the lateral nasal wall provides an additional measure of safety. The majority of patients are discharged to home later that same day on saline nasal spray and oral antibiotics for 10 days.

■ Results

A total of 78 endoscopic drillout procedures (NF 2–4) were performed on 53 patients between May 1991 and March 1999. Average follow-up time by office visit or telephone interview was 46 months (range 6–92 months, average = 29 months). Follow-up time was defined as the time interval from the most recent frontal sinus procedure.

The index endoscopic drillout procedure for the treatment of severe frontal sinus disease was successful in 77% of patients with severe frontal sinus disease. The endoscopic approach was even effective for patients who had previously undergone external proce-

dures. While offering success rates comparable with external procedures, the complication rate was very favorable: no major complications, and two patients with postoperative epistaxis not requiring transfusion (Fig. 14–8).

■ Conclusion

Frontal sinus surgery requires precision diagnosis and surgical planning using the history, endoscopic exam, and CT scans. The philosophy presented allows increasing aggressiveness to deal with the most difficult problems. However, lesser techniques including the use of frontal sinus trephine will hopefully lead to fewer iatrogenic frontal sinus problems.

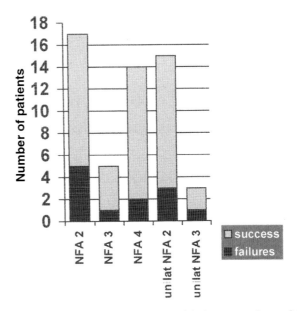

FIGURE 14–8 Success rate of index procedure of frontal sinus drillout.

REFERENCES

1. Kasper KA. Nasofrontal connections: a study based on 100 consecutive dissections. *Arch Otolaryngol.* 1936;23:322–343.

2. Stammberger H, Hawke M. *Essentials of Functional Endoscopic Sinus Surgery.* Philadelphia: Mosby Year Book; 1993.

3. Schaeffer JP. The genesis, development and adult anatomy of the nasofrontal region in man. *Am J Anat.* 1916;20:125–146.

4. Van Alyea OE. Frontal sinus drainage. *Ann Otolaryngol.* 1946; 55:267–278.

5. Kuhn FA, Bolger WE, Tisdal RG. The agger nasi cell in frontal recess obstruction: an anatomic, radiologic and clinical correlation. *Op Tech Otolaryngol Head Neck Surg.* 1991;2:226–231.

6. Messerklinger W. On the drainage of the frontal sinus in man. *Acta Otolaryngol.* 1967;63:176–181.

7. Setliff R. New Concepts and the use of powered instrumentation for functional endoscopic sinus surgery. In: Stankiewicz JA, ed. *Advanced Endoscopic Sinus Surgery.* St. Louis: Mosby; 1995.

8. Bent JP, Cuilty-Sillers C, Kuhn FA. The frontal cell as a cause of frontal sinus obstruction. *Am J Rhinol.* 1994;8:185–191.

9. Lothrup HA. Frontal sinus suppuration with results of a new procedure. *JAMA.* 1915;65:153–160.

10. Draf D. Endonasal micro-endoscopic frontal sinus surgery: the Fulda Concept. *Op Tech Otolaryngol Head Neck Surg.* 1991; 2:234–240.

11. May M, Schaitkin B. Frontal sinus surgery: endonasal drainage instead of an external osteoplastic approach. *Op Tech Otolaryngol Head Neck Surg.* 1995;6:184–192.

12. Metson R, Gliklich R. Clinical outcome of endoscopic surgery for frontal sinusitis. *Arch Otolaryngol Head Neck Surg.* 1998;124: 1090–1094.

13. Gross W, Gross C, Becker D, et al. Modified transnasal endoscopic Lothrop procedure as an alternative to frontal sinus obliteration. *Otolaryngol Head Neck Surg.* 1995;113:427–434.

14. Schaefer S, Close L. Endoscopic management of frontal sinus disease. *Laryngoscope.* 1990;100:155–160.

15. Hoseman W, Kuhnel T, Held P, et al. Endonasal fronal sinusotomy in surgical management of chronic sinusitis: a critical evaluation. *Am J Rhinol.* 1997;11:1–9.

16. Wigand M, Hosemann W. Endoscopic surgery for frontal sinusitis and its complicatons. *Am J Rhinol.* 1991;55–89.

17. Metson R. Endoscopic treatment of frontal sinusitis. *Laryngoscope.* 1992;102:712–716.

15a

Lasers and Nasal and Sinus Surgery: KTP/532 Laser and Nasal and Sinus Surgery

HOWARD L. LEVINE

Lasers have become part of the standard operating room armamentarium for all types of surgical procedures. They are used selectively as an adjunct to nasal and sinus surgery but are not the primary surgical tool for most nasal and sinus surgeons. For some types of pathology, the laser is appropriate and ideal, providing rapid, efficient, and exacting management. For other types of pathology, the laser is tedious, producing excessive edema and tissue trauma, and is a poor substitute for other nasal endoscopic surgical modalities. When contemplating using the laser, one should consider several aspects, such as safety unique to intranasal use, instrumentation for intranasal use, the type of the pathology to be treated, the energy dosage for that pathology, and the results that might be expected.

There are several lasers that are used for nasal and sinus surgery. These include the potassium titanyl phosphate (KTP/532), neodymium:yttrium aluminum garnet (Nd:YAG), holmium:yttrium aluminum garnet (Ho:YAG), and carbon dioxide (CO_2). These lasers differ in their wavelength, power range, absorption length, and absorbing chromophobe. They have different features that relate to endoscopic sinus surgery, such as quality of handpiece, surgical access, hemostatic capability, and precision (Table 15a–1).

The KTP/532 laser has flexible fibers and handpieces that make access relatively easy into the recesses and spaces of the nose and sinuses. By keeping the power constant and varying the working distance between the fiber tip and the tissue, coagulation, vaporization, or cutting is achieved.

The Nd:YAG laser is effective for turbinate dysfunction and ostiomeatal complex surgery; however, it is

cumbersome to use. There is marked thermal reaction, which often causes tissue edema.

The Ho:YAG laser causes minimal thermal reaction and minimal charring when used in a water medium. When used in an air medium, there are miniature explosions that make surgery difficult.

The CO_2 laser has a rigid articulating arm, making it cumbersome to use.

The KTP/532 laser is preferred by the author because of its ease and efficiency of use. It is a suitable tool for vascular tissue, such as the nasal and paranasal sinus mucosa. It works best for turbinate dysfunction, vascular disorders, and intranasal/intrasinus scarring.

■ Surgical Lasers

History of Use of the Laser for Nasal and Sinus Surgery

In the mid-1970s I began using the CO_2 laser for laryngeal lesions. The great success of this laser led me to look for an efficient laser for the nasal and sinus cavities. The KTP/532 laser was being tested at the time as part of the U.S. Food and Drug Administration's requirements for new instruments and seemed promising for nasal and sinus use. It had flexible fibers and a reasonable depth of penetration, scatter, and zone of injury. Handpieces were developed that had various curves to reach the lateral walls of the nose and into the sinuses. Several types of pathologic entities were treated with the laser.

TABLE 15a–1   Comparison of Different Common Lasers

	KTP/532	*Nd:YAG*	*Ho:YAG*	*CO_2*
Wavelength	532 nm	1064 nm	2140 nm	10600 nm
Power range	<1 to 40 W	<1 to <100 W	<1 to 80 W	<1 to >100 W
Absorption length	2–3 mm	3–4 mm	0.5 mm	0.02 mm
Absorption chromophobe	Hemoglobin, melanin	Dark-colored tissue	Water	Water
Quality of handpiece	Excellent	Poor	Poor	Poor
Surgical access	Excellent	Fair	Good	Poor
Hemostasis	Excellent	Very good	Excellent	Poor
Precision	Excellent	Good	Very good	Poor

Modified from Bhatt NJ. *Endoscopic Sinus Surgery.* San Diego and London: New Horizons; 1997:67.

Laser Safety

As with any use of the laser for management of otolaryngologic pathology, there are several safety precautions. There must be familiarity with the laser by both the surgeon and the laser operator. Both must understand all aspects of safety, energy dosage, fiber management, and instrumentation. Many of the general principles of safety for laser endonasal use are the same as those for other laser uses.

The surgeon and the laser operator must communicate consistently and frequently about whether the laser is "on" or "off," as well as the wattage and exposure time. The surgeon should clearly and succinctly state "laser on" (or "standby"), wattage, and exposure time. When this is accomplished, the laser operator should repeat the instruction to be clear on how the laser is set. This avoids confusion and minimizes the chance for error.

Proper signage outside the laser suite must include a warning that the laser is being used, the laser wavelength, and the type of eye protection needed. Many surgeons and laser suite staff now wear eye protection when the laser is being used in an open wound, but they wear eye protection optionally when working in a closed cavity such as the nose, sinus, or oral cavity.

Patient protection should include eye protection with goggles for patients under local anesthesia or monitored sedation, and moistened eye pads for patients under general anesthesia.

When coupling the laser with nasal endoscopes for use within the nose and sinuses, a proper eye safety filter is used and inserted between the endoscope and the beam splitter or camera.

Endonasal Laser Instrumentation

Many intranasal laser procedures can be performed with headlight, laser safety glasses, nasal speculum, and laser fiber with the appropriate handpiece. This is especially true for anterior nasal pathology and much of the inferior and anterior middle turbinate surgery.

For most other intranasal and endonasal laser surgery, the nasal endoscope provides visualization for the surgeon.

One of several laser handpieces (Fig. 15a–1) is used depending on the area to be operated.

Energy Dosage

Energy dosage is determined like any other laser procedure. Spot size, wattage, and exposure time are all-important.

$$\text{Energy density} = \text{power} \times \text{time}/\text{Area [watts/sec/cm}^2]$$

Cutting requires high-energy density achieved with small spot size, high wattage, and variable exposure. Coagulation requires low-energy density achieved with large (defocused) spot size, low to intermediate wattage, and variable exposure. Vaporization requires high-energy density, achieved with intermediate spot size, high energy, and variable exposure.

Endonasal Pathology

TURBINATE DYSFUNCTION

Vasomotor and allergic rhinitis frequently are challenging problems to manage. Medical management with antihistamines and/or decongestants and various steroid and anticholinergic nasal sprays is often effective. In spite of adequate medical management, nasal obstruction and/or congestion may persist. In these instances, laser photocoagulation of the inferior turbinate is often an appropriate adjunctive or complete management option.

Several different laser wavelengths have been used for nasal turbinate dysfunction. Mittelman[1] used the CO_2 laser to perform partial turbinectomy for severe, obstructive, chronic perennial rhinitis. He vaporized the anterior

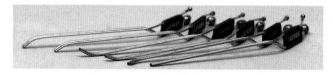

FIGURE 15a–1   Laser handpieces, allowing the flexible fiber to be inserted through them, and an additional port for smoke evacuation.

one-fourth to one-half of the inferior turbinate with excellent success.

Kawamura et al[2] described the use of the CO_2 for allergic rhinitis. The laser was used at 12 W and 0.1 second at weekly intervals for 5 weeks to reduce the turbinate. Inferior turbinates of 389 patients with perennial allergic rhinitis were vaporized by a defocused CO_2 laser. One month after surgery, 78% of the 389 patients had excellent or good results, whereas 21 had no improvement, subjectively. Seventy-two of the 389 patients were followed for over 2 years, and 61 of the 72 had excellent or good results. Twenty-seven of the 72 patients needed revaporization. In a previous report, Futatake et al[3] described histologic studies that showed a layer of scar tissue forming beneath the submucosa. It has been thought that the scar tissue prevents the turbinate from expanding when stimulated by external irritants. The laser probably decreases the number of goblet-secreting cells and the autonomic innervation of the turbinate.

A group of 1003 patients who underwent KTP/532 reduction of the turbinate has been followed for 9 years, 9 months by the author. Eight hundred and ninety-six of these were available for follow-up. These patients had laser reduction performed under attended local anesthesia or general anesthesia if the procedure was associated with a septoplasty. Septoplasty was performed in 645 (72%) of the 896 patients. The laser was used at 8 W and continuous to "crosshatch" the anterior two-thirds of the inferior turbinate. This allowed the nasal mucosa to regenerate, preserving a "normal" surface while creating a layer of scar tissue in the submucosa. Four hundred and ninety-eight (55.5%) of the 896 patients had extensive improvement in breathing. One hundred and ninety-seven (22.0%) of the 896 patients had moderate improvement in breathing. One hundred and thirteen (12.6%) of the 896 patients had mild improvement in breathing. Eighty-eight (9.8%) of the 896 patients had no improvement in their breathing. Three hundred and eighty-nine (43.4%) of the 896 patients had extensive reduction in their nasal drainage. Two hundred and sixty-nine (30.0%) of the 896 patients had moderate reduction in their nasal drainage. One hundred and thirty-two (14.7%) of the 896 patients had mild reduction in their nasal drainage. One hundred and six (11.8%) of the 896 patients had no change in their nasal drainage. No patient was worse.

The laser appears to provide adequate turbinate reduction without crusting or atrophy.[4,5] Healing is rapid and morbidity low. The laser improves the airway and reduces secretions in most instances.

VASCULAR DISORDERS

Hereditary hemorrhagic telangiectasia is an autosomal dominant disorder affecting the smooth muscle of blood vessels. Though bleeding may occur from any mucosal surface, it occurs most often from the nasal mucosa. The laser is used to photocoagulate the telangiectatic blood vessels. It is rarely, if ever, curative, but rather controls the bleeding by either sealing bleeding vessels or creating a layer of scar over the vessels to toughen the surface, thereby minimizing mucosal trauma and subsequent bleeding.

Over the years, both the Nd:YAG and KTP/532 lasers have been used. Both have controlled bleeding by lessening the frequency and severity of epistaxis. Most patients have had laser photocoagulation using the KTP/532 laser because of its more superficial depth of penetration compared with the Nd:YAG laser. This lessens the potential injury to the underlying perichondrium of the nasal septum.

The laser is used at low-energy density of 1.5 to 3.0 W, defocused spot size, and intermittent mode of 0.1 second on and 0.1 second off. This allows for the greatest degree of coagulation.

Patients are operated on under general anesthesia to avoid the need for topical and/or injectable local anesthesia with vasoconstriction. This allows easy visualization of blood vessels and reduced chance of aspiration of blood. Blood vessels are photocoagulated beginning with smaller vessels peripherally and working toward the larger vessels centrally. If bleeding occurs while working, suction cautery is used briefly to dry the field and then proceed with laser photocoagulation.

Approximately 70% of patients report reduced frequency and severity of epistaxis 12 months after laser photocoagulation.

Chronic epistaxis is not an entity usually managed by laser. On occasion, individuals will present with frequent epistaxis secondary to aggregates of blood vessels on the mucosal surface of the nose. Traditional cautery or nasal packing in the office does not control the bleeding, and therefore laser is an option. The laser is used in the same manner as with management of hereditary hemorrhagic telangiectasia.

NASAL POLYPOSIS WITH EOSINOPHILIA

The laser is not an efficient surgical tool to remove nasal polyposis. It is slow and tedious. A moderate amount of mucosal edema occurs most likely from thermal damage. However, it may have some value for certain kinds of polypoid disease.

Nasal polyposis with eosinophilia is one of the most difficult problems facing the rhinologist because of the high incidence of recurrence in spite of the best of medical or surgical management. Patients frequently have asthma and/or aspirin sensitivity associated with their nasal polyposis. The asthma is often more difficult to manage because of ongoing rhinosinusitis secondary to the nasal polyposis, causing postnasal drainage and irritating the lower respiratory tract.

Those patients with massive polyps are placed on high-dose steroid (40 mg each day for 1 week before surgery).

TABLE 15a–2   KTP/532 Laser Photocoagulation of Nasal Polyps with Eosinophilia*

	Medical Management	No Treatment
No symptoms	13	8
Improved	19	2
No better	8	0
Worse	2	0

*Follow-up = 48 months. N = 52.

They are managed with endoscopic sinus surgery using powered instrumentation, removing all of the polypoid tissue and preserving normal mucosa. Nasal septal obstruction and/or middle meatal obstruction is corrected to better allow the use of topical nasal steroids in the late postoperative period. Once the nose and sinus cavity is fairly well healed with minimal edema and moderate restoration of the mucosa and crusting is minimal, a topical nasal corticosteroid spray is used. At the earliest sign of recurrence, systemic steroids are used. If it appears as if systemic steroids are either ineffective or must be used for a lengthy time, laser photocoagulation of the sinus cavity is undertaken.

The laser is used under nasal endoscopic control to photocoagulate the entire sinus cavity where polyposis appears. The laser is used at 6 to 10 W (depending on the depth of polypoid tissue), slightly defocused, and in an intermittent mode (0.1 second on and 0.1 second off) to cool the underlying tissue between laser bursts.

Fifty-two patients have been observed for 48 months. Some patients have required medical management in addition to the laser photocoagulation. This medical management was often effective when it had previously failed (Table 15a–2).

Success was measured by those who had either no symptoms or improved symptoms with or without medical management. Forty-two (80.8%) of 52 patients were in this category. Although this number is encouraging, it very well may decrease with longer follow-up.

ANTRAL CHOANAL POLYPS

Antral choanal polyps generally arise on the lateral or inferior wall of the maxillary sinus and expand and exit through an accessory sinus ostium. They enlarge and fill the ostiomeatal complex and occupy the nasal choana. Traditional sinus surgery has involved a Caldwell-Luc procedure through a gingivobuccal sulcus incision to gain access to the base of the polyp to minimize the chances of recurrence.

Antral choanal polyps can be removed endoscopically with less morbidity to the patient. The laser is used to amputate the polyp near the accessory ostium of the maxillary sinus. The accessory ostium (if present) is interconnected to the natural ostium, and a large maxillary antrostomy is created. The polyp can then be extracted from the maxillary sinus, usually leaving a small pedicle from which it arose. The laser is then used to photocoagulate the base of the polyp within the maxillary sinus. The KTP/532 laser is used at 8 to 12 W.

INTRANASAL/INTRASINUS SCAR FORMATION

No matter how careful the endoscopic surgeon may be, there will be some surgical patients who develop scar tissue in the ostiomeatal complex and sinus cavities. For some, the scar will merely occur between the middle turbinate and lateral nasal wall. This is often asymptomatic, but on occasion it may obstruct the outflow from the frontal, anterior ethmoid, or maxillary sinus into the nose. In these instances the synechiae are removed endoscopically with the KTP/532 laser. If the middle turbinate seems to be in a reasonable medical position, nothing more is done. If it seems to want to lateralize with the possibility of reforming the synechia, Gelfilm is rolled like a "window shade" (the roll in the middle meatus and the hanging, leading edge extending out of the middle meatus, down over the inferior turbinate) and placed into the ostiomeatal complex. It is left in place for a few weeks and may be replaced in the outpatient.

POSTOPERATIVE MANAGEMENT

Most patients will have some crusting and edema following laser nasal and sinus procedures. All patients are given saline nasal spray to be used at least 4 to 6 times a day. Steroids and antibiotics have been used in the past but have not appeared to make a difference in the healing or postoperative discomfort. Patients are allowed gentle nose blowing about 1 week after surgery.

REFERENCES

1. Mittelman H. CO$_2$ laser turbinectomy for chronic obstructive rhinitis. *Lasers Surg Med.* 1982;2:29–36.
2. Kawamura S, Fukutake T, Kubo N, Yamashita T, Kumazawa T. Subjective results of laser surgery for allergic rhinitis. *Acta Otolaryngol Suppl.* 1993;500:109–112.
3. Fukatake T, Yamashita T, Tomoda K, Kumazawa T. Laser surgery for allergic rhinitis. *Arch Otolaryngol Head Neck Surg.* 1986;112:1280–1282.
4. Goldsher M, Joachims HZ, Golz A, et al. Nd:YAG laser turbinate surgery animal experimental study: preliminary report. *Laryngoscope.* 1995;105:319–321.
5. Kass EG, Massaro BM, Komorowski RA, Toohill RJ. Wound healing of KTP and argon laser lesions in the canine nasal cavity. *Otolaryngol Head Neck Surg.* 1993;108:283–292.   ◂

15b
∎∎∎

Nd:YAG Laser and the Treatment of Nasal and Sinus Pathology

MICHEL JAKOBOWICZ

This chapter presents an innovative concept for the management of nasal sinus disorders: the coupling of a flexible fiberoptic endoscope with the neodymium: yttrium-aluminum-garnet (Nd:YAG) laser. This provides a video image of the interior of the nose and sinuses and delivers laser energy to manage many different types of pathology. This chapter describes the equipment, technique, and results accumulated over the author's many years of experience.

In 1914, Albert Einstein[1] discovered the principle of light amplification by stimulated emission of radiation: the laser. With the Nd:YAG laser, the emission originates from the active center, the neodymium crystal, which is a garnet crystal, composed of yttrium and aluminum. The krypton lamp power can reach 100 watts, allowing for crystal stimulation. The Nd:YAG laser emits energy at 1060 nm, which is about the speed of infrared light. This wavelength allows the emission to be transported intact by fiberoptics without damaging the fiber. It is an excellent laser for flexible fiberoptic intranasal surgery and has been used since 1987 by the author to treat benign lesions of the nasopharynx of adults and adolescents.

In popular culture, laser is associated with mythical futuristic significance and endowed with extraordinary powers. In medicine, however, it remains a surgical tool and nothing else. Its applications are now precisely defined. The otolaryngologist using the laser needs to have specific training and in-depth clinical experience as with any surgical technique.

∎ Biophysical Notions: Nd:YAG Laser and Tissue

The laser's applications in medicine are based on the conversion of light energy into heat in the irradiated tissue. The extent and the degree of the thermal effect depend on beam geometry and the energy of incident light, as well as the optical and thermal tissue properties. The laser beam is emitted in visible light such as argon and dye lasers or in invisible light such as Nd:YAG or CO_2 laser.

The Nd:YAG Laser Beam Differentiated from the CO_2 Laser Beam

The differences between the Nd:YAG and CO_2 laser determine the condition in which the laser is used. The CO_2 laser emits light at 10,600 nm, penetrating the tissue surface and its depths. All tissues absorb it. It is used essentially as a scalpel, but it can vaporize and coagulate tissue.

The Nd:YAG laser emits light at 1060 nm and is moderately absorbed by water, glass, and plastic. It can be transported by a quartz fiber without being changed. The proteins of all opaque tissues absorb it. The more pigmented the tissues, the more absorbed the light is. For this reason, the superficial cell layers do not absorb the beam, as is the case with the CO_2 laser. The energy absorbed becomes effective at a depth of 2 or 3 nm. At this particular depth, Nd:YAG distributes its heat uniformly. The heat makes a pear-shaped coagulation effect that extends to a depth of 2 to 6 mm, as a function of the power irradiation time and tissue properties. This deep pear-shaped thermal effect causes very little damage to the surface. This is confirmed by electronic microscopic examination that reveals good preservation of the surface tissue. A thin fibrin sheet covers the surface tissue after the Nd:YAG irradiation, without any contact between the fiber and the mucosa.

Interaction between Nd:YAG Laser and Tissue

In 1979, Frank and colleagues[2] showed that the Nd:YAG laser irradiation of the bladder wall, with 40 W of power, created several different findings in the tissue.

In the superficial layers, there is a zone of edema. In the deeper layers, there are protein drops or clusters deposited in cellular interstices and on sections of smooth muscles. On the deeper layers, there is necrosis of 2 to 4 mm, without elevation of the surface temperature above 100°C. This is observed only on histological sections. Even deeper, there is heat distribution in the bladder wall that never reaches the critical temperature of 58°C on the external bladder wall.

These observations have been seen in animals and humans with the help of thermocameras and thermometric probes during laser irradiation. These methods give valuable information with the following histological conclusions.

1. There is coagulation and destruction of lesions without any significant alteration of surface tissues.
2. The mechanical stability of the irradiated wall is preserved.
3. Several laser-irradiated sessions at 40 W by the Nd:YAG laser during a period of 2 seconds did not produce any intestinal perforation.

In 1979, Halldorson showed that the interaction between the Nd:YAG laser and tissue could be easily controlled. The risks are far less than with the CO_2 or the argon laser all the more before the exposure of tissue to the CO_2 laser at 0.5 W over 4 seconds produces a thermal elevation equivalent to that provoked by 40 W with the Nd:YAG, which is even slower.

In general, the Nd:YAG laser beam can be transmitted by a quartz fiber without being absorbed until the energy reaches the tissue. Only there does energy emission take place. The Nd: YAG laser is a defocused beam that produces a pear-shaped shot similar to an explosive bullet, producing a deep tissue disintegration and a retraction by a cicatricial phenomenon.

These experiments were conducted at the same time by other researchers, notably Buiter[3] in Groningen, Germany, who used the Nd:YAG laser with various rigid tubes. At the end of the 1970s, he used rigid fiberoptics or surgical microscopes under general anesthesia to ensure palliative treatment of head and neck cancers, to vaporize and destroy mucosa, to manage choanal atresia, and to coagulate the epistaxis caused by hereditary hemorrhagic telangiectasia (Rendu-Osler-Weber syndrome).

■ Advantages of the Nd:YAG Laser as Compared with the CO_2 Laser

The Nd:YAG laser is relatively easy to use after appropriate training and after the operator gains experience.

Because of the flexible fibers through which the Nd:YAG laser energy is passed, there is better accessibility to various lesions in the nasal cavity, paranasal sinuses, and nasopharynx. An eye safety filter prevents any eye injury that may occur by transmission of energy from the operative site. Surgical precision is in the order of tenths of a millimeter. In addition, the deep retractile scarring is definitive and consistent. This is not always the case with the CO_2 laser, which has more surface action.

The Nd:YAG laser has a superior hemostatic and sterilizing effect resulting from the thermal energy compared with the CO_2 laser.

The postoperative effects are practically nonexistent: There is minimal postoperative edema. Postoperative infections rarely occur. Therefore, there is little justification for the use of systematic antibiotics. Postoperative hemorrhage also rarely occurs.

■ Preoperative Preparation

A meticulous history is obtained to clarify patients' complaints and to be certain they are candidates for fiberoptic office laser management. Care is taken to look for the etiology of continuous or intermittent nasal obstruction that is position dependent or the presence of anterior or posterior nasal drainage and its character (serous or purulent). It is important to understand what type of previous medical or surgical treatment had been tried. Any surgical contraindications are evaluated.

A complete ear, nose, and throat examination is performed, including nasal endoscopy that gives precise details on anatomical abnormalities and pathology within the nasal cavity and sinus recesses. Appropriate laboratory examinations may be necessary to determine if there is any allergy infection present.

Rhinomanometry is occasionally used. It measures the degree and location of obstruction. The airflow of each nasal fossa before and after vasoconstriction is measured to help determine the degree of turbinate involvement in the nasal obstruction.

A sinus CT scan completes the evaluation before any treatment. The CT scan helps to determine the extent of disease, the patency of outflow pathways into the nasal cavity, and the extent of a polyposis and to eliminate a possible tumor etiology.

■ Therapeutic Indications of the Nd:YAG Laser

There are several different indications for the use of the fiberoptic laser in the management of nasal and sinus pathology. In the nasal cavity, this includes hypertrophic rhinitis that can be caused by allergic rhinitis, vasomotor rhinitis, postoperative compensation after septoplasty or rhinoplasty, nasal fracture, endoscopic sinus surgery, nasal polyposis, membranous choanal atresia, synechiae, and recurrent epistaxis (e.g., hereditary hemorrhagic telangiectasia, superficial vessels in Kiesselbach's area, and pyogenic granuloma). In rhinopharynx pathology, adenoid residues, cicatricial adhesions, inflammation, and nasopharynx cysts can benefit from fibroscopic therapy. The same is true for edema, cyst, or nodulus on the posterior pad of the eustachian tube.

■ Equipment

Therapeutic fiberoptic Nd:YAG laser therapy employs a flexible fiber and flexible endoscope with an internal operating channel (Fig. 15b–1). Imaging is either through the endoscope or from an attached camera and video monitor, depending on the comfort of the operator.

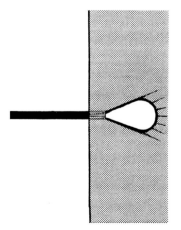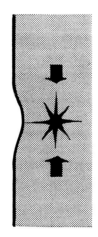

FIGURE 15b–1 YAG effect. The energy absorbed becomes effective at a depth of 2 or 3 mm. The absorption draws a pear-type coagulation to a depth of 2 to 6 mm, then a retraction by a cicatricial phenomenon.

The Nd:YAG Laser

Although the Nd:YAG laser has maximum power ranging from 40 to 100 W, depending on the model, the customary power in otolaryngology is generally less 30 W. Because the Nd:YAG laser beam is invisible, a helium neon-aiming beam is available on the system. This second red coaxial ray permits accurate aiming of the Nd:YAG beam.

There are several Nd:YAG models available for surgical use. The 100 W model is the oldest and needs cooling by water under high pressure. The slightest fall in water pressure will set off the automatic security blocking system, preventing its use. This model is found in many surgery centers where colleagues from other specialties require higher power and may have been using the system for many years.

The 40 to 60 W model is a more recent addition to surgical armamentarium. It is air cooled, has sufficient power for otolaryngology, is generally simple to operate, and is easily movable. Its small size and lower price make it a popular laser.

The Fiber

The Nd:YAG fiber is typically a bare quartz fiber and is 3 m long. The fiber has a thin Teflon sheath, giving it more strength. The fiber diameter is either 400 or 600 micron, depending on the size of the endoscopic operating channel. Most of the time, the 600-micron fiber is chosen because it is less brittle and enables more powerful delivery of laser energy. However, being less flexible, it is more difficult to handle.

When introducing the bare quartz fiber into the operating channel of the endoscope, care must be taken to avoid damage to the inner channel liner. The Teflon sheath, which increases the diameter of the fiber, helps to prevent such injury. This protective sheath is a flexible tube inserted into the operating channel of the endoscope to protect it. The bare quartz fiber slides into the sheath. It can be reused and changed at very little cost.

The Endoscope

A flexible fiberoptic endoscope is used, and viewing is done either through the scope itself or from a small monitor. The flexibility of the endoscope facilitates nontraumatic access to lesions that otherwise would be difficult to approach with a rigid endoscope or nasal speculum.

Several different endoscopes have been used. A 3.6 mm diameter endoscope with a 1.1 mm operating channel delivers an inadequate picture on the monitor, and the choice of fibers available is insufficient. A 4.1 mm diameter endoscope with an operating channel of 1.1 mm gives a better image, but the operating channel permits only 400-micron bare fibers. This fiber can only deliver the necessary power for treatment with energy so high that there is retrograde heat production, which can damage the endoscope. A 4.8 mm diameter endoscope equipped with an operating channel of 2 mm is most often used. This allows the passage of a 600-micron bare fiber.

Of course, the best fiberoptic endoscope is one that gives the best image, has the smallest external diameter, and offers the most precise handling. From year to year, the fiberoptic endoscope forges a better image quality thanks to the scope's fiberoptic amelioration and smaller diameter, which enable greater image definition.

The Light Source

Although a 250 W light source can be used with the fiberoptic endoscope, a xenon light source is much better.

Imaging

A video camera is fitted onto the endoscope, and a video screen and a video recorder are used for observation and documentation.

■ Considerations

For the Patient

Laser nasal and sinus surgery is nearly always an ambulatory procedure. Occasionally a light sedative may be necessary.

For the Surgeon

On occasion, anatomical abnormalities make access to the entire nasal fossa difficult. This plus the size of the fiberoptic endoscope can make it difficult to access the lesions, especially when they are on the lateral nasal walls.

For Operating Room Personnel

For safety reasons, it is absolutely necessary for all those in the operating room to wear special protective goggles that are adapted to the wavelength of the used laser emission.

It is important to keep the laser in "standby" mode when it is not being used.

For the Equipment

Applied too long, corrosive sterilization can oxidize and desiccate the fiberoptic endoscope's flexible sheaths, which can then split the scope. (Manufacturers must solve these numerous problems with respect to patient health and safety.)

Equipment manipulations can be hard on the life of the equipment. Forced curves and twisting of the fiberop-

tic endoscope can break the optical fibers in the scope, spoiling the image quality. The camera cable can be broken or even pulled off due to excessive and uncontrolled twisting. The economic consequences of such poor handling should not be neglected.

■ Limiting Factors and Contraindications

For some nasal fossae, the fiberoptic endoscope's diameter can be too large because of anatomical abnormalities. This may provoke irritation of the mucosa and epistaxis by friction. Though bleeding may be managed by the Nd:YAG laser, which is a coagulation laser, some patients may require topical vasoconstrictors on the site or traditional silver nitrate cautery. Obstructive septal deviations that do not allow the passage of any endoscope will need a septoplasty either prior to or at the time of laser treatments.

This treatment is reserved for adults and adolescents. Children younger than 12 years old may be difficult to manage during an office laser procedure and therefore are rarely accepted as patients for this technique under local anesthesia.

A rhinopharyngeal infection, either evolving or present, is a temporary contraindication because of the increased inflammation, causing bleeding and the potential for spread of infection. Allergic reaction or contraindication to lidocaine or adrenaline does not exclude laser treatment but may preclude local anesthesia. Depending on the pathology, many patients are treated without any anesthesia.

Patients with high blood pressure and those on anticoagulants if not medically controlled are not candidates for this procedure. Malignant nasopharyngeal lesions are generally managed by methods other than office laser techniques.

■ Technique

General Modalities

The patient is seated and anesthetized with local anesthesia. Topical anesthesia is applied using nasal tampons. The areas where the laser will be used are injected with an anesthetic containing adrenaline.

Skill using the combination fiberoptic endoscope and laser fiber system requires apprenticeship and use in a laboratory to minimize problems and for the surgeon to gain proficiency. An instrument can be misused, especially if the surgeon does not know it well. The Nd:YAG laser has particular characteristics of destruction, coagulation, and retraction. It is not an ideal scalpel, unlike the CO_2 laser. It should be used for what it is and not for what it is not.

The Nd:YAG laser can be used under direct sight control without any other endoscopic support, but access is limited to the front of the nasal cavity. Penetrating further appears inadvisable when the surgeon cannot see further. The use of rigid hollow tubes is possible if the anatomy permits.

For the author, the fiberoptic endoscope is the preferred tool because it circumnavigates many of these problems. It enables traversing the nasal cavity from anterior to posterior. The laser shots are precise, and the patient feels secure because the treatment is relatively painless (except on the synechiae).

The technique involves the introduction of the bare quartz fiber into the 1.6 mm diameter Teflon sheath. The fiber end is maintained within the recess of the sheath while the fiberoptic endoscope is introduced into the nasal cavity. Because the operating channel of the endoscope has a 120-degree angle, the quartz end of the laser fiber can damage the endoscope's internal sheath when passed through at this angle.

In this way, the endoscope holds the Nd:YAG laser fiber in the Teflon sheath, but at a distance from the distal endoscope's extremity. It is only when the endoscope is eventually in view of the lesion that the fiber is slid out of the channel just enough so that it can be seen in the eyepiece or on the video screen.

The fiber makes contact with the lesion, then is moved back to be absolutely sure to avoid any direct contact between the fiber and the mucous membrane. For certain lesions, such as synechiae, it is necessary to work in contact with the lesion. In such cases, the carbonization of the fiber tip inhibits the penetration of the Nd:YAG laser beam that is absorbed by the mucosa surface, reducing its effectiveness.

Without contact, the Nd:YAG laser is able to create its characteristic pear-type coagulation effect while sparing the surface tissue. The crater created by the Nd:YAG laser beam has different diameters, depending on the tissue coloration.

After the initial laser firing, the carbonized tissues absorb more energy than clear tissues. It is therefore necessary to modulate the power from 15 to 30 W, depending on the observed tissue reaction. Three to six sessions are often necessary. Laser irradiation time must be adapted as a function of the target tissue. To obtain the same effect with 15 W as with 30 W, the time of the laser exposure must be longer, being a function of the formula

$$W = P \times t,$$

where the work (W), measured in joules, is equal to the power (P), measured in watts, applied during a precise time (t), measured in seconds. An energy of 150 to 300 J is delivered for each nasal cavity at every session. For example, nasal polyposis may require a total of 1000 J for effective treatment.

The laser causes fumes that may impair the visibility of the operator, but because the nose is not a confined space, a simple expiratory breath is sufficient to disperse the fumes and to cool the quartz fiber at the same time. A smoke evacuator can be used.

Healing is allowed to occur between sessions. The Nd:YAG laser session is not repeated for 3 weeks.

Technical Aspects Relating to Clinical Indications

Therapeutic fiberoptic laser surgery is an effective modality for accessing and treating nasal and sinus pathology under only local anesthesia as an office procedure. The ease of use of the endoscope enables accurate surgical precision to manage benign lesions of the nose, sinuses, and nasopharynx with good visual control. Sometimes, if the nasal cavity does not allow the passage of the endoscope, the nasopharynx is approached through the other nasal cavity.

Local anesthesia does not easily create perfect nasal and sinus analgesia for an office procedure. The patient may feel the laser shot, but generally, there is no substantial pain. No patient has ever had aborted treatment for this reason.

Hypertrophic Rhinitis

The fiberoptic endoscope is introduced and passed from anterior to posterior in the nasal fossa. The quartz fiber is then advanced out from the endoscope, and the laser energy is applied from posterior to anterior to photocoagulate the inferior turbinate from the posterior tip to the anterior head. This tangential laser photocoagulation is applied in continuous contact for a period of 5 to 10 seconds and delivers energy of 150 to 300 J per nasal cavity at 20 to 30 W to ensure one or two stripes parallel to the medial surface of the inferior turbinate.

Particular care is taken at the posterior tip of the inferior turbinate, especially if the patient complains of airway obstruction when lying down because, in that position, venous blood stagnates in that portion of the turbinate. Treatment in this region may cause excessive bleeding.

The laser treatment is relatively painless when performed under local anesthesia. Generally, three sessions are necessary for the best result (Fig. 15b–2).

Anterior Nasal Polyposis

Anterior nasal polyposis is initially generally treated with topical and/or systemic corticosteroids. Well-established polyps that have become fibrotic often need traditional endoscopic ethmoidectomy. Invasive and proliferating polyposis is not a good indication for the Nd:YAG laser,

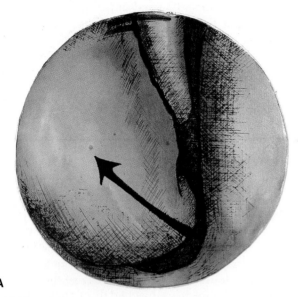

A

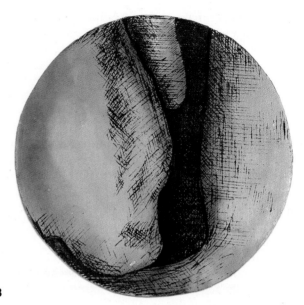

B

FIGURE 15b–2   Hypertrophic rhinitis in the nasal cavity. (A) The shooting is applied from the back to the front on the low turbinate (one or two stripes). (B) The result after three sessions shows the amelioration of the nasal permeability.

but the laser may become useful after ethmoidectomy if the polyps appear to recur. Often a brief corticosteroid treatment will shrink the polyps enough to allow the Nd:YAG laser treatment.

Medical treatment complements the surgery. The patient is advised to avoid food containing arachidonic acid, shellfish, and tannins of certain wines or beers, aspirin and penicillin, and public swimming pools because of the irritation from chlorine.

Prior to treatment, it is necessary to treat any kind of respiratory infection medically with decongestants, mucolytics, or antibiotics, as needed or by the method of displacement of Proetz. Allergy management with antihistamines, topical steroids, and immunotherapy is used if needed.

The fiberoptic flexible endoscope is inserted into the nasal cavity under the polyps until the deepest one is reached, at which point the quartz fiber is slid out of the channel to make contact with the polyps. With this endoscopic control, the laser is extremely precise and absolutely painless on the polyps. Only the patient may discern the characteristic smell of burning mucus, especially as the patient reacquires his or her sense of smell.

If the base of the polyp is accessible, a polypectomy is performed with the laser with minimal bleeding by excising the polyp from its base.

The laser lesion created by the Nd:YAG laser beam will have different diameters as a function of the color of the polyps, from white to gray to red, according to their age, their degree of infection, or the inflammatory process. The power and the exposure time of the laser irradiation as a function of the target are modulated. Most often it is 20 to 30 W for a period of 5 to 10 seconds, with

or without contact. Three to six sessions of treatments with 3-week intervals appear to provide the best results except on scarred tissue (Fig. 15b–3).

Recurrent Epistaxis

The Nd:YAG laser acts generally to manage the symptoms of epistaxis, not necessarily the cause. The anesthetic techniques depend on the etiology. Hereditary hemorrhagic telangiectasia (Rendu-Osler-Weber syndrome) can be treated with injectable local anesthesia with a spray of 10% lidocaine. Ten percent of patients with severe medical conditions justify a general anesthesia with intubation and nasal packing to protect the airway from bleeding.

Ectatic vessels are photocoagulated under local anesthesia with a spray of 10% lidocaine. Pyogenic granuloma (unless small) usually requires general anesthesia. It is important to soften crust and scabs with saline and for the patient to be relaxed.

The Nd:YAG laser should be set at low-power levels, 10 to 50 W, for 0.1 to 0.5 second (Figure 15b–4).

The patient is sitting, and we operate under local anesthesia with the operating microscope or by sight. The laser is used in the noncontact mode, in a circumferential application from the periphery to the center. If photocoagulation is successful, packing is avoided postoperatively. A surgical dressing with an antibiotic ointment and topical saline spray is occasionally necessary if an ablation of a vascular malformation or a pyogenic granuloma was performed. There is minimal, if any, postoperative pain.

Three to six sessions with 3-week intervals are usually necessary.

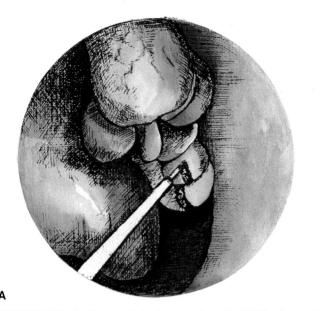
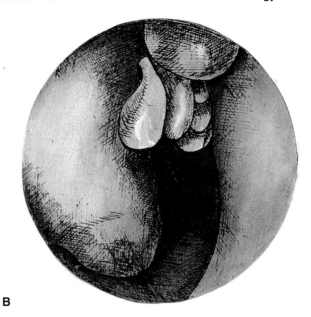

A   **B**

FIGURE 15b–3   Polyposis in the nasal cavity. (A) The laser shot is precise on every polyp. (B) After three sessions, the patient regains a permeable nose.

Synechiae

A synechia disappears with the Nd:YAG laser in one or occasionally two sessions.

A continuous mode is used with a power of 30 W, in contact, progressing from anterior to posterior to vaporize the synechia (Figure 15b–5). It is unusual for the synechia to recur.

Choanal Atresia

Many surgical methods have been proposed to correct choanal atresia by the transpalatal, transnasal, or transmaxillary approach. Access is relatively easy, approaching the membranous choanal atresia anteriorly endoscopically. This can be performed under general anesthesia using endoscopic guidance (either rigid or flexible).

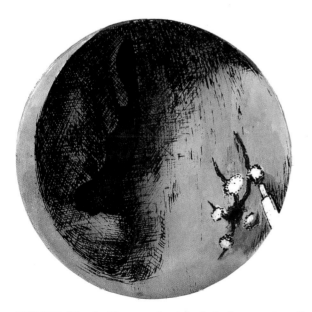
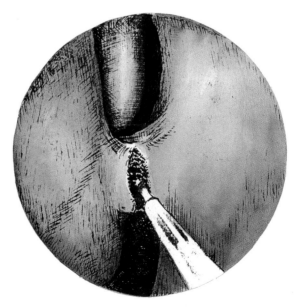

FIGURE 15b–4   Recurrent epistaxis in the nasal cavity. The Nd:YAG laser is set at low power levels in a circumferential application from the periphery to the center of the vascular lesion in the noncontact mode.

FIGURE 15b–5   Synechiae in the nasal cavity disappear in the contact mode. We advance from front to back until there is complete destruction.

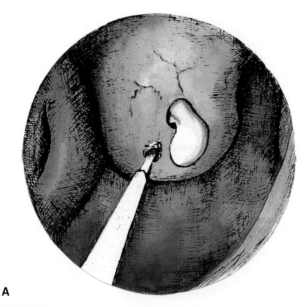

A

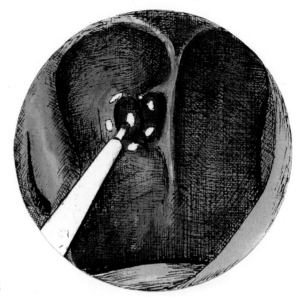

B

FIGURE 15b–6   A nasopharynx cyst in the cavum. (A) Here, on the posterior wall, we evacuate the cyst. (B) Three weeks later, the laser shot ensures the studding of the superficial wall to the deep one. We draw a crown around the cicatricial crater.

Nd:YAG energy is applied at 30 W, in continuous mode, in contact with the mucosa. It is well tolerated by the patient, usually with minimal postoperative pain.

Posterior Nasopharyngeal Wall

Small adhesions discovered under fiberoptic examination can accumulate debris and become symptomatic. These need to be lysed. This can be easily done with the Nd:YAG laser. Thornwaldt's bursa of 1 to 2 mm in diameter can be marsupialized with the laser, preventing symptoms. Adenoid tissue that is symptomatic is removed by laser vaporization. Several sessions may be needed. Nasopharyngeal cysts are rare. Initially, the cyst is evacuated; then, using the Nd:YAG laser, the cyst is opened, liberating its mucoid, purulent, or hematic contents, which are aspirated with a suction connected to the fiberoptic endoscope. Three weeks later, another laser treatment will ensure adherence by studding of the superficial wall to the deep wall if the cyst is not completely removed (Fig. 15b–6).

Eustachian Tube Pathology

Cysts, nodules, and cicatracial adhesions around the eustachian tube can be treated with the laser and endoscope. Care should be taken to avoid injury to the torus tubarius that could lead to a secondary stenosis. The laser shot is pointed, discontinuous, in pulse mode, with 15 to 30 W power, depending on the desired effect. Three sessions are usually necessary for a complete treatment.

■ Complications

Complications with the laser flexible fiberoptic method have been unusual.

Ocular lesions can occur if the eyes are not protected with special goggles specific to the Nd:YAG laser wavelength. All those present in the procedure room must wear them.

Papilloma virus can be spread through the plume after laser vaporization of the papilloma. Therefore, a special laser mask is worn, and the procedure must be done in a well-ventilated room. A smoke evacuator should be used. This enables safe removal of papilloma and avoids papilloma virus intoxication.

Hemorrhage can occur from the fiberoptic endoscope irritating the mucosa or the laser beam injuring a moderate-sized blood vessel. This may require cauterization with the Nd:YAG laser or on occasion nasal packing. Following the procedure, excessive nose blowing may cause bleeding.

Local secondary infections are easily controlled with antibiotics.

Edema or serous rhinorrhea can disturb the patient during the first 2 or 3 days following the laser procedure. Three days of steroid therapy can minimize such edema.

The author did have one case of a secondary myelitis after a pinpoint shot was applied too long on the nasopharynx.

■ Results

From 1987 to 1999, 1576 patients with intranasal pathology and 646 patients with benign lesions of the sinus were treated with the Nd:YAG laser and flexible fiberoptic endoscope.

Hypertrophic Rhinitis

The results of the laser treatment can be judged by subjective criteria in the form of a questionnaire in which the patient reports the improvements in respiratory comfort and objective criteria are determined by the improvement shown on rhinomanometry. Those patients who experienced complete or nearly complete subjective and objective improvement are considered classified as very good. Those patients who have partial subjective or objective improvement only or whose improvement has been insufficient are considered good.

Of 958 patients treated, 638 were labeled very good (66.6%), 191 were good (19.9%), 47 failed (4.9%), and 82 (8.6%) were lost to follow-up. These results are generally maintained over the course of time.

Polyposis

In the case of polyposis, the Nd:YAG laser sessions are considered as part of the usual treatments in which an attempt was made to manage the patient initially medically and surgery was performed when this failed.

From 1987 to 1998, 549 patients suffering from polyposis were treated. Many had associated nasal polyps, asthma, and aspirin sensibility. They were evaluated at 3 months, 6 months, and 1 year following the laser treatment, then at regular intervals one or two times a year.

The following criteria were used in the analysis of the data. Those patients who regained their sense of smell and developed a patent airway (in subjective terms and rhinomanometric examination), in whom nasal spray usage ceased and polyps retracted, were classified very good. Those patients who could breathe normally and have a dry nose but had not regained their sense of smell were classified as good.

Immediate results were encouraging. Five hundred and forty-nine patients were treated with the Nd:YAG laser. Of them, 62.4% were very good, 31.2% were good, and 6.4% failed. When these immediate results were analyzed more carefully, additional information was found. Of the 360 patients who were never operated before, 68% were very good, 24% were good, and 8% failed.

TABLE 15b–1   Recurrence Rates of Nasal and /or Sinus Polyposis Following Nd:YAG Laser Treatment

Recurrences	3 Months	6 Months	12 Months	>12 Months
Entire group (549 patients)	5.8%	7.25%	7.25%	21.2%
Without prior ethmoidectomy (360 patients)	2.3%	4.6%	6.0%	16.2%
With prior ethmoidectomy (133 patients)	7.4%	9.3%	10.2%	27.8%
Samter's triad (56 patients)	22.9%	17.1%	5.7%	31.4%

Of the 133 patients operated previously with ethmoidectomy, 57% were very good, 39% were good, and 4% failed. Of the 56 patients with asthma, nasal polyposis, and aspirin sensitivity, 46% were very good, 51% good, and 3% failed.

In all cases, more than 90% of patients acquired a good nasal airway with a dry nose; however, these spectacular and immediate results were not maintained. As expected with nasal polyposis disease, there was recurrence. Out of 549 patients treated by the Nd:YAG laser, 41.5% relapsed with nasal and/or sinus polyposis (Table 15b–1).

Of the 360 patients without prior ethmoidectomy, 29 (1%) relapsed after the Nd:YAG laser treatment, less than 13% within 1 year, and slightly more than 16% after 1 year.

Almost 55% of the patients operated by endoscopic sinus surgery before the Nd:YAG laser treatment relapsed, half of them before 1 year. It should be noted that there are more relapses in the group of patients with polyposis who had laser polyp surgery preceded by endoscopic sinus surgery. Two explanations are possible. Perhaps patients with recurrent polyposis develop a more fibrotic polyp or have a different etiology for the polyps. Another possibility suggests caution and thought. Endoscopic sinus surgery perhaps opens the door to spreading the polyps when it opens intersinusnasal walls. However, more than likely, the recurrences after sinus surgery suggest the presence of more severe disease.

Finally, aspirin triad disease provides the poorest results, with 77% of relapses in the first year, while 23% succeed in maintaining their improved status more or less beyond 1 year.

False hopes have been conjured up so frequently with respect to the treatment of nasal and sinus polyposis that caution is necessary whenever new therapy is developed. The author has been employing Nd:YAG laser treatment on polyposis for more than 12 years, and the results now have some meaning. This treatment has become a part of the therapeutic arsenal active against polyposis.

There is no unique therapeutic answer when confronted with sinus and nasal polyposis. It is a benign and recurrent disease whose pathophysiology is not understood. Recurrence is the rule in more than 50% of all cases. All the different treatments must be evaluated or reevaluated. This evaluation cannot be guided only by criteria of recurrence and cure.

Although polyposis is a disturbing disease, it is a benign disease where risks of major surgery should be considered. It is important to weigh the cost, effectiveness, and risk of surgery versus medical management.

The Nd:YAG laser at least is a supplementary treatment for polyposis. Even if it does not completely eradicate the polyposis, it restricts the need for steroid therapy and minimizes the need for surgery.

Membranous Choanal Atresia

The Nd:YAG laser treatment permits the creation of an opening in the membranous choanal atresia with minimal risk. The Nd:YAG laser is the easiest technique and can be done on an outpatient basis with minimal morbidity to the patient.

Synechiae

These lesions are essentially of an iatrogenic nature and are very awkward for the patient and for the surgeon. Treatment is generally successful, but failure can occur with the reformation of the synechiae. Fifty-two patients have been treated. Normal airway was regained in 82.7%. Bone abnormalities (deviated nasal septum, septal spur, or turbinate deformity) influenced nasal obstruction, and therefore synechia removal had little effect in 7.7% of patients. Dense synechiae were present in 5.8%, and these patients failed. There were 3.8% of patients lost to follow-up.

These 90% good results are the consequence of the Nd:YAG laser effect causing retraction, vaporization, and coagulation of the synechiae.

Recurrent Epistaxis

Hereditary hemorrhagic telangiectasia (Rendu-Osler-Weber syndrome) was managed, with 80% of patients showing good results initially, but their long-term results still remained in question. There were failures in 20% of patients and these patients needed a septal dermoplasty.

Pyogenic granulomas and recurrent epistaxis with ectatic vessels for which the Nd:YAG laser was used led to a successful result with no relapse.

Nasopharyngeal Pathology

There were 652 patients who had some type of nasopharyngeal pathology managed with the Nd:YAG laser and fiberoptic endoscope.

Adenoid tissue was treated in 196 patients who presented with symptoms causing posterior rhinorrhea, a congestive mucosa, or pharyngeal paresthesias. Symptoms disappeared in 73% of patients who had a normal fiberoptic nasopharyngeal exam.

There were reduced symptoms in 15% of patients even though the fiberoptic examination still revealed residual adenoid tissue. There was failure in 9% of patients, and 3% were lost to follow-up.

Cicatricial adhesions of the nasopharynx were seen and treated in 56 patients. There were excellent results in 75%, 4% were better, 17% failed, and 4% were lost to follow-up.

Lutschka bags and Thornwaldt's bursae were treated in 43 patients. Of these, 72% resulted in a normal nasopharynx, and 19% had improvement in their symptoms even though the fiberoptic examination showed persistence of the lesion. Ten percent of patients either failed or were lost to follow-up.

Nasopharyngeal cysts were seen and treated in 108 patients. To date, there is no failure, but 1% of the patients have not had a postoperative evaluation.

Chronic inflammation (nasopharyngitis) was seen in 100 patients who had postnasal drainage with pharyngeal paresthesias, some of which were quite painful. Of the 100 patients treated, 54% of them had resolution of their symptoms and normal endoscopic examination results. There was improvement in 25% of the patients, failure in 14%, and 7% were lost to follow-up.

These results need few comments. The surgical studding of the nasopharyngeal posterior wall and alteration of the pharyngeal nerve plexus may cause enough scar formation to decrease secretions. However, the poorest results are the epipharyngitis failures occurring in older patients. This may occur because of the decreased secretions that already occur in older patients caused by mucosal atrophy.

These were many patients with pathology in and around the torus tubarius. One hundred and forty-nine patients had eustachian tube problems, with either a closed or patulous tube. Cysts, nodules, or edema were seen on the torus.

Edema causing hearing loss as seen on audiometric testing was seen and treated in 74 patients. The symptoms disappeared, and there was a return to normal hearing in 80% of patients after three treatments with the Nd:YAG laser. There was audiometric improvement but persistent ear symptoms in 9%, failure in 8%, and 3% were lost to follow-up.

Nasopharyngeal cysts were treated in 32 patients. Very good results were seen in 84% of patients with resolution of symptoms and a normal fiberoptic examination, good results in 9% with resolution of symptoms but some pathology still seen on fiberoptic examination, and 6% failed.

Otorrhea involving the eustachian tube was treated in 14 patients. There was improvement in hearing on audiometric testing and drainage in 71% and failure in 29% of patients.

Cicatricial adhesions were treated, and there were very good results in 76% (improved symptoms and a normal fiberoptic examination), good results in 7% (improved symptoms yet with persistent pathology on fiberoptic examination), and failure in 17%.

■ Conclusion

Flexible fiberoptic endoscopes can be combined with the Nd:YAG laser to treat pathology in the nose, paranasal sinuses, and nasopharynx. This can be accomplished under local anesthesia as an ambulatory procedure that has little if any bleeding. The technique requires specific training and control of the technique.

Hypertrophic rhinitis, synechiae, choanal atresia, and recurrent epistaxis can be treated with good results. The Nd:YAG laser provides good management of nasal polyposis, minimizes the need for steroid therapy, and lessens the need for surgical intervention.

Procedures can be repeated three or four times without any additional medical management, minimal interruption of activity, and no hospitalization generally (except on occasion for Rendu-Osler-Weber syndrome and choanal atresia management).

REFERENCES

1. Einstein A. Quantum theorie der Strahlung. *Phyz. Zeit.* 1917;18:121.
2. Hofstetter FF, Keiditsche BR. Endoscopic application of the Nd:YAG laser in urology: biophysical fundamentals and instrumentation. *Soc Photo-op Instrum Eng.* 1979;211(36–40):26–30.
3. Buiter CT. *Endoscopic and YAG laser therapy in the uppper ways.* Groningen, Netherlands: Department of Oto-Rhino-Laryngology, University Hospital of Groningen.

16

Outcome and Results in the Surgical Management of Rhinosinusitis

HOWARD L. LEVINE

Staging systems and outcome results for head and neck neoplasms have long been important to the otolaryngologist in determining future treatment and advising the patient and family. Staging systems and statistical and outcome analysis for rhinosinusitis have greatly lagged behind that which exists for other disease entities. Most reports discuss surgical technique and relate to the author's method of assessing and evaluating disease. Some staging systems use various aspects of patient symptoms, and others incorporate aspects of the physical examination. Most staging systems use some features of CT scan findings because CT scans provide information about volume and location of disease. Because there is no standardized or uniform method of reporting results, there is difficulty in comparing techniques and results from one author to another. Even the definition of the various types of rhinosinusitis has been debated. There have been discussions and agreement by the American Academy of Otolaryngology Head and Neck Surgery (AAO-HNS), Rhinology and Paranasal Sinus Committee about definitions of rhinosinusitis (acute, subacute, recurrent acute, chronic, and acute exacerbation of chronic).[1]

The desire to have outcome data and uniform definitions of disease and staging of disease is stimulated by the growing interest in the diagnosis and management of rhinosinusitis, the number one chronic disease in the United States. There is prognostic value in having any staging system and evaluating outcome. With a higher stage, there should be worsening of disease and therefore a greater and more intense level of management. It is not clear whether the ideal staging system, however, is best based on nasal endoscopic findings,

patient history, CT abnormalities, or some combination of these.

■ Staging Systems

In 1993, the International Conference on Sinus Disease: Terminology, Staging, and Therapy, was held in Princeton, New Jersey.[2] The purpose of the conference was to bring together leading authorities in nasal and sinus disease representing otolaryngology, radiology, family medicine, internal medicine, and pediatrics from around the world to discuss anatomical nomenclature, sinus staging, and medical management of rhinosinusitis. The conference stressed the diagnostic categories of rhinosinusitis, symptom score, related systemic diagnoses, radiologic staging, surgical score, and endoscopic appearance score. This was an attempt to bring together several different patient symptoms and signs to create a staging system. (Demographic information presented in this chapter is based on the American Academy of Otolaryngology Head and Neck Surgery Rhinology and Paranasal Sinus Committee Classification of Rhinosinusitis, modified since the conference.[1])

Systemic diagnoses with disease are included in the discussion in this chapter. Diseases included are abnormalities of mucociliary clearance (primary ciliary dyskinesia and Young's syndrome), asthma (with or without aspirin sensitivity and acetylsalicylic acid triad), bronchiectasis, diabetes mellitus, immune deficiency, multiple myeloma, sarcoidosis, and other conditions predisposing to infection. Underlying factors to be included are atopy and smoking.

Radiologic staging requires CT scan assessment. Plain radiographs have no role in the staging process. Each sinus group (maxillary, anterior ethmoid, posterior ethmoid, sphenoid, and frontal) is graded as 0 (no abnormality), 1 (partial opacification), or 2 (total opacification). The ostiomeatal complex is scored as either 0 (no occlusion) or 2 (total opacification). Anatomical variants are noted as absent (0) or present (1) but do not contribute to scan score. Variants include concha bullosa, paradoxical middle turbinate, infraorbital ethmoid cells (Haller's cells), everted uncinate process, agger nasi pneumatization, and absence of frontal sinus. These variants have little impact on staging but are important for planning surgery. Anatomical variants with normal mucosa are probably inconsequential.

When a CT scan is obtained is important. If there is to be consistent methods of staging, and CT scan is part of this, then there must be agreement about when the scan is obtained. It is best obtained after adequate medical management and a period in which there is no acute infection (possibly 3–4 weeks after acute or subacute infection).

A surgical score was created but not considered an essential part of the staging.

The International Conference also used patient-perceived symptom data. The patient, using a visual analogue [0 (not present) to 10 (present and most severe)] scale, assessed symptom scores. Symptoms included nasal blockage, nasal congestion, nasal pressure, headache, facial pain, facial pressure, olfactory disturbance, and nasal discharge. Patients were asked to rank in order their three worst symptoms.

The nasal endoscopic examination was quantified by looking for polyps, discharge, edema, scarring or adhesions, and crusting. Absence of polyps was 0; presence of polyps confined to the middle meatus was 1; presence of polyps beyond the middle meatus was 2. No discharge was 0; clear and thin discharge was 1; and thick and purulent discharge was 2.

Other authors have looked at different aspects of CT scans as a staging tool. Friedman and Katsantonis,[3] for example, have used a staging system since 1984 that is based on their experience in assessing and evaluating sinus disease and provides a statistical basis for sinus surgery:

Stage I: Single-focus disease radiographically, either unilaterally or bilaterally

Stage II: Discontiguous or patchy areas of disease radiofrequency, either unilateral or bilateral

Stage III: Contiguous disease throughout the ethmoid labyrinth, with or without other major sinus opacity, with symptomatic response to medication

Stage IV: Contiguous hyperplastic disease involving all sinuses, with minimal or no symptomatic response to medication

In this system, structural abnormalities, including hypertrophic uncinate process, deviated nasal septum, concha bullosa, and paradoxically bent middle turbinate, are all recognized as causes of rhinosinusitis but are not classified unless they are part of a roentgenographic picture of rhinosinusitis. Asthma and immunologic abnormalities were not classified as part of the staging system.

For the most part, patients with stage I disease were treated medically. Most patients in stage II underwent surgical intervention (intranasal sphenoethmoidectomy, endoscopic sinus surgery, Caldwell-Luc or intranasal antrostomy). Patients with stage III or stage IV disease underwent intranasal sphenoethmoidectomy with endoscopic control.

The distribution of chronic sinusitis patients was stage I, 14.28%; stage II, 43%; stage III, 27.35%; and stage IV, 15.35%. The recurrence rates in stages I and II were similar, 7.7% and 8.9%, respectively. Stages III and IV disease showed progressive increases in recurrence rates, with 16.1% in stage III and 25.6% in stage IV.

The presence of asthma was an important and independent indicator of recurrence. In stage III, 14.25% of nonasthmatics sustained recurrence, compared with 21.61% of asthmatics who had recurrence. In the stage IV group, this was even more dramatic: There was a 34.23% recurrence in asthmatic patients. This was nearly double the 17.26% of nonasthmatic stage IV patients.

A regression analysis was performed that showed a correlation coefficient of 0.99 with progression of disease by stage.

Metson et al,[4] at the request of the Rhinology and Paranasal Sinus Committee of the AAO-HNS, attempted to establish a protocol to evaluate CT staging systems. Four otolaryngologists at six international sites according to five established sinus CT staging systems rated fifty identical scans.[5–8] Twenty of the 24 reviewers repeated the rating 1 week later to determine the intrarater reliability. Their study found that two of the systems (Gliklich and Metson, Lund and McKay) were the most favorable with regard to clinical applicability. The Gliklich and Metson system ranked the highest for ease of use, with good intrarater and interrater agreement. The Lund and McKay system had the least number of unclassifiable scans and was best able to distinguish subtle differences between disease states; however, it had the lowest intrarater and interrater agreement.

Gliklich and Metson System

Stage 0: less than 2 mm mucosal thickening on any sinus wall

Stage 1: all unilateral disease or anatomical abnormalities

Stage 2: bilateral disease limited to the ethmoid or maxillary sinuses

Stage 3: bilateral disease with involvement of at least one sphenoid or frontal sinus

Stage 4: pansinus disease

Lund and McKay System

The Lund and McKay System using a scoring and localization system. Points are given for degree of opacification for each sinus on each side.

0 points = no abnormality
1 point = partial opacification
2 points = total opacification

Sinuses are identified as:

Maxillary
Anterior ethmoid
Posterior ethmoid
Sphenoid
Frontal
Ostiomeatal complex (only 0 or 2 points)
0 points = normal
2 points = obstruction

Each side is scored separately.

Results In the author's previous textbook,[9] an attempt was made to report results, classify, and stage different types of sinus disease. This was done at a time when very little was available about definitions of types of sinus disease or staging of sinus disease. Levine and May looked at anatomical variations, type, severity (graded by CT scan), and causes of inflammatory disease (determined by history and endoscopy). They determined the presence of allergy, presence of polyps and severity by extent, and presence of unfavorable prognostic factors (previous sinus surgery, reactive airway disease, triad asthma, allergic aspergillosis, Kartagener's syndrome, dysmotility syndrome, cystic fibrosis, and immune disorder). The goals of the classification system were to (1) identify the patient for whom sinus surgery is appropriate, (2) choose the surgical approach that will provide the best results for each patient, (3) predict the success of endoscopic sinus surgery in relieving sinus disease symptoms, and (4) evaluate success or failure in a systematic and reproducible way. Patients were assessed following surgery and classified as

I. Symptom-free

II. Symptom-free after one additional therapy
  A. Medical treatment
  B. Minor revision surgery (synechiae removal, single polyp removal, turbinate surgery)

III. Improved (three most prominent symptoms)

IV. Improved with maintenance
  A. Medical treatment
  B. Major revision surgery

V. Same or worse (surgical failure)

VI. Lost to follow-up

Since the author's previous reporting of results, an additional 1868 patients underwent endoscopic sinus surgery from March 1991 to March 1999 and had a mean follow-up of 5 years, 2 months.

Of the 1868 patients, 710 (38%) underwent only a primary operation, and 1158 (62%) underwent revision surgery. Of the 710 patients undergoing a primary operation, 128 (18%) had asthma, nasal polyps, and aspirin sensitivity. Of the 1158 patients undergoing revision surgery, 834 (72%) had asthma, nasal polyposis, and aspirin sensitivity.

In the 582 nonasthmatic patients undergoing primary nasal sinus surgery, the symptoms were facial pressure or pain in 537 (92.3%), nasal obstruction or blockage in 514 (88.3%), nasal discharge or purulence or postnasal drip in 467 (80.2%), and headache in 443 (76.1%), taste or smell change in 385 (66.2%), fatigue in 206 (35.4%), and cough in 193 (33.2%).

In the 734 nonasthmatic revision patients undergoing sinus surgery, the symptoms were nasal discharge or purulence or postnasal drip in 631 (87.2%), facial pressure or pain in 606 (83.7%), nasal obstruction or blockage in 597 (82.5%), cough in 583 (80.5%), taste or smell change in 570 (78.7%), and asthma requiring additional medications in 540 (74.6%). Headache was present in 526 (72.7%) and fatigue in 186 (25.7%).

In the 582 nonasthmatic patients undergoing endoscopic sinus surgery, 132 (22.7%) were symptom free (category I). Eighty-one (13.9%) were improved after one additional medical therapy (antibiotics, short course of systemic steroids) (category IIA). Sixteen patients (2.7%) were improved after minor revision surgery (category IIB). One hundred and nineteen (20.4%) had their three most prominent symptoms improved (category III). One hundred and seven (18.4%) were improved with medical maintenance (ongoing nasal steroids, decongestants, mucolytics) (category IVA), and 52 (8.9%) required revision surgery (category IVB). Seventy-five patients (12.9%) were the same or worse (category V). This gave an overall success of symptom-free patients (group I) 22.7%. There was improvement with patients either symptom free with surgery alone, one additional treatment, or improved (groups I–IV) at 87.0%.

In the 724 nonasthmatic patients undergoing revision endoscopic sinus surgery, 99 patients (13.7%) were symptom free (category I). Fifty-nine patients (8.2%) were symptom free after one additional medical treatment (category IIA). Sixteen patients (2.2%) were symptom free after one additional surgical treatment (category IIB). One hundred and one patients (14.0%) had their three most prominent symptoms improved (category III).

One hundred and fifteen patients (15.9%) were improved but required ongoing medical management (category IVA). Two hundred and one patients (27.7%) required revision surgery (mostly to remove additional polyps and correct sinusitis) (category IVB). One hundred and thirty-two patients (18.3%) were the same or worse. This gave an overall success rate of symptom-free patients (group I) 13.7%. There was improvement with symptom free with surgery alone, one additional medical or surgical treatment or improvement (groups I–IV) in 81.7% of patients.

There were 662 asthmatic patients (228 primary surgical and 434 revision surgical). Of these, 404 (61%) had triad asthma with nasal polyps, aspirin sensitivity, and asthma.

As might be expected, asthmatic patients with nasal and sinus disease have a disease different from nonasthmatic patients. Following endoscopic sinus surgery, 628 patients (75.3%) felt that their asthma was easier to control, requiring less medication (steroid inhalers, systemic steroids), and there were fewer acute attacks. Even though a large number of asthmatic patients felt their asthma was easier to manage, there was the need for significant ongoing additional management in 396 patients (59.8%). This included systemic and topical steroids, numerous courses of antibiotics, nearly continuous use of systemic mucolytics, intermittent nasal irrigations, and many with multiple surgical procedures.

■ The Difficulty in Reporting Results

The reporting of results for sinus surgery is difficult for several reasons. There is yet to be a uniform, accepted definition of the disease that uses consistent nomenclature to define the different types of sinusitis. The AAO-HNS Rhinology and Paranasal Sinus Committee has attempted to do this.[1] There is no accepted staging system for disease. A few of the several different methods appear in the literature as discussed in this chapter. There is also no agreed upon definition of success in treatment. Should success be relief of some or all symptoms? Should success be the improvement or resolution of disease on CT scan? Should success be a normal (other than surgical changes) nasal endoscopic exam?

What makes this all so difficult is that sinus disease, unlike other disease entities, is dynamic. At any moment the patient is experiencing and the physician is observing merely a "snapshot" of the disease. The symptoms, nasal endoscopy, and CT scan constantly fluctuate as internal and external stimuli alter the nasal and sinus cavity.

This author looked at symptoms and the relationship to additional treatment. While recognizing this is far from perfect, hopefully it gives the general practitioner of nasal and sinus disease an indication of the behavior of the disease as it is managed by endoscopic sinus surgery.

REFERENCES

1. Lanza DC, Kennedy DW. Adult rhinosinusitis defined. *Otolaryngol Head Neck Surg.* 1997;117:S4–S5.
2. Kennedy DW. International Conference on Sinus Disease: Terminology, staging, therapy. *Ann Otol Rhinol Laryngol.* 1995;10410 (suppl, pt 2):167.
3. Friedman WH, Katsantonis GP. Staging systems for chronic sinus disease. *Ear Nose Throat.* 1994;73:480–484.
4. Metson R, Gliklich RE, Stankiewicz JA, et al. Comparison of sinus computed tomography staging systems. *Otolaryngol Head Neck Surg.* 1997;117:372–379.
5. Kennedy DW. Prognostic factors, outcomes and staging in ethmoid sinus surgery *Laryngoscope.* 1992;102:1–18.*
6. Friedman WH, Katsantonis GP, Sivore M, Kay S. Computed tomography staging of paranasal sinuses in chronic hyperplastic rhinosinusitis. *Laryngoscope.* 1990;100:1161–1165.
7. Gliklich RE, Metson R. A comparison of sinus computed tomography (CT) staging systems for outcomes research. *Am J Rhinol.* 1994;8:291–297.
8. Lund VJ, McKay IS. Staging in rhinosinusitis *Rhinology.* 1993; 31:183–184.
9. Levine HL, May M. *Rhinology and Sinusology: Endoscopic Sinus Surgery.* New York: Thieme Medical Publishers; 1993:261.

17

Revision Endoscopic Sinus Surgery

JAMES A. STANKIEWICZ, HANJO NA, AND JAMES M. CHOW

Success in endoscopic sinus surgery (ESS) occurs in 85 to 95% of patients. About 5 to 15% of patients fail and require revision sinus surgery. Some of the same problems that cause failure for primary ESS will also be a problem for revision surgery. Nasal polyps, extensive disease, and previous surgery are problematic cases. Underlying problems such as cilia abnormalities, immunodeficiency, and cystic fibrosis need to be taken into consideration in surgical planning. The most common symptoms noted in the failure patient are headache and symptoms of recurrent infection. The most common anatomical problems related to failed surgery are a retained or intact uncinate process and a lateralized or destabilized middle turbinate. Pathophysiology noted on objective evaluation includes anterior and posterior ethmoid disease, frontal recess obstruction or stenosis, an obstructed, blocked, or closed antrostomy, recirculation phenomenon, recurrent or persistent fungal disease, and sphenoid obstruction or closure. Surgical decision making designed to treat these problems is carefully planned and targeted with other surgical alternatives ready as backup. A working knowledge of paranasal sinus surgical anatomy is imperative. Surgical revision can be performed safely after careful preoperative study in a systematic sinus-by-sinus fashion. Stereotactic computerized ESS is extremely helpful in finding disease and identifying the orbit and skull base. Making note of the anatomical landmarks and sinus disease via radiography and examination will prepare the surgeon for the endoscopic diversity and challenge of revision sinus surgery.

Initial endoscopic sinus surgery results have proven to be successful in 75 to 95% of cases. However, the definition of success varies from surgeon to surgeon. In most studies, it is defined appropriately as the resolution or improvement of symptoms. However, Kennedy[1] has shown that symptoms do not correlate well with resolution of disease; therefore, one must evaluate the patient with the objective results taken in light of subjective complaints. Not all failures need nor undergo revision surgery. Revision surgery occurs in 5 to 15% of patients, with success rates of 63% or better.

Evaluation of postoperative failure should involve a multidisciplinary approach. Obviously, a history and physical examination are paramount. To understand decision making in revision sinus surgery, it is necessary to know why we have failed and what has occurred to make the patient again symptomatic. Several studies over the years have discussed symptoms requiring revision surgery. Usually the most common symptoms are recurrent infection and/or headache. A detailed history is important to help sort out this common complaint. Objective evaluation with endoscopic exam and CT scanning will help determine which sinuses are problematic. Seeing the patient when the patient is sick can help further focus attention to troubled sinus problems. Some underlying problems play such an important role that nothing further surgically can be done, and only symptomatic treatment is warranted.

When looking at failures, several causes have to be analyzed prior to any treatment planning (refer to Table 14–1 in Chapter 14). The patient may have the wrong diagnosis. For instance, surgery may have been performed for a diagnosis of headache. When the surgery fails to cure the symptoms even though objectively everything looks great, other causes for the headaches may become apparent. The patient may have an underlying problem that is mucosal and goes beyond infection or surgery. Suggested poor prognostic indicators include allergy, asthma, aspirin triad, esophageal reflux, immunodeficiency, cystic fibrosis, cilial disturbances, and postoperative smoking. All may cause persistent symptoms despite good objective results. Inappropriate or inadequate surgery may have been performed where too much or too little has been removed, allowing for nonphysiologically working sinus passages or persistence of disease. Poor technique may have been used, causing synechiae, turbinate instability or lateralization, and/or persistence of sinus anatomy and disease, which should have been removed. Poor postoperative observation and care may have occurred, allowing for middle turbinate or middle turbinate remnant lateralization, scarring, adhesion, synechia, or persistent disease. In some instances preserved uncinate processes, lateralized turbinate, and an uncorrected septal deviation may contribute to disease. Nasal polyps, especially with asthma and/or aspirin sensitivity, recur with the reappearance of symptoms in a high percentage of patients. Patients with extensive disease, especially with allergic fungal sinusitis or a history of previous surgery, have a high rate of recurrent disease despite the most aggressive of surgeries.[2] This is probably due to the marked changes in mucosa, cilia, and, overall, surgery.

Specific anatomical areas where failure most commonly occurs are noted (refer to Table 14–2 in Chapter 14). These areas are retained uncinate process, lateralized middle turbinate, blocked or missed natural ostia, blocked frontal recess, and blocked sphenoid. Chu et al[3] noted four sites of disease in at least one-quarter of patients. Ramadan[4] looked at cases of failed ESS in 52 out of 398 total surgery patients (13%). He found that 31% had residual ethmoid air cells, 28% had maxillary ostia stenosis, 26% had frontal recess stenosis, and 15% had recirculation or missed ostia. Twenty-nine out of 56 patients (52%) had adhesions with a lateralized middle turbinate. Moses et al[5] reported a 67% success rate of revision ESS in 90 patients out of 753 consecutive functional ESS (FESS) cases (12%). Extent of disease, nasal polyps, allergy, previous traditional surgery, male gender, chronic steroid use, and deviated septum all appeared to adversely affect outcome, which differs from the data from Marks and Shamsa.[2]

Symptoms that occur heralding recurrent or persistent disease include headache, purulent drainage, congestion, cough, bad breath, loss of smell, and "bad" smell. Symptoms in isolation to be wary of include postnasal drainage, which may be related to esophageal reflux, and nasal obstruction, which may be due to turbinate, septum, and/or nasal valve problems. Revision sinus surgery in these patients will not be successful (refer to Table 14–3 in Chapter 14).[3]

The patient with chronic sinusitis or recurrent infection after initial surgery is treated aggressively with prolonged broad-spectrum antibiotics as well as oral, topical, and sometimes injected steroids. Limited office procedures, including lysis of synechiae, correction of recirculation, limited local polypectomy, and polyp injection, may be combined with the initial aggressive medical management. On completion of this initial trial, if the patient is without relief, a CT scan is obtained to identify the source of infection. If the patient presented without indication of active disease but has chronic or recurrent complaints, obtain a coronal CT scan of the sinuses. Sometimes 1 mm coronal and axial CT scans can uncover small areas of obstruction. A reconstructed sagittal CT scan can be helpful in sorting out problems in the frontal recess. Patients with a relatively good objective examination can have hidden areas of disease, such as frontal or sphenoid sinusitis, which otherwise are overlooked unless careful CT evaluation is performed. However, patients also can have CT scans that appear relatively normal, especially if the scans are done after recent treatment with medication, so it may be important to see the patient when symptomatic. This strategy serves two purposes. First, it allows soft tissue and bone evaluation in regions that clinically appear obstructed or perhaps disease free. One should look for normal variants compromising drainage, including concha bullosa, sphenoethmoid cells (Onodi cells), agger nasi, and infraorbital (Haller's) cells, or the persistence of infection. A retained uncinate with missed natural ostia may be more apparent on CT than clinical examination (Fig. 17–1). Second, this strategy offers a road map in a previously operated field. One should specially evaluate the lamina papyracea, the region of the cribriform plate, and the fovea ethmoidalis for dehiscence, as well as the proximity of the neurovascular anatomy of the sphenoid sinus.

Anatomy is the cornerstone of surgery. Without adequate knowledge of normal and the many variations of normal, primary FESS is high-risk surgery and revision

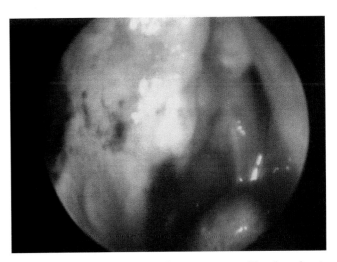

FIGURE 17–1 Retained uncinate process with missed natural ostia, right-sided.

surgery more so. To decrease the risk of complication and improve results in revision surgery, a working knowledge of fundamental anatomy is necessary. In many revision cases, patients have marked alterations in the integrity of the lateral nasal wall or severe polyposis, making it exceedingly difficult to determine where to begin safely. The first surgical step of the procedure should therefore be a complete reassessment of the lateral wall to identify any remaining landmarks.

May et al[6] describe six friendly landmarks in revision FESS that offer the surgeon the ability to sort out confusing anatomy (refer to Table 14–4 in Chapter 14). The *anterior arch* is formed by the remnant of the middle turbinate medially, the anterior ethmoids and agger nasi cells superiorly and anterolaterally, and the lamina papyracea laterally. It protects the surgeon from staying medially in the cribriform plate. Identifying the anterosuperior attachment of the middle turbinate during revision endoscopic sinus surgery is helpful in maintaining orientation because this attachment marks the boundary between the ethmoid complex and the space between the middle turbinate and the septum. The latter space should not be manipulated because of its proximity to the floor of the cribriform plate, which is vulnerable to penetration at this point. The *lamina papyracea*, when previously seen on CT, guides the surgeon along the most lateral portion of the dissection, protecting the eye from inadvertent injury. The lamina is identified by finding the maxillary antrostomy immediately. The *maxillary antrostomy* should include the natural ostium to avoid failure. The lamina papyracea lies just lateral and superior to the maxillary antrostomy. Looking superior into the maxillary antrostomy, the floor of the orbit can be seen and followed medially to join with the lamina papyracea. The *ridge* formed by the border between the superior aspect of the maxillary antrostomy and the inferior edge of the lamina papyracea represents the level of the orbital floor. The posterior ethmoid is located above this ridge, and the sphenoid sinus lies below it. If the lamina papyracea and maxillary sinus floors are traced posteriorly, the ridge will define the air cells superior to it as the posterior ethmoids and inferior to it as the *sphenoid sinus*. For pure orientation, the sphenoid sinus will be in a plane perpendicular to a line parallel to the maxillary antrostomy. Because the location of the antrostomy is important to finding the lamina, so too is the sphenoid sinus in establishing the skull base. It is always best to find the sphenoid by locating the natural ostia if it can be visualized or is not scarred over. The sphenoid location is most commonly isolated by going superiorly 1 to 1.5 cm to the top of the *choanal arch*, bordered medially by the septum and laterally by the superior turbinate. The lower third of the superior turbinate either covers or is just lateral to the sphenoid ostia and is the easiest way to find the sphenoid sinus ostia. The

sphenoid is also located by using a measurement source for distance reference. The anterior face is usually 7 cm from the nasal spine in the normal adult, and the posterior wall measurement approximates the back wall of the nasopharynx, which is usually ~9 cm. Once the sphenoid is opened, the front wall leads to the skull base and posterior ethmoids. This offers a landmark for the most superior limit of the posterior ethmoid cells. Dissection can then proceed from a posterior dissection to an anterior dissection to the frontal recess.

The revision surgical field may have atypical mucosa. If mucosa was stripped in the primary procedure, the replacement mucosa may have blood vessels lacking normal hemostatic mechanisms or healed mucosa with scarring and few working cilia. As a result, the patient may bleed more than at the initial surgery, and healing will be problematic.

In children, second-look procedures in most cases are unnecessary, with little or no difference in outcomes. Each case, though, should be individualized as to the need for a second-look procedure or revision surgery. Reasons to perform a second-look endoscopy include the use of nonabsorbable stenting, inability to complete surgery, inability to visualize the patient postoperatively, and obvious evidence of synechiae, turbinate lateralization, or persistent disease.[7,8]

Image-guided (stereotactic computerized) surgery is beneficial during ESS, especially in revision cases, because it can help the surgeon identify critical contiguous vital structures such as the carotid arteries and optic nerves and skull base. It provides a third dimension, adding field orientation to the two-dimensional viewing plane of the endoscope. This integration is particularly important during revisions in which normal surgical landmarks are often not visible through the endoscope or in which frequent anatomical variation exists. Any failed sinus surgery case requiring a revision surgery should be looked upon as a difficult surgery. There are no easy revisions because more often than not more disease or scarring is found than was initially noted. The stereotactic computerized surgery performed in conjunction with ESS can identify all pockets of disease, answer questions of anatomy, and identify the orbit and skull base. This new technology allows for a more complete and safe surgery. Care should always be taken to not rely totally on the computerized systems. Most units have accuracy to within 2 mm. However, calibration errors can occur that affect accuracy, and if not questioned, serious injury could occur.

■ Medical and Surgical Failures

Any group of surgeons who acquire enough sinus surgical experience will have a small percentage of patients who simply will not heal and have persistent disease. These patients are our most frustrating group and require frequent debridements, irrigations, inhalations, antibiotic steroids, occasional repeat surgeries, and a second opinion. Sometimes an experienced colleague may be able to find an overlooked problem. Often there is an underlying mucosal or mucociliary problem, such as cystic fibrosis, immune deficiency, primary cilial dysfunction, allergy (including allergic fungal problems, foods, inhalants, and environmentals), atrophic rhinitis, or genetic problems. Medical therapies that are directed at these causes could be helpful. Culture may show extraordinary organisms such as *Pseudomonas, Proteus, Serratia, Escherichia coli, Enterococcus,* and methicillin-resistant *Staphylococcus.* Topical antibiotic and antifungal solutions/irrigations and oral and IV antibiotics/antifungal may be necessary to control mucosal and bone infection. Despite these efforts, some patients' cases cannot be improved, and they have to live with their disease. Some patients undergo very aggressive surgery with removal of or opening of almost all nasal and sinus structures, including all turbinates, causing chronic rhinitis, and in some cases a dysfunctional nose, which should be treated as such. Patience, encouragement, counseling, and local care are most helpful in this group.

■ Specific Issues for Revision Surgery

A workable general approach to revision endoscopic sinus surgery is the following:

1. Observe available landmarks both radiographically and clinically.
2. Moving first from anterior to posterior, check each sinus for abnormality.
3. Define or create landmarks necessary to operate safely on a sinus-by-sinus basis as the surgeon moves posteriorly.
4. The two most important landmarks are the following:
   - The maxillary antrostomy to define the lamina papyracea and sphenoid sinus
   - The sphenoid sinus to define the skull base
5. Repair abnormalities of the maxillary, lower ethmoid, and sphenoid sinus first.
6. Once skull base landmarks are defined, repair the upper ethmoid and frontal sinuses in a posterior-to-anterior direction, ending with the frontal sinus.
7. The same safety techniques for primary ESS apply for revision ESS.
8. There is no easy revision surgery.
9. Revision surgery is a situation where part of or the whole middle turbinate may need removal.
10. Stenting may be necessary.
11. Traditional sinus surgery procedures are done, if needed, in combination with the endoscopic procedure or alone.
12. Stereotactic computerized surgery is very helpful.

■ Maxillary Sinus Considerations

The most common reasons for failure of FESS resulting in persistent maxillary sinus disease are middle turbinate lateralization blocking the ostia, failure to remove the uncinate process, never finding the natural ostia, ostia stenosis, recirculation, any cause of cilial dysfunction, persistent fungal ball or crust, and chronic osteitis or osteomyelitis, as previously noted. Removal of the lateralized turbinate allows the ostia to drain properly. Proper removal of the uncinate process opens the infundibulum, allows for proper identification of the natural ostia and, if need be, permits the creation of an appropriate antrostomy that includes the natural ostia. Synechiae large enough to cause drainage problems are removed. Maxillary ostia stenosis needs to be reopened and perhaps stented. In most case of significant synechiae, the middle turbinate is partially resected because it is destabilized or itself scarred.

Parsons et al[10] talked about the missed natural ostia and its relation to the surgical approach in revision endoscopic sinus surgery. The uncinate process requires complete removal to find the natural ostia. An antrostomy created without including the natural ostia can lead to persistent sinus disease. Scar banding with partial obstruction at the area of the natural ostia of the maxillary or ethmoid sinuses can potentially prevent restoration of mucociliary flow and normal drainage of the sinus. It is extremely important to include the natural ostia in the maxillary antrostomy during FESS and revision ESS. It is also important to revise those sinuses and remove any scarring at the natural ostia.

Recirculation is often very obvious, with thick mucoid drainage apparent from separate maxillary openings after the uncinate has been removed (Fig. 17–2). Sometimes, the recirculation cannot be noted with even a 30-degree telescope. A flexible or 70-degree endoscope can be very helpful in identifying and correcting the problem. Careful coordination between endoscopic examination, including palpation and coronal CT, is important in locating these cells. Remember that the endoscopic view is an anteroposterior view and not coronal, as per CT scans. Mental adjustments for the surgeon sometimes are required to make these corrections. In patients with ciliary dysfunction in which a wide antrostomy is apparent with inclusion of the natural ostia, it is sometimes necessary to place an inferior window to remove inferior disease and allow gravity drainage to assist the healing of the cilia.[11] Also, check the frontal sinus for disease draining

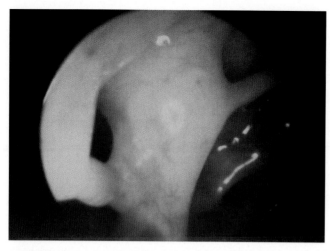

FIGURE 17–2 Recirculation left maxillary sinus.

into the maxillary sinus from above. Sometimes an unsuspected fungal ball is located inferiorly in the maxillary sinus that is contributing to the persistent polypoid disease, maxillary crusting, or active infection.[12]

■ Ethmoid Revision Consideration

Persistent ethmoid disease is usually caused by inadequate removal of ethmoid cells, mucoceles, polypoid disease such as allergic fungal sinusitis, scarring, crusting due to an exposed nonhealing area of bone created by cautery or remnants of ethmoid cells, and lateralization of the middle turbinate with obstruction anywhere in the ethmoids (Fig. 17–3). Polypoid disease is treated medically with oral, topical, or injected cortisone, which may be very helpful. Culture and appropriate antifungal medications may also be necessary for fungal sinusitis. Beware of the formation of mucoceles in the ethmoid sinus. Mucoceles may occur after previous polyp surgery owing to scarring, aberrant reforming of ethmoid cells, and polypoid obstruction creating pockets of isolated infection. Although often not obviously apparent on CT scans, any rounded appearance in the ethmoid cells should alert the surgeon to the possibility of a mucocele. Removal or marsupialization is usually mandatory, but it can be difficult in some heavily scarred osteitic multiply operated ethmoid cells. In this circumstance, a drill is sometimes necessary to remove thickened osteitic or fibrous dysplastic bone to create an open ethmoid. Specific areas of crusting, especially with what appears to be pseudomonas-like debris, should be examined closely with an endoscope. Often, the surgeon will uncover demucosalized, devitalized bone or bone fragments that when removed will solve the problem. The middle turbinate if compromised should be partially removed so that it cannot lateralize and obstruct. All persistently diseased ethmoid cells noted endoscopically, radiographically, or with a computer need to be opened. Any residual uncinate process requires removal to free the infundibulum and agger nasi cells.

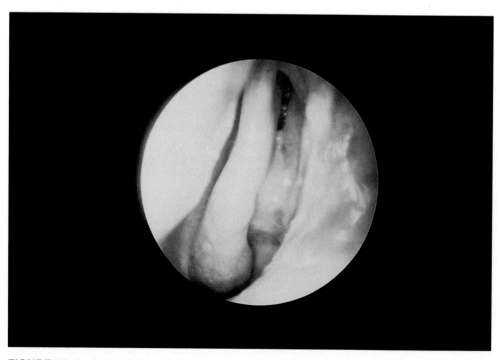

FIGURE 17–3 Lateralized middle turbinate with obstruction, anterior ethmoid, maxillary sinus, and frontal recess.

■ Sphenoid Sinus Revision Surgery

In many instances, the sphenoid is not actually opened but, instead, a posterior ethmoid cell or Onodi (sphenoethmoid) cell is opened in error. Actual disease is not removed, creating a need for revision surgery. Even when the sphenoid is opened, the natural ostia may not be included, creating a recirculation. Repeated surgery causes increased scarring. Circumferentially opened sphenoid sinuses tend to close, especially in revision cases. Polypoid disease and fungal balls tend to block an open sphenoid from within, creating a need for revision surgery. Special punch forceps, the microdebrider, and occasionally a drill may be necessary to create a wider opening. Axial views on CT scan show the carotid artery in the lower and midsphenoid to be posterior lateral (not lateral or anterolateral), which allows room to work inferiorly and laterally and which avoids injury to the carotid and optic nerve. Great care needs to be taken superiorly to avoid injury to the skull base and optic nerve. A microdebrider that cuts from the side and not straight ahead can be used in the sphenoid for removal of polypoid disease anteriorly, inferiorly, and anterolaterally. The anterior face of the sphenoid may need to be lowered parallel to the floor of the sphenoid.

Of special difficulty is the location and opening of the obstructed sphenoid, where no landmarks are present (Fig. 17–4). Again, as described, available landmarks must be sought out. These include measurement of the nasal spine to the choana (7 cm guideline), knowledge that the ostia is usually 1 to 1.5 cm above the choana medially against the septum, the reference plane 20 to 30 degrees above the superior part of the inferior turbinate or parallel to the lower part of the middle turbinate in maxillary sinus anstrostomy, radiographic evaluation

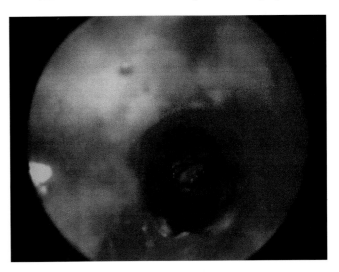

FIGURE 17–5   Opened sphenoid sinus seen in Figure 17–4.

(fluoroscopy or cross-table lateral images), and image-guided surgery, which are used to find the sphenoid. The lower one-third of a persistent superior turbinate usually has the ostia just medial to it. Once found with a probe, the sphenoid opening can be dilated and opened (Fig. 17–5). If enlargement is necessary, inferior dissection is safe. Stenting to prevent sphenoid closure may be necessary (Fig. 17–6).

If the mucosa is polypoid beneath the sphenoid ostium, it is electrocauterized rather than avulsed, to reduce the risk of an arterial injury. If the middle turbinate is removed, the posterior cut end of the middle turbinate is also cauterized to prevent bleeding from the lateral branch of the sphenopalatine artery. Careful dissection is performed in Onodi posterior ethmoid cells above the face of the sphenoid sinus to prevent injury to the

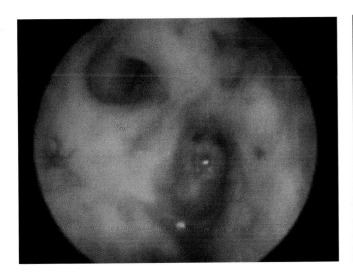

FIGURE 17–4   Obstructed sphenoid sinus.

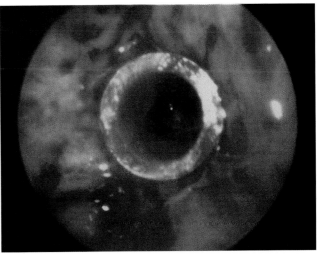

FIGURE 17–6   Stent in sphenoid sinus seen in Figure 17–4.

optic nerve and carotid artery and to lessen the risk of intracranial entry.

■ Frontal Sinus Revision Surgery

The best way to avoid revision frontal sinus surgery is to perform truly functional surgery and avoid the frontal recess. Knowing that the frontal sinus drains in most cases medial to the uncinate process and infundibulum allows the surgeon to realize that the frontal sinus is spared of disease affecting the anterior ethmoid ostiomeatal complex in 80% or more of cases. Therefore, the surgical philosophy in primary FESS surgery of the frontal sinus is based on close examination of the CT scan and frontal recess, leaving it inviolate if no evidence of disease is present. In essence, the uncinate process is removed, anterior ethmoids, including the agger nasi cells, are opened, and nothing more is done. If disease is present, removal of the agger nasi cells opens the frontal recess adequately in most cases. Sometimes actual enlargement of the frontal ostia or frontal cell drainage is necessary but should only be performed anteriorly, medially, or laterally, never circumferentially. Surely more unwarranted revision surgery has been created in the frontal recess owing to injudicious surgical intrusion in the normal frontal sinus than necessary. Patency of frontonasal opening and the frontal recess is largely dependent upon the superior articulation of the uncinate process, the agger nasi cells, and the presence or absence of frontal cells. Persistent disease in the anterior ethmoid cells can lead to frontal sinus obstruction. The upper aspect of the uncinate process must be removed to visualize the anterior ethmoid cells. Occasionally, the ethmoid cell may pneumatize the orbital plate of the frontal bone posterior to the frontal sinus. This supraorbital ethmoid cell may narrow the opening of the frontal sinus into the frontal recess, but perhaps more significantly, its opening may be mistaken for that of the frontal sinus. The supraorbital ethmoid cell usually opens more posterior and lateral, whereas an opening to the frontal sinus is noted more anteriorly and medially. These openings need to be found if disease is present; left alone if there is no disease. Stereotactic guidance is very helpful, especially in the revision case. A lateralized middle turbinate and inadequate removal of agger nasi cells are probably the major causes of frontal sinus revision surgery[9] (Fig. 17–7). The frontal recess is very narrow, especially when approaching the ostia, such that any aggressive removal of mucosa or bone can lead to scarring (often in the horizontal plan) and osteitis with new bone growth.

The surgical plane for frontal sinus revision involves removal of obstructing disease and scar, with preservation of as much functional mucosa as possible. With this in

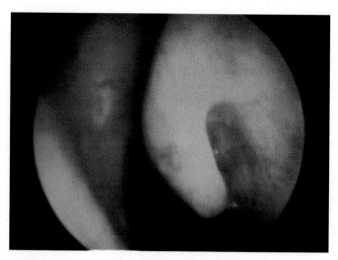

FIGURE 17–7   Lateral middle turbinate frontal recess.

mind, instrumentation is key. Without adequate frontal sinus instruments, including probes, curettes, one-sided rasps, giraffe forceps, punch forceps, and the microdebrider, frontal sinus revision surgery is very difficult. In some cases, it is simple enough to just punch away a lateralized middle turbinate remnant or remove an obstructing agger nasi cell. Removal of the middle turbinate may lead to lateralization and frontal recess stenosis.[9] The lateralized middle turbinate may require total removal to free the frontal recess. In the multiply operated-upon frontal recess, the frontal ostia may be difficult to locate or is only a few millimeters in size, making postoperative stenosis a real possibility. Any ostia under 4 mm is at risk for closure with or without stenting. In these circumstances, depending on endoscopic and radiographic findings, a game plan should be prepared ahead of time that might include a trephination, stenting, medial frontal osteoplasty (Draf 1 or 2), or even an endoscopic Lothrop procedure. Postoperative endoscopic observation, debridement, and dilatation are the key to success in many of these patients. For surgeons with less endoscopic experience, the external frontal ethmoidectomy with stenting or flap reconstruction (Sewall-Boyden procedure) may provide a suitable alternative.

Osteoplastic flap surgery with or without obliteration for extensive recurrent disease is the final procedure for disease control. This approach does have certain advantages, including unparalleled visualization of both frontal sinuses, ability to directly address problems of the posterior table and dura, and elimination of the need to establish a frontonasal communication.[13,14] Obliterating the frontal sinus also has several disadvantages. Increased cost and morbidity, with poor patient acceptance, are the most glaring problems. Wide expo-

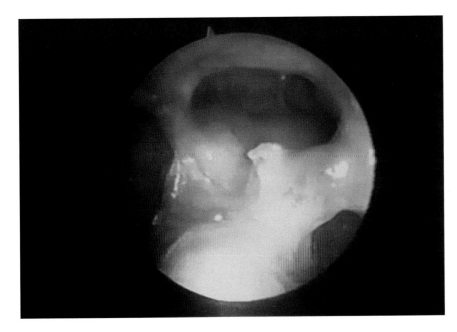

FIGURE 17–8 Postoperative view of a healed frontal sinus opening after undergoing modified Lothrop procedure.

sure is required, along with a donor site and its potential risk of infection. Frontal bossing may occur due to implanting too much fat or an inadequate periosteal closure that allows separation of the bone flap from the frontal skull, and may lead to frontal prominence or depression of the bone fragment. Sometimes extensive pneumatization of the frontal sinus may make obliteration impractical. Although recurrence rates are reportedly low, there are several reasons for failure, such as the incomplete removal of mucosa, inadequate occlusion of the frontonasal opening, persistent disease in the frontal recess, and fat suppuration. If a patient should develop recurrent disease, the most likely symptom will be pain. Unfortunately, following an obliterative procedure, such a complaint can be very difficult to evaluate, largely because several patients will experience postoperative pain in the absence of any underlying infection.[13] The true dilemma is trying to determine which patient has recurrent infection versus postoperative pain. In fact, nasal symptoms typical of sinusitis are usually lacking because the frontal sinus is no longer accessible to the nose. Frontal sinus evaluation in the obliterated sinus is very difficult, requiring MRI or even exploration in the worst-case scenario.

In the modified transnasal endoscopic Lothrop procedure or frontal drillout described by Gross et al,[15] a single common opening that includes both natural frontal ostia is created that provides an alternative to an osteoplastic flap (Fig. 17–8). This maneuver should theoretically decrease the potential for mucus recirculation. Advanced powered drill technology with protective sheathing and suction, performed under endoscopic guidance, has en-

abled the development of this improved procedure. The beveled sheath protects the posterior table and its mucosa, helping to avoid both circumferential mucosal injury and base of skull violation. Coupled with stereotactic computerized guidance, the frontal floor can be entered more easily. Advantages over osteoplastic frontal sinus obliteration include decreased morbidity, improved cosmesis, and cost reduction. It must be remembered that this procedure is very technically difficult and requires practice dissections. It is not for the inexperienced surgeon.

When all else fails, cranialization frontal sinusectomy with a pericranial flap and hydroxyapatite reconstruction, or revision of an osteoplastic flap with a modified Lothrop procedure, may prove helpful.

■ Conclusion

Failures of sinus surgery that need revision require astute diagnostic evaluation to uncover the true source of the problem. Once done, surgical correction proceeds in an orderly fashion from anterior to posterior and then superior posteriorly to the frontal recess. All necessary landmarks or measurements are noted or uncovered before any opening of a sinus to ensure safety. Radiographic localization, which may include image-guided computer technology, may be very important on the more difficult revision patient. In some cases, despite our best efforts, a sinus will not heal and respond physiologically. An underlying medical cause for persistent infection should be sought. Irrigation, intubations, and reassurance may give temporary relief.

■ Acknowledgment

Special thanks to Susan Whelton for her valuable assistance in the preparation of this chapter.

REFERENCES

1. Kennedy DW. Prognostic factors, outcomes and staging in ethmoid sinus surgery. *Laryngoscope.* 1992;102:1–18.
2. Marks SC, Shamsa F. Evaluation of prognostic factors in endoscopic sinus surgery. *Am J Rhinol.* 1997;11(3):187–191.
3. Chu CT, Lebowitz FA, Jacobs JB. An analysis of sites of disease in revision endoscopic sinus surgery. *Am J Rhinol.* 1997;11(4):287–291.
4. Ramadan HH. Surgical causes of failure in endoscopic sinus surgery. *Laryngoscope.* 1999;109(1):22–29.
5. Moses RL, Cornetta A, Atkis JP, et al. Revision endoscopic sinus surgery: the Thomas Jefferson University Experience. *Ear Nose Throat.* 1998;77(3):193–195, 199–202.
6. May M, Schaitkin B, Kay SL. Revision endoscopic sinus surgery: six friendly surgical landmarks. *Laryngoscope.* 1994;104:766–767.
7. Mitchell RB, Rareira KD, Yonnis RT, et al. Pediatric functional endoscopic sinus surgery: is a second look necessary? *Laryngoscope.* 1997;107(9):1267–1269.
8. Walner DL, Fabriglia M, Willging JP, et al. The role of second look endoscopy after pediatric functional endoscopic sinus surgery. *Arch Otolaryngol Head Neck Surg.* 1998;125(4):425–428.
9. Fried MP, Kleefild J, Tayor R. New armless image-guidance system for endoscopic sinus surgery. *Otolaryngol Head Neck Surg.* 1998;119(5):528–532.
10. Parson DS, Stivers FE, Talbot A. The missed ostium sequence and the surgical approach to revision functional endoscopic sinus surgery. *Otolaryngol Clin North Am.* 1996;29(1):169–183.
11. Duncavage J. Maxillary sinus revision surgery. In: Stankiewicz JA, ed. *Advanced Endoscopic Sinus Surgery.* Philadelphia: CV Mosby; 1995:ch 7.
12. Kuhn FA. Chronic frontal sinusitis: the endoscopic frontal recess approach. *Op Tech Otolaryngol Head Neck Surg.* 1996;7:222–229.
13. Seiden AM, Stankiewicz JA. Frontal sinus surgery: the state of the art. *Am J Otolaryngol.* 1998;19(3):183–193.
14. Jacobs JB, Lebowitz RA, Lagmay VM, et al. Conservative approach to inflammatory nasofrontal duct disease. *Ann Otol Rhinol Laryngol.* 1998;107:658–661.
15. Gross WE, Gross CW, Becke DG, et al. Modified transnasal endoscopic Lothrop procedure as an alternative to frontal sinus obliteration. *Otolaryngol Head Neck Surg.* 1995;113:427–434.

18

Complications, Management, and Avoidance

HEINRICH RUDERT

The endonasal sinus surgery developed by Halle[1-4] and Hajek[1,2,5-7] at the beginning of the 20th century was abandoned in the 1930s due to severe complications. Mosher,[8] a pioneer of this surgical technique in the United States, wrote in 1929 "Theoretically the operation is easy. In practice, however, it was proved to be one of the easiest operations with which to kill a patient." Because of this, the endonasal operation techniques were not found and described in surgical textbooks. Heermann[9] was one of the few who never gave up the endonasal technique. He was also the first to revive the endonasal technique by introducing the surgical microscope for endonasal sinus surgery, in 1958. Without a doubt, however, the revitalization of the endonasal operation method is due solely to Messerklinger[10-15] and his constant application of Hopkins's optical devices in rhinological diagnosis, as well as the development of the later-named infundibulotomy. Wigand and colleagues,[16,17] Kennedy,[18] Stammberger,[19-21] and Draf[22] helped this idea become accepted at last.

Currently, extranasal operative techniques no longer play a major role in the surgical treatment of inflammatory sinus diseases. Complications peculiar to this technique, such as swelling of the cheek, scar abscess, and symptomatic trigeminal neuralgias, are no longer observed. But the expectations of endoscope- and microscope-assisted endonasal operative techniques reducing the number of orbital or endocranial complications have not been met. One reason is because the absolute number of paranasal sinus interventions has increased greatly since the reintroduction of the endonasal technique due to the significantly expanded number of indications for surgery. Between 1982 and 1985, 1204 patients were operated on at the ENT department of the University of Kiel, during which time the operations were in part performed extranasally. Between 1991 and 1994, 2178 patients underwent endonasal sinus surgery.[23] Most complications are caused by beginning and inexperienced surgeons, because the supervision by an experienced surgeon is limited by a narrow surgical approach. There is no doubt that the individual number of complications is decreasing as the surgeons become more experienced.[24] While performing more than 1000 endonasal surgeries, the author personally caused only one slight lesion of the dura, whereas the injury rate of the remaining surgeons at the ENT department at Kiel University was 0.85%.[23] There are published papers, however, that maintain that the complication rate of surgeons with a great deal of experience can increase again.[25-27]

The increase of published intra- and postoperative complications may be caused by the increasing number of medicolegal conflicts during the last years. In the meantime, it seems that endonasal surgery constitutes the largest group of medicolegal conflicts in otorhinolaryngology.[28]

■ Classification of Complications

The classification can be performed according to different aspects, for example, the location of the injury in the sinus system or according to the injured organs. Often complications are classified as major or minor.[29] The category temporary, requires no treatment includes periorbital emphysema and chemosis as well as sensitivity disturbances of the teeth and lips. The category temporary, correctable with treatment includes adhesions, bleeding, bronchospasm, and postoperative infections of the sinuses. The third group consists of any change that is permanent if it persists beyond 1 year. These are dental or lip pain or numbness, and anosmia. May et al[29] divide the group of major complications into correctable with treatment and permanent. The category correctable with treatment consists of orbital hematoma (postseptal), loss of vision, diplopia, CSF leakage, meningitis, brain abscess, focal brain hemorrhage, hemorrhage requiring transfusion, carotid artery injury, and epiphora. Permanent major complications are blindness, diplopia, central nervous system deficit, and death.

The above-mentioned complications are usually early complications. Late complications are recurrences, mucoceles,[30–33] and myospherulosis due to ointments and foreign bodies.[34–36] Of course, also orbital and endocranial complications can occur as late complications.

Meanwhile, the literature about the complications of endonasal surgery is very extensive and is growing from month to month. A comparison of complication rates of single authors is complicated because of the lack of general standards. For this reason, no table showing such a comparison is given here. The relevant literature is published by May et al,[29] Levine,[37] Stammberger,[38] Rudert,[23] and Hosemann and colleagues.[39,40] We will start with the orbital complications and the injuries of the lacrimal duct, including bleeding, then turn to the endocranial complications.

Lid Hematoma

Of the minor complications, the most frequent is bleeding into the anterior parts of the orbit. This manifests itself shortly after the operation as a lid hematoma (black eye). It is caused by unintentionally opening the orbit in its anterior part. It happens during either the removal of the uncinate process or the exploration of the maxillary ostium in the anterior rising part of the infundibulum. In most cases, the lid hematoma heals without residuum, if no orbital fat is removed.

THERAPY

Special therapy is not necessary. Repositioning or sealing a potential prolapsus of orbital fat into the nose is not necessary. We also refrain from doing this during the orbital decompression in case of endocrine orbitopathy. Because the opening of the orbit is in the very anterior parts of the orbit in the extraconal space and the medial rectal muscle is not injured, no functional disturbances are expected.

Injury of the Lacrimal Duct and Sac

Injuries of the lacrimal duct are much more frequent than actually diagnosed, because they rarely cause drainage problems. But of 195 patients sent to us for a dacryocystorhinostomy, 29 (14.8%) had a history of one or more sinus surgeries.[23] Bolger et al[41] performed a fluorescein rinse of the lacrimal duct in 46 patients directly after endonasal sinus surgery. In seven patients, they found lesions of the lacrimal duct by detecting fluorescein in the middle nasal duct. In three of the seven cases, a fluorescein drainage into the middle nasal duct was observed even some months after surgery. None of the patients showed a stenosis of the lacrimal duct.

Injuries of the lacrimal sac occur during the removal of the uncinate process, whose insertion at the lateral nasal wall is just a few millimeters behind the lacrimal sac. They also occur during the enlargement of the maxillary ostium in the anterior direction. According to Lang and Papke,[42] the distance from the lacrimal sac to the maxillary ostium measures ~4.35 mm (range 1.3 to 11.5 mm) (Fig. 18–1). In the case of a good pneumatization, 30% of the anterior ethmoid cells lie as lacrimal cells and 77% as agger cells above the lacrimal sac.[43] Therefore, the sac can also be damaged during the exposition of the frontal recess.

THERAPY

A therapy in the form of an endonasal dacryocystorhinostomy is necessary only when a stenosis with epiphora occurs as a late result of the lacrimal duct injury.

Intraconal Injuries of the Orbit

Injuries of the eye muscles were seen more frequently during the days when predominantly extranasal operations were performed. This is definitely true for disturbances of the superior obliquus muscle after extranasal frontal sinus operations (Killian and Lothrop procedures). During endonasal surgery, only the medial rectal

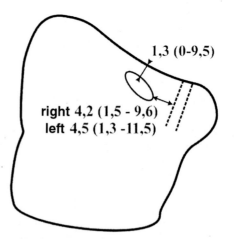

FIGURE 18–1 The maxillary ostium is located fairly high and anterior in the maxillary sinus (mean distance to the orbit: 1.3 mm, mean distance to the lacrimal sac: 4.3 mm). The lacrimal sac and the orbit are at high risk if the maxillary ostium is not probed carefully, as described in Figure 14–8.

muscle is more endangered. The circumstance that mostly injuries to the right orbit are observed is explained by the fact that the surgeon is usually positioned on the right side of the patient.[44–49]

Damage to the medial rectal muscles is more frequently caused by injuries to the lamina papyracea and the periorbit during surgery of the middle and posterior parts of the ethmoid sinuses than by injuries in the anterior parts of the ethmoid sinuses, because the extraconal layer of fatty tissue beyond the insertion of the medial rectal muscle at the bulb is relatively thin.[50] The medial rectal muscle is injured either directly by a surgical instrument (e.g., ethmoid forceps) or indirectly by an injury of the blood or nerve supply. Not recognizing a fat hernia bulging into the ethmoid sinus is another form of damage, if it is interpreted as a nasal polyp. During the removal of this "polyp," the eye muscle is caught and injured.[51–53]

Injury to the contents of the orbit occur in cases of anatomical variants of the ethmoid such as Onodi cells, a missing ethmoid bulla, or when the lamina papyracea is missing due to operations or a strong polyposis of the ethmoid. The optic nerve can be injured in the apex of the orbit or in the optic nerve canal if it is bulging medially into the posterior parts of the ethmoid sinuses or is without bony layers (Onodi cell).

THERAPY

The injury of the medial rectal muscle needs urgent therapy in cooperation with the ophthalmologist. Exploring the medial bony orbital wall and the injury of the periorbit through an extranasal approach (Killian procedure) and finding the medial rectal muscle under the surgical microscope is recommended, along with stitching the two remaining bodies of the muscle if necessary. Interventions later on are usually unsuccessful, because the muscles cannot be separated from the surrounding scar tissue.[50]

An injury of the optic nerve is always associated with an irreversible blindness. There is no therapy.

Retrobulbar Postseptal Hematoma

The occurrence of a retrobulbar hematoma with subsequent blindness is one of the most severe complications of endonasal surgery. According to Stankiewicz,[54] there are two types: the slowly developing venous hematoma and the arterial retrobulbar hematoma that develops quickly even during the operation. The venous type develops through a direct injury of intraorbital veins, which means the lamina papyracea and the periorbit must already have been opened. The quickly developing arterial hematoma usually happens when the severed anterior ethmoid artery running through the anterior ethmoid is retracted back into the orbit without opening the lamina papyracea or the periorbit. The symptoms are a significant proptosis, mydriasis, edema of the lid, chemosis, massive increase of bulb pressure, and loss of vision. In case of a venous hematoma, the symptoms develop over a few hours. The sequelae are the same.

The anterior ethmoid artery runs anteriorly to the insertion of the ground lamella of the middle turbinate at the skull base either in the roof of the ethmoid or in a form of a bony mesenterium from the anterior ethmoid foramen obliquely from lateral in the back to medial in the front, where it runs into the olfactory fossa. A smooth cut of the artery leads to heavy bleeding into the anterior ethmoid, which usually stops spontaneously, or by coagulation. This is much easier to perform using the surgical microscope than by endoscope, because you can work bimanually under the surgical microscope. A retrobulbar hematoma develops if the anterior ethmoid artery is not cut sharply, but with dull ethmoid forceps (e.g., ripped out of the surrounding bone), and the remnants of the artery retract themselves into the orbit. The developing retrobulbar hematoma causes choking of the ophthalmic artery. We know from the ophthalmological literature that blindness will be irreversible after 90 minutes unless the pressure is relieved immediately. The loss of vision is caused by the compression of the ophthalmic artery and the posterior short ciliar arteries and by the additional compression of the retinal blood vessels if the inner eye pressure increases to above 80 mm. In a few publications, the incidence of a retrobulbar orbit hematoma is described as being between 0.05 and 0.5%. This was observed 3 times in our patient contingency of 1172 patients between 1986 and 1990, or 0.25% of the cases.[23]

THERAPY

Because the neurosensoric retina can tolerate an ischemic phase for a maximum of 90 minutes without irreversible damage, the therapy must occur immediately. All therapeutic steps are geared to acutely decompressing the orbit. Therefore, massaging the bulb, as recommended by a few authors,[54] is strictly rejected by our ophthalmologists. It is extremely unlikely that a hematoma can be moved outside the orbit, because the periorbita is not opened, and therefore the hematoma cannot be drained. The emergency treatment in the form of a lateral canthotomy should be performed immediately, especially because there are no cosmetic or functional disturbances remaining after this intervention. Therefore, the following steps are necessary (Fig. 18–2)[55]:

1. Extended lateral canthotomy. Because the bulb is encapsulated through the orbital septum like an hourglass and there is a risk of injuring it, the bulb should be protected by a spatula positioned in the outer corner of the eye. The cut is performed down to the bone under a complete horizontal dissection

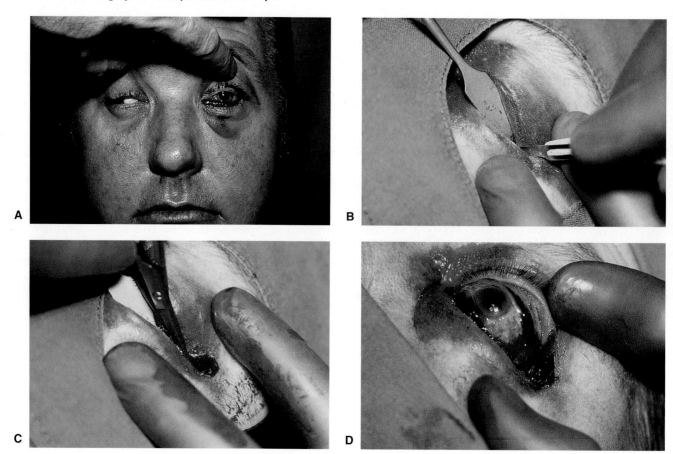

FIGURE 18–2 (A) Patient with a left-sided retrobulbar hematoma. There is a massive protrusio of the left bulb and chemosis. The eyeball is fixed and does not move. The pupil is dilated and does not react to light. (B) Lateral canthotomy. The bulb is protected by a spatula. The cut is carried down to the bone under a complete horizontal dissection of the lateral corner of the eye. (C) The lateral canthal ligament is then cut vertically at the bone edge (upper and lower cantholysis). (D) The bulb is now soft, and the pupil reacts to light again.

of the lateral lid, either with a scalpel or with straight pointed scissors.

2. The lateral tendon of the lid is then cut vertically with the scissors at the bone edge to the top and to the bottom (upper and lower cantholysis). It needs to be proven by palpation that the canthotomy goes down to the bone and that the lateral canthal ligament is cut. Canthotomy is sufficient if you can see the orbital fat in the depth when you separate the upper and lower lids with the fingers.

With these measures, sufficient decompression is usually achieved. Should this not be the case, the next step must follow: a wide transcutaneous cut in the area of the temporal lower lid in the region of the bony orbital limitation, with consecutive separation of the orbital septum with bowed dull scissors, until orbital fat tissue is bulging forward.

The attempt to try decompression by removing the lamina papyracea either endonasally or extranasally and separating the periorbita before lateral canthotomy is frequently not sufficient and leads to a delay of therapy. Of course, this intervention can be performed additionally.

The ligation or coagulation of the ethmoid artery causing the retrobulbar bleeding is not possible, because the vessel is retracted into the orbit. Subsequently, a high-dosage steroid treatment and dehydrating therapy (e.g., with mannitol), should be performed.

Injuries of the Ethmoid Roof and the Cribriform Plate

Iatrogenic lesions of the dura are observed despite the best optical and technical aids, and also despite the good education of the surgeons. The incidence reported in the literature is somewhere between 0.2 and 2.5%.[23,25,38,47,49,56–60] In our own patient contingency, the risk, with a large number of surgeons, was 0.85% per patient and 0.5% per operated side. Between 1986 and 1996, 527 patients and 949 sides were operated on by the author himself, with only one CSF fistula. The risk therefore was 0.19% per patient and 0.1% per operated side, respectively.[23]

The danger to the skull base has several reasons:

1. In a prone patient, the skull base is turned completely toward the surgeon. Therefore, he or she is working perpendicularly to the skull base.

2. The basal lamella of the middle turbinate creates an angle with the roof of the ethmoid, an angle that is dull toward the front and peaked toward the back. The higher the basal lamella is perforated during the opening of the posterior ethmoid, the shorter the distance is to the roof of the ethmoid. The roof of the ethmoid can easily be mistaken for a bony septum of a posterior ethmoid cell.

3. During the attempt to remove a cell septum located close to the skull base with a dull instrument, a piece of the skull base could be removed and the thin dura torn.

4. Depending on the pneumatization, the roof of the ethmoid might be situated higher than the roof of the sphenoid. In this case, the skull base could be injured during the attempt to open the sphenoid sinus transethmoidally (Fig. 18–3).

5. Another danger zone is the lateral lamella of the cribriform lamina plate in the case of a low rima olfactoria, which is nevertheless, according to Keros,[61] 4 to 16 mm in 89% of cases (Fig. 18–4). The lateral lamella of the cribriform plate is, at 0.05 mm, thinner than the neighboring roof of the ethmoid at 0.5 mm.[62] The lateral lamella is injured if one is working too medial or if the middle turbinate is resected too close to the skull base or is fractured. According to Keros,[61] the danger of an injury is extremely high in a Type III case, because the lateral

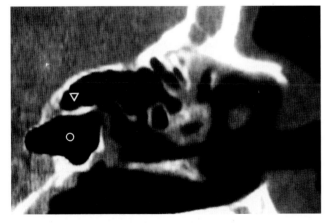

FIGURE 18–3 CT (sagittal reconstruction) of the paranasal sinuses. In this case, the roof of the ethmoid *(triangle)* stands higher than the roof of the sphenoid sinus (circle). Therefore, the sphenoid sinus should only be opened transnasally, never transethmoidally.

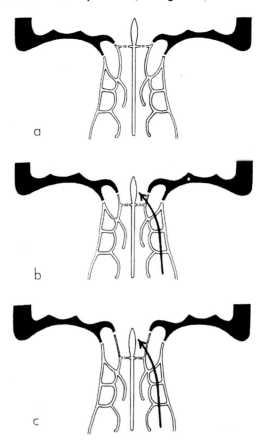

FIGURE 18–4 The three different positions of the lamina cribrosa. (A) High level: no lateral lamella of the lamina cribrosa. (B,C) The lower the position of the lamina cribrosa, the longer the very thin lateral lamella and the higher the risk of injuring.

lamella is very long (up to 16 mm). A low or high level of the lamina cribrosa can be identified on the preoperative coronal CT through the location of the anterior ethmoid arteries, because these and the fossa olfactoria have the same level. If the anterior ethmoid artery should be located in the ethmoid roof, the lamina cribrosa is also high (Type I, according to Keros). If the ethmoid artery runs in a bony mesenterium through the ethmoid, a low level of the cribriform plate must be expected (Type III, according to Keros). That means that the ethmoid roof is significantly higher than the cribriform plate and the lateral lamella and offers a much larger area of potential injury.

6. Another cause for potential harm to the dura can be gaps in the skull base. Ohnishi[63] detected in human cadavers a significant percentage of bony gaps in the medial wall of the ethmoid sinus (lateral lamella of the lamina cribrosa), along the anterior and posterior ethmoid nerves, in the area of the filae olfactoriae, and at the medial wall of the middle turbinate, as well as in the anterolateral as-

pect of the ethmoid roof. Around these gaps, the nasal mucosa is fixed to the dura, so that the dura can be injured without perforation of the bony ethmoid roof.

DIAGNOSTIC

Fresh injuries of the skull base during the course of an ethmoid sinus operation can usually be identified with the consequent application of optical aids (endoscope or microscope). Their prompt localization and treatment do not cause any problems. The diagnosis of old skull base defects is much more problematic. First of all, it must be clarified whether the liquid secretion is cerebrospinal fluid. Nowadays, this can be done with the determination of the β-2-transferrin in the nasal secretion.[59,64,65] To locate the defect, a high-resolution CT scan (2 mm slices) of the frontal basis is performed in coronal levels. If it is not possible to detect the location of the injury with CT or a T2 weighted MRI, a fluorescein nasal endoscopy is performed, according to Messerklinger.[12] Usually, 5% sodium fluorescein is employed, according to Stammberger.[66] After lumbar puncture and injection of 0.25–0.50 mL of 5% sodium fluorescein solution specifically for intrathecal use, diluted with 10 mL of the patient's CSF, the patient must lie face down, and the bottom end of the bed is lifted so that the patient's head is lower than his or her feet. Because of the higher specific weight, the fluorescein sinks down the ventricle and runs through the dura

leakage into the nose. After only a few minutes, the presence of an intensely yellow-green cerebrospinal fluid in the nose can be identified. The nose is examined intraoperatively with the 30-degree endoscope and under blue light. Slight marked CSF traces can be identified as bright white-green areas. The fluorescence can be detected in a dilution of 1:10 million. The marked cerebrospinal fluid shows the way to the lesion of the dura with a high degree of certainty (Fig. 18–5).

According to Stammberger et al,[66] it is a safe method. The complications that occur are caused by

1. Applying too much of the fluorescein solution. According to body weight, only 0.5 to a maximum of 1 mL of the 5% fluorescein solution should be injected.
2. Wrong concentration. Only the application of a 5% sodium fluorescein solution produces the same osmolarity as the cerebrospinal fluid.
3. Fluorescein used for external application is not allowed. Nor should ampullas for IV application be used, due to preservatives in this material.

THERAPY

We are of the opinion that a lesion of the dura definitely needs a surgical closure, because the direct connection of the nasal mucosa contaminated with bacteria with the intracerebral space leads to the danger of lethal inflam-

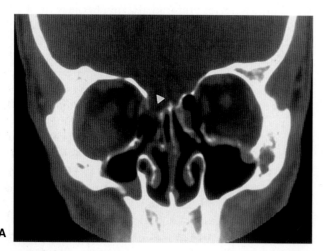

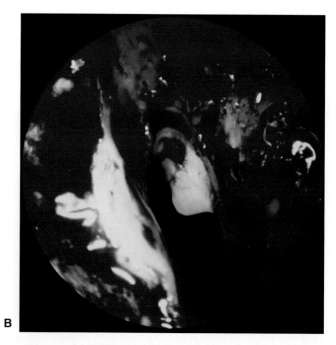

FIGURE 18–5 Lesion of the lateral lamella of the right lamina cribrosa in a patient who suffered from meningitis several weeks after endonasal surgery. (A) CT scan. The lesion is marked with a triangle. (B) Endoscopic view after lumbar puncture and intrathecal injection of 1.0 mL of 5% sodium fluorescein solution. The prolapse of the brain shows the greenish color of the fluorescein. The defect was closed transnasally with lyodura.

matory complications such as meningitis and intracerebral abscess. The risk of experiencing such an infection is ~20 to 50% in untreated traumatic defects of the frontal base.[67] The closure of the defect is usually performed through an endonasal approach. We usually take homologous tissue (fascia lata) or lyodura, if possible in two layers with the underlay and overlay technique. Transplants are fixed with fibrin glue. An additional covering with nasal or turbinate mucosa is not absolutely necessary. The transplant tissue is covered with Gelfoam, then the ethmoid is filled with oxidiced cellulose, which is supported in the case of a larger defect by cottonwool tamponade. The tamponade is removed in stages after the eighth day.

It is not possible to use the underlay technique to cover a defect in the sphenoid sinus. Therefore, the overlay technique, with the removal of the mucosa and the closure of the sphenoid sinus, is usually successful. Also defects of the cribriform plate and its lateral lamella can be closed only using the overlay technique.

Bleeding

The number of cases of bleeding that need transfusions has been greatly reduced since the introduction of endonasal surgery.[23,68] In 10 of 1172 cases in our patient contingency, blood transfusions were necessary. In all cases, it was late bleeding. Intraoperative bleeding that needed to be taken care of was usually observed in the area of the sphenopalatine artery and its branches, especially during the dissection in the area of the posterior ends of the middle turbinate (arteria nasalis posterior lateralis) and in the area of the frontal wall of the sphenoid sinus and floor (injuries of the posterior medial nasal arteries).

Intraoperative bleeding is controlled by the use of postoperative dressing of oxidized cellulose (Oxycel cotton) by creating small strips and inserting them into the sinus cavity. Use of saline spray and irrigation over the first postoperative week causes the material to become soft and can be suctioned from the sinus at the first postoperative visit.

Bleeding often stops spontaneously or can be coagulated with the bipolar forceps. The same is true for injuries of the anterior ethmoid artery. Late bleedings in the first days after the operation are usually easy to locate and can be stopped by coagulation or by packing. There are rare single bleedings from the lateral posterior parts of the nose that are resistant to therapy. In these cases, a coagulation of the sphenopalatine artery has proven useful.[69] We like to use the surgical microscope for these, as well as the self-retaining nasal speculum,[70] so that the surgeon can work bimanually, aspirating with one hand and coagulating with the other hand (Fig. 18–7).

Bleeding into the orbit was discussed in the section Retrobulbar Postseptal Hematoma.

Bleeding of the Internal Carotid Artery

Injuries of the internal carotid artery occur due to anomalies and aneurysms of the artery, and in the case of a missing bony covering of the artery in the sphenoid sinus, if the sphenoid sinus is not opened strictly transnasally and paraseptally. The internal carotid artery can be compressed with a tamponade of the sphenoid sinus or with a balloon occlusion of the internal carotid artery, but frequently, hemiplegia or death is the result.

Intracerebral Bleeding of the Anterior Ethmoid Artery and Branches of the Anterior Cerebral Artery

These bleedings are very rare but difficult to control. Neurosurgical decompression of the brain by applying a trephination in the skull can avoid a fatal ending. We had to give a testimonium in one such case in which an injury of the skull happened between the roof of the ethmoid and the sphenoid sinus. The patient died despite neurosurgical decompression of the brain.

Different Complications

MYOSPHERULOSIS

A myospherulosis with formation of granulomas in the orbit or the eyelids develops through a foreign body reaction in the orbit, probably caused by ointment tamponades or nasal emulsions containing paraffin.[34–36,71,72] These unpleasant, difficult-to-treat alterations in the area of the eyelids are probably explainable by the transportation of ointment into the orbit. Also, recurrences of chronic sinusitits are sometimes caused by foreign body reactions. After operating on recurrences, we were able to detect light-breaking foreign bodies in our pathologic specimens. Therefore, we do not use any kind of ointment, either in the form of tamponades or for postoperative care.

CONTROVERSY

This author has used mupirocin (Bactroban) ointment as a water-soluble antibiotic preparation to cover dressings placed in the sinus cavity. No evidence of foreign body reaction has been seen.

FRONTAL SINUSITIS AFTER PARANASAL SINUS SURGERY

Difficult-to-treat frontal sinusitis after ethmoid operations was observed more frequently in the early years of endonasal operations. Frontal sinusitis is usually caused by unnecessary operating in the frontal recess, in the case of a normal frontal sinus drainage, or in the case of a frontal sinus involvement, the opening of the frontal recess was not extended consequently to the frontal ostium. Since we began paying attention to this matter, frontal sinusitis caused by an operation is rarely observed.

THERAPY

After the operation of the ethmoid together with the frontal recess, we proceed as described in the following section. The frontal recess is dissected by removing the ethmoid bulla and the suprabullar cells to the skull base, as well as removing potentially existing agger nasi cells. Employing a 30- or a 45-degree endoscope, anterior to the anterior ethmoid artery, the frontal foramen is reached by removing the thin eggshell-like cell septs of frontal ethmoid cells. During this procedure, the frontal sinus spoon and the bowed ethmoid forceps are used consequently in a posteroanterior direction. After the frontal ostium is exposed, special attention is paid to preventing injury to the mucosa in this area, to avoid stenoses in the frontal ostium itself. Afterward, the patient is treated with antibiotics and steroids. In most cases, the problem is solved. In isolated cases, however, this procedure is not sufficient. The only option left is to remove the frontal sinus floor and establish a frontal sinus drainage Type II or a median drainage (Type III, according to Draf).[22,73] Attention must be paid throughout this procedure to preserving at least the mucosa of the posterior circumference of the frontal ostium, so that the epithelialization of a new frontal ethmoid canal can develop from it. The technique is explained in the following section. We never insert a spacer, after having seen foreign body reactions again and again. In cases of disease in the lateral parts of the frontal sinus, which cannot be reached by an endonasal approach, we combine the endonasal procedure with an external osteoplastic frontal sinus operation, whereby we prefer the coronal incision. Obliterating the frontal sinus has not proven effective in chronic inflammatory processes of the frontal sinus.

■ Avoiding Complications

To avoid surgical complications, the following preconditions must be met:

1. Explicit knowledge of the surgical anatomy
2. Adequate preoperative imaging
3. Appropriate instruments, including optical aids
4. Adjusting the operative strategy to the specific goal

If these preconditions are not met, the feasibility of many paranasal sinus surgeries must be questioned because of the many possibilities of complications, taking into consideration that ~90% of the cases are elective operations. The endonasal operation technique developed in the 1920s by Halle[1–4] and Hajek[5–7] were not abandoned without reason in the 1930s.

Preconditions for Endonasal Sinus Surgery

KNOWLEDGE OF THE ANATOMY OF THE LATERAL NASAL WALL

The first and most important precondition for endonasal sinus surgery is an explicit knowledge of the anatomy of the lateral nasal wall. The best way to acquire this is to explore a sagitally cut head of a cadaver, which also shows the position of the frontal skull base. The skull base and the floor of the nose are two levels running nearly parallel. The floor of the nose is an important reference level for the surgeon that can be viewed during the total length of the operation. The skull base is not endangered as long as the instruments are kept parallel to the nasal floor. This is especially important at the beginning of the operation, when the skull base is not yet dissected. As early as 1929, Mosher[8] indicated an imaginary line running through both inner corners of the eyes as an approximate borderline to the neurocranium. A virtual plane through the inner corners of the eyes and the outer ear canals illustrates even more the position of the frontal skull base. The frontal skull base is not in danger as long as the operation is performed between this plane and a second one through the floor of the nose (Fig. 18–6).

At the lateral nasal wall of the skull of a cadaver cut in the median, two more landmarks are always visible: the middle turbinate and, lateral from this, the ethmoid bulla.

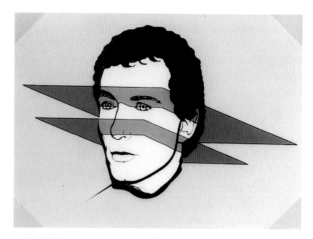

FIGURE 18–6 An imaginary plane through the inner corners of the eyes and the ear canals indicates the borderline of the ethmoid to the endocranium. This plane runs parallel to the visible plane of the floor of the nose. The skull base is not in danger as long as the instruments are working between these planes parallel to the floor of the nose.

Keeping both structures preserved as long as possible is extraordinarily helpful during the operation. This will be explained in detail later. Exposing the lateral nasal wall step by step from medial to lateral should best be done in an anatomical institute. The book written by Johannes Lang[43] is recommended as a textbook or atlas. To acquire the surgical technique, one should use fresh cadavers in a pathological institute or participate in a surgical course on heads in an anatomical institute, working through the external nasal openings on complete heads and employing optical aids such as endoscopes and microscopes.

ADEQUATE IMAGING

The next precondition for a safe surgery is adequate imaging. It has been shown that the CT scan for preoperative diagnostics is superior to all other imaging techniques. Patients should be treated for 1 week before the CT with antibiotics and, in the case of polyposis, with additional systemic steroids, so that only the irreversible alterations of the paranasal sinuses are shown.[74] This way, unpleasant surprises can be avoided at the time of the operation when those reversible changes that showed up on a CT scan performed in the acute phase often regress. The operation itself is also made easier by the pretreatment. A coronal imaging is the routine technique. But spinal CT performed with axial 1 mm sections is the ideal for CT imaging today. Coronal reconstruction with 2 or 3 mm sections are sufficient for most endonasal surgery. Coronal reconstruction from spinal axial sections avoids any dental artifacts. An axial level is also wanted, in addition to an explicit description of the posterior wall of the frontal sinus, of the frontal recess, and of the posterior wall of the sphenoid sinus. In lesions of the frontal sinus and of the sphenoid sinus, a sagittal reconstruction has proven useful, on which the transition between the roof of the ethmoid and the sphenoid sinus and the condition in the frontal recess can be illustrated. The radiologist should comment on several points, the best way being a checklist[74]:

1. The insertion of the uncinate process at the lamina papyracea (nondangerous variation) or at the middle turbinate or the lateral lamella of the cribriform plate (dangerous variations)

2. High or low level of the cribriform plate, which also indicates the location of the anterior ethmoid artery, either protected in the ethmoid roof or running unprotected through the ethmoid

3. Relation of the optic nerve to the wall of the posterior ethmoid (the potential presence of Onodi cells) and to the sphenoid sinus

4. The course of the internal carotid artery in the lateral wall of the sphenoid sinus (protected or unprotected)

5. The potential presence of bony gaps in the area of the lamina papyracea or the ethmoid roof or the walls of the sphenoid sinus

The anatomical knowledge acquired from the cadaver skulls needs to be fused with the individual measurements illustrated by the CT scan to form a three-dimensional model by the surgeon to replace a navigational system for as long as such a system is not routinely available.

APPROPRIATE INSTRUMENTS

Another important precondition is the availability of appropriate instruments. Along with the classical nasal specula developed by Hartmann, Killian, and Cottle, we use the self-retaining nasal specula[75] with a long end lying on the septum and a short, serrated end inserted in the piriform apertura (Fig. 18–7A). These specula are mounted on the operating table with a flexible tension arm so that the surgeon can work bimanually (Fig. 18–7B). This is especially advantageous when a surgical microscope is used (focus 300 or 350 mm).[70] The surgeon can operate bimanually as he or she would during microsurgery of the ear or the larynx. Absolutely essential is the availability of 0- and 30-degree endoscopes. The 45-degree endoscope developed by Stammberger has proven useful in operations of the maxillary sinus and the frontal recess.

Most instruments used for endonasal sinus surgery were developed at the end of the 19th and the beginning of the 20th centuries. The ethmoid forceps developed by Weil and Blakesley are still standard instruments. During the last few years, cutting forceps and punches have been accepted along with dull ethmoid forceps. These were developed as early at the beginning of the 20th century. We use the cutting forceps developed by Grünwald and Williams-Watson, as well as the cutting punches developed by Kofler and Hajek. By using these instruments, we can avoid resecting nonaffected mucosa and loosening or breaking bony septs unintentionally, minimizing the danger of injuring the dura or vessels and nerves.

Among the new developments, the powered shavers must be mentioned. In the hand of an experienced operator, the shavers have many advantages. But they can cause irreversible damage if the orbit or the skull base is unintentionally perforated, because they aspirate the contents of the orbit or the brain in a very short amount of time. Therefore, we think that it is too dangerous for a beginner or even an average paranasal sinus surgeon to use them, and we cannot recommend them without restriction. The advantage is that they rinse and aspirate simultaneously. When shavers are used together with a surgical microscope, a 350 mm lens is recommended instead of a 300 mm lens.

It is also evident that the use of image-guided instruments is growing.

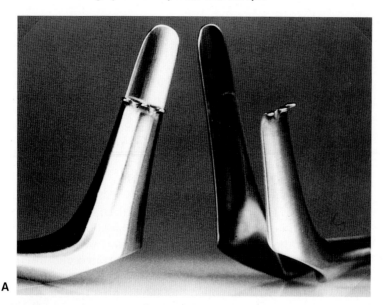

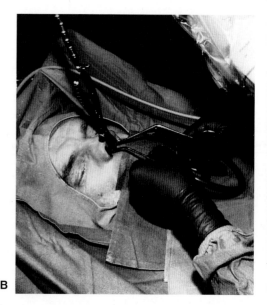

FIGURE 18–7 (A) Self-retaining specula, used by the author, with the long end lying on the septum and the short, serrated end inserted in the piriform aperture. (B) The specula are mounted on the operating table with a flexible tension arm so that the surgeon can work bimanually. This is especially advantageous when a surgical microscope is used.

ADEQUATE STRATEGY OF SURGERY

The most important preconditon to minimize iatrogenic harm is an adequate strategy when the operation is performed. The goals are always to restore the drainage of the affected sinuses and to give the diseased mucosa the chance to heal. Of course, there are cells that must be opened that are positioned in front of the affected cells. The start of the approach is therefore nearly always the anterior ethmoid. The exception is an isolated disease of the sphenoid sinus (e.g., a mucocele) that is always opened paraseptally through the upper nasal duct without touching the ethmoid.

In the case of diseases of the ethmoid, the maxillary sinus, or the frontal sinus, the operation always starts with the resection of the uncinate process. The uncinate process forms the anterior lip of the bow-shaped groove of the infundibulum. According to the extension and the depth of this groove, the lacrimal duct and the orbit are endangered during the removal (Fig. 18–1). The distance from the lacrimal sac to the insertion of the uncinate process measures ~3 mm (range 1–8 mm). The lateral wall of the infundibulum forms the medial wall of the orbit above the mouth of the maxillary ostium. Because the extension of the infundibulum groove toward the front, medial to the uncinate process, can vary quite a bit and measures sometimes only a few millimeters, the lacrimal sac as well as the orbit can be damaged when the sickle knife is inserted into the uncinate process. To avoid an injury of the lacrimal sac or the orbit, the edge of the uncinate process must be sounded with the bowed ball probe from the semilunar hiatus. The insertion line of the uncinate process along the lateral nasal wall must be felt before it is removed.[23,76] Another possibility is to use a Hajek punch instead of a sickle knife. This way, the uncinate process can be caught and removed from the hiatus semilunaris without endangering the lacrimal sac or the orbit.

The ethmoid bulla is the most important landmark on the way to the anterior ethmoid after the removal of the uncinate process. The lower and the anterior edge of the bulla mark the original position of the infundibulum. As long as the bulla is intact, it is fairly easy to locate the maxillary ostium and the entrance into the frontal recess. Therefore, the anterior wall of the bulla must be preserved as long as possible.

CONTROVERSY

This author enters the anterior, inferior, and medial aspect of the bulla as the initial starting point for endoscopic sinus surgery. From this entry it is possible to remove the entire bulla and identify the lateral wall, the lamina papyracea, and then the sinus roof. The basal lamina is next identified and entered if there is posterior ethmoid sinus disease. This difference only points out the need for the surgeon to develop a method that provides comfort and consistency and a method where there is understanding of the anatomy.

The maxillary ostium should be probed before opening and removing the ethmoid bulla. The maxillary ostium is situated fairly far to the front and fairly high in the maxillary sinus, and is therefore located directly below the floor of the orbit. According to Lang and Bressel,[77] it

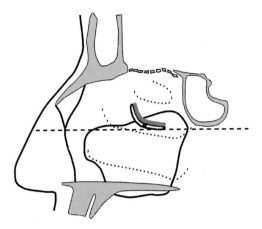

FIGURE 18–8 Projection of the maxillary sinus on the lateral nasal wall. The maxillary ostium is normally located in the posterior horizontal part of the infundibulum. It is safely probed on an imaginary line drawn parallel to the floor of the nose through the deepest point of the bulla. Otherwise the orbit could be violated. Searching the ostium is recommended before dissecting the ethmoid bulla.

is located in the posterior two-thirds of the infundibulum, that is, in its horizontal part. The safest way to locate the maxillary ostium is to search for it on an imaginary horizontal line parallel to the floor of the nose through the deepest point of the bulla (Fig. 18–8). To do this, we use a 30-degree, wide-angle endoscope and a curved aspirator, or the spoon developed by Messerklinger, with which remnants of the uncinate process can be removed. The rise of air bubbles shows that the maxillary ostium has been found. The risk of injury to the orbit increases greatly if the surgeon leaves this imaginary horizontal line in a cranial direction, because the lateral wall of the ascending crus of the infundibulum is part of the medial

wall of the orbit. The orbit can be opened unintentionally if the ostium is searched too far to the front and too high in the ascending crus of the infundibulum. Bleeding into the lower eyelid, which is already visible shortly after the operation, is a reversible effect that, fortunately, usually has no consequences if the injury to the orbit is realized in time.

If one is not sure whether the orbit is injured, it is very useful to try the bulb-pressure test developed by Draf, in which mild external pressure on the bulb causes the orbital fat to move. This is visible under the surgical microscope or the endoscope. In this and in other critical phases of the operation, it is useful to let the assisting operation nurse watch the eye of the patient. The eye registers every touch, or even the opening of the orbit, by movement.

The next step after the identification of the maxillary sinus serves to identify the frontal recess. This step should also be done before the bulla is opened. A horizontal gap, which shows strong interindividual variations, between the insertion of the middle turbinate at the agger nasi and the anterior wall of the ethmoid bulla, leads into the frontal recess (Fig. 18–9).

Anteroposterior Dissection of the Lower Level of the Ethmoid

After identification of both entrances, the maxillary ostium, and the frontal recess, the operation is continued in an anteroposterior direction into the ethmoid.

For the next steps of the operation, it seems to be useful to divide the ethmoid, not only into the anterior and posterior part of the ethmoid separated by the lamina basilaris of the middle turbinate, but also horizontally into a lower level more distant to the skull base and an upper level close to the skull base. Again, one draws

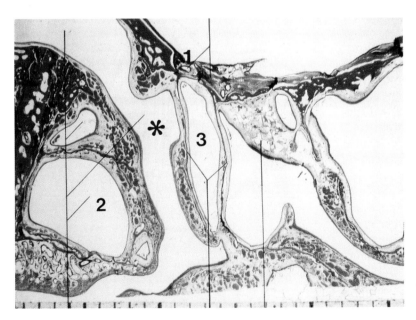

FIGURE 18–9 Sagittal cut through the lateral nasal wall. The frontal recess (asterisk) borders anteriorly on the agger nasi cells (2) and posteriorly on the ethmoid bulla (3). The bulla is a reliable landmark for identification of the entrance into the frontal recess. It therefore should be preserved as long as possible. L.A. ethmoidalis anterior (1). (From Lang J. Clinical Anatomy of the Nose, Nasal Cavity, and Paranasal Sinuses. New York: Thieme; 1989. Used with permission.).

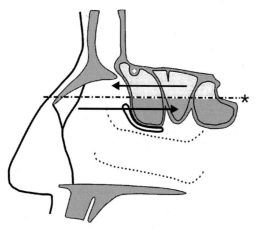

FIGURE 18–10 For reasons of safety, it is advisable to divide the ethmoid horizontally by an imaginary line (asterisk) drawn parallel to the floor of the nose 5 mm above its deepest point (lower edge of the bulla ethmoidalis) into an upper level close to the skull base and into a lower level more distinct to the skull base. Surgery of the ethmoid should always be started in the lower level in an anteroposterior direction parallel to the skull base. After having removed the posterior wall of the ethmoid or the anterior wall of the sphenoid sinus, the operation is continued in the upper level in a posteroanterior direction under vision of the roof of the ethmoid. In this way it is nearly impossible to violate the skull base.

another imaginary line parallel to the floor of the nose through the ethmoid bulla approximately 7 mm above its deepest point toward the back (Fig. 18–10). The surgical approach at the beginning of the operation should always take place in the lower level to ensure that an injury to the ethmoid roof is avoided.

The ethmoid bulla is opened at its deepest point in an anteroposterior direction. The upper part of the anterior wall of the bulla at the entrance of the frontal recess is preserved during this phase of the operation. The perforation of the inferior part of the anterior wall of the bulla is performed with closed ethmoid forceps parallel to the nasal floor and parallel to the septum in an anteroposterior direction. The closed ethmoid forceps are opened in the bulla and withdrawn in an open position. This way, the catching and removing of tissue are avoided. Additionally, the open forceps enlarge the opening of the bulla so much that the contents of the bulla are easily visible. Moreover, when the forceps are removed in an open position, the catching and removing of fat because of misorientation (e.g., unintended opening of the orbit) become impossible. Using the ethmoid forceps as described, perforating a separation wall with them closed and removing them when they are opened, should also be part of all the other steps of dissection in the deeper compartments of the ethmoid.

The next frontal separation wall that is breached during the anteroposterior approach is the lamina basilaris of the middle turbinate, which divides the anterior from the posterior ethmoid. This wall must also be perforated at its

deepest point parallel to the nasal floor and as medially as possible with a closed Blakesley forceps, which is then opened and retracted. The posterior ethmoid usually consists of one large cell, whose posterior wall, along with the anterior wall of the sphenoid sinus, forms the sphenoethmoidal angle, which extends laterally in varying degrees. Approaching the low ethmoid level as medially as possible prevents an unintentional opening of the orbit in the postbulbar parts, in which the medial rectal muscle runs parallel to the periorbit. Additionally, when the surgery is performed medially, the cauda of the middle turbinate and its insertion on the lateral nasal wall remain intact. If the opening in the lamina basilaris of the middle turbinate is not too large, its stability is not affected, so that the danger of lateralization of the middle turbinate remains fairly small. Another advantage is that the larger branches of the sphenopalatine artery, the lateral posterior nasal arteries, are not damaged. The violation of smaller branches can easily be stopped by bipolar coagulation.

Opening of the Anterior Wall of the Sphenoid Sinus

The next step of the anteroposterior approach is to open the anterior wall of the sphenoid sinus, which is done only if the sphenoid sinus is affected. The opening of the anterior wall of the sphenoid sinus must always be performed in the upper nasal duct transnasally and paraseptally through the sphenoid ostium, never over a transethmoid way (Figs. 18–11, 18–12). We categorically refuse the transethmoid opening of the sphenoid sinus and orient ourselves paraseptally and medially to the middle turbinate, again parallel to the nasal floor, until we reach the anterior wall of the sphenoid sinus above the choana.

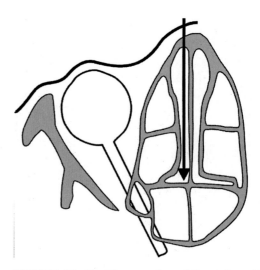

FIGURE 18–11 The opening of the sphenoid sinus should always be performed transnasally, never transethmoidally. Otherwise the optic nerve (see Fig. 18–12) and the carotid artery or the skull base (see Fig. 18–3) are at risk.

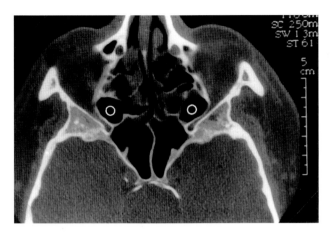

FIGURE 18–12 CT scan of a bilateral Onodi cell (circles). The optic nerves would be at high risk in case of transethmoidal approach to the sphenoid sinuses.

CONTROVERSY

This author opens the sphenoid sinus through the posterior ethmoid sinus by working in the medial inferior aspect of the front face of the sinus. The posterior aspect of the medial turbinate is medialized to safely enter into the sphenoid sinus.

The sphenoid ostium can now easily be reached by dissecting the mucosa of the anterior wall of the sphenoid sinus and can be carefully probed. It is safest to enlarge the ostium in a mediocaudal direction with Stammberger's round punch. As much of the medial and lower edge of the sphenoid ostium is removed as needed for a 30-degree endoscope to be introduced into the sphenoid sinus. With the endoscope, the lateral wall of the sphenoid sinus is controlled to identify a bulging optical nerve or the internal carotid artery. Subsequently, the anterior wall of the sphenoid sinus is carefully removed with Hajek's punch. During the removal of the anterior wall in a caudal direction, one must be careful not to injure a branch of the medial posterior nasal artery. If this happens despite the precautions, the artery must be caught and coagulated with the bipolar forceps.

If a probe of the sphenoid ostium cannot be successfully managed, one can open the anterior wall of the sphenoid sinus with a diamond bur, then the sphenoid sinus can be opened carefully with the closed Blakesley forceps. The entire approach takes place medially to the middle turbinate and laterally to the septum. The beginning surgeon can also use the transseptal way in the same way as it is used for the transsphenoid hypophysectomy.

After a paraseptal opening of the sphenoid sinus, the situation can now be controlled again from the opened ethmoid. One can now connect the ethmoid and the sphenoid sinus after removing the posterior wall of the ethmoid and the lateral parts of the frontal wall of the sphenoid sinus. In this situation, you are always surprised by the fairly high position of the posterior ethmoid cells, which in some cases can even be located above the roof of the sphenoid sinus (Fig. 18–3). The transition between the roof of the ethmoid and the sphenoid is characterized by a visible step. The transethmoid opening of the sphenoid not only risks injuring the orbital apex and any optical nerve lying unprotected in the Onodi cells, but also risks perforating the skull base above the sphenoid sinus. With the removal of the anterior wall of the sphenoid sinus as described, and later of the posterior wall of the ethmoid, we can now view the roof of the ethmoid and the sphenoid sinus without any risk to the skull base. The more whitish color of the skull base usually contrasts with the other paranasal sinus walls.

Posteroanterior Dissection of the Upper Ethmoid Level

With the removal of the frontal wall of the sphenoid sinus and posterior wall of the ethmoid sinus, we left the lower level of the ethmoid and reached the upper level. Although we use Hajek's punch to remove the cell septs, which are affixed to the skull base, in a predominantly posteroanterior direction (Fig. 18–10), it is nearly impossible to injure the skull base during the operation. The posterior part of the punch is guided behind the cell septs, and they are then removed step by step until the roof of the ethmoid is reached. This rises slowly from the back to the front until it turns into the posterior wall of the frontal sinus. The cell septs affixed to the lamina papyracea of the orbit can also be punched in a posteroanterior direction without harming the orbit.

When we reach the anterior ethmoid artery in a posteroanterior direction, the remnants of the anterior wall of the bulla, which was left intact during the anteroposterior approach, obstruct the view into the depth of the frontal recess. Removing the upper remnants of the anterior wall of the bulla with the punch is now recommended to hereby enlarge the frontal recess. Very often, the anterior wall of the bulla reaches the ethmoid roof directly behind the frontal ostium. Preserving the anterior wall of the bulla as long as possible also protects the skull base in its frontal parts. In those cases in which the bulla does not reach the skull base, the suprabullar recess is opened after the removal of the anterior wall of the bulla. By removing the anterior wall of the bulla and the suprabullar cells, the frontal recess is exposed up to the anterior ethmoid artery. The anterior ethmoid artery should always be identified as an important landmark. According to the degree of pneumatization of the ethmoid, the artery either lies in the roof of the ethmoid itself or, in the case of an extended pneumatization, runs through the anterior ethmoid in a kind of bony mesenterium laterally from the back to medially in the front. Its position can be viewed in the coronal projection of the preoperative CT. On the 2 mm slices of the ethmoid, you can recognize in the medial orbit wall the entrance of the anterior ethmoid artery from the orbit into the ethmoid. Its course through the ethmoid is rarely seen on the CT slices, because the oblique course from the back to the front is not seen on the coronal levels. Important is that the ethmoid artery shows the position of the cribriform plate. When the anterior ethmoid artery runs below the skull base through the ethmoid, the lamina cribrosa is also low and has a large lateral lamella, which is significantly thinner than the bone of the ethmoid roof. In this case, one must be careful that the manipulations in the ethmoid are not performed too far medially. Injury to the anterior ethmoid artery must also be avoided. A smooth cut with a sharp instrument is less dangerous, because the bleeding is stopped early on, or can be stopped by bipolar coagulation. It is dangerous if the artery is caught by a dull instrument and torn out of its channel. The stump is then torn either laterally into the orbit, resulting in a retrobulbar hematoma, or medially with subsequent bleeding into the olfactoria fossa. In most cases the retrobulbar hematoma can be treated by a lateral canthotomy. Bleeding in the olfactoria fossa, with all its consequences, is difficult to treat.

Surgical Approach to the Frontal Sinus

The anterior ethmoid artery is also a good indicator for the position of the frontal ostium. According to the insertion of the uncinate process, this opens either into the infundibulum or directly into the frontal recess. In this phase of the operation, the ostium, in case of a lower pneumatization of the uncinate process and of the agger nasi cells, can be viewed with a 30- or a 45-degree endoscope. In case of a strong pneumatization, it must be exposed by carefully removing agger nasi cells from the back to the front with a spoon (Fig. 18–13). In this way,

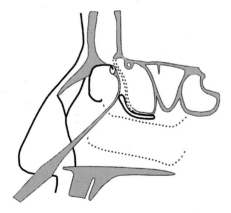

FIGURE 18–13 In resistant frontal sinusitis it is necessary to remove a cellula frontalis or an agger nasi cell by a spoon, working in an anterior direction (Draf type I operation). The ethmoid artery and the remnants of the anterior wall of the ethmoid bulla (parallel broken lines) are safe guidelines to the frontal ostium.

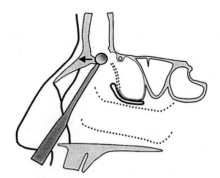

FIGURE 18–14 If the freeing of the frontal ostium (Draf type I) is not sufficient, the ostium must be enlarged by resection of the superior frontal spine (Draf types II and III). The best way to do this is to use a diamond bur. The head of the bur has to be hooked behind the frontal spine and moved toward the front. The skull base is not at risk if one proceeds again in a strict posteroanterior direction.

the bottleneck formed by the cells of the frontal recess below the frontal ostium is enlarged. An enlargement of the frontal ostium itself is not necessary and, to avoid a scar stenosis, should not be attempted. The exposure of the frontal ostium as described is equivalent to a frontal sinus operation Type I as described by Draf. An enlargement of the frontal ostium is only necesarry if a Draf Type I is not sufficient, and should be performed in the case of a recurrence operation. In this case, the Type II or Type III must be applied, whereby the frontal recess is reached by removing the insertion of the middle turbinate at the agger nasi. Exposing the blue line of the lacrimal sac with a diamond bur under the surgical microscope eases the approach. The frontal process and the superior nasal spina are thinned out above the lacrimal sac. This all happens without risk to the frontal skull base when the bur is hooked into the anterior edge of the frontal recess and moved upward and toward the front (Fig. 18–14). This way, it is possible to create a large ostium that can be viewed without an angled endoscope, merely with a microscope or a 0-degree endoscope. This Draf Type II, if performed as described on both sides, can be connected to a Type III in the form of a median drainage. Here, the interfrontal septum and the anterior upper part of the septum itself are removed. This work can be performed without any risk to the skull base if one proceeds in a posteroanterior direction, because the posterior wall of the frontal sinus is not touched.

■ Conclusion

The strategy of endonasal sinus operations to avoid intraoperative complications can be summarized in this way:

1. The paranasal sinuses with the exception of the sphenoid sinus are approached through the anterior ethmoid.

2. The insertion of the middle turbinate at the lateral nasal wall needs to be preserved as long as possible.

3. The ethmoid bulla is the most important landmark for the localization of the frontal recess and the maxillary ostium. The bulla should also be preserved as long as possible.

4. A line drawn through the middle of the ethmoid bulla parallel to the nasal floor and at the same time also approximately parallel to the skull base divides the ethmoid into an upper and a lower level.

5. The opening of the anterior and the posterior ethmoid is always performed in an anteroposterior direction in the lower level of the ethmoid. The risk of harm to the skull base and the orbit is extremely low if one works medially and parallel to the septum and as low as possible parallel to the nasal floor.

6. The sphenoid sinus is never opened transethmoidally, but always transnasally, medial to the middle turbinate, approximately in the area of the sphenoid ostium. This way, the internal carotid artery and the optic nerve in the lateral wall of the sphenoid sinus are protected against injury.

7. The upper level of the ethmoid, including the frontal recess, is dissected in a posteroanterior direction while keeping the skull base and the lamina papyracea in view. The frontal sinus ostium is exposed if necessary with a curette in a posteroanterior direction and in a medial direction by removing the cell walls in the frontal recess.

8. A frontal sinus operation Type II and III is performed in a posteroanterior direction by removing the frontal process and the superior nasal spina with a diamond bur.

REFERENCES

1. Halle M. Externe oder interne Operationen der Nebenhöhlen I. *Berliner klin Wochenschr.* 1906;42:1369–1372.

2. Halle M. Externe oder interne Operationen der Nebenhöhlen II. *Berliner klin Wochenschr.* 1906;43:1404–1407.

3. Halle M. Die intranasale Eröffnung und Behandlung der chronisch kranken Stirnhöhlen. *Arch f Laryngol Rhinol.* 1911;24:249–265.

4. Halle M. Die intranasalen Operationen bei eitrigen Erkrankungen der Nebenhöhlen der Nase. *Arch f Laryngol Rhinol.* 1915;29:73–112.

5. Hajek M. *Pathologie und Therapie der entzündlichen Erkrankungen der Nebenhöhlen der Nase.* Leipzig, Germany: Deuticke; 1915.

6. Hajek M. Indikation der verschiedenen Behandlungs: und Operationsmethoden bei den entzündlichen Erkrankungen der Nebenhöhlen der Nase. *Z Hals-Nasen-Ohrenheilk.* 1923;4:511–522.

7. Hajek M. Pathology and treatment of the inflammatory diseases of the nasal accessory sinuses. London: Henry Kimpton; 1926.

8. Mosher HP. The surgical anatomy of the ethmoid labyrinth. *Trans Am Acad Ophthalmol Otolaryngol.* 1929;31:376–410.

9. Heermann H. Über endonasale Chirurgie unter Verwendung des binokularen Mikroskops. *Arch Ohren Nasen Kehlkopfheilkd.* 1958;171:295–297.

10. Messerklinger W. Über die Drainage der menschlichen Nasennebenhöhlen unter normalen und pathologischen Bedingungen. *Mitteilung. Monatsschr Ohrenheilkd.* 1966;100:56–68.

11. Messerklinger W. Über die Drainage der menschlichen Nasennebenhöhlen unter normalen und pathologischen Bedingungen. 2. Mitteilung: Die Stirnhöhle und ihr Ausführungssystem. *Monatsschr Ohrenheilkd.* 1967;101:313–326.

12. Messerklinger W. Nasenendoskopie: Nachweis, Lokalisation und Differentialdiagnose der nasalen Liquorrhoe. *HNO.* 1972;20:268.

13. Messerklinger W. *Endoscopy of the Nose.* Baltimore: Urban & Schwarzenberg; 1978.

14. Messerklinger W. Über den Recessus frontalis und seine Klinik. *Laryng Rhinol Otol.* 1982;61:217–223.

15. Messerklinger W. Die Rolle der lateralen Nasenwand in der Pathogenese, Diagnose und Therapie der rezidivierenden und chronischen Rhinosinusitis. *Laryngol Rhinol Otol.* 1987;66:293–299.

16. Wigand ME, Steiner W, Jaumann MP. Endonasal sinus surgery with endoscopic control: from radical operation to rehabilitation of the mucosa. *Endoscopy.* 1978;10:255–260.

17. Wigand ME. Transnasal ethmoidectomy under endoscopic control. *Rhinology.* 1982;92:1038–1041.

18. Kennedy DW. Functional endoscopic sinus surgery: technique. *Arch Otolaryngol Head Neck Surg.* 1985;111:643–649.

19. Stammberger H. Unsere endoskopische Operationstechnik der lateralen Nasenwand: ein endoskopisch-chirurgisches Konzept zur Behandlung entzündlicher Nasennebenhöhlenerkrankungen. *Laryngorhinootologie.* 1985;64:559–566.

20. Stammberger H. Endoscopic endonasal surgery—concepts in treatment of recurring rhinosinusitis: 1. Anatomic and pathophysiologic considerations. *Otolaryngol Head Neck Surg.* 1986;94:143–147.

21. Stammberger H. Endoscopic endonasal surgery—concepts in treatment of recurring rhinosinusitis: 2. Surgical technique. *Otolaryngol Head Neck Surg.* 1986;94:147–156.

22. Draf W. Endonasal micro-endoscopic frontal sinus surgery, the Fulda concept. *Op Tech Otolaryngol Head Neck Surg.* 1991;2:234–240.

23. Rudert H. Complications of endonasal surgery of the paranasal sinuses: incidence and strategies for prevention. *Laryngorhinootologie.* 1997;76:200–215.

24. Stankiewicz JA. Complications in endoscopic intranasal ethmoidectomy: an update. *Laryngoscope.* 1989;99:686–690.

25. Weber R, Keerl R, Hosemann W, et al. Complications with permanent damage in endonasal paranasal sinus operations—more frequent in experienced surgeons? *Laryngorhinootologie.* 1998;77:398–401.

26. Schick B, Weber R, Keerl R, et al. Orbital hematomas. *Laryngorhinootologie.* 1996;75:363–367.

27. Keerl R, Stankiewicz JA, Weber R, et al. Surgical experience and complications during endonasal sinus surgery. *Laryngoscope.* 1999;109:546–550.

28. Neugebauer A, Nishino K, Neugebauer P, et al. Effects of bilateral orbital decompression by an endoscopic endonasal approach in dysthyroid orbitopathy. *Br J Ophthalmol.* 1996;80:58–62.

29. May M, Levine HL, Mester SJ, et al. Complications of endoscopic sinus surgery: analysis of 2108 patients—incidence and prevention. *Laryngoscope.* 1994;104:1080–1083.

30. Benninger MS, Marks S. The endoscopic management of sphenoid and ethmoid mucoceles with orbital and intranasal extension. *Rhinology.* 1995;33:157–161.

31. Kennedy DW, Josephson JS, Zinreich J, et al. Endoscopic sinus surgery for mucoceles: a viable alternative. *Laryngoscope.* 1989;99:885–895.

32. Marks SC, Latoni JD, Mathog RH. Mucoceles of the maxillary sinus. *Otolaryngol Head Neck Surg.* 1997;117:18–21.

33. Rudert H, Harder T, Werner JA, et al. Giant mucocele of the paranasal sinuses, extending into the contralateral posterior cranial fossa and causing reversible sensorineural hearing impairment. *Laryngorhinootologie.* 1993;72:247–251.

34. Godbersen GS, Kleeberg J, Lütges J, et al. Sphärulocytose (Myosphärulose) der Nasennebenhöhlen. *HNO*. 1995;43:552–555.

35. Tasman AJ, Faller U, Moller P. Sclerosing lipogranulomatosis of the eyelids after ethmoid sinus surgery: a complication after ointment tamponade. *Laryngorhinootologie*. 1994;73:264–267.

36. Bütler S, Grossenbacher R. Cholesterol granuloma of the paranasal sinuses. *J Laryngol Otol*. 1989;103:776–779.

37. Levine HL. Functional endoscopic sinus surgery: evaluation, surgery, and follow-up of 250 patients. *Laryngoscope*. 1990;100:79–84.

38. Stammberger H. Komplikationen entzündlicher Nasennebenhöhlenerkrankungen einschließlich iatrogen bedingter Komplikationen. *Eur Arch Otorhinolaryngol Suppl*. 1993;1:61–102.

39. Hosemann W, Wigand ME, Wessel B, et al. Medico-legale Probleme in der endonasalen Nasennebenhöhlenchirurgie. *Eur Arch Otorhinolaryngol Suppl*. 1992;2:284–296.

40. Hosemann W. Die endonasale Chirurgie der Nasennebenhöhlen—Konzepte, Techniken, Ergebnisse, Komplikationen, Revisionseingriffe. *Eur Arch Otorhinolaryngol Suppl*. 1996;155–269.

41. Bolger WE, Parsons DS, Mair EA, et al. Lacrimal drainage system injury in functional endoscopic sinus surgery: incidence, analysis, and prevention. *Arch Otolaryngol Head Neck Surg*. 1992;118:1179–1184.

42. Lang J, Papke J. Über die klinische Anatomie des Paries inferior orbitae und dessen Nachbarschaftsstrukturen. *Gegenbaurs morphol Jb*. 1984;130:1–47.

43. Lang J. *Clinical Anatomy of the Nose, Nasal Cavity, and Paranasal Sinuses*. New York: Thieme; 1989.

44. Buus DR, Tse DT, Farris BK. Ophthalmic complications of sinus surgery. *Ophthalmology*. 1990;97:612–619.

45. Dessi P, Castro F, Triglia JM, et al. Major complikations of sinus surgery: a review of 1192 procedures. *J Laryngol Otol*. 1994;108:212–215.

46. Freedman HM, Kern EB. Complications of intranasal ethmoidectomy: a review of 1000 consecutive operations. *Laryngoscope*. 1979;89:421–434.

47. Lawson W. The intranasal ethmoidectomy: an experience with 1077 procedures. *Laryngoscope*. 1991;101:367–371.

48. Maniglia AJ. Fatal and other major complications of endoscopic sinus surgery. *Laryngoscope*. 1991;101:349–354.

49. Weber R, Draf W, Keerl R, et al. Endonasal microendoscopic pansinusoperation in chronic sinusitis: 2. Results and complications. *Am J Otolaryngol*. 1997;18:247–253.

50. Penne RB, Flanagan JC, Stefanyszyn MA, et al. Ocular motility disorders secondary to sinus surgery. *Ophthal Plast Reconstr Surg*. 1993;9:53–61.

51. Flynn JT, Mitchell KB, Fuller DG, et al. Ocular motility complications following intranasal surgery. *Arch Ophthalmol*. 1979;97:453–458.

52. Mark LE, Kennerdell JS. Medial rectus injury from intranasal surgery. *Arch Ophthalmol*. 1979;97:459–461.

53. Rosenbaum AL, Astle WF. Superior oblique and inferior rectus muscle injury following frontal and intranasal sinus surgery. *J Ped Ophthalmol Strabismus*. 1985;22:194–202.

54. Stankiewicz JA. Two faces of orbital hematoma in intranasal (endoscopic) sinus surgery. *Otolaryngol Head Neck Surg*. 1999;120:841–847.

55. Rochels R. Emergency therapy of traumatic orbital hematoma with acute visual impairment. *Laryngorhinootologie*. 1995;74:325–327.

56. Wigand ME, Hosemann WG. Endoscopic surgery for frontal sinusitis and its complications. *Am J Rhinol*. 1991;5:85–89.

57. Küttner K, Siering U, Eichhorn M. Ergebnisse und Erfahrungen bei der endoskopisch-chirurgischen Behandlung entzündlicher Nasennebenhöhlenaffektionen. *HNO-Prax*. 1990;15:45–52.

58. Vleming M, Middelweerd RJ, De Vries N. Complications of endoscopic sinus surgery. *Arch Otolaryngol Head Neck Surg*. 1992;118:617–623.

59. Simmen D, Bischoff T. Rhinosurgical concept in management of fronto-basal defects with cerebrospinal rhinorrhea. *Laryngorhinootologie*. 1998;77:264–271.

60. Rauchfuss A. Komplikationen der endonasalen Chirurgie der Nasennebenhöhlen. *HNO*. 1990;38:309–316.

61. Keros P. Über die praktische Bedeutung der Niveauunterschiede der Lamina cribrosa des Ethmoids. *Laryngorhinootologie*. 1965;41:808–813.

62. Kainz J, Stammberger H. Das Dach des vorderen Siebbeins: ein Locus minoris resistentia an der Schädelbasis. *Laryngorhinootologie*. 1988;67:142–149.

63. Ohnishi T. Bony defects and dehiscences of the roof of the ethmoid bone. *Rhinology*. 1981;19:195–202.

64. Oberascher G. A modern concept of cerebrospinal fluid diagnosis in oto- and rhinorrhea. *Rhinology*. 1988;26:89.

65. Oberascher G. Diagnostik der Rhinolquorrhoe. *Eur Arch Otorhinolaryngol Suppl*. 1993;1:347–362.

66. Stammberger H, Greistorfer K, Wolf G, et al. Surgical occlusion of cerebrospinal fistulas of the anterior skull base using intrathecal sodium fluorescein. *Laryngorhinootologie*. 1997;76:595–607.

67. Gjuric M, Goede U, Keimer H, et al. Endonasal endoscopic closure of cerebrospinal fluid fistulas at the anterior cranial base. *Ann Otol Rhinol Laryngol*. 1996;105:620–623.

68. Maune S. Indication, incidence and management of blood transfusion during sinus surgery: a review over 12 years. *Rhinology*. 1997;35:2–5.

69. Rudert H. Endonasal coagulation of the sphenopalatine artery in severe posterior epistaxis. *Laryngorhinootologie*. 1997;76:77–82.

70. Rudert H. Mikroskop- und endoskopgestützte Chirurgie der entzündlichen Nasennebenhöhlenerkrankungen. *HNO*. 1988;36:475–482.

71. Armengot M, Barona R, Garin L, et al. Ethmoid cholesterol granuloma. *Otolaryngol Head Neck Surg*. 1993;109:762–765.

72. Geiger K, Witschel H, Buttner C. Chronic lipogranuloma (paraffin granuloma) of the eyelids and orbits after endonasal paranasal sinus operation. *Laryngorhinootologie*. 1993;72:356–360.

73. Draf W. Endonasale mikro-endoskopische Pansinusoperation bei chronischer Sinusitis. III. Endonasale mikro-endoskopische Stirnhöhlenchirurgie: eine Standortbestimmung. *Otolaryngol Nova*. 1992;2:118–125.

74. Simmen D, Schuknecht B. Computertomographie der Nasennebenhöhlen—eine präoperative Checkliste. *Laryngorhinootologie*. 1997;76:8–13.

75. Rudert H. Mikroskop—und endoskopgestützte Chirurgie der entzündlichen Nasennebenhöhlenerkrankungen. *HNO*. 1988;36:475–482.

76. Schaefer STD. An anatomic approach to endoscopic intranasal ethmoidectomy. *Laryngoscope*. 1998;108:1628–1634.

77. Lang J, Bressel S. Über den Hiatus semilunaris, das Infundibulum und das Ostium des Sinus maxillaris, die vordere Ansatzzone der Concha nasalis media und deren Abstände zu Landmarken an der Aussen- und Innennase. *Gegenbaurs morphol Jb*. 1988;134:637–646.

19

Ophthalmologic Complications of Endoscopic Sinus Surgery

MARK LEVINE

Successful endoscopic sinus surgery requires a thorough knowledge of the area. The intimate anatomical relations between the orbit and ethmoid sinus is of paramount importance in the management of paranasal sinus disease. Vital structures supporting visual function pass adjacent to nasal and sinus passages with little more then mucosal lining and the thin bony lamina separating them. These barriers may be breached by inflammatory reactions, neoplastic processes, or trauma. Because of the importance of the orbit and its contents and this relationship, this chapter discusses the anatomy of the region and the potential complications and their management.

The ethmoid is an unpaired midline bone situated between the orbits. In the coronal view, the central portion of the ethmoid is shaped like a cross. The vertical arm is formed by the nasal septum inferiorly and the crista galli superiorly. On either side, the horizontal arm forms the cribriform plate and fovea ethmoidalis. Suspended from the horizontal arms are the pneumatized ethmoid sinus labyrinth.[1]

The lateral wall of each labyrinth is composed of the lamina papyracea separating the air cells from the orbit. Along the orbital surface of the lamina papyracea lie the medial rectus muscles and above it the superior oblique muscle. In the posterior orbit, the optic nerve passes close to the lamina papyracea adjacent to the posterior ethmoid air cells. Bansberg et al[2] found that 8% of the posterior ethmoid sinus air cells override the ipsilateral sphenoid sinus and are juxtaposed to the optic nerve on the medial side and that the intracanalicular optic nerve is at risk during extirpation of these air cells. In addition, the optic nerve is relatively fixed in position as it enters the bony optic nerve canal at the orbital apex. Therefore, the optic

nerve cannot easily be pushed aside and escape direct mechanical injury from surgical instruments introduced into the area. Surgical trauma to the vascular supply of the optic nerve may result in ischemic optic neuropathy.

The medial wall of the ethmoid labyrinth is formed by the thin lamina of the bone surrounding each air cell. The uppermost air cells are capped by the orbital process of the frontal bone forming the roof or fovea ethmoidalis.

The middle turbinate is suspended from each horizontal ethmoid arm. Anteriorly, the origin of the turbinate separates the cribriform plate medially from the fovea ethmoidalis laterally. The anterior and posterior ethmoid arteries arise from the ophthalmic artery as it courses through the superior medial orbit. The vessels pass through the foramina within the frontal ethmoid suture lines at the upper edge of the lamina papyracea. The ethmoid arteries pass across the superior ethmoid sinus, enter the anterior cranial fossa, and pass into the nose just below the cribriform plate. Injury to the ethmoid arteries as they penetrate the periorbita is the major cause of orbital hemorrhage during ethmoid sinus surgery.

Anteriorly, the lacrimal fossa and sac lie in the medial orbit between the anterior and posterior lacrimal crests. The most anterior ethmoid air cells lie anterior to the middle turbinate and may invade the lacrimal bone and frontal process of the maxillary bone. Intranasally, the lacrimal fossa and canal are situated behind the thin vertical ridge of bone just anterior to the tip of the middle turbinate, the membranous portion of the middle meatus and bulla ethmoidalis. The bony nasal lacrimal canal passes within the frontal process of the maxillary bone and along the medial antral wall, exiting into the inferior meatus near the junction of the anterior and middle thirds of the inferior turbinate. The canal is accessible to damage from surgery in the medial antral wall or the most anterior ethmoid air cells.

Preoperative evaluation is important in preventing complications. Patients should be screened for potential risk of hemorrhage. Appropriate laboratory studies, including prothrombin time, partial thromboplastin time, platelet count, and bleeding time, are required in the presence of a history of bleeding disorders. All aspirin, ibuprofen, and other drug products that impair clotting should be discontinued at least 2 weeks before surgery. Medical problems such as hypertension and diabetes should be controlled. Preoperative CT scans should be reviewed for the presence of possible dehiscence in the lamina papyracea, as well as for study of the architecture of the ethmoidal labyrinth, the orbits, and their contents.

A screening history for eye disease as well as documentation of visual acuity and extraocular motility is most helpful. At the time of surgery, the eyes should not be covered or draped so that the globe may be palpated. This may be helpful in identifying defects in the lamina papyracea.

PEARL

For the patient having surgery under general anesthesia, the eyes are taped closed with a small strip of $\frac{1}{2}$-inch hypoallergenic tape. The globe is palpated prior to injecting any local anesthesia and starting the surgery. This gives the surgeon a baseline to the tension of the orbit. The globe is palpated periodically during surgery and at the conclusion.

Traditional ethmoidectomy and sinus surgery are relatively safe procedures, but major and fatal complications may occur. In 1000 intranasal ethmoidectomies, Freedman and Kern[3] report a low incidence of complications (2.8%), most of them of a minor type. In 1990, Friedman and Katsantonis[4] also reported a low incidence of complication secondary to intranasal ethmoidectomies, (2.08% minor, 0.94% major). Intracranial and orbital complications are rare.

In 1987, Stankiewicz[5] reported his experience with endonasal sinus surgery and indicated a complication rate of 28% in 90 patients (17% in 150 ethmoidectomies). In 1989, Stankiewicz[6,7] again discussed complication rates in 3000 ethmoidectomies performed in 180 patients. His overall complication rate had dropped to 9.3%. Most complications were minor. However, two cases had cerebrospinal fluid leaks, and one case of temporary blindness occurred. The author credits the low incidence of complications in the latter group of patients to experience.

Schaefer et al[8] reported an incidence of 14% minor complications and 0% major. In 458 procedures, Levine[9]

had 8.3% minor complications and 0.7% major. Most major complications reported are CSF leaks.

In a study by May et al,[10] the incidence of complications of endoscopic sinus surgery in 2108 patients was compared with complications in 11 other series of patients grouped together (2583 total) and with a series of patients who underwent traditional endonasal sinus surgery (2110 total). The overall incidence of major complications in all three groups were not statistically different. There was, however, a statistically significant difference in the incidence of orbital complications. Retrobulbar hematoma was significantly higher for traditional sinus surgery (0.47%) compared with endoscopic sinus surgery (0.05% May et al, 0.12% other ESS). It is possible that the higher incidence of this complication associated with traditional surgery is due to the greater extent of surgery for more advanced disease based on touch rather than direct visualization in the posterior ethmoid compartment with greater risk of posterior penetration.

The incidences of minor complications were significantly different for the three groups. The most common minor complication was orbital violation that occurred most frequently during the time of uncinectomy as was manifested as ecchymosis, emphysema, or was asymptomatic.

Table 19–1 lists the reported complications found in this study.

TABLE 19–1   Complications from Sinus Surgery

Minor
  Temporary, requiring no treatment
    Subcutaneous periorbital emphysema
    Periorbital ecchymosis (preseptal)
    Dental or lip pain or numbness
  Temporary, corrected with treatment
    Bronchial asthma
    Adhesions (symptomatic)
    Epistaxis requiring packing
    Infection: -frontal, maxillary, sphenoid sinus
  Permanent and not correctable (present beyond 1 year)
    Dental or lip pain or numbness
    Loss of smell
Major
  Corrected with treatment
    Orbital hematoma (postseptal)
    Loss of vision
    Diplopia
    Ephiphora (requiring dacryocystorhinostomy)
    Carotid artery injury
    Hemorrhage requiring transfusion
    Cerebrospinal fluid leak
    Meningitis
    Brain abscess
    Focal brain hemorrhage
  Permanent despite treatment
    Death
    Blindness
    Diplopia
    Stroke
    Central nervous system deficit

The most common major orbital complication is formation of an intraorbital retrobulbar hematoma. This can occur when the anterior and posterior ethmoidal artery is damaged or small vessels in the orbital fat are torn and can develop quickly perioperatively or postoperatively, with sudden pain around or behind the eye followed by proptosis, decreased vision, pupil dilation and an afferent pupillary defect. The increased intraorbital or intraocular pressure can lead to blindness secondary to ischemia or vascular occlusion. There is a 60 to 90 minute window of opportunity to institute appropriate medical and surgical therapy to avoid ischemic optic neuropathy and optic atrophy.

If the visual function is intact, ice compresses, elevation of the head of the bed, and close observation are indicated in the recovery room. If the visual function is compromised, intranasal packing must be removed. This will decrease intraocular and intraorbital pressure by allowing orbit hemorrhagic soft tissue to prolapse through the medial wall defect into the previous space occupied by the intranasal packing. In addition, the lateral canthotomy with lysis of the superior-inferior canthal tendon should be performed. The released lateral canthal tendon will allow forward displacement of the eyelids and globes with a subsequent decrease in intraocular and intraorbital pressure. This frequently leads to a rapid recovery of visual acuity and reversal of the previous afferent pupil defect. If the visual function continues to be compromised, blunt orbital dissection may release entrapped air or blood under high pressure for the orbital soft tissues. Frequently these maneuvers can be quickly accomplished with local anesthesia at the bedside in the recovery room in those patients who have lost vision after endoscopic sinus surgery. To control continued active bleeding or persistent decreased vision, further orbital surgery is indicated in the operating room. This may include an orbital apex decompression by further removal of the medial orbital wall and orbital floor with inspection of the intranasal space to control bleeding.

PEARL

An endoscopic orbital decompression is performed. Clots are suctioned from the nasal and sinus cavity. A fracture is made in the lamina papyracea, and the lamina papyracea is removed in an "eggshell" fashion using a Freer elevator. The bone is removed superiorly to the orbital roof and inferiorly to the infraorbital nerve. If necessary, incisions are made in the periorbital to decompress the globe.

For patients with major orbital or nasal hemorrhage, surgical exploration should be initiated directly to the anteroposterior ethmoid arteries as the probable source.

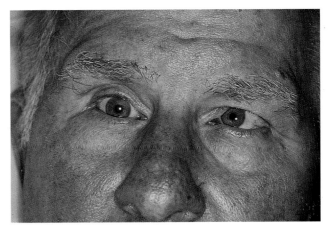

FIGURE 19–1 Status postendoscopic sinus surgery with left esotropia in primary gaze secondary to muscle trauma and resultant cicatricial esotropia.

Surgical repair of a lateral canthotomy and lateral canthal attachment to the lateral orbital rim should be delayed several days until the orbital edema has subsided and adequate tissue approximation is possible. The use of corticosteroids to reverse optic nerve damage should be considered adjunctive therapy to adequate control of the orbital hemorrhage and anatomical decompression of the compromised orbital soft tissue. Medical treatment can consist of acetazolamide (Diamox) 500 mg and mannitol 0.5 to 1.0 mg/kg, both administered intravenously to decrease the intraocular pressure at the first sign of visual compromise and proptosis.

Diplopia may be caused by damage to the medial rectus or superior oblique muscle either by direct damage to the muscle itself or by involvement of the nerve (Figs. 19–1, 19–2).

During the ethmoidectomy portion of endoscopic sinus surgery, the medial orbital wall frequently cannot be identified as a distinct surgical boundary separating

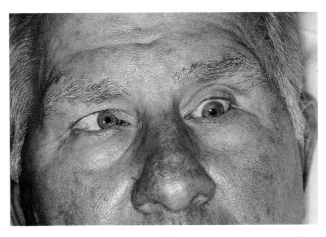

FIGURE 19–2 Looking left with inability to abduct left eye and a positive forced duction test.

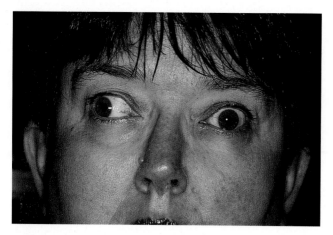

FIGURE 19–3 Status postendoscopic sinus surgery with right exotropia in primary gaze.

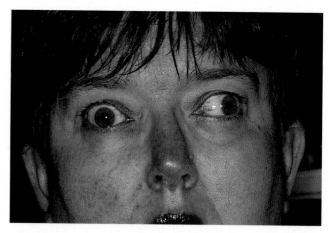

FIGURE 19–4 Looking left with inability to adduct right eye beyond midline and negative forced duction test.

the orbital soft tissues from the ethmoid air cells and intranasal space. This may be due to edematous, inflamed ethmoid sinus mucosa, ethmoid air cell polyposis, adherent inflammatory mucoid material, or intraoperative hemorrhage. In addition, chronic ethmoid sinusitis may result in attenuation or absence of the normal thin medial orbital wall. As the ethmoid sinus surgery precedes the normal orbital soft tissues, prolapse in the surgical area may not be recognized as such. Subsequent direct surgical trauma to the medial rectus muscle, adjacent orbital fat, or superior oblique may occur. Frequently trauma to the extraocular muscles would be associated with a subconjunctival hemorrhage in the bulbar conjunctiva along the medial aspect of the globe. If this is recognized intraoperatively, further endoscopic surgery in this area should be immediately discontinued. The degree of orbital hemorrhage frequently is quite minimal compared with the extent of intraorbital manipulation and destruction that may occur to the extraocular muscles. Postoperatively, the management of extraocular muscle dysfunction requires an accurate diagnosis of either entrapment with tethering of the extraocular muscles or paresis of the muscle secondary to cranial nerve injury. The clinical examination will usually show restrictive strabismus and a positive forced duction test, suggesting muscle entrapment or paralytic strabismus, and a negative forced duction test, suggesting nerve injury. Forced generation testing may be needed to establish the correct diagnosis (Figs. 19–3, 19–4, 19–5).

Surgical exploration of the extraocular muscle entrapment in the orbital fracture should be attempted if no spontaneous resolution of the diplopia has occurred within 2 weeks after the endoscopic sinus surgery. However, extraocular muscle paralysis secondary to nerve injury may recover significantly with observation over 6 to 12 months. If spontaneous neurologic improvement has ceased and strabismus measurements have stabilized,

extraocular muscle surgery is indicated to minimize residual strabismus.[11]

Optic nerve injury with secondary decreased visual acuity and/or visual field deficit can occur during the posterior ethmoidectomy phase of endoscopic sinus surgery. The lateral wall of the posterior ethmoid air cells is immediately adjacent to the optic nerve near the orbital apex.

A thorough ophthalmic evaluation is indicated in those patients who have suspected optic nerve injury after endoscopic sinus surgery. Frequently, other signs of orbital injury will be presen, including medial rectus

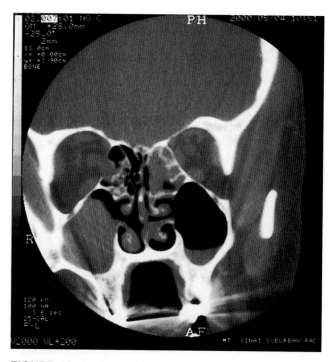

FIGURE 19–5 Coronal CT scan showing injury to the right medial rectus muscle and its nerve.

muscle dysfunction or subconjunctival hemorrhage. Computed tomography will define the extent of surgical trauma and hemorrhage into the orbital apex. Guidelines for the optimal management of optic nerve trauma, which is secondary to intraoperative direct contusion or ischemia, have not been firmly established. However, recent reports suggest that high-dose systemic corticosteroids may reverse vision loss secondary to indirect optic nerve injury after closed head trauma. When the visual loss is noted postoperatively, the institution of dexamethasone and an initial loading dose of 1 mg/kg followed by 0.5 mg/kg every 6 hours are indicated. Optimally, medical management is begun as soon as possible after optic nerve injury is recognized. However, reversible optic nerve injury may be present up to 1 week after indirect optic nerve trauma. If the vision improves with corticosteroids, therapy is continued for 5 more days and then rapidly tapered. If visual acuity fails to respond within 24 to 36 hours of continued corticosteroids, consideration should be given to transethmoid sphenoid decompression of the intracanalicular optic nerve. However, the most successful series of surgical managed cases have been those patients with closed head trauma with indirect optic nerve injury.

A strong case for surgical decompression of the optic canal can be made for those patients who have had initial recovery of vision while on corticosteroids, but had recurrent decreased vision with either maintaining or tapering of corticosteroids. In this subset of patients, the corticosteroids may have had a beneficial effect in reducing optic nerve edema or microcirculatory spasm at or near the optic nerve canal. Subsequent recurrent decreased vision may be related to further compromise of the optic nerve by compression with ischemia at the optic nerve canal. Decompression of the optic nerve along the canal by partially removing the bony confines of the optic nerve in this location would theoretically restore vision and nerve function. However, this procedure may be inappropriate in those patients who have already had extensively disrupted anatomical relationships adjacent to the orbital and intracanalicular optic nerves.

Finally, although injury to the nasolacrimal system is less severe than other complications, it is susceptible to injury in enlarging the maxillary sinus ostium. As the maxillar sinus ostium is enlarged anteriorly, the bony canal of the nasolacrimal duct is encountered. The potential for injury of the lacrimal sac can be high during any operation in the region of the superior aspect of the uncinate process. At this level, the lacrimal sac and fossa lie only 2 to 3 mm anterior to the free edge of the uncinate process.

REFERENCES

1. Dutton JJ. Orbital complications of paransal sinus surgery. *Ophthal Plast Reconstr Surg.* 1986;2(3):119–127.
2. Bansberg SF, Harner SG, Forbes G. Relationship of the optic nerve for the paransal sinuses as shown by computed tomography. *Otolaryngol Head Neck Surg.* 1987;96:331–335.
3. Freedman HM, Kern EB. Complications of intranasal ethmoidectomy. *Laryngoscope.* 1979;89:421–434.
4. Friedman WH, Katsantonis GP. Intranasal and transantral ethmoidectomy. *Laryngoscope.* 1990;100:343–348.
5. Stankiewicz JA. Complications of endoscopic intransal ethmoidectomy. *Laryngoscope.* 1987;97:1270–1273.
6. Stankiewicz JA. Complications in endoscopic intransal ethmoidectomy: an update. *Laryngoscope.* 1989;99:686–690.
7. Stankiewicz JA. Complications of endoscopic sinus surgery. *Otolaryngol Clin North Am.* 1989;22(4):749–758.
8. Schaefer SD, Manning S, Close LG. Endoscopic paransal sinus surgery, indications and considerations. *Laryngoscope.* 1989;99:1–5.
9. Levine HL. Functional endoscopic sinus surgery: evaluation, surgery, and follow-up of 250 patients. *Laryngoscope.* 1990;100:79–84.
10. May M, Levine HL, Mester SJ, et al. Complications of endoscopic sinus surgery: analysis of 2108 patients, incidence and prevention. *Laryngoscope.* 1994;1–4:1080–1083.
11. Neuhaus RW. Orbital complications secondary to endoscopic sinus surgery. *Ophthalmology.* 1990;97(11):1512–1518.

20

The Diagnosis of Allergic Fungal Sinusitis

BERRYLIN J. FERGUSON

Appropriate medical therapy for allergic fungal rhinosinusitis is predicated on recognition of the disease process. Up until 1981, patients with allergic fungal sinusitis (AFS) were mistakenly diagnosed as "immunocompetent hosts" with invasive fungal sinusitis, or the presence of the fungus was unappreciated and the diagnosis of chronic inflammatory sinusitis was given. In 1981, Millar and colleagues[1] published an abstract that highlighted the similarity of the sinus histopathology to allergic bronchopulmonary aspergillosis (ABPA). Because this similarity was the basis for the original recognition of AFS, early authors assumed the causative fungus in the rhinosinusitis form of the disease was *Aspergillus*, just as in the pulmonary form of the disease. No fungal cultures were obtained to support this diagnosis. Nevertheless, for over half a decade, AFS was known as allergic *Aspergillus* sinusitis. Katzenstein, a pathologist in St. Louis, Missouri, a location that turned out to be a hotbed for AFS, also noted the distinctive sinus histopathology and its similarity to ABPA. Along with her colleagues, she published the first papers on the unique histopathology of the entity.[2] Even after the recognition of the similarity of the disease process pathologically to ABPA, many authors continued to mistake this entity as infectious.[3]

■ Spectrum of Fungal Manifestations within the Paranasal Sinuses

The various manifestations of fungal sinusitis depend on the immunologic competence of the host. Prognosis and treatment vary dramatically depending on whether the fungal sinusitis is invasive, noninvasive, or secondary to a hypersensitivity reaction.[4]

At one end of the spectrum are immunosuppressed patients, who suffer invasive fungal sinusitis from a variety of organisms, most commonly the *Aspergillus* species, and mucormycosis, frequently from *Rhizopus* species. Invasive fungal rhinosinusitis is often relentlessly fatal unless the underlying cause of immunocompromise can be reversed. Appropriate therapy includes systemic antifungal therapy and surgery.

Rarely, immunocompetent patients develop invasive fungal rhinosinusitis. In these individuals, the disease is chronic, persisting for months or years, and in some situations it is fatal. It is exceedingly rare in the United States. The largest series was reported in Sudan.[5]

Fungus balls may grow in any sinus. They occur in immunocompetent patients, and the treatment is surgical removal. They seldom recur. They differ from AFS histologically in the presence of matted hyphae without mucin, rather than scattered hyphae in allergic mucin.

At the allergic end of the immunocompetency spectrum lies AFS. An IgE-mediated hypersensitivity to the fungus or fungi is the presumed cause of the disorder. AFS is frequently recurrent, chronic, almost never life threatening, and best treated with surgery, steroids, and probably postoperative immunotherapy. Because the same fungus can cause any of these disease manifestations, one sees how patients in whom the diagnosis of AFS is unappreciated may be mistakenly treated as if they have an invasive form of the disease and inappropriately subjected to the toxicities of systemic antifungal therapy and radical exenterative surgery. Figure 20–1 details the variety of fungal manifestations along an immunologic spectrum.

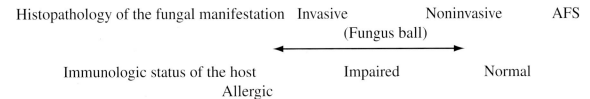

Histopathology of the fungal manifestation   Invasive   Noninvasive   AFS
(Fungus ball)

Immunologic status of the host   Impaired   Normal
Allergic

FIGURE 20–1   The spectrum of fungal manifestations in the paranasal sinuses depends on the immunologic status of the host.

■ Histopathology

The distinctive histopathology of AFS was most likely overlooked for many years because it lies not in the polypoid tissue but rather in the tenacious inspissated mucin. This allergic mucin is often characterized as being "peanut buttery."[6] I find it more like rubber cement in its thick elastic properties that often cast the shape of the nasal or sinus cavity from which it is extracted. Under the microscope, this mucin reveals necrotic eosinophils, frequently in wavelike concentric layers. On higher power, Charcot-Leyden crystals are seen. On cross section, they may appear hexagonal, whereas on longitudinal section they are thick splinters with tapered ends. They are thought to be a product of eosinophil degranulation[2] (Fig. 20–2A) Most important diagnostically is the finding of hyphal fragments scattered throughout the eosinophilic mucin. Special stains for fungi such as Gomori methenamine–silver are frequently required to see these hyphae, although they may occasionally be appreci-

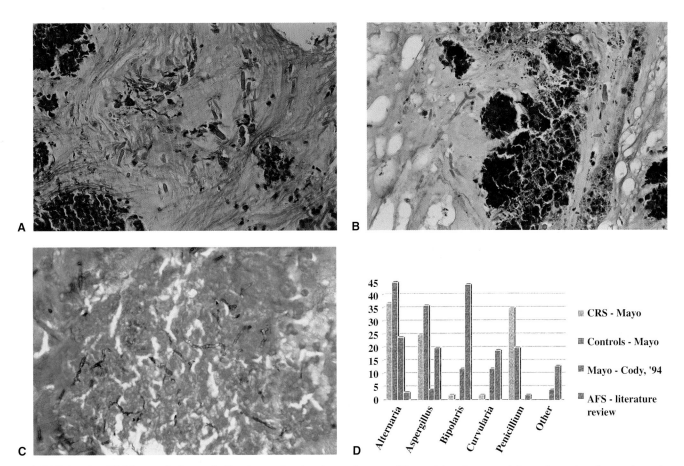

FIGURE 20–2   (A) Histopathology of allergic mucin showing necrotic eosinophils and abundant Charcot-Leyden crystals on hematoxylin and eosin stain. (B) Histologic pathology of allergic fungal mucin showing dense inflammatory infiltrate, rare Charcot-Leyden crystals, and hyphae present. Note branching of hyphae and length, which helps distinguish hyphae from a Charcot-Leyden crystal on hematoxylin and eosin stain. (C) Gomori methenamine–silver nitrate stain of mucin showing hyphae. (D) Graph of fungal species incidence in four patient groups: CRS,[35] normals,[35] AFS at the Mayo Clinic reported by Cody et al (1994),[16] and AFS reported in the literature.[36]

ated on hematoxylin and eosin stain (Fig. 20–2B,C). One cannot differentiate among the many fungi that cause AFS based on histopathological appearance. Most cases are not caused by the *Aspergillus* species, in contradistinction to the early assumptions by Millar et al[1] and Katzenstein et al,[2] who initially designated AFS as allergic *Aspergillus* sinusitis. Rather, several types of fungi, including *Aspergillus*, are responsible. Ultimate attribution to a particular fungal species depends on fungal culture results.[7]

Preoperative steroids may sometimes obscure the diagnosis, as detailed in one case of a man with characteristic clinical findings for AFS treated with 5 days of prednisone 60 mg daily preoperatively. Histologic examination revealed fungal hyphae, but no allergic mucin or eosinophils. The patient was diagnosed as having a sphenoid fungus ball, but 2 weeks later, his symptoms returned, and endoscopic removal of sphenoid mucin now showed characteristic allergic mucin with eosinophils, Charcot-Leyden crystals, and fungal forms.[8]

Eosinophilic Mucin Sinusitis without Fungus: A Difficulty in the Histopathological Diagnosis of AFS

Occasionally, patients with clinical characteristics of AFS are noted to have characteristic eosinophilic mucin but no evidence of hyphae, despite special stains. In the initial report of nine patients by Katzenstein et al,[2] two cases lacked fungi. One went on to have fungi noted on subsequent surgery. Allphin et al[9] reported on 13 patients with this polypoid histopathology and eosinophilic mucin but absent fungi and negative fungal cultures. Interestingly, all patients in both reports had moderate to severe asthma and were aspirin sensitive. These aspirin sensitive asthmatics with nasal polyposis are sometimes referred to eponymously as having Samter's triad. Aspirin-sensitive asthmatics frequently have severe asthma, unlike most patients with AFS, who either do not have asthma or the asthma is mild.[10,11,35] This group of patients, with eosinophilic mucin sinusitis without hyphae and severe asthma that is often aspirin sensitive, represent a group of patients with a different pathophysiologic basis for their sinus disease than patients with AFS. The most probable cause of AFS as already stated is a hypersensitivity reaction to fungi. That is why the fungi are present in the mucin. They are the driving force for the inflammatory reaction. Those with eosinophilic mucin sinusitis without fungus probably have a systemic immunologic abnormality, which would account for their asthma and the involvement of all sinuses. In a review of 431 AFS patients compared with 69 eosinophilic mucin rhinosinusitis (EMRS) patients, significant differences were present between the two groups. The EMRS patients were statistically older (mean age 48 compared with 30),

more likely to have asthma (93% vs. 41%), more likely to have aspirin sensitivity, also known as Samter's triad, (54% vs. 13%), and, most significantly, never had unilateral disease. In AFS, unilateral sinus disease is present ~50% of the time.[35] Patients with AFS may show unilateral disease, because the fungal stimulus is only present unilaterally, thus sparing the remaining sinuses. Patients with eosinophilic mucin sinusitis without fungus have bilateral disease because the driving force is a more systemic abnormality that accounts for their asthma and upper airway polyposis.

Ramadan and Quraishi[13] noted that their four cases of such patients all had asthma and were significantly older than the AFS population. Rather than terming this entity *allergic mucin sinusitis without fungus*, as they did, I prefer the term *eosinophilic mucin sinusitis without fungi*, thus avoiding reference to the word *allergic* for an entity in which the underlying pathophysiology is unknown. Further investigation regarding possible differences between these two groups of patients is required, because they may respond differently to antifungal therapy and recurrence rates may differ. It certainly is true that steroid therapy is effective in both groups of patients because of its anti-inflammatory activity. Most likely steroids act by downregulating the eosinophilic activity common to both groups. Steroids act to induce apoptosis in eosinophils. Eosinophil survival is prolonged in specimens from bronchoalveolar lavages of Samter's triad patients.[14]

Further Controversies in the Diagnosis of AFS: The Mayo Clinic Experience

In 1999, the Mayo Clinic reported the presence of eosinophilic histopathology with fungi present by culture or histology in 94 of 101 (93%) patients undergoing surgery for any form of chronic rhinosinusitis (CRS). Histologic evidence of fungi, using the criterion fungal elements, further defined as hyphae, destroyed hyphae, conidia, and spores, was found in 81% of this group. The high yield of positive fungal cultures (96%) in patients with CRS in this series is difficult to interpret, because 14 of 14 normal volunteers all had fungus present when undergoing this fungal nasal/sinus collection technique. The collection technique is a nasal wash with 20 mL of saline, which is plated for mold. Those patients with eosinophilic CRS and fungi present by culture or histology in the Mayo Clinic series had a much-reduced incidence of allergy, including mold allergy, compared with other series of AFS.[15] Thus, Ponikau et al[15] believed that IgE-mediated inflammation is not crucial to the development of AFS, and that eosinophilic chemotaxis and activation may result from a T lymphocyte–mediated inflammatory cascade triggered by certain fungi, especially *Alternaria*.

Are there differences in mold found in patients in Ponikau's series with eosinophilic rhinosinusitis with fungus compared with AFS?

In an analysis of frequency of species of fungi found in four populations, differences and similarities are apparent. The four populations illustrated in Figure 20–2D are

1. Patients with CRS with eosinophilia undergoing nasal washes by Ponikau et al[15]

2. Normals undergoing nasal washes by Ponikau et al[15]

3. Patients with AFS reported by Cody et al 5 years earlier also at the Mayo Clinic[16]

4. Fungi reported in the literature associated with AFS

Differences can be seen even within the same institution. Cody et al[6] reported that a far larger number of patients with AFS grow *Bipolaris* or *Curvularia*, two fungi frequently implicated in other series of AFS, but rarely seen in the more recent Ponikau et al[15] series. Distribution of other fungal species, such as *Alternaria* and *Aspergillus*, for example, are fairly high in both of Ponikau's groups, CRS and normals, with no pattern emerging. In the literature, *Bipolaris* is the most frequently reported mold associated with AFS. This could reflect the greater publication on AFS from authors in Texas, where *Bipolaris* is the most common cause, than *Bipolaris* truly being responsible for most cases of AFS worldwide.

Saprophytic Fungal Colonization in EMRS Non-AFS patients

It is possible that the EMRS patients previously discussed can become colonized with a small amount of fungus, but the fungus is not driving the disease process. As Ponikau et al[15] have shown, normals also have mold in their nose. For AFS to exist, it may be important that the fungi germinate and grow in the mucin, further fueling an IgE-mediated allergic reaction. Green and colleagues[17] showed that IgE-mediated response to fungi is increased with germination. This same antigenic stimulation may not be present if just a few ungerminated mold spores are present in the nose.

■ Fungal Cultures

Fungal cultures are positive in ~70 to 80% of patients diagnosed with AFS.[18] Unlike all other areas of the country, the Mayo Clinic reports virtually 100% positive fungal cultures on all patients, irrespective of pathology.[15] This points out the possibility of false positives if one relies on fungal cultures, given the ubiquity of fungal spores. Why all patients with histopathologic evidence of AFS do not grow a fungus on fungal cultures has been attributed to overhomogenization of the specimen prior

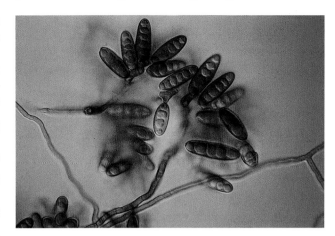

FIGURE 20–3 Photomicrograph of *Bipolaris*.

to plating, which disrupts the fragile hyphal walls, a delay in plating and incubating the culture, and inappropriate culture techniques to separate the fungi from the thick mucin in which they grow. Some advocate immediate culture to Sabouraud's agar at the time of harvesting with incubation.[19] Even if the fungus grows, it may be impossible to speciate it. Speciation requires the production of spores, and if the fungus remains in an asexual form, this may be impossible.

Dematiaceous fungi are the most common based on culture data and account for 84% of the total positive cultures.[7,20] *Dematiaceous fungi* is a term referencing the darkened color of these fungi on histopathologic examination in tissue. It does not refer to the color of the fungi when growing in vitro. The most common fungi were *Bipolaris* species, followed by *Curvularia, Alternaria,* and *Exserohilum* (Fig. 20–3). *Aspergillus* species accounted for 13% of all fungal cultures (Table 20–1).

Unusual causes of AFS include *Epicoccum nigrum*[20] and *Schizophillum commune*,[21] as well as a *Nodulisporium* species.[22] The clinical manifestations, response to therapy, and histopathology are similar no matter which fungus is

TABLE 20–1   Summary of Allergic Fungal Sinusitis Cases with Positive Cultures

Organism	Positve Cultures (n)	% of Total*
Dematiaceae family	141	84
Bipolaris (Drechslera)	75	45
Curvularia	43	26
Alternaria	12	7
Exserohilum	9	5
Fusarium	1	<1
Fonsecaea pedrosa	1	<1
Aspergillus species	22	13
Other (*Rhizomucor*)	1	<1

*Total cases = 168
Used with pemission from Manning SC, Holman M. Further evidence for allergic pathophysiology in allergic fungal sinusitis. Laryngoscope. 1998;108:1485–1496.

associated with the process. If immunotherapy directed to the fungus causing the hypersensitivity response is important, then culture information will be increasingly important. Unfortunately, no commercial antigens to *Bipolaris* or to many of these unusual fungi are available.

There does appear to be geographic variability in incidence of AFS and in fungal organisms associated with the disease process. In the United States, the Mississippi River area and the South have the largest number of cases. The entity is quite uncommon in the Northwest and Rocky Mountain states. While dematiaceous fungi are most common in the United States, *Aspergillus* species cause most cases reported in the Middle East.[36]

■ Pathophysiology

Fungal Serology

AFS was first recognized because of its histopathologic similarity to ABPA. Thus, it is reasonable that a similar pathophysiologic mechanism was initially attributed to AFS. In the pulmonary form of the disease, ABPA, histopathologic confirmation was difficult to obtain. However, serologic tests were available and demonstrated extremely high levels of IgE, ranging from normal to as high as 50,000 IU/mL.[23] These total IgE levels fluctuated with disease activity. In ABPA, *Aspergillus* species were the usual suspects, although other fungal species were occasionally shown to be associated with the disease process. In patients with classic ABPA, both elevated IgE and IgG to either *Aspergillus fumigatus* or *A. flavus* are present. Both Gell and Combs Type I (mast cell activation via specific IgE antibody–antigen interaction) and Type III (IgG antibody and antigen complex) reactions have been postulated in the pathogenesis of ABPA. Because of both elevated IgG and IgE to a particular fungus, the concept that ABPA was an immune-complex disorder became commonplace. There is only one case report that raises the specter of ABPA acting as a true immune-complex disorder.[24] In 1983, Katzenstein et al[2] documented specific IgE antibodies to *A. flavus* in two of nine cases of the sinus form of the disease and postulated a Type I Gell and Combs sensitivity similar to ABPA.

Manning and Holman[19] added further evidence to the allergic pathophysiologic basis of AFS by showing that all eight patients with culture-positive *Bipolaris* AFS demonstrated skin test positivity to *Bipolaris* as well as RAST IgE to *Bipolaris* and ELISA IgG antibodies for *Bipolaris*. In 10 controls, only 1 patient had a positive skin test for *Bipolaris*, as well as IgE and IgG antibodies to *Bipolaris*.

More recently, Kuhn and colleagues[25] studied whether specific IgE to fungal species was superior to

total IgE in predicting persistence or recurrence of the pathophysiologic process. They found that generally a total IgE was most specific and sensitive. Only in a few cases was a specific IgE to a fungus able to predict recurrence better than total IgE.[25] Many of the fungi that cause AFS are not commercially available for skin or in vitro testing. This may account for some of the lack of sensitivity for specific fungal antigens. In other words, the patient could not be tested for the causative fungus. The most common fungi associated with AFS are the *Bipolaris* species. However, this may vary with geography. *Bipolaris* species are most similar antigenically to *Helminthosporium* species, and in allergy testing *Hlminthosporium* antigen testing is used as a surrogate for *Bipolaris*.[34] Some investigators have advocated serologic screening with *Helminthosporium, Aspergillus, Alternaria,* and *Curvularia* fungal antigens because these represent the most common etiologic fungal agents for which commercial assays exist.[34]

Immunologic Evaluation

Initial laboratory evaluation frequently reveals a peripheral eosinophilia in the range of 7 to 15%. Total IgE is frequently elevated, with a mean of 668 IU/mL, with normal being less than 125 IU/mL.[19,35] As already described under serologic evaluation, most patients demonstrate a Class II or higher RAST to multiple fungi. Total IgE fluctuates with disease activity. In a review of 67 patients followed in their practice in Arizona, Schubert and Goetz[27] found that total serum IgE correlated significantly with the severity of disease. Importantly, an increase of 10% or more in total serum IgE during follow-up was a strong predictor of recurrence and need for surgical intervention. Unlike other investigators, Schubert and Goetz were unable to demonstrate elevated specific fungal IgEs in their patients despite positive skin tests, although they did find elevated specific fungal IgGs in these patients. Fungal IgGs fluctuated with disease activity but was less predictive of recurrence than total IgE. Ninety-two percent of their 67 patients had normal total IgGs, and 8% demonstrated low quantitative immunoglobulins, which nevertheless showed normal function.[26,27] No other studies have shown an immunologic deficiency in these patients, but in most reports, a full immunologic investigation was not performed.

Lower Airway Association

Although ABPA is probably the lower airway representation of the upper airway process, it is peculiar how uncommonly the upper and lower airway pathologies occur concurrently; but they do occur. Katzenstein et al,[2] in their initial report of the pathophysiologic process of AFS, noted that, in retrospect, a case described by Safirstein in 1976 of a patient with ABPA and chronic nasal obstruction probably represented the first reference to AFS.[2,28]

Proposed Mechanism

It is presumed that a susceptible allergic individual inhales the causative fungal spores, and an allergic reaction to the antigenic spore occurs. Increased mucus is produced, trapping the spore(s) within the already edematous and boggy nasal mucosa. The spore(s) cannot be transported easily from the sinonasal tract because of this thickened mucus, and the continued presence of the fungi within the mucus in the nasal cavity perpetuates the allergic reaction and mucus production. An intense inflammatory response continues.

Why are allergic patients more predisposed to AFS than nonallergic subjects? It is most likely that the normal individual's mucociliary defenses transport inhaled spores along with all other small, trapped elements toward the nasopharynx, where they are swallowed, thus clearing the sinonasal cavity and ending the possibility of perpetuation of the process. If not transported, the fungi could continue to grow as a tangled mat of hyphae and manifest as a fungus ball, without any associated allergic mucin.

Manning et al[19] showed that the histopathologic specimens from patients with AFS had elevated major basic protein and eosinophil-derived neurotoxin compared with normal sinus controls. Nasal polyps develop as a result of the increased inflammatory mediators within the nose, further trapping the inflammatory mucin containing the spores behind them. The spores germinate into hyphae. In the absence of removal, the disease process continues, and the hyphal agents in the inspissated mucin involve the contiguous sinuses. Here they remain, continuing to fuel the allergic flame. The inflammatory eosinophilic mucin is produced, and the fungi continue to grow within it. This mucus becomes increasingly tenacious and rubbery as it is aged. As the process enlarges, it may block the outflow tract of any of the sinuses, resulting in postobstructive mucoceles. These in turn result in bony remodeling and erosion as they enlarge. Alternatively, the allergic fungal mucin enlarges the involved sinus cavity and in a similar manner may cause bony erosion and proptosis or intracranial expansion.

Because the process is not an invasive one, it does not infiltrate contiguous structures; rather, it pushes them away as it expands. Therefore, while there is intracranial expansion, the dura remains intact. At least one series purported to show an invasive character to AFS; however, the representative histopathology in the article did not clearly show invasion, and the clinical course of the patients was in line with a noninvasive process such as AFS.[29]

Tsimikas et al[30] described a patient who developed an *Aspergillus* frontal lobe abscess 8 days after undergoing a frontoethmoidectomy for AFS with associated mucopyocele. It is reasonable to postulate that the initial surgery violated the dura and seeded the frontal lobe. No subsequent reports have shown an invasive aspect to AFS. Theoretically, it would certainly be possible for patients afflicted with active AFS to develop an invasive fungal rhinosinusitis if they became markedly immunosuppressed. One of the common adjunctive therapies for AFS and ABPA is high and prolonged systemic steroid use. Systemic steroids are known to be a risk factor for invasive fungal sinusitis. Therefore, the degree of immunosuppression required to promote invasion must be in excess of the commonly recommended steroid suppressive doses and would probably require a profound leukopenia.

■ Clinical Presentation

Patient Characteristics

Patients with AFS initially present with nasal congestion secondary to nasal polyposis. Nasal obstruction is a symptom that is often ignored. This is understandable, because these patients are atopic and have probably experienced a lifetime of intermittent nasal congestion. The vast majority of patients have nasal polyps. Polyps may be unilateral or bilateral, and the disease process may afflict one or many sinuses. Polyps are a nonspecific consequence of inflammation and do not represent the distinctive pathophysiology of AFS. It is the presence of allergic fungal mucin that is the physical finding that makes one most suspicious of the presence of AFS. The mucin is characteristically rubbery and frequently difficult to suction out, but often visibly nestled within the polyps (Fig. 20–4). The patient may

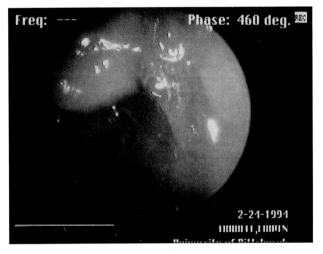

FIGURE 20–4 Endoscopic photo demonstrating translucent green allergic mucin nestled in nasal polyps.

give a history of blowing out thick tenacious rubbery mucus on occasion. They are never able to completely expel the mucin, and the disease persists.

Manning and Holman[19] cataloged the patient characteristics of AFS based on a literature review of AFS cases defined by the presence of allergic mucin with histologic evidence of fungal forms or by allergic mucin with positive fungal cultures. They did not give the number of cases that met the former criteria, although 168 cases had positive fungal cultures. Other reviews had noted an equal male-to-female ratio and a mean age of 26 years.[10] Manning and Holman[19] found a male predominance with a male-to-female ratio of 1:6. They also found a slightly younger average age of 23.3 years. Ages ranged from a low of 7 years to a high of 62 years.

Allergic Rhinitis

In a review of the cases in the literature, only 63% of patients with AFS give a history of allergic rhinitis.[19] However, many of these series never rigorously evaluated the subjects for allergies. Mabry et al[31] specifically assessed 16 consecutive patients with histologic evidence of AFS. They found that 15 of 16 (90%) had a Class II or greater response to at least one antigen by in vitro testing. Because *Bipolaris* antigen is not available commercially for skin or in vitro testing, even the one nonreactor might have been positive if the pertinent fungi had been assayed. There are no studies that definitively document the absence of allergy in patients with AFS. By and large most patients show a marked Type I hypersensitivity to multiple fungi as well as other allergens. Table 20–2 shows the fungal hypersensitivity found by Mabry and colleagues[31] in nine patients with AFS. All patients were allergic to multiple fungal antigens.

TABLE 20–2   Fungal Antigens Included in Testing and Treatment Protocol

Antigen	Patients Testing Positive/Total Patients
Alternaria	9/9
Aspergillus	8/9
Cladosporium	5/9
Curvularia	8/9
Epicoccum	7/9
Fusarium	7/9
Helminthosporium	9/9
Mucor	7/9
Penicillium	4/9
Pullularia	5/9
Stemphyllium	8/9

Used with permission from Mabry RL, Manning SC, Mabry CS. Immunotherapy in the treatment of allergic fungal sinusitis. *Otolaryngol.* 1997;116:31–35.

■ Asthma

Asthma was present in 41% of patients in the most recent comprehensive review.[35] Detailed reading of the original sources reveals that the asthma when present is usually mild and not steroid dependent. Other series report asthma rates ranging from 33 to 54%.[10,19]

Rarely are patients with the "triad syndrome" of nasal polyposis, aspirin sensitivity, and asthma diagnosed with AFS. Cody et al[16] reported a 27% incidence of triad syndrome in a series of patients from the Mayo Clinic; however, when patients without culture or histopathologic evidence of fungi are excluded from this series, then no classic AFS patients demonstrated aspirin-sensitive asthma.

■ Ocular Findings

Growth of polyps and continued accumulation of the allergic fungal mucin may cause nasal widening and proptosis, especially in the younger population. In some series, the incidence of proptosis approaches 20%.[32] Reversible blindness secondary to sphenoid involvement has been reported in several case reports. Prompt surgical decompression with systemic steroid therapy is advocated in these cases.

■ Intracranial Findings

Generally, intracranial extension is asymptomatic and discovered only when imaging is performed. As mentioned under the pathophysiology section, there is one case reported of intracranial fungal infection following surgery for a mucopyocele associated with AFS.

■ Staging System

Kupferberg et al[18] developed a staging system with which to follow patients for recurrence of AFS following surgery. They found that these physical findings appear before the return of subjective clinical symptoms (Table 20–3).

Occasionally, AFS may be diagnosed in patients who have had previous sinus surgery in which recurrent polyps are not present; rather, the distinctive translucent green mucin is noted in an opened maxillary sinus, and removal

TABLE 20–3   AFS Endoscopic Staging System

Stage 0	No evidence of disease
Stage 1	Edematous mucosa/allergic mucin
Stage 2	Polypoid mucosa/allergic mucin
Stage 3	Polyps and fungal debris

Used with permission from Kupferberg SB, Bent JP III, Kuhn FA. Prognosis for allergic fungal sinusitis. *Otolaryngol Head Neck Surg.* 1997;117(1):35–41.

TABLE 20–4   Endoscopic Grading System for AFS

Stage 0	No evidence of disease
Stage 1	Edematous mucosa/no allergic mucin
Stage 2	Polyps/no allergic mucin
Stage 3	Presence of allergic mucin

Modified with permission from Kupferberg SB, Bent JP III, Kuhn FA. Prognosis for allergic fungal sinusitis. *Otolaryngol Head Neck Surg.* 1997;117(1):35–41.

with histopathologic examination reveals AFS. In addition, it is unclear from Kupferberg et al's article how one distinguishes allergic mucin from fungal debris. Certainly, if the allergic mucin is subjected to histopathologic examination, one finds evidence of AFS. For these reasons, I propose the following modifications of the Kupferberg et al endoscopic staging system outlined in Table 20–4.

Geography and Exposure to Fungal Sources

Many have noted that AFS appears more common in the warm humid climates of the southern United States and along the Mississippi River. The mold counts in these areas are also significantly greater than in other locations. The greatest number of reported cases and published reports come from central Texas and Arizona.[19,27] The initial series by Katzenstein et al[2] from St. Louis reported a 7% incidence of AFS among all sinus cases. Cases of AFS have been reported from desert areas, including Saudi Arabia. A large surge in the number of AFS cases in San Diego

occurred in personnel involved in Operation Desert Storm who returned to their home base in San Diego. A few years after the conflict, the number of cases of AFS seen in San Diego in the military population was markedly decreased (D. Hunsaker, personal communication, 1999).

Numerous fungi are responsible for AFS. The causative organism is frequently recovered from air samples of the residences of the affected patients. No association between fungi causing AFS and the fungi cultured from suspected sick buildings has been established.[20]

Imaging

Computed tomography of the sinuses in patients with AFS shows characteristic findings, which, though not diagnostic, are sufficient that the diagnosis should be strongly considered. These findings are hyperattenuation of the intrasinus contents, multiple sinus involvement, and bony erosion. In a retrospective review of the CTs of 45 patients with AFS, all patients had intrasinus high-attenuation areas. Multiple sinus involvement was present in 43 of 45 patients. Bilateral sinus involvement occurred in 51%, and the remaining 49% had unilateral disease.[12] These areas of high attenuation represent thick allergic mucin. Surrounding the mucin is the lower-attenuation soft tissue densities of the hyperplastic mucosa lining the sinuses and the nasal polyps (Fig. 20–5) Bony remodeling or erosion is common (91%)[12];

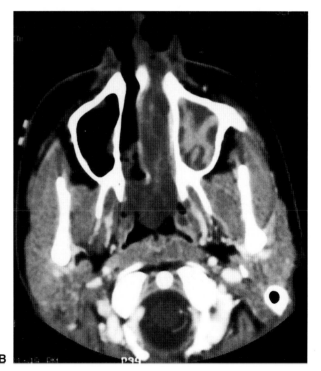

A

B

FIGURE 20–5   (A) Coronal sinus CT demonstrating absent bone between the cranial cavity and ethmoids secondary to bony erosion from AFS. (B) Axial sinus CT of same patient demonstrating hyperattenuation of mucin in central cavity of maxillary sinus. Nasal polyposis produced the soft tissue density obstructing the right nasal airway.

it is thought to be secondary to pressure atrophy or the release of inflammatory mediators that dissolve bone, and is not due to fungal invasion. Invasive fungal sinusitis requires histologic documentation. I know of no cases where histologic invasion is convincingly demonstrated in a patient with AFS, despite the common finding of bony erosion.

Enhanced sinus CTs are unnecessary and rarely add to the diagnosis. The mucin does not take up the contrast agent.[12]

Magnetic resonance imaging of the sinuses is inferior to CT in diagnosing and assessing patients with presumed AFS. MRI is not able to give important information regarding bony landmarks, and if interpreted without CT scan information, it may fool the clinician into thinking that no abnormality is present. The proteinaceous allergic fungal mucin may show up as a signal void, particularly on T2-weighted images. In 1988, Jay et al[32] were the first to note these characteristic MRI findings and compare them to CT. The higher attenuation areas in the central areas of the sinuses correlated to areas of diminished signal on both T1 and T2 MRI. The surrounding sinus mucosa reflected an increased signal on T2 MRI.

Criteria for Diagnosis of AFS

Bent and Kuhn[33] defined the criteria necessary to diagnose of AFS as: (1) Type I hypersensitivity confirmed by history, skin tests, or serology; (2) nasal polyposis; (3) characteristic CT scans; (4) eosinophilic mucus without fungal invasion into sinus tissue; and (5) positive fungal stain of sinus contents or culture. Other investigators have suggested similar requirements with a few changes, such as omitting the requirement of a history of Type I hypersensitivity, while requiring absence of immunologic suppression.[6] Although all of these are usually found in patients with AFS, I have had a few patients who did not fit these criteria, yet they would clearly be diagnosed as having AFS, based on the histopathologic appearance of the mucin extracted from their sinuses. For example, I have treated two patients who had had previous surgery and became symptomatic. Allergic mucin was noted to be present in the absence of polyps, and histopathologic examination revealed eosinophilic mucin with hyphae. They had no CT scan or polyps. We do not know whether AFS becomes invasive if occurring in a patient who is subsequently immunosuppressed. It seems to me that the simplest criteria that allows one to diagnose this entity without including often-associated findings is the most prudent. Therefore, I agree with the criteria used by Manning and Holman[19] in their comprehensive review of cases with AFS, which was to include those patients with the characteristic histopathology of eosinophilic mucin containing hyphae. In addition, I require the presence of Type I (IgE)–mediated response

to the cultured fungus. Thus, the simplest, most straightforward requirement for defining patients as having AFS is

1. Presence of eosinophilic mucin with hyphae from the nose or sinuses
2. Demonstration of IgE-mediated allergy to the fungus

Occasional difficulties with these strict criteria include those patients with negative fungal cultures who have hyphae present in the mucin. This is usually attributed to inappropriate handling, collection, or plating. In addition, demonstration of IgE-mediated fungal hypersensitivity may be difficult due to lack of available commercial antigens for testing certain fungi, such as *Bipolaris* species. However, most patients with AFS demonstrate moderately high reactivity to multiple fungal antigens. By in vitro RAST testing, Mabry et al found some degree of sensitivity to almost every fungal antigen tested, with most fungal allergens demonstrating a Class II or greater.[34] Although there was a predictable correlation between RAST and intradermal dilutional testing, skin testing frequently indicated a greater sensitivity than predicted by RAST.

■ Conclusion

Although AFS was recognized only two decades ago, there are over 400 well-documented cases in the literature. It is a distinctive form of fungal sinusitis characterized by an IgE-mediated hypersensitivity reaction to the fungus. AFS is diagnosed by its characteristic histopathology of eosinophilic mucin with hyphal presence. Many fungi may cause the entity, with the most common being the *Bipolaris* species. The disease process is similar irrespective of the causative fungal agent. A very high degree of suspicion for AFS can be entertained if the patient is young, allergic, and has nasal polyps, and sinus CT shows increased attenuation in the central sinus cavities or bony remodeling or erosion. Serologic evaluation that supports the diagnosis is a total IgE in excess of 600 IU/mL, a peripheral eosinophilia, and elevated specific IgE or IgG to various fungi.

REFERENCES

1. Millar JW, Johnston A, Lamb D. Allergic aspergillosis of the maxillary sinuses *Thorax.* 1981;36:710.
2. Katzenstein ALA, Sale SR, Greenberger PA. Allergic aspergillus sinusitis: a newly recognized form of sinusitis. *J Allergy Clin Immunol.* 1983;72:89–93.
3. Washburn RD, Kennedy DW, Begley MD, et al. Chronic fungal sinusitis in apparently normal hosts. *Medicine (Baltimore).* 1988;67:231–247.
4. Ence BK, Gourley DS, Jorgenson NL, et al. Allergic fungal sinusitis. *Am J Rhinol.* 1990;4:169–178.
5. Milosev B, Mahboub ES, Aal OA, et al. Primary aspergilloma of paranasal sinuses in the Sudan: a review of seventeen cases. *Br J Surg.* 1969;56(2):132–137.

6. DeShazo RD, Chapin K, Swain RE. Fungal sinusitis. *N Engl J Med.* 1997;337(4):254–259.

7. Manning SC, Shaefer SD, Close LG, et al. Culture-positive allergic fungal sinusitis. *Arch Otolaryngol Head Neck Surg.* 1991;117:174–208.

8. Graham SM, Ballas ZK. Preoperative steroids confuse the diagnosis of allergic fungal sinusitis. *J Allergy Clin Immunol.* 1998;101(1, pt 1): 139–140.

9. Allphin AL, Strauss M, Abdul-Karim FW. Allergic fungal sinusitis: problems in diagnosis and treatment. *Laryngoscope.* 1991;101: 815–820.

10. Corey JF, Delsupehe KG, Ferguson BJ. Allergic fungal sinusitis: allergic, infectious, or both? *Otolaryngol Head Neck Surg.* 1995;113: 110–119.

11. Waxman JE, Spector JG, Sale SR. Allergic *Aspergillus* sinusitis: concepts in diagnosis and treatment of a new clinical entity. *Laryngoscope.* 1987;97:261–266.

12. Mukherji SK, Figueroa RE, Ginsberg LE, et al. Allergic fungal sinusitis: CT findings. *Radiology.* 1998;207(2):417–422.

13. Ramadan HH, Qurishi HA. Allergic mucin sinusitis without fungus. *Am J Rhinol.* 1997;11(2):145–147.

14. Vignola AM, Chanes P, Chiappara G, et al. Evaluation of apoptosis of eosinophils, macrophages, and T lymphocytes in mucosal biopsy specimens of patients with asthma and chronic bronchitis. *J Allergy Clin Immunol.* 1999;103:563–573.

15. Ponikau JU, Sherris DA, Kern EB, et al. The diagnosis and incidence of allergic fungal sinusitis. Mayo Clin Proc 1999:74(9):877–844

16. Cody DT, Neel HB, Ferreiro JA, et al. Allergic fungal sinusitis: the Mayo clinic experience. *Laryngoscope.* 1994;104:1074–1079.

17. Green BJ, Mitakakis TZ, Tovey ER. Allergen detection from 11 fungal species before and after germination. *J Allergy Clin Immunol.* 2003; 111:285–289.

18. Kupferberg SB, Bent JP III, Kuhn FA. Prognosis for allergic fungal sinusitis. *Otolaryngol Head Neck Surg.* 1997;117(1):35–41.

19. Manning SC, Holman M. Further evidence for allergic pathophysiology in allergic fungal sinusitis. *Laryngoscope.* 1998;108:1485–1496.

20. Noble JA, Crow SA, Ahearn DG, et al. Allergic fungal sinusitis in the Southeastern USA: involvement of a new agent *Epicoccum nigrum Ehrenb. Ex Schlects.* 1824. *J Med Vet Mycol.* 1997;35(6):405–409.

21. Clark S, Campbell CK, Sandison A, et al. Schizophyllum commune: an unusual isolate from a patient with allergic fungal sinusitis. *J Infect.* 1996;32(2):147–150.

22. Cox GM, Schell WA, Scher RL, et al. First report of involvement of *Nodulisporium* species in human disease. *J Clin Immunol.* 1994; 32(9):2301–2304.

23. Ricketti AJ, Greenberger PA, Patterson R. Serum IgE as an important aid in management of allergic bronchopulmonary aspergillosis. *J Allergy Clin Immunol.* 1984;74:68–71.

24. Geha RS. Circulating immune complexes and activation of the complement sequence in acute allergic bronchopulmonary aspergillosis. *J Allergy Clin Immunol.* 1997;60:357.

25. Kuhn FA, Javer A. Utilizing fungal specific IgE levels as a serological marker for allergic fungal sinusitis (AFS) activity [abstract]. American Rhinologic Society Spring Meeting, 1999.

26. Schubert MS, Goetz DW. Evaluation and treatment of allergic fungal sinusitis: II. Treatment and follow up. *J Allergy Clin Immunol.* 1998; 102(3):395–402.

27. Schubert MS, Goetz DW. Evaluation and treatment of allergic fungal sinusitis: I. Demographics and diagnosis. *J Allergy Clin Immunol.* 1998;102(3):387–394.

28. Safirstein BH. Allergic bronchopulmonary *Aspergillosis* with obstruction of the upper respiratory tract. *Chest.* 1976;70:788–790.

29. Zieske L, Koopke R, Hamill R. Dematiaceous fungal sinusitis. *Otolaryngol Head Neck Surg.* 1991;105:567–577.

30. Tsimikas S, Hollingsworth HM, Nash G. *Aspergillus* sinusitis with concurrent allergic bronchopulmonary *Aspergillus* sinusitis. *J Allergy Clin Immunol.* 1994;94:264–267.

31. Mabry RL, Manning SC, Mabry CS. Immunotherapy in then treatment of allergic fungal sinusitis. *Otolaryngol Head Neck Surg.* 1997; 116:31–35.

32. Jay WM, Bradsher RW, Snyderman N, et al. Ocular involvement in mycotic sinusitis caused by *Bipolaris. Am J Ophthalmol.* 1988;105: 366–370.

33. Bent JP III, Kuhn FA. Antifungal activity against allergic fungal sinusitis organisms. *Laryngoscope.* 1996;106:1331–1334.

34. Mabry RL, Marple B, Mabry CS. Mold testing by RAST and skin test methods in patients with allergic fungal sinusitis. *Otolaryngol Head Neck Surg.* 1999;121:252–254.

35. Ferguson BJ. Eosinophilic mucin rhinosinusitis—a distinctive clinicopathological entity. *Laryngoscope.* 2000;110(5):799–813.

36. Ferguson BJ, Barnes L, Bernstein JM, et al. Geographic variation in allergic fungal rhinosinusitis. *Otolaryngol Clin North Am.* 2000;33: 441–449

21

Meningoencephaloceles and Cerebrospinal Fluid Leak

HOWARD L. LEVINE

Although cerebrospinal fluid (CSF) leaks and meningoencephaloceles are uncommon problems facing the nasal sinus surgeon, their consequences are significant and may even be catastrophic. These intracranial and sinus-related problems may be congenital, idiopathic, traumatic, or iatrogenic. Many nasal and sinus surgeons have the ability and technology to endoscopically diagnose and manage meningoceles, meningoencephaloceles, and cerebrospinal fluid leak. Office nasal endoscopy and intraoperative endoscopy with image-guided triplanar localization surgery have advanced the success in managing these problems and reduced the morbidity and mortality for the patient. Many physicians now feel that an intranasal endoscopic approach is warranted as a first try for the majority of patients with pathology arising in the anterior cranial fossa and extending into and involving the paranasal sinuses.

■ Cerebrospinal Fluid Leak

Since World War I CSF leakage has been described as traumatic or nontraumatic.[1] Approximately 90% of CSF rhinorrhea is traumatic in origin, and the trauma may be surgically or nonsurgically induced. Nonsurgical trauma is usually from blunt or projectile injury and is generally associated with other intracranial injuries. Surgical trauma is usually from intracranial surgery, pituitary surgery, or paranasal sinus surgery. One to 3% of head trauma will have CSF leaks.[2] Over two-thirds of traumatic CSF leaks stop within the first month. CSF otorrhea has a greater chance of spontaneous resolution than sinus and/or paranasal rhinorrhea.[2–4] Consideration

is given to repairing post-traumatic CSF leaks if there is still active leaking after 14 days especially because prophylactic antibiotics do not always prevent meningitis.[5] The most common nasal and paranasal sinus locations for CSF leakage are the frontal sinus, cribriform plate, and sphenoid sinus.

Nontraumatic sources of CSF leak are from the cribriform plate, sella turcica, sphenoid sinus, or posterior ethmoid sinus. Nontraumatic causes of CSF leak are divided into normal pressure and high pressure. Females are more affected than males, and most often the spontaneous rhinorrhea begins with a sneeze, cough, or straining. About 45% of spontaneous leaks are from high pressure. High pressure in the subarachnoid space probably forces spinal fluid through a weakened area such as the cribriform plate. Slow-growing tumors (usually pituitary) account for 84% of high-pressure CSF rhinorrhea. The remaining cases of CSF rhinorrhea are related to hydrocephalus.[6]

Normal-pressure CSF leaks account for 55% of spontaneous leaks. These are usually caused by slow erosion of the skull base associated with intracranial tumors, mucoceles, osteomata, and nasal and/or sinus neoplasms (nasopharyngeal angiofibromaa, nasopharyngeal carcinomas), or through congenital pathways (craniopharyngeal canal, meningoencephaloceles), hydrocephalus, or low-pressure flow as with bony erosion, seller atrophy, olfactory atrophy, congenital anomalies, and idiopathic.[6]

The preoperative CT scan provides data helpful in the prevention of CSF leaks. Critical areas to look at are the roofs of the ethmoid sinus and the cribriform plate. It is important to look at the level of the cribriform plate and the relationship to the roof of the ethmoid sinus. The cribriform plate is generally lower than the roof of the ethmoid sinus but may be lower by several millimeters. Ideally, axial, coronal, and sagittal CT scans are needed to have the most complete views of the sinuses. The axial CT provides valuable information about the anteroposterior dimension of the frontal and sphenoid sinuses. The sagittal view provides information about the height and roof of the ethmoid and sphenoid sinus. For difficult cases where the pathology has altered the anatomy or in revision surgery, image-guided technology is helpful in minimizing the chances of trauma.

To minimize the chances of intraoperative trauma causing CSF leak, it is important to consider the areas to avoid, proper instrumentation, and surgical technique.

There are a few common places where intracranial violation of the nasal sinus cavity occurs during sinus surgery. Each of these relates to the anatomical features of that area. One of the most common areas is the junction between the middle turbinate and the roof of the ethmoid sinus. Here the bone is generally quite thin (Fig. 21–1). It is apparent on many CT scans that there is a thicker bony plate forming the majority of the middle turbinate; however, the bone becomes very thin superiorly near the attachment. The roof of the ethmoid

sinus is generally higher than the nasal cavity roof (cribriform plate) (Fig. 21–2). The attachment of the middle turbinate to the roof of the fovea ethmoidalis is not a simple vertical attachment. Rather, the middle turbinate tends to slope slightly laterally in this area, narrowing the region. This puts this bone at risk because of the sloping and thinness and because there frequently are polyps present in this region that may have altered the anatomy.

The area of the cribriform plate is a potential area for injury. Although the bone is generally thicker than the fovea ethmoidalis, it is perforated by the olfactory fibers, and the dura is tightly adherent. The lateral cribriform plate is especially vulnerable in the region of the anterior ethmoid artery. This is one of the areas of least resistance in the anterior skull base.[7]

Another area at risk for injury is the junction of the posterior ethmoid sinus air cells and the front wall of the sphenoid sinus. The bone of the anterior sphenoid wall is generally very thin, making this region vulnerable to injury. This area may be injured in following the ethmoid sinus air cells posteriorly and inadvertently working superiorly (Fig. 21–3). Injury also may occur in trying to open the front face of the sphenoid sinus.

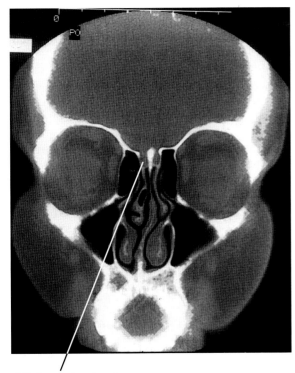

Thin bone at junction of
middle turbinate and ethmoid
sinus roof

FIGURE 21–1 Thin bone at the junction of the fovea ethmoidalis of the ethmoid sinus and the middle turbinate is an area of injury causing CSF leak.

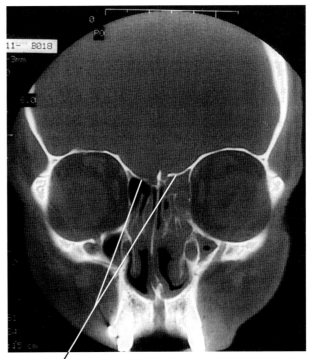

Different heights of
foula ethmoidalis

FIGURE 21–2 Care must be taken when operating in the region of the ethmoid sinus roof and cribriform plate. The roof of the ethmoid sinus is higher than the cribriform plate; therefore, knowing the location of one does not ensure knowing the location of the other.

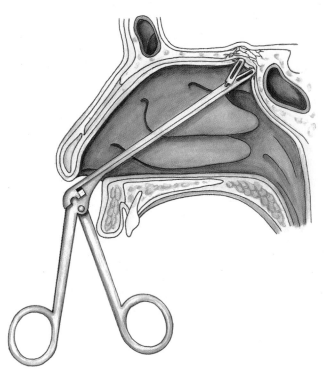

FIGURE 21–3   Injury may occur at the junction of the ethmoid sinus roof and the anterior face of the sphenoid sinus, causing CSF leak.

Proper choice and use of surgical instruments help to avoid trauma to the roof of the sinus and nasal cavity. Typical instruments for traditional and endoscopic sinus surgery have been grasping forceps and curettes. Curettes have been used in the removal of the air cell partitions of the ethmoid sinus. Removal of bone with curettes can inadvertently fracture the bone into the roof either exposing dura or lacerating dura and creating a CSF leak.

CONTROVERSY

This author does not use curettes because of the seemingly increased risk for injury when working along the fovea ethmoidalis. In this region, small spicules of bone extending down from the fovea ethmoidalis from ethmoid air cell partitions may be fractured with a curette and cause injury to the sinus roof. In the past, soft tissue–type cup forceps have been used to remove polyps and thin bony partitions. These have the tendency to tear mucosa. This has the potential of tearing bone along with the mucosa and creating an injury. Newer micro-powered endoscopic instruments preserve mucosa and create a delicacy when coupled with endoscopes and accuracy when combined with image-guided triplanar surgical localization.

The diagnosis of a CSF leak is made clinically and roentgenographically. Cerebrospinal fluid is a watery clear, nonsticky fluid that is low in protein and high in sugar and has a low specific gravity. The normal volume of cerebrospinal fluid is ~150 mL. It is formed at the rate of ~0.35 mL/minute (~150 mL three times a day). A ring or halo sign may diagnose a CSF leak. If drops of CSF are mixed with blood and are placed on gauze or found on bed linens, a lighter halo forms around the bloodier central area. Glucose determination of the nasal secretions is helpful in making the diagnosis of CSF rhinorrhea. Glucose oxidase paper is generally unreliable. Although CSF contains glucose generally in a concentration greater than 30% per mg and the glucose oxidase paper is sensitive to glucose of less than 5% per mg, there is a false-positive rate of 45 to 75%, especially when there is blood contaminating the fluid.[8] The absence of a positive test is probably more helpful. Quantitative glucose measurements identify CSF if it contains more than 30 mg per 100 mL of glucose. Protein analysis of the fluid is more reliable if there is greater than 45 % per mg.

More recently β_2-transferrin has been considered as the most definitive test to determine the presence of CSF rhinorrhea.[9,10] This protein is highly specific for human CSF. About 1 cc of fluid is needed.

There are several tests that are used to determine the actual presence and site of CSF leakage from within the sinus or nasal cavity.

Fluorescein is one of several intrathecal dyes that have been used.[11] Five to 10 mL of cerebrospinal fluid are used to dilute 0.25 to 1.0 mL of 5% fluorescein. This is injected intrathecally. The appearance of fluorescein is visualized either directly or through the placement of neurosurgical cotton pledgets. The cotton pledgets are placed in the nasal and/or sinus cavity and can be located in several different sites in the nose (eustachian tube orifice, sphenoethmoid recess, anterior ostiomeatal complex, and cribriform plate). The patient is put in a head-down position. The nose can be examined endoscopically, and the pledgets also can be examined to determine the site of leakage. Radioactive scanning has also been used. Pledgets are inserted into similar areas. A lumbar puncture is performed, and an isotope is injected. The pledgets are removed after an appropriate time and scanned.

A great advance in diagnosis has been the use of intrathecal contrast (metrizamide) combined with CT scanning.[12,13] This has become the most accurate and appropriate method of testing. This is best for making the diagnosis of CSF leak when there is active leaking. A slow or intermittent leak may not be detected. Several contrast materials are used such as Isovue Omnipaque, a nonionic material that has decreased reactions. This is injected through a lumbar puncture. Thin-sectioned CT

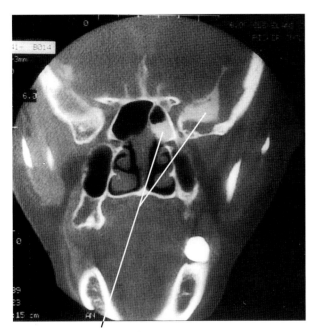

Intrathecal contrast intracranial
and in left sphenoid sinus

FIGURE 21–4 Intrathecal contrast material identifying CSF leakage in the anterior ethmoid sinus.

scan is performed usually in a coronal, but occasionally also an axial, view (Fig. 21–4).

Management of CSF leak may be conservative or invasive. About 70% of traumatic leaks will resolve spontaneously within the first week.[12] Meningitis occurs in ~20% of patients with CSF rhinorrhea.[14] There is a higher incidence in spontaneous and postoperative CSF rhinorrhea than nonsurgical post-traumatic CSF.[15] Over 50% of patients with meningitis from CSF rhinorrhea had their meningitis over 1 year after their traumatic event.[16] *Streptococcus pneumoniae* is the organism seen in over 83% of patients with meningitis from trauma.[17]

Sinus or nasal meningoencephaloceles may be confused with sinus or nasal polyps. The intranasal or intrasinus meningoceles are pale gray pulsatile masses that are compressible and slightly translucent. Meningoceles most commonly arise from the sinus roof, whereas polyps arise from the lateral nasal wall. If a meningocele or meningoencephalocele is suspected, an MR image is obtained. Because the density of brain parenchyma and neoplasms or polyps appears the same on CT scans, MRI is helpful in distinguishing inflammatory, neoplastic, and intracranial tissue.[18] MRI has advantages over CT such as direct orthogonal scanning in virtually any plane, improved soft tissue resolution, and the choice of various acquisitions to distinguish various tissues. A T1-weighted coronal and/or sagittal MR image through the cribriform plate will optimally display brain herniation into

the ethmoid sinus or nasal cavity. An isolated soft tissue mass adhering to the cribriform plate and fovea ethmoidalis should raise the suspicion of a meningocele.[18]

Conservative management of CSF leaks involves repeated lumbar puncture or insertion of an indwelling subarachnoid drainage catheter for several days. Although this is advocated by many authors, there is some controversy in the use of lumbar drainage because of the theoretical risk of promoting a retrograde CSF infection or pneumocephalus.[19] Patients are kept at bed rest with the head slightly elevated. Cerebrospinal fluid is removed at ~50 mL per shift to lessen the pressure and hopefully allow the leak to seal. A parental antibiotic that crosses the blood-brain barrier is usually given. All efforts are made to reduce any straining or significant Valsalva's maneuver, as well as sneezing and coughing. Stool softeners are used. If flow continues after 10 to 12 days, or if there is incomplete resolution of symptoms or intermittent leak after 3 to 4 weeks, meningitis, or compromised tissue causing potentially poor healing (radiation, immune-compromised state), then surgical intervention is considered.[20]

There are several surgical approaches to consider. The traditional approach has been a bifrontal craniotomy with galeal flap to line the anterior cranial fossa.[20] This is effective and is used when more conservative nonsurgical and surgical approaches have failed. It has greater morbidity and cost than other, newer surgical approaches.

In the past, otolaryngologists have used several external and transnasal approaches in an attempt to extracranially repair CSF leaks. With the recent advances in endoscopic sinus surgical techniques and also with image-guided endoscopic sinus surgery, repairs are now done intranasally and endoscopically with greater accuracy and success.

Septal mucoperichondrial flaps can be created. These are based posteriorly in the nasal cavity. Generally, a common cavity is created in the nose and sinuses. The flap is rotated into the defect and packed in place. Another flap used is the osteomucoperichondrial flap. It is created from the medial ethmoid sinus wall and middle turbinate. It is also rotated into the defect and packed in place.

Several authors have used a free muscle, fascia, cartilage, or mucosal flap from the middle turbinate, depending on the defect.[21–23] If a sizable defect is present and there is herniation of the dura and/or the brain, a free graft of cartilage is obtained from the nasal septum. It is shaped to fit into the defect. It is secured with "tissue glue" made from fibrin and cryoprecipitate.[24–27] Generally, muscle and/or fascia are placed over this. For smaller defects, fascia alone is used. It is placed over the defect and if possible tucked under the edges of the defect (much like an underlay technique used in tympanoplasty). This graft is also secured with "tissue glue," and muscle is

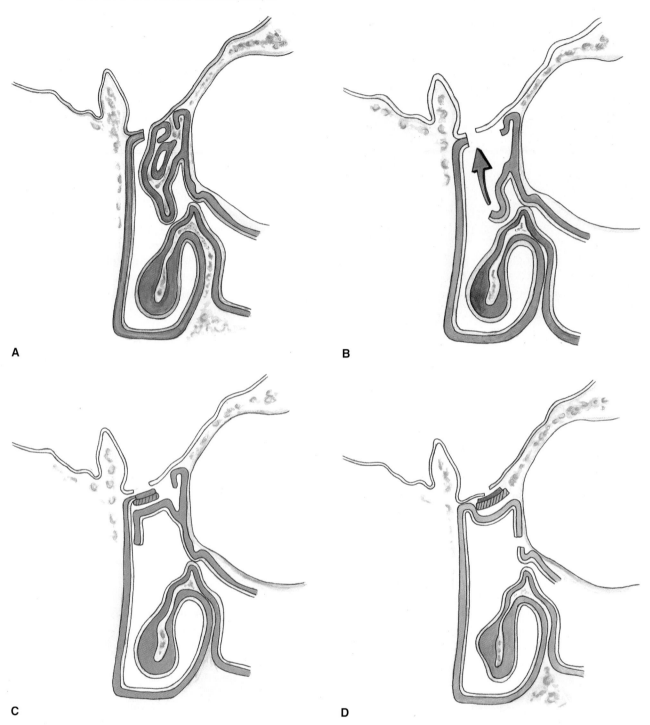

A

B

C

D

FIGURE 21–5   Rotation of the middle turbinate flap over the fovea ethmoidalis defect.

placed over it. If any of the middle turbinate is left from a previous surgery or previous attempts at repair, the lateral mucosa and bone (for ethmoid defects) or the medial mucosa and bone (for cribriform plate defects) is rotated over the repair to give a mucosal lining over the nasal/sinus side (Fig. 21–5). The graft or flap is packed into place with Gelfoam, and a sponge tampon is used to hold the tissue and packing in place. This is left in place for several days with the patient at bed rest and an indwelling subarachnoid catheter drain.

Surgical management of meningoceles depends on the size. Small masses may be gently pushed back intracranially and the defect repaired with a fascia or cartilage graft using methods similar to CSF leak repair.

Larger meningoceles are excised using bipolar cautery, and the defect is repaired just as the bony defect from the CSF leak was repaired.

REFERENCES

1. Calcatera TC. Extracranial surgical repair of cerebrospinal rhinorrhea. *Ann Otolaryngol.* 1980;89:108–116.
2. Brisman R, Hughes JE, Mount L. Cerebrospinal rhinorrhea. *Arch Neurol* 1970;22:245–252.
3. Dandy WE. Treatment of rhinorrhea and otorrhea. *Arch Surg.* 1944:4975–4985.
4. Lewin W. Cerebrospinal fluid rhinorrhea in closed head injuries. *Br J Surg.* 1954;42:1–18.
5. Leech PJ, Paterson A. Conservative and operative management for cerebrospinal fluid leakage after closed head injury. *Lancet.* 1973; 1:1013–1015.
6. Shugar JMA, Som PM, Eisman W, et al. Non-traumatic cerebrospinal fluid rhinorrhea. *Laryngoscope.* 1981;91:114–120.
7. Kaintz J, Stammberger H. The roof of the anterior ethmoid: a place of least resistance in the skull base. *Rhinology.* 1990;3:191–199.
8. Katz RT, Kaplan PE. Glucose oxidase sticks and cerebrospinal fluid rhinorrhea. *Arch Phys Med Rehabil.* 1985;66(6):391–393.
9. Yokoyama K, Hasegawa M, Shiba KS, et al. Diagnosis of CSF rhinorrhea: detection of tau-transferrin in nasal discharge. *Otolaryngol Head Neck Surg.* 1988;98(4):328–332.
10. Oberascher G. A modern concept of cerebrospinal fluid diagnosis in oto- and rhinorrhea. *Rhinology.* 1988;26(2):89–103.
11. Kirchner FR, Proud GO. Method for the identification and localization of cerebrospinal fluid, rhinorrhea and otorrhea. *Laryngoscope.* 1960;70:921–931.
12. Park JI, Strelzow VV, Friedman WH. Current management of cerebrospinal fluid rhinorrhea. *Laryngoscope.* 1983;93:1293–1300.
13. Luotonene J, Jokinen K, Laitinen J. Localization of CSF fistula by metrizamide CT cisternography. *J Laryngeal Otolaryngol.* 1986;100: 955–958.
14. Spetzler RF, Zabramski JM. Cerebrospinal fluid fistula. *Contemp Neurosurg.* 1986;8(1):1–5.
15. Ommaya AK. Cerebrospinal fluid rhinorrhea. *Neurology.* 1964;14: 106–113.
16. Laun A. Traumatic cerebrospinal fluid fistulas in the anterior and middle cranial fossa. *Acta Neurochir (Wien).* 1982;60:215–222.
17. Hand WL, Sanford JP. Posttraumatic bacterial meningitis. *Ann Intern Med.* 1970;72:869–874.
18. Zinreich SJ, Borders JC, Eisele DW, Mattox DE, Long DM, Kennedy DW. The utility of magnetic resonance imaging in the diagnosis of intranasal meningoencephaloceles. *Arch Otolaryngol Head Neck Surg.* 1992;118:1253–1256.
19. Graf CJ, Gross CE, Beck DW. Complications of spinal drainage in the management of cerebrospinal fluid fistula. *J Neurosurg.* 1981; 54(3):392–395.
20. Davies MA, Teo C. Management of traumatic cerebrospinal fluid fistula. *J Craniomaxillofac Trauma.* 1995;1(2):9–17.
21. Papay FA, Benninger MS, Levine HL, Lavertu P. Transnasalendoscopic repair of sphenoidal cerebral spinal fluid fistula. *Otolaryngol Head Neck Surg.* 1989;101(8):595–597.
22. Papay FA, Maggiano H, Dominquez S, Hasselbusch SJ, Levine HL, Lavertu P. Rigid endoscopic repair of paranasal sinus cerebrospinal fluid fistulas. *Laryngoscope.* 1989;99:1195–1201.
23. Stankiewcz JA. Cerebrospinal fluid fistula and endoscopic sinus surgery *Laryngoscope.* 1991;101:250–256.
24. Sponitz WD, Mintz PD, Avery N, Bitchell TC, Kaul S, Nolan SP. Fibrin glue from stored human plasma. *Am Surg.* 1987;53(8): 460–462.
25. Sierra DH, Nissen AJ, Welch J. The use of fibrin glue in intracranial procedures: preliminary results. *Laryngoscope.* 1990;100:360–363.
26. Dodson EE, Gross CW, Swerdloff JL, Gustafson LM. Transnasal endoscopic repair of cerebrospinal fluid rhinorrhea and skull base defects: a review of twenty-nine cases. *Otolaryngol Head Neck Surg.* 1994;111:600–605.
27. Persky MS, Rothstein SG, Breda SD, Cohen NL, Cooper P, Ransohoff J. Extracranial repair of cerebrospinal fluid otorhinorrhea. *Laryngoscope.* 1991;101:134–136.

22

Endoscopic Orbital Decompression

RALPH B. METSON AND MATHEW COSENZA

Graves' disease is an autoimmune disorder that most commonly affects the thyroid gland and *orbit*. The term *dysthyroid* orbitopathy is used to describe the ocular manifestations of Graves' disease, which include orbital congestion with enlargement of extraocular muscles and fat. This discrepancy between the volume of the bony orbit and its contents results in proptosis, which can have both cosmetic and vision-threatening consequences.

Dysthyroid orbitopathy appears to follow a clinical course independent of thyroid gland dysfunction or treatment. The severity and stage of the eye findings often bear little relation to the degree of the thyroid abnormalities. Thyroid gland treatment affects only one end-organ of this disease process and does not alter the fundamental autoimmune process causing the orbitopathy. Surprisingly, 10% of patients with dysthyroid orbitopathy display no endocrine function abnormality at any period throughout their life.

The initial acute phase of dysthyroid orbitopathy typically lasts 6 to 18 months and is associated with inflammation and congestion of the orbital contents.[1] An increase in the volume of soft tissue leads to elevated intraorbital pressure, with a resultant anterior displacement of the globe. In severe cases, exposure keratitis, diplopia, and optic neuropathy with visual impairment can result. The typical progression of signs and symptoms has been described by the acronym NOSPECS (Table 22–1). Corticosteroids may be useful for the initial treatment of these inflammatory symptoms; however, the symptoms generally recur unless the steroids are continued long term. Low-dose irradiation with ~20 Gy can be effective in limiting the lymphocytic

process leading to the orbital congestion and optic neuropathy.

A chronic, stable phase of dysthyroid orbitopathy occurs as much as 3 years after the onset of the orbital findings. Enlargement and fibrosis of the extraocular muscles and an increase in the amount of orbital fat are permanent changes that may require surgical therapy. Surgery is usually performed once the orbital process has stabilized. Surgical treatment includes strabismus repair for diplopia, eyelid adjustments for lid retraction, and orbital decompression for exophthalmos with optic neuropathy or exposure keratitis.

Surgical decompression of the orbit has traditionally been performed by the otolaryngologist through a transantral approach, known as the Walsh-Ogura procedure. A large maxillary antrostomy allows for removal of the entire orbital floor with preservation of the infraorbital nerve. The medial orbital wall is removed through a transantral ethmoidectomy. This approach can result in inferior globe displacement and is associated with the morbidity of a Caldwell-Luc procedure. Furthermore, limited visibility along the orbital apex and ethmoid roof can result in incomplete surgery or serious operative complications.

The endoscopic intranasal approach for orbital decompression has grown in popularity since it was introduced by Kennedy et al[2] and Michel et al[3] in the early 1990s. Over the past decade, its safety and efficacy for the treatment of dysthyroid orbitopathy have been clearly demonstrated. The endoscopic approach allows for reduction of proptosis in patients with Graves' disease, while affording the surgeon excellent visualization and avoiding the need for an external or intraoral incision.

TABLE 22–1   Classification of Dysthyroid Orbitopathy*

Class	Description
0	**N**o signs or symptoms
1	**O**nly signs (eyelid retraction, lid lag, edema)
2	**S**oft tissue signs and symptoms (e.g., resistance to retropulsion, injection)
3	**P**roptosis (mild, 21–23 mm; moderate, 24–27 mm; severe, >28 mm)
4	**E**xtraocular muscle involvement (minimal to frozen globe)
5	**C**orneal involvement (superficial to necrosis and perforation)
6	**S**ight loss by optic neuropathy (visual field defects, color vision, acuity)

*Adapted from descriptions by Werner SC. Modification of the classification of eye changes of Graves' disease. *Am J Ophthalmol.* 1977;83:725.

■ Surgical Technique

The patient is placed in a supine position on the operating table with the head slightly elevated. Packing soaked in a 4% cocaine solution is placed in the nasal cavity to initiate mucosal vasoconstriction.

CONTROVERSY

Cocaine is an excellent choice for the patient undergoing surgery under local or sedation type anesthetics because of its properties as a topical anesthetic and decongestant. However, when performing surgery under general anesthesia, HLL uses oxymetazoline to achieve vasoconstriction. The cost is less, and there is less chance of cocaine interaction with anesthetics and vasoconstrictors.

Both eyes are draped in the surgical field. If general anesthesia is used, the corneas are covered with protective shells. Under endoscopic visualization, submucosal injections of 1% lidocaine with epinephrine 1:100,000 are placed along the lateral nasal wall and middle turbinate. If a septal deviation precludes endoscopic access to the middle meatus region, a septoplasty is performed before the decompression.

Orbital decompression is begun with an incision in the uncinate process. This incision is made just posterior to the maxillary line, a bony eminence that extends from the anterior attachment of the middle turbinate to the root of the inferior turbinate (Fig. 22–1). The maxillary ostium should be generously enlarged to provide optimal exposure of the orbital floor and to prevent obstruction of the maxillary sinus by the decompressed globe. Bone is removed in a posterior direction to the level of the back wall of the sinus (Fig. 22–2). Anterior

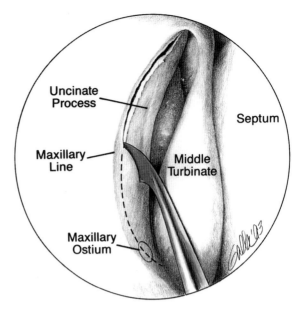

FIGURE 22–1   The uncinate process is incised just posterior to the maxillary line, an eminence that extends from the anterior attachment of the middle turbinate to the root of the inferior turbinate.

removal stops at the thick bone of the frontal process of the maxilla, which protects the nasolacrimal duct. The ostium is enlarged superiorly to the level of the orbital floor and inferiorly to the root of the inferior turbinate. A 30-degree endoscope is used to identify the infraorbital nerve along the roof of the sinus.

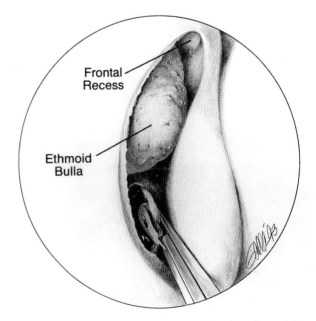

FIGURE 22–2   The maxillary sinus ostium is enlarged in a posterior direction until it is flush with the back wall of the sinus. A large ostium is necessary to optimize exposure and removal of the medial orbital floor.

An endoscopic sphenoethmoidectomy is then performed with identification of the anterior and posterior ethmoid arteries along the ethmoid roof.

CONTROVERSY

Although in theory the anterior and posterior ethmoid arteries should be identified in every endoscopic sphenoethmoidectomy, this is often difficult because the vessels are small or are covered in bone. Successful endoscopic ethmoidectomy can be performed without identification of these blood vessels.

The middle turbinate that serves as a landmark during the sphenoethmoidectomy is removed before opening the lamina papyracea to optimize exposure to the medial orbital wall and facilitate postoperative cleaning.

The skeletonized lamina papyracea is gently penetrated with a small spoon curette (Fig. 22–3). Bony fragments of the lamina are lifted in a medial direction to avoid perforation of the underlying periorbita. This elevation may also be performed with a periosteal elevator or delicate Blakesley forceps (Fig. 22–4). If surgery is being performed with the patient under local anesthesia, additional injections may be necessary to desensitize the medial orbital wall.[4] Anesthetic agent is injected just

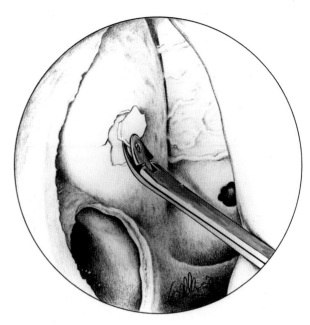

FIGURE 22–4   A fine Blakesley forceps removes the elevated bony fragments of the medial orbital wall to expose the underlying periorbita.

deep to the periorbita through the bony opening in the lamina.

Bone of the lamina papyracea is removed in a superior direction to the level of the ethmoid roof. Lamina papyracea within the frontal recess is preserved to prevent postoperative obstruction of the frontal sinus. As dissection continues in a posterior direction toward the orbital apex, thicker bone and underlying periorbita are generally encountered within 2 mm of the sphenoid face. This thickening represents the anulus of Zinn, from which the extraocular muscles originate and through which the optic nerve passes. This bone represents the posterior limit of dissection and need not be removed.

Fragments of bone are cleared from the anterior end of the lamina papyracea where it joins the lacrimal bone. Dissection in this region may be facilitated by use of an angled spoon curette and 30-degree endoscope. The thick white fascia of the lacrimal sac may be uncovered but should not be opened. Firm bone anterior to the maxillary line protects the majority of the sac and should not be removed.

Removal of bone along the medial orbital floor can be the most technically challenging aspect of this surgery. A spoon curette is used to fracture the bone in a downward direction (Fig. 22–5). This bone may break apart in several small fragments, or it may fracture in one large piece with a natural cleavage plane along the infra-orbital canal. Frequently, this bone is too thick to fracture with the same curette used to remove the more delicate lamina papyracea, in which case a larger spoon or mastoid curette is used. A 30-degree endoscope may facilitate

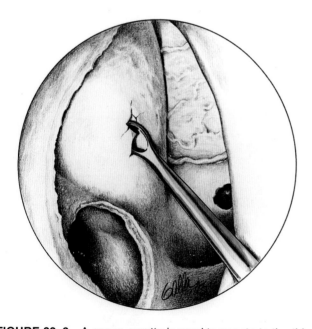

FIGURE 22–3   A spoon curette is used to penetrate the thin bone of the lamina papyracea along the medial orbital wall. Bony fragments are lifted away from the underlying periorbita. An exposed ethmoid roof is visible after completion of a sphenoethmoidectomy. Enlarged maxillary and sphenoid sinus ostia are also seen.

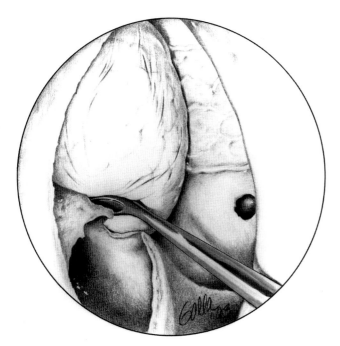

FIGURE 22–5 Fragments of the orbital floor are fractured downward with a spoon curette. Only bone that is medial to the infraorbital nerve is removed.

visualization within the maxillary sinus and aid in the identification of the infraorbital nerve. This nerve serves as the lateral limit of bone removal.

After the periorbita has been fully exposed and cleared of bony fragments, it is opened with a sickle knife (Fig. 22–6). The incision is usually begun in front

of the sphenoid sinus, because orbital fat will immediately begin to prolapse through the incision and obstruct visualization of the more posterior structures. Care must be taken to keep the tip of the blade superficial so as not to injure the underlying orbital contents. This concept is particularly important when working in the region of the medial rectus muscle, which may be enlarged from Graves' disease.

Incision of the periorbita is extended along the ethmoid roof and the orbital floor. A horizontal strip of periorbita overlying the medial rectus muscle is preserved. This fascial sling serves to decrease prolapse of the muscle and is thought to reduce the incidence of postoperative diplopia.[5] However, in patients with optic neuropathy, maximal decompression is needed and the fascial sling is sacrificed to allow for a wider excision of periorbita. After the periorbita is adequately incised, fragments can be removed with angled Blakesley forceps. The sickle knife is used to incise remaining fibrous bands, which are often seen coursing superficially between lobules of fat. At the completion of the procedure, the generous prolapse of orbital fat into the opened ethmoid and maxillary sinuses should be observed (Fig. 22–7).

A lateral orbital decompression may be performed at this time, depending on the extent of the patient's disease and the degree of additional decompression desired. Because of the prior medial decompression, the orbital contents are easily retracted in a medial direction to provide excellent exposure of the lateral bony wall, which is removed or contoured (Fig. 22–8). Concurrent excision of excess intraconal fat may also be performed if necessary.

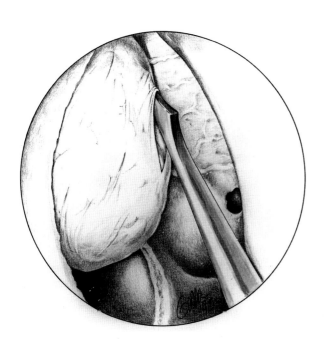

FIGURE 22–6 The exposed layer of periorbital fascia is incised with a sickle knife and removed.

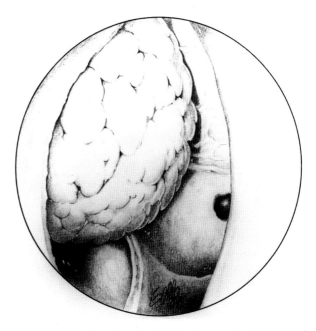

FIGURE 22–7 Herniated orbital fat is seen bulging into the ethmoid and maxillary sinuses at the completion of the decompression.

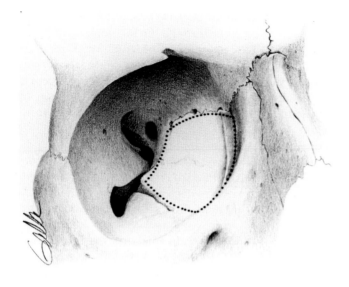

FIGURE 22–8 View of right orbit showing area of bone removed (dotted line) by endoscopic orbital decompression. Resected bone includes the lamina papyracea and the orbital floor medial to the infraorbital canal.

At the conclusion of surgery, no nasal packing is placed to avoid compression of the vulnerable optic nerve. Patients are discharged the morning after surgery with oral antibiotics and instructions to begin twice-a-day nasal saline irrigations with a bulb syringe. Residual debris is cleared from the nasal cavity under endoscopic visualization 1 week later at the first postoperative visit. Bilateral orbital decompressions may be done concurrently or as a staged procedure.

■ Discussion

Endoscopic orbital decompression affords the surgeon excellent visualization for safe removal of orbital bone, particularly in the regions of the ethmoid roof and orbital apex. In contrast to transantral decompression, the endoscopic approach avoids postoperative infraorbital nerve hypoesthesia. It also results in less intraoperative blood loss and shorter hospitalization.

The authors' experience with over 100 orbital decompressions for Graves' orbitopathy has demonstrated the safety and efficacy of this procedure. Endoscopic medial decompression, under either general or local anesthesia, results in an average reduction in proptosis of 3.5 mm (range 2–12 mm). The addition of a concurrent lateral orbital decompression performed through an external incision yields ~2 mm of additional decompression.

Endoscopic orbital decompression affords a maximal posterior orbital decompression at the orbital apex,

an area often not fully accessible via the external or transantral routes. Orbital apex decompression is of particular importance in cases of optic neuropathy that can result from compression of the optic nerve or its vasculature by the enlarged extraocular muscles and orbital fat. Optic neuropathy produces progressive visual loss that manifests as a decrease in acuity, color vision, and visual fields. In a series of endoscopic orbital decompressions, Kennedy et al[2] demonstrated an improvement in 9 of 16 orbits (56%) and a decrease in visual acuity in 1 of 16 orbits (6%) after orbital decompression. Metson et al[6] reported an improvement in visual acuity in 4 of 22 orbits (18%) with no patients showing a decrease in visual acuity.

Double vision that is present prior to orbital decompression is generally not improved by this surgery. Such patients require subsequent eye muscle surgery to correct their strabismus. Because the position and pull of the extraocular muscles are affected by decompression, such surgery can cause new onset diplopia. This double vision is not considered a complication of surgery, but a natural sequela to repositioning of the globe. The preservation of a strip of periorbita overlying the medial rectus muscle during endoscopic decompression appears to decrease the incidence of diplopia following surgery.[6] The use of a balanced decompression technique is also thought to decrease postoperative double vision. This technique involves performing external lateral wall decompression at the time of endoscopic medial wall decompression to reduce pressure on the medial rectus muscle while simultaneously increasing the degree of ocular recession.[7] All patients must be informed of the possibility of diplopia prior to undergoing orbital decompression.

We favor endoscopic removal of the medial orbital wall and floor as an initial step for decompression in the patient with dysthyroid orbitopathy. A concurrent lateral decompression is performed if additional decompression is desired. Simultaneous medial and lateral decompressions appear to result in less postoperative hypoglobus than an equivalent degree of decompression achieved by transantral removal of the entire orbital floor. This factor makes the endoscopic approach particularly suitable to the patient with unilateral proptosis.

Endoscopic decompression has proven amenable to local anesthetic techniques.[5] In addition to allowing a more rapid postoperative recovery, the use of local anesthetic enables the surgeon to monitor the patient's vision on a continual basis during the surgery and reduces the likelihood of occult injury to the optic nerve. Additional experience with the use of local anesthesia for this surgery may demonstrate the suitability of performing endoscopic decompression on an ambulatory basis.

Endoscopic orbital decompression should be performed only by those surgeons with extensive experience in endoscopic intranasal techniques. Decompression surgery inherently places the orbital contents, including the extraocular muscles, lacrimal sac, and optic nerve, at greater risk for injury than routine endoscopic sinus surgery. A team approach is advocated that uses the skills of both the otolaryngologist and the ophthalmologist during the performance of this procedure.

REFERENCES

1. Dallow RL, Netland PA. Management of thyroid ophthalmopathy (Graves' disease). In: Albert DM, Jacobiec FA, eds. *The Principles and Practice of Ophthalmology.* Philadelphia: WB Saunders; 1993.

2. Kennedy DW, Goodstein ML, Miller NR, et al. Endoscopic transnasal orbital decompression *Arch Otolaryngol Head Neck Surg.* 1990;116:275–282.

3. Michel O, Bresgen K, Russmann W, et al. Endoskopish kontrollierte endonasale Orbitadekompression beim malignen Ophthalmus. *Laryngorhinootologie.* 1991;70:656–662.

4. Metson R, Shore JW, Gliklich RE, et al. Endoscopic orbital decompression under local anesthesia. *Otolaryngol Head Neck Surg.* 1995;113(6):661–667.

5. Metson R, Samaha M. Reduction of diplopia following endoscopic orbital decompression: the orbital sling technique. *Laryngoscope.* 2002;112:1753–1757.

6. Metson R, Dallow R, Shore JW. Endoscopic orbital decompression. *Laryngoscope.* 1994;104:950–957.

7. Kacker A, Kazim M, Murphy M, Trokel S, Close LG. "Balanced" orbital decompression for severe Graves' orbitopathy: technique with treatment algorithm *Otolaryngol Head Neck Surg.* 2003;128(2):228–235.

23

Dacryocystorhinostomy

RALPH B. METSON

Contemporary surgical techniques developed for the treatment of patients with obstructed paranasal sinuses can be similarly applied for the treatment of patients who present with epiphora or dacryocystitis from lacrimal obstruction. West[1] first described intranasal drainage of an obstructed lacrimal sac in 1914. Since that time a variety of intranasal dacryocystorhinostomy (DCR) approaches have been utilized for the successful treatment of lacrimal obstruction.[2,3] Until recently, however, the clinical applicability of intranasal DCR has remained limited because of difficulty with visualization and exposure of the lacrimal sac when operating in the narrow confines of the superior nasal cavity. With the introduction of endoscopic instrumentation for nasal surgery, technical difficulties with intranasal access to the lacrimal sac have been largely overcome.[4–7] In addition to avoiding a skin incision, endoscopic DCR enables the surgeon to identify and correct common intranasal causes of DCR failure, such as adhesions, an enlarged middle turbinate, or an infected ethmoid sinus.

■ Endoscopic Anatomy

From an endoscopic intranasal perspective, the lacrimal sac can be found beneath the bone of the lateral nasal wall just anterior to the attachment of the middle turbinate (Fig. 23–1). The superior border of the sac may extend above the level of the turbinate attachment. The posterior edge of the sac often extends beneath the middle turbinate, behind a landmark referred to as the maxillary line. The maxillary line is an important landmark for endoscopic DCR. It is readily identified as a

curvilinear eminence along the lateral nasal wall that runs from the anterior attachment of the middle turbinate to the root of the inferior turbinate. Its location corresponds to the suture line between the maxillary and lacrimal bones that runs in a vertical direction through the lacrimal fossa. Exposure of the posterior half of the sac typically requires removal of the thin uncinate process and underlying lacrimal bone located posterior to the maxillary line. In contrast, exposure of the anterior sac necessitates removal of thicker bone located just anterior to the maxillary line. As the nasolacrimal duct courses inferiorly, it passes an average of 10 mm (range 8–17 mm) anterior to the natural ostium of the maxillary sinus. Injury to the duct can occur if the maxillary ostium is enlarged too far in an anterior direction. In clinical practice this injury is relatively uncommon because the hard surrounding maxillary bone protects the duct.

The inferior end of the lacrimal sac tapers as it enters the nasolacrimal canal formed by the maxillary, lacrimal, and inferior turbinate bones. The nasolacrimal duct runs within this osseous canal for a distance of ~12 mm. It continues beneath the inferior turbinate as a membranous duct for an additional 5 mm before opening into the inferior meatus. The duct orifice is found at the junction of the middle and anterior thirds of the meatus ~8 mm behind the anterior tip of the inferior turbinate and 29 mm from the anterior nasal spine. It is often covered by a flap of mucosa, known as Hasner's valve, which is thought to prevent reflux of nasal secretions. Gentle pressure over the medial canthal region will often produce fluid or bubbles at the duct orifice to confirm its location.

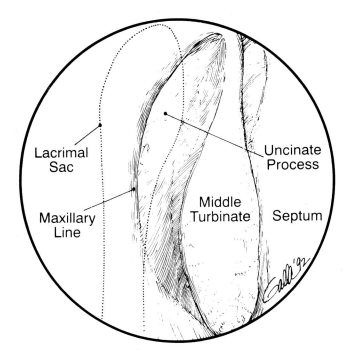

FIGURE 23–1 Endoscopic view of right nasal cavity shows location of the lacrimal sac (dotted outline) underlying the lateral nasal wall. The maxillary line, a bony eminence that originates at the attachment of the middle turbinate, corresponds to a vertical suture line that runs through the lacrimal sac.

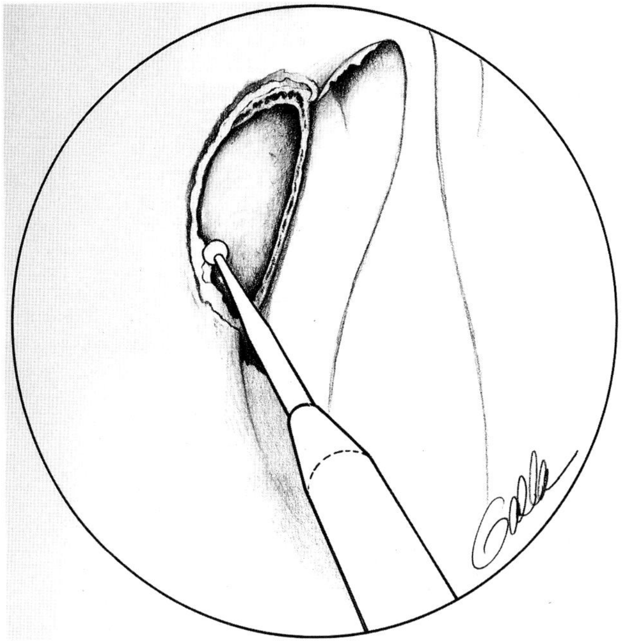

FIGURE 23–2 Once mucosa has been excised from the lateral nasal wall in the region of the maxillary line, a drill is used to remove thick bone overlying the lacrimal sac. It is important that bone anterior to the maxillary line is removed to expose the entire medial sac wall.

■ Surgical Technique

Endoscopic DCR may be performed under either local or general anesthesia, depending on the condition of the patient and the preference of the surgeon. The operation is typically performed with a video camera attached to the endoscope, so that the assistant surgeon can observe the entire procedure on a video monitor. With the patient supine and the head slightly elevated to decrease venous pressure at the operative site, nasal packing soaked in a 4% cocaine solution is placed along the lateral nasal wall to initiate mucosal decongestion. The nose and affected eye are draped in the operative field. A 0-degree, 4 mm diameter nasal endoscope is used for visualization, as submucosal injections of 1% lidocaine HCl with epinephrine 1:100,000 are placed in the middle turbinate and the lateral nasal wall just anterior to the attachment of the turbinate.

Surgical dissection is begun with removal of an ∼1 cm diameter circle of mucosa and bone along the lateral nasal wall overlying the lacrimal sac. Initial tissue removal usually includes a portion of the uncinate process located posterior to the maxillary line. An air space is often entered that corresponds to the infundibulum or an anterior ethmoid air cell overlying the lacrimal sac. As dissection is carried more anteriorly, the lacrimal bone is opened, and the underlying medial wall of the sac will be exposed.

Next, the maxillary bone, which forms the anterior aspect of the lacrimal fossa, must be removed. Removal of this relatively thick bone is technically the most difficult step of the surgery. Bone removal may be accomplished with a curette, bone-biting forceps, microdebrider, or drill (Fig. 23–2). The surgical laser also has been used for endoscopic DCR because of its ability to remove bone with excellent hemostasis.[8] After the medial sac wall has been exposed, it is entered with an angled Blakesley forceps. Use of the laser provides for a more hemostatic sac opening, whereas the forceps allow for a tissue specimen to be obtained for pathologic examination to rule out occult neoplasm. It is often helpful to use a lacrimal probe within the sac to tent up the medial sac wall as it is opened. This maneuver serves to isolate the medial wall and prevent inadvertent injury to the underlying structures. Once the sac is entered, the probe will be visible.

PEARL

A light pipe may be inserted into the punctum, illuminating the sac and overlying bone and making the identification of the sac easier. The light pipe also serves to tent up the lacrimal sac mucosa.

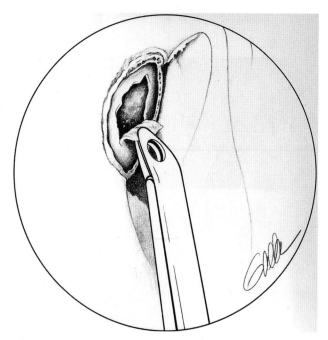

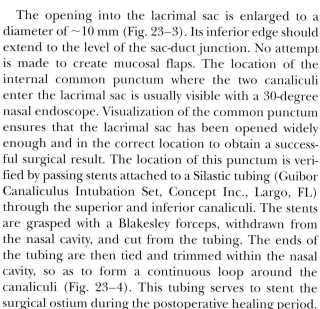

FIGURE 23–3 Once the medial wall of the lacrimal sac has been incised with a sickle knife, it is removed with an angled Blakesley forceps. This specimen is always sent for pathologic examination to ensure that an occult neoplasm is not the cause of the lacrimal obstruction.

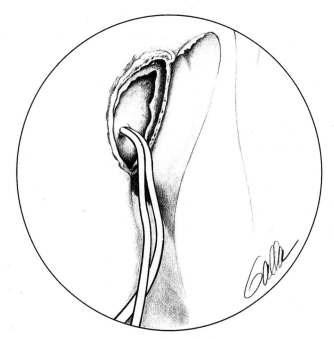

FIGURE 23–4 At the completion of surgery, lacrimal probes threaded with Silastic tubing are passed through the canaliculi and into the lacrimal sac. The tubing is trimmed and tied within the nasal cavity, where it serves as a stent during the healing period.

The opening into the lacrimal sac is enlarged to a diameter of ~10 mm (Fig. 23–3). Its inferior edge should extend to the level of the sac-duct junction. No attempt is made to create mucosal flaps. The location of the internal common punctum where the two canaliculi enter the lacrimal sac is usually visible with a 30-degree nasal endoscope. Visualization of the common punctum ensures that the lacrimal sac has been opened widely enough and in the correct location to obtain a successful surgical result. The location of this punctum is verified by passing stents attached to a Silastic tubing (Guibor Canaliculus Intubation Set, Concept Inc., Largo, FL) through the superior and inferior canaliculi. The stents are grasped with a Blakesley forceps, withdrawn from the nasal cavity, and cut from the tubing. The ends of the tubing are then tied and trimmed within the nasal cavity, so as to form a continuous loop around the canaliculi (Fig. 23–4). This tubing serves to stent the surgical ostium during the postoperative healing period.

Endoscopic revision DCR is performed in a similar fashion to endoscopic primary DCR; however, bone of the lateral nasal wall overlying the lacrimal sac has already been removed.[9,10] Revision DCR is therefore usually easier to perform than primary DCR. This factor makes revision DCR patients who have already failed an external DCR approach very appropriate initial candidates for the surgeon who wishes to learn endoscopic DCR techniques.

■ Postoperative Care

If nasal packing is placed for hemostasis at the conclusion of surgery, it is removed the following day. Patients are discharged with instructions to begin twice-a-day nasal saline irrigations with a bulb syringe. Any remaining intranasal debris is removed from the operative site at the first postoperative visit 1 week following surgery. The Silastic tubing used to stent the surgical ostium is typically removed 2 months after surgery by cutting the exposed tubing at the medial canthus and withdrawing it through the nose. It may be removed sooner if excessive granulation tissue formation is seen to occur around the tube at the ostium. Patency of the lacrimal drainage system is verified by endoscopic observation of fluorescein dye flowing from the eye through the surgical ostium into the nose.

■ Discussion

Over the past decade endoscopic DCR has proved itself to be a safe and effective technique for the treatment of lacrimal duct obstruction. The author's results and those of others demonstrate a greater than 90% surgical success rate for patients who undergo primary endoscopic DCR[11,12] These results are similar to those described for conventional external DCR techniques[13,14]; however, the endoscopic approach avoids the morbidity of a facial incision. Furthermore, endoscopic techniques have the potential to reduce patient morbidity through improved intraoperative hemostasis, greater utilization of local anesthesia, and shorter hospitalization as compared with conventional techniques. As more otolaryngologists and ophthalmologists become trained in the endoscopic DCR, it is likely that this approach will become the most commonly utilized technique for the treatment of patients who present with epiphora and dacryocystitis from lacrimal obstruction.

REFERENCES

1. West JM. A window resection of the nasal duct in cases of stenosis. *Trans Am Ophthalmol Soc.* 1914;12:654.
2. Berryhill BH, Dorenbusch AA. Twenty years experience with intranasal transseptal dacryocystorhinostomy. *Laryngoscope.* 1982;92:379–381.
3. Jokinen K, Karja J. Endonasal dacryocystorhinostomy. *Arch Otolaryngol.* 1974;100:41–44.
4. Gonnering RS, Lyon DB, Fisher JC. Endoscopic laser-assisted lacrimal surgery. *Am J Ophthalmol.* 1991;111:152–157.
5. Massaro BM, Gonnering RS, Harris GJ. Endonasal laser dacryocystorhinostomy: a new approach to nasolacrimal duct obstruction. *Arch Ophthalmol.* 1990;108:1172–1176.
6. McDonogh M. Endoscopic transnasal dacryocystorhinostomy—results in 21 patients. *S Afr J Surg.* 1992;30:107–110.
7. Metson R. Endoscopic surgery for lacrimal obstruction. *Otolaryngol Head Neck* Surg 1991;104:473–479.
8. Metson R, Woog JJ, Puliafito CA. Endoscopic laser dacryocystorhinostomy. *Laryngoscope.* 1994;104:269–274.
9. Orcutt JC, Hillel A, Weymuller EA. Endoscopic repair of failed dacryocystorhinostomy. *Ophthal Plastic Recon Surg.* 1990;6:197–202.
10. Metson R. Endoscopic revision dacryocystorhinostomy. *Laryngoscope.* 1990;100:1344–1347.
11. Bernal Sprekelsen M, Barberan MT. Endoscopic dacryocystorhinostomy: surgical technique and results. *Laryngoscope.* 1996;106:187–189.
12. Onerci M, Orhan M, Erdener U. Intranasal endoscopic surgery with silicone intubation for lacrimal obstruction. *Am J Rhinol.* 1996;10:93–95.
13. Welham RAN, Henderson PH. Results of dacryocystorhinostomy: analysis of causes for failure. *Trans Ophthalmol Soc UK.* 1973;93:601–609.
14. McLachlan DL, Shannon GM, Flanagan JC. Results of dacryocystorhinostomy: analysis of reoperations. *Ophthalmic Surg.* 1980;11:427–430.

24

Anesthesia for Sinus Surgery

DOUGLAS MAYERS AND MARGARET M. HILDEBRANDT

The success of endoscopic sinus surgery is greatly dependent upon properly administered anesthesia. The physical and emotional well-being of the patient, not to mention a safe field for the surgeon to work, can be positively or negatively influenced by the anesthetic. Disastrous anesthesia-related complications have been reported in patients undergoing endoscopic sinus surgery.[1-5] The goal of the anesthesiologist must be to minimize the chances for complications while providing the best surgical field possible.

■ Preoperative Evaluation

The goal of the preoperative evaluation of a patient should be to eliminate negative outcomes as much as possible. Every patient must have an appropriate history and physical examination documenting the major medical problems and reasons for the surgery. Ideally, laboratory tests would be ordered based on the history and physical of the specific patient. This would be possible where the preadmission testing process is part of an anesthesia preoperative clinic. However, when this is not possible, the laboratory testing is usually done by a predetermined protocol. The protocol successfully used by our ambulatory surgery facility in several thousand patients is as follows:

1. Under age 16: – no laboratory tests required
2. 16 to 40 years: hemoglobin/hematocrit for women
3. 40 to 59 years: in addition to the above, blood urea nitrogen (BUN), glucose, and electrocardiogram
4. 60 years and older: in addition to the above, hemoglobin/hematocrit for men

5. Pregnancy test for women of childbearing age

For those patients with a history of pulmonary disease, a chest x-ray is obtained.

Most of our ESS is done in a freestanding ambulatory surgery center. Because the surgery center is not attached to the hospital, some patients with certain medical problems are not candidates for surgery and anesthesia at the freestanding ambulatory surgery center. If, as part of the preoperative evaluation, a patient is found to have one of these conditions, the surgery is scheduled for the hospital setting. There are very few patients in this category. In our practice, where 200 to 300 ESS procedures are done in the ambulatory surgery center each year, fewer than 1% are done in the hospital. Often the sicker patients will still have ambulatory surgery, but their conditions dictate a setting where more intense medical resources are easily available. Many of these patients will stay 1 or more nights in the hospital to be treated or observed for problems related to their underlying medical conditions. These underlying medical conditions include

1. Serious cardiac conditions where congestive heart failure or angina is a significant possibility
2. Severe pulmonary compromise where extubation after general anesthesia or intubation for respiratory failure is a significant possibility
3. Documented malignant hyperthermia (MH) or a first-degree relative with MH
4. Known or significant suspicion that the patient will present a difficult endotracheal intubation
5. Massive obesity (greater than twice ideal weight), mainly because of respiratory and airway problems

6. A medical or physical problem that would stretch the resources of the ambulatory surgery center (e.g., a stable but demented total-care nursing home patient is not a good candidate for a freestanding ambulatory surgery center)

■ Anesthetic Management

There are two main choices in anesthetic management for ESS: general anesthesia or monitored anesthesia care (MAC). The decision in favor of one type of anesthetic over another is based on many factors. The anesthesiologist and surgeon must work together to provide the best conditions for the surgery in this area of shared responsibility. Those who favor MAC cite the simplicity and safety that have been demonstrated for this modality.[6–8] In addition, some nasal and sinus surgeons believe that MAC decreases the chances of the surgeon going through the upper segment of the ethmoid sinus through the cribriform plate into the cranium because of patient feedback. Thus, if the patient suddenly feels pain while working on the ethmoid sinus, the surgeon would be instantly alerted to the possibility of being too close to the cribriform plate. At least one study has found lower blood loss in MAC compared with general anesthesia.[9] The average blood loss for MAC compared with general anesthesia was not dramatically lower and would not have significant clinical consequences.

Practitioners who favor general anesthesia do so for several reasons. Airway control is easier under general anesthesia. This is especially important for patients with asthma, chronic obstructive pulmonary disease (COPD), bronchitis, or bronchiectasis. Patients who have had previous sinus surgery may be difficult to regionally block with local anesthesia because of the difficulty of the anesthetic flowing through the scar tissue. Anxious patients are also difficult patients for MAC, requiring a great deal of sedation, obtunding the patient, and limiting the patient's ability to manage secretions.

A general anesthetic requires either an endotracheal tube placement or laryngeal mask airway (LMA) (Fig. 24–1).

> **CONTROVERSY**
>
> LMA is now the surgeon's (HLL) choice for nearly all ESS patients. No patient has had aspiration of blood or secretions. Blood pressure is easier to control. There is less chance of bronchospasm at the time of anesthetic emergence and in the immediate postoperative period.

Thus, concerns with MAC of inadequate spontaneous respiration or aspiration of blood that might come down from the sinuses are largely eliminated with general anesthesia. The general anesthetic is also often believed to allow better control over physiological parameters such as blood pressure. No clear-cut advantage of general anesthesia over MAC has been demonstrated,[10] but our practice favors the general anesthetic for the reasons mentioned above.

Whatever the anesthetic choice, adequate monitoring is required. Minimally, each patient must be monitored with electrocardiogram, noninvasive blood pressure, pulse oximetry, inhaled oxygen concentration, and exhaled CO_2 concentration. In addition, if temperature is not monitored, the ability to monitor temperature must be readily available. These monitoring standards are outlined in the American Society of Anesthesiologists's *Standards, Guidelines and Statements.*[11] The ability to monitor breath-by-breath major inhalation anesthetic concentration, although not required, certainly adds useful information. Watching the decline of anesthetic concentration on emergence from general anesthesia is helpful to the clinician. For example, if a patient is slow to emerge and the exhaled inhalation anesthetic has reached a concentration near zero, we know to look for other reasons and do not need to speculate about the degree of retained inhalation agent.

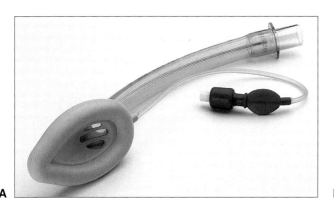

A

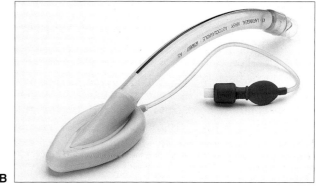

B

FIGURE 24–1   (A,B) Views of the laryngeal mask airway (LMA).

Typically, the drugs used for MAC include a tranquilizer (midazolam, diazepam, lorazepam, etc.) a narcotic (morphine, meperidine, fentanyl, alfentanyl, etc.), and a sedative (almost always propofol). The key is the judicious use of these drugs so that the patient is sedated and calm but easily arousable, breathing adequately, and able to protect his or her own airway.[11] We do not have extensive experience with MAC for ESS, but we commonly use it for other elective procedures in this area of the body. Our usual regimen includes midazolam, fentanyl, and propofol in small incremental doses until the patient reaches the desired level of sedation. Then the sedation is maintained with a low dose (25–100 μg/kg/min) of propofol and small intermittent doses of fentanyl (0.5–1.0 mL). Supplemental oxygen is supplied through a nasal cannula that is placed in the mouth. The patient is continually reminded to breathe through his or her mouth. While the anesthesiologist is sedating the patient, the surgeon uses a combination of injected and topical local anesthetics to make the nasal tissue insensitive to the surgical stimulus. Usually 1% lidocaine with diluted epinephrine (1:100,000) is injected into specific sites, and 4% cocaine-soaked pledgets are strategically placed in the nose to produce numbness and vasoconstriction.

The usual principles for any general anesthetic in the head and neck region apply to anesthesia for ESS. After induction of the anesthetic, the patient's trachea is intubated or an LMA is inserted through the mouth for airway protection and ventilatory support. Induction is accomplished with an ultra-short-acting barbiturate (usually thiopental) or propofol. We prefer propofol because it is eliminated faster. A muscle relaxant facilitates the intubation. Often succinylcholine is used for this purpose, but an intermediate-acting nondepolarizing muscle relaxant (atracurium, cisatracurium, mivacurium, rocuronium, or vecuronium) can be used. If succinylcholine is used for intubation, it usually will need to be followed with a nondepolarizing muscle relaxant for maintenance of the anesthetic. If an LMA is used, no muscle relaxant is required for either insertion of the LMA or maintenance of anesthesia, and the patient is allowed to breathe spontaneously with assistance (if needed) throughout the case.

PEARL

LMA insertion can be accomplished using many different techniques, but the one that works the best for us is to extend the neck as if going to intubate the patient, use a tongue depressor to retract the tongue as far out of the oropharynx as possible, and slide the lubricated, partially inflated LMA into position (Fig. 24–2). Occasionally, the tip of the LMA curves cephalad, and we need to insert a finger into the oropharynx to guide it into position.

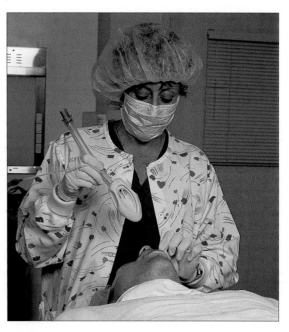

FIGURE 24–2   Insertion of the LMA is done standing at the head of the patient, partially inflating the LMA to create rigidity, moving the patient's tongue out of the way, and sliding the LMA into place. On occasion, a finger is inserted into the mouth to guide the LMA into place.

A small dose of glycopyrrolate (0.005–0.2 mg/kg) is given prior to induction to prevent excessive salivary secretions. The anesthetic maintenance is accomplished with small intermittent doses of narcotic (fentanyl or alfentanyl) or a continuous drip of remifentanil, nitrous oxide, oxygen, and either a major inhalation agent or continuous infusion of propofol. Any of the major inhalation agents (halothane, enflurane, isoflurane, sevoflurane, and desflurane) in common use would probably be adequate.[12] We stay away from halothane because it sensitizes the myocardium to arrhythmia, and our surgeons often use small doses of epinephrine in injected local anesthetics for vasoconstriction. We most commonly use isoflurane with sevoflurane reserved for the shorter procedures and mask inductions in small children. With LMA, we almost exclusively use sevoflurane, as the rate of spontaneous respiration with isoflurane is more rapid than sevoflurane and the time of emergence is quicker. Our experience with desflurane is very limited, but there does not seem to be any contraindications to its use. There is some evidence that using propofol for maintenance instead of an inhalation agent decreases the amount of intraoperative bleeding.[13] The emergence and extubation must be monitored carefully because excessive coughing before the endotracheal tube is removed can increase bleeding from the sinuses by increasing venous pressure. If needed, the muscle relaxant is reversed with neostigmine (or another cholinesterase inhibitor) and glycopyrrolate. The use of neostigmine in patients with reactive airway disease is sometimes mentioned as relatively contraindicated because it induces increased acetylcholine, which in turn can exacerbate or even induce bronchoconstriction. We have never seen this complication even though we often have reversed the muscle relaxant in an asthmatic patient. Coughing and bucking on the endotracheal tube can be minimized by not stimulating the airway once the anesthetic emergence has started. For example, moving the endotracheal tube or excessive suctioning should be avoided. Small doses of intravenous lidocaine (up to 1.5 mg/kg) can be helpful in reducing coughing.[14]

When the LMA is used, the anesthetic gases are terminated very close to the end of the surgical procedure, and the oropharynx is suctioned as quickly as possible with a Yankauer tonsil suction, reaching as far into the oropharynx as possible on both sides of the LMA. When the patient is awake and responding, the LMA is removed. The patient rarely coughs and/or "bucks," as the LMA is so well tolerated, even in the almost fully awake patient.

CONTROVERSY

One of the biggest concerns in converting to LMA from endotracheal intubation for ESS was the possibility of blood and/or secretions accumulating in the back of the throat and being aspirated into the lungs. With a proper-fitting LMA, there seems to be a good enough seal, preventing the seepage of blood below the LMA. After suctioning over 200 patients undergoing ESS, we have not found there to be large amounts of blood accumulating from the surgical site. There is still the concern of aspiration of stomach contents as with the use of the LMA for any type of surgery, but we have not experienced this complication so far in our practice. Because of the benefits of LMA over endotracheal tube intubation for ESS, we even prefer to use LMA on patients with a history of hiatal hernia or gastroesophageal reflux, provided they are being treated for their condition and their symptoms are not of a constant nature.

Although there is little or no literature to document, it is commonly believed that increased blood pressure induces increased bleeding. We have noticed on many occasions that when bleeding increases during an endoscopic procedure, the blood pressure has also increased, and correspondingly when the pressure is lowered, the bleeding decreases. Thus, it is now our routine practice to maintain a patient's blood pressure in the low end of an acceptable range. From a practical standpoint, we attempt to keep the pressure at ~ 80% of the preoperative blood

pressure. The first line of blood pressure control is to deepen the anesthetic. In some patients this will not be adequate, and other pharmacologic modalities need to be used, including β-adrenergic blockers (propranolol, labetalol, esmolol, etc.) vasodilators (hydralazine, diltiazem, nifedipine, etc.). With the use of the LMA, we have found very little need to treat increased blood pressure with anything other than deepening the anesthetic. In extreme cases nitroglycerin or nitroprusside may be needed. It may be that vasodilators are not the best agent for lowering blood pressure, because in one study, esmolol use was associated with less blood loss at the same blood pressure when compared with nitroprusside.[15] However, in the ambulatory setting, the procedure will often be abandoned before these last two drugs are used.

Pain relief in the immediate postoperative period is extremely important, both emotionally and physically. Patients are often concerned that they will not be given enough. Pain can also induce increased blood pressure, which in turn may lead to increased bleeding. Thus, it is important to give adequate pain relief without giving too much medication, which in turn can lead to respiratory and cardiovascular complications. Small, intermittent intravenous doses of narcotics (morphine up to 0.1 mg/kg in divided doses IV or meperidine up to 1 mg/kg IV in divided doses) are the standard therapies in this situation. Friedman et al[16] found that the pain associated with ESS was less than they expected and was not significantly diminished by an intraoperative sphenopalatine ganglion block using the local anesthetic bupivacaine when compared with patients who received lidocaine for the block. All patients are sent home with a prescription for an oral analgesic medication (usually a narcotic mixed with acetaminophen).

Nausea and vomiting continue to be an area of concern. Many articles have been published on the topic, mainly dealing with attempts to prevent nausea and emesis.[17] The reported incidence of nausea and vomiting is not zero, and in some studies it is over 50%. Patients should be told that every effort will be made to prevent nausea and vomiting, but there is always a chance that they will occur. Our regimen is varied but usually includes metoclopramide (0.15–10 mg/kg) prior to induction to empty the stomach of any accumulated fluids (gastric secretions and blood) during surgery. Other common intraoperative medications for prevention of nausea and emesis include ondansetron, dolasetron, granisetron, and dexamethasone. Commonly, after induction an 18 French Salem sump is inserted into the stomach orally to help empty the stomach of fluids and gas. After surgery, if nausea occurs, several different drugs are used. These include ondansetron, dolasetron, granisetron, perphenazine, prochlorperazine, promethazine, droperidol, and trimethobenzamide. All seem to be effective, but none are 100%; also, all have potential side effects, although the 5-HT3 receptor antagonists (dolasetron, ondansetron, granisetron) are the least sedating but the most expensive.

Once the surgical procedure is completed, the anesthetic emergence should be accomplished as efficiently as possible. When the patient has been extubated (for general anesthesia) and in all cases breathing adequately with stable vital signs, he or she is transported to the postanesthesia recovery unit (PACU). In PACU the patient is monitored, including electrocardiogram, blood pressure, respirations, and pulse oximeter, in addition to being observed for adequate improvement in level of consciousness, and for surgical complications (especially excessive bleeding). An anesthesiologist and the surgeon must be readily available for consultation if any complications or potential complications are found by the PACU nursing staff.

When appropriate criteria[18] are met, the patient is discharged in the care of a responsible adult. Postoperative instructions and follow-up are reviewed with the patient and responsible adult. It has become common practice to give printed instructions for each surgical procedure to the patient upon discharge from the unit.[19]

■ Coexisting Clinical Situations

Many patients will have coexisting diseases that could complicate their care. One of the most common is cardiac disease with or without hypertension. The preoperative clinical management of the patient with cardiovascular disease is the most important factor in a successful intra- and postoperative course for ESS. The preoperative care must delineate the cardiovascular problems and functional level of the patient. The patient should be in the best possible functional status. Then, for the surgery, the anesthesiologist's job is to maintain that "tuned up" status. The workup and anesthetic management of patients with cardiovascular disease have been extensively reviewed[20] and occupies chapters in the frequently cited standard anesthesia texts.

A common coexisting condition is pulmonary disease. Chronic pulmonary disease (chronic obstructive pulmonary disease, chronic bronchitis, and emphysema), analogous to cardiovascular diseases, should be treated so that the patient is in the best possible shape prior to the surgery. Well-understood techniques are then used to anesthetize the patient without worsening the pulmonary disease. A significant number of patients having ESS will also suffer from asthma or reactive airway disease. In addition, there is the well-known correlation between nasal polyps, asthma, and aspirin use.[21] A patient actively wheezing should not be electively anesthetized. From a practical standpoint, a patient who preoperatively manifests some asthmatic symptoms that are cleared with a few puffs of an albuterol inhaler or one treatment of albuterol mist by mask can usually be safely anesthetized. Short-term use in the perioperative period of corticosteroids, such as cortisone, prednisone, and methylprednisolone, is often helpful in controlling symptoms. The anesthetic management of these patients centers on minimizing airway stimulation that can induce bronchospasm. With general anesthesia, mainly this means making sure the patient is in an adequate anesthetic depth before the endotracheal tube or LMA is inserted and maintaining the anesthetic until the surgery is completed.

There are many other medical problems that pose significant anesthetic problems. Some of these diseases are diabetes, renal failure, liver disease, and endocrine disease. The anesthetic management related to these and other problems has been discussed in many settings and need not be reviewed here.[21]

■ Conclusion

Endoscopic sinus surgery has become one of the most common head and neck surgical procedures performed. A successful outcome depends on many factors, but one of the most important is properly conducted anesthetic management of the patients. By providing the best possible surgical field and appropriately controlled vital signs with stable cardiovascular and pulmonary status, the anesthesiologist can positively affect outcomes for these patients.

REFERENCES

1. Hill JN, Gershon NI, Gargiulo PO. Total spinal blockade during local anesthesia of the nasal passages. *Anesthesiology.* 1983;59(2):144–146.
2. Lormans P, Gaumann D, Schwieger I, Tassonyi E. Ventricular fibrillation following local application of cocaine and epinephrine for nasal surgery. *ORL J Otorhinolaryngol Relat Spec.* 1992;54:160–162.
3. Maniglia AJ. Fatal and major complications secondary to nasal and sinus surgery. *Laryngoscope.* 1989;99:276–283.
4. Reinhart DJ, Anderson JS. Fatal outcome during endoscopic sinus surgery: anesthetic manifestations. *Anesth Analg.* 1993;77:188–190.
5. Walton SL. Postextubation foreign body aspiration: a case report. J Am Assoc Nurse Anesth. 1997;65(2):147–149.
6. Jonathan DA, Violaris NS. Comparison of cocaine and lignocaine as intranasal local anaesthetics. *J Laryngol Otol.* 1988;102:628–629.
7. Lee WC, Kapur TR, Ramsden WN. Local and regional anesthesia for functional endoscopic sinus surgery. *Ann Otol Rhinol Laryngol.* 1997;106:767–769.
8. Thaler ER, Gottschalk A, Samaranayake R, Lanza DC, Kenndey DW. Anesthesia in endoscopic sinus surgery. *Am J Rhinol.* 1997;11(6):409–413.
9. Jorissen M, Heulens H, Peters M, Feenstra L. Functional endoscopic sinus surgery under local anesthesia: possibilities and limitations. *Acta Otorhinolaryngol Belg.* 1996;50:1–12.

10. Gittelman PD, Jacobs JB, Skorina J. Comparison of functional endoscopic sinus surgery under local and general anesthesia. *Ann Otol Rhinol Laryngol.* 1993;102:289–293.

11. American Society of Anesthesiologists. *ASA Standards, Guidelines, and Statements, October 1997.* Author; 1998.

12. Yoshikawa T, Sano K, Kanri T. Clinical assessment of anesthesia and estimated blood loss during maxillary sinus surgery. *Anesth Prog.* 1989;36:242–243.

13. Blackwell KE, Ross DA, Kapur P, Calcaterra TC. Propofol for maintenance of general anesthesia: a technique to limit blood loss during endoscopic sinus surgery. *Am J Otolaryngol.* 1993;14(4): 262–266.

14. Steinhaus JE, Gaskin L. A study of intravenous lidocaine as a suppressant of cough reflex. *Anesthesiology.* 1963;24(3):285–290.

15. Boezaart AP, van der Merwe J, Coetzee A. Comparison of sodium nitroprusside- and esmolol-induced controlled hypotension for functional endoscopic sinus surgery. *Can J Anaesth.* 1995;42(5): 373–376.

16. Friedman M, Venkatesan TK, Lang D, Caldarelli DD. Bupivacaine for postoperative analgesia following endoscopic sinus surgery. *Laryngoscope.* 1996;106:1382–1385.

17. Haynes GR, Bailey MK. Postoperative nausea and vomiting: review and clinical approaches. *South Med J.* 1996;89(10):940–949.

18. Mecca RS, Durkin P. Postanesthesia care after ambulatory surgery: is there a difference? *Curr Rev Clin Anesth.* 1998;18(18):165–176.

19. DiLima SN,. Weavers SB, eds. *Ambulatory Surgery Patient Education Manual.* Gaithersburg, MD: Aspen Publishers; 1997.

20. Mangano DT, Goldman L. Preoperative assessment of patients with known or suspected coronary disease. *N Engl J Med.* 1995; 333(26):1750–1756.

21. Stoelting RK, Dierdorf SF. *Anesthesia and Co-Existing Disease.* 3rd ed. New York: Churchill Livingstone; 1993.

25

Postoperative Care of the Patient Undergoing Endoscopic Sinus Surgery

HOWARD L. LEVINE

Although the method used, technology employed, and technical skill of the surgeon are important to achieving an excellent result, of equal importance is the care given to the patient following surgery. Postoperative care may be considered as immediate (in the recovery and ambulatory surgery center) and later as both home care and office care.

The author performs nearly all endoscopic sinus surgery in the ambulatory surgery facility. Patients remain in the facility until their vital signs are stable, there is reasonable level of consciousness, bleeding is minimal, and there is as much certainty as possible that no serious complications have occurred. (Details of the care given in the ambulatory surgery facility are reviewed in Chapter 26.)

Patients are given detailed instructions at the time of scheduling of their surgery. These instructions include a brief description of endoscopic sinus surgery in addition to information in preparation for surgery and expectations for the day of surgery.

The instruction brochure describes how to prepare for surgery, what to expect on the day of surgery and the first week after surgery, and includes information about physical activity, rest, nasal care, sneezing, moisturizing the nasal cavity, and pain. It describes the first postoperative office visit and the nasal endoscopy that is performed at that time.

Patients are discharged with a "postoperative home-going bag." This includes 2 × 2 inch gauze nasal dressings and nonallergic tape. They are instructed to wear the dressing for comfort to catch any blood or mucus, which usually lasts for ~24 hours. If the dressing becomes saturated more often than every 10 minutes, they

are told to contact the surgeon. If excessive bleeding is present while at home, patients are advised to use oxymetazoline or neosynephrine nasal spray every 10 minutes for 30 minutes. If the bleeding persists in spite of this, they either return to the surgeon's office or go to the nearest emergency room.

The postoperative home-going bag also includes a sample bottle of nasal saline spray. Patients begin the spray the next day and use it 4 or 5 times a day. Cotton-tipped applicators are included. These are dipped in hydrogen peroxide to remove any dry blood in the nares of the nose. Patients are told not to blow their nose until after the first postoperative visit because this may stimulate bleeding.

Patients are sent home with a prescription for an analgesic, usually acetaminophen with codeine (Tylenol with codeine) or oxycodone HCl (Oxycontin). Antibiotics are given only if there is active infection found at the time of surgery. These antibiotics are modified over the first several postoperative days depending on the results of intraoperative obtained cultures. Prophylactic antibiotics are not used. Methylprednisolone in a Medrol Dosepak is given to patients who have extensive polyps or asthma out of control, or those who had been on preoperative steroids. Systemic steroids begin to reduce the chances of recurrence of polyp reformation and protect asthmatic patients from bronchospasm caused by nasal drainage during the immediate postoperative period. No other postoperative medications are routinely used.

During the first week, activity is kept to a minimum, with no heavy lifting, straining, or exertion. After the first week patients return to all activity, including aerobic activity and swimming.

■ The First Postoperative Visit

The first postoperative visit is usually 5 or 6 days after surgery. At that visit, the nose is sprayed with Boyette's solution to decongest and anesthetize it. (Boyette's solution is 4% lidocaine, phenylephrine, and sodium chloride, with sterile water added to make 200 mL.) The nasal cavity is examined with a 0-degree, 4 mm endoscope. Various straight and angulated suctions (7–12 French) (Fig. 25–1) are used to remove old blood, mucus, and Surgicel Fibrillar (oxydized regenerated cellulose) (Ethicon Inc, Sommerville, NJ) nasal dressing if it was used. Depending on the degree of mucosal edema, each of the sinus cavities that are accessible is inspected, suctioned, and debrided. If crusts are present, they are removed with alligator forceps. Crusts and eschar that are adherent are left and allowed to separate on their own.

During endoscopic sinus surgery, intraoperative photographs are taken before the surgery is started. These endoscopic photographs are a record of any significant pathology seen. A photograph is also obtained at the conclusion of the procedure. Image-guided triplanar localization technology with the InstaTrak system (Visualization Technology, Inc., Wilmington, MA) permits an intraoperative image showing the endoscopic operative field, as well as axial, coronal, and sagittal CT scan views. All of these photographs are kept as part of the patient's office record. In addition, an operative data sheet is completed and is part of the patient's office record. The intraoperative photographs and the data sheet become valuable pieces of information in recalling what was found and what occurred during the surgery. It is helpful in the short- and long-term management of the patient.

After the first postoperative visit, patients are allowed to resume all activity. They are permitted to blow their nose gently, which helps in the ongoing evacuation of blood clots, crusts, and retained mucus from the surgery. Saline spray irrigation is continued if there is excessive crusting in the nasal cavity or persistent remnants of the Surgicel Fibillar dressing.

■ Long-term Care

Subsequent postoperative visits are determined by the pathology found at the time of surgery and/or the appearance of the nasal and sinus cavity at the time of the first postoperative visit.

If a great deal of crusts, mucus, and retained nasal dressing is present or if there is a tendency for lateralization of the middle turbinate, a second postoperative endoscopic sinus debridement is performed about 1 week later. If there is minimal material to remove endoscopically or if the ostiomeatal complex appears to remain open, the next endoscopic examination may be 2 to 3 weeks later. All subsequent visits are based on similar criteria.

Healing of the sinus cavity may take from 3 to 8 weeks, depending on the operative pathology. Those patients with anatomical obstruction to the outflow of the sinuses into the nasal cavity (i.e., middle turbinate concha bullosa, uncinate bullosa, or Haller's cells) have healing within a 3-week period. Those patients with extensive nasal and sinus polyposis (especially those undergoing revision surgery) have healing over a 6- to 8-week period. During this time there is crusting, retained secretions, eschar, and mucosal edema.

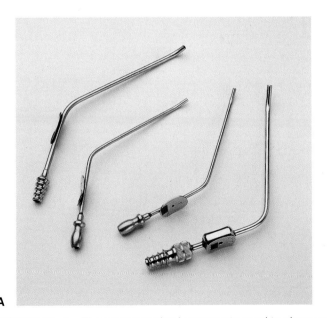
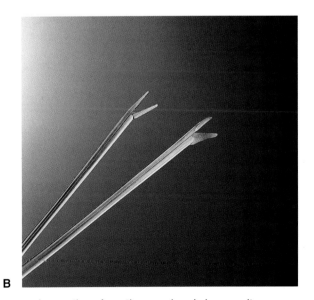

A   **B**

FIGURE 25–1   The postoperative instruments used to clear mucus and secretions from the nasal and sinus cavity.

As the nasal sinus cavity heals, few or no medications are used. For those patients with chronic or atrophic rhinosinusitis, ongoing humidification of the nasal and sinus cavity is needed. This is accomplished in several ways. A simple nasal saline spray or saline gel is used. In dry environments, a humidifier or vaporizer is used. It is important to keep these free of mold and mildew so that spores are not spread thoughout the environment. Steam acquired in a shower, over a steaming pot of water, or through some of the newer facial steam devices is effective.

Patients with chronic or atrophic rhinosinusitis often have thick, discolored secretions. These secretions seem to accumulate within the sinuses due to poor ciliary function. The secretions are most common in the morning upon first awakening and when in drier environments. Mucolytics such as guaifenesin help thin the stagnating secretions (2400 mg/day must be used for the guiafenesin to be effective). Nasal douching with one of several products helps to wash away the retained stagnant secretions. Some of the more effective irrigants are saline, saline with sodium bicarbonate, Alkalol (The Alkalol Co., Taunton, MA), Oasis Nasal Spray and irrigation (www.oasisnasalspray.com) and ENTsol (Kenwood Laboratories, Fairfield, NJ). These are usually instilled into the nose and sinuses with a bulb syringe, nasal irrigating bottle, WaterPik, or RhinoFlow, (distributed by Respironics Inc., Murrysville, PA).

Topical and/or systemic steroid are occasionally used, depending on the pathology found at the time of surgery and/or during the postoperative visits. Topical nasal steroids are initiated for patients with recurrent or extensive nasal polyposis. These are started once the nasal and sinus cavity is nearly healed and there is reasonable remucosalization. The steroids are continued indefinitely, often for months or years. If there is no recurrence of the polyposis after several months, the topical steroids are stopped. Systemic steroids are used only in the first several days following surgery. If there is any evidence of polyp recurrence, a short course of systemic steroids is given, usually in the form of methylprednisolone in a Medrol Dosepak. Topical nasal steroids are given concurrently.

■ Consultation

From time to time, there are additional related problems, such as allergy, asthma, or headaches, that worsen the nasal sinus symptoms. Allergy evaluation and management are often needed. If asthma is out of control, sinusitis may be the cause. Patients undergoing sinus surgery with significant asthma need to have the asthma managed as best as possible prior to any surgical intervention.

Many patients come to the nasal sinus physician with headaches believing that the headaches are from the sinuses. Most of these patients have headaches of another cause. Consultation with a headache specialist is frequently needed.

26

Nursing Care for Outpatient Endoscopic Sinus Surgery

BARBARA R. BILSKI, CINDI L. DAVIS, AND HOWARD L. LEVINE

Modern treatment of paranasal sinus diseases has undergone significant advancement over the past decade. Contemporary techniques and endoscopic sinus surgery, with its specially trained personnel and specialized instrumentation, are ideally suited for the outpatient surgery center because of the relatively short anesthesia and generally overall good health of the patients. Although some patients still require an inpatient setting for their surgery because of significant medical problems, especially uncontrolled asthma, the rhinologist has become generally comfortable operating in ambulatory facilities that have become the mainstay site for this type of surgery.

Effective and safe outpatient ESS relies significantly on appropriate case selection, preoperative teaching by experienced personnel, and proper surgical instrumentation. In addition to an experienced surgeon, a well-trained surgical team whose members are familiar with ESS ideally includes the surgical nursing staff in charge of instrumentation and the patient in the operating room, the anesthesia team, pre- and postoperative nurses who manage the patient before and after surgery, and a nurse from the surgeon's office who coordinates office activity with ambulatory surgical facility.

■ Preoperative Evaluation

As with most other outpatient surgical procedures, patient selection and preparation take place during the initial surgical consultation. Patients with significant medical problems, especially cardiac or pulmonary disease, may not be candidates for outpatient surgery or may require special preoperative assessment by primary care physicians, medical subspecialists, and/or anesthesiologists well in advance of the planned surgery. This assessment may preclude surgery in an ambulatory surgical facility.

Another group of patients who should not be treated in an ambulatory facility are those with intracranial or intraorbital complications of sinusitis who will require monitoring of their disease complications and sequelae by skilled nursing personnel, often in intensive care or step-down observation units.

Endonasal and paranasal tumors should be biopsied endoscopically in a surgical suite. Although biopsy of these tumors is usually performed successfully in the outpatient setting, definitive excision is often reserved for an appropriate inpatient facility.

A history of previous surgery and intraoperative problems should be obtained. Past experiences of severe nausea and vomiting following anesthesia should be noted. Family history of bleeding problems and atypical anesthesia events should be obtained.

■ Preoperative Teaching

Ideally, postsurgical instructing should begin during the preoperative office visit. Written material that details the operative recovery period and provides answers to many of the most commonly asked questions and concerns for postsurgical sinus patients is provided to the patient by the physician, nurse clinician, and/or surgery scheduling personnel well in advance of the proposed surgery date (Fig. 26–1). This provides the patient ample opportunity

325

ENDOSCOPIC SINUS SURGERY

You deserve a breath of fresh air ®

Recurrent sinus problems are often caused by nasal polyps, recurrent infection or a blockage in the area where the sinuses should drain into the nose. These problems can be corrected with ENDOSCOPIC SINUS SURGERY. This delicate surgery is accomplished through your nose by reestablishing the normal air circulation and drainage of your sinuses. The same endoscopic equipment used to examine your sinuses during your office visit is used in the operating room.

Using the nasal endoscopes gives the physician a brightly illuminated and magnified view of the inside of the nose and sinuses. This permits a thorough removal of your sinus disease and the preservation of many of the normal nasal and sinus structures. In this way, much of the normal function of the nose and sinuses can be restored.

Even though you will have no visible incisions and the post-operative swelling and discomfort are minimal, you are undergoing a major sinus surgical procedure. Therefore, you will be required to take certain precautions. This information is provided to help you have a comfortable and successful recovery. No matter what is said in these guidelines, if you have any question about your postoperative care, please do not hesitate to call the doctor.

PREPARING FOR SURGERY

MEDICATIONS YOU MUST AVOID BEFORE SURGERY: ASPIRIN, IBUPROFEN PRODUCTS (Advil®, Nuprin®, Motrin®, other NSAIDS). **You must not take any of these products for one week before and one week following your surgery.** A list of medications to avoid is given to all Dr. Levine's patients. If you do not have this list, please call Dr. Levine's office.

SPECIAL MEDICATIONS. Bring medication taken regularly with you. If you use medications for high blood pressure, heart problems, asthma or diabetes, check with your surgeon about taking them the morning of your surgery.

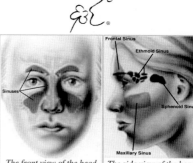

The front view of the head showing the location of the sinuses.   *The side view of the head showing the location of the sinuses.*

WHAT TO BRING TO SURGERY. Most patients go home the same day. Since there is a small chance you will need to stay overnight, bring a few personal items such as toothbrush, slippers, and robe. Most patients find it easier to use the hospital gowns rather than personal bed clothes. If you usually wear contact lenses, you will be more comfortable wearing your eye glasses after surgery.

SURGERY SCHEDULE. You will be told by the hospital or surgery center when to arrive for your surgery.

EATING & DRINKING BEFORE SURGERY. Most anesthetics require a time period with no food or drink. You will be advised about your eating and drinking schedule.

LEAVE VALUABLES AT HOME.

ARRANGE YOUR TRANSPORTATION. Since you should not drive for 24 hours after your surgery, you must have someone available to drive you home.

THE DAY OF SURGERY

ANESTHESIA. You will discuss your anesthesia with a member of the anesthesia department before surgery. Also, the doctor will see you before surgery to answer any last minute questions.

FIGURE 26–1 The patient brochure containing preoperative and postoperative instructions.

to review this material and to share it with others who will assist in providing care following surgery. Clinical staff should be available to answer questions that may arise from this material. For selected patients, the process of informed consent is reinforced by use of videotape education materials such as "Functional Endoscopic Sinus," produced by the American Academy of Otolaryngology Head and Neck Surgery.

Specific instructions are provided to patients regarding the avoidance of aspirin, nonsteroidal anti-inflammatory drugs, certain vitamin and herbal medications, and anticoagulants for 2 weeks prior to surgery. An updated list of these medications should be kept by physicians, nurses, and surgery-scheduling personnel to minimize the risk that these medications are used by patients prior to surgery. This list should also be made available to each patient.

Successful preoperative teaching also necessitates instructing patients about their recovery period. Each patient is informed that several visits are required following

surgery for removal of any intranasal dressings and debridement of eschar and exudate that are nearly always present following surgery. Patients may be advised to take pain medication ½ hour prior to each visit. They may choose to be accompanied by a friend or relative who is responsible for transportation should they feel the need. Patients must understand that significant resolution of their sinus symptoms may not occur until 6 to 8 weeks following surgery. They are informed that "recovery is a process, not an event."

The authors generally use a nasal and sinus outpatient facility consisting of a freestanding ambulatory surgery center that is part of a larger group of independent office suites. This building also has CT scanning equipment and laboratory facilities in association with a designated presurgical testing area. After patients have had the opportunity to schedule their procedure with the surgical scheduling staff, they are directed to the testing area for the appropriate preadmission testing.

THE HOSPITAL STAY. Following surgery, you will remain in the hospital several hours to be sure you have recovered from surgery and anesthesia.

PAIN. Because there is some discomfort after surgery, there will be pain medication for you at the hospital and a prescription for your home use. You may take acetaminophen (Tylenol®) as directed on the label.

INFORM YOUR FAMILY. Although your family does not need to be in the hospital while you are having your surgery, the doctor will want talk with them immediately after—either in person at the hospital or by telephone at work or home.

NASAL DRESSINGS. After surgery there may be a small, soft dressing or sponge-like tampon in your nose which will be removed before you leave the hospital. There will be a mustache-like dressing on your upper lip to absorb any drainage. It is common to change this dressing often immediately after surgery. Before you leave the hospital, you will be given any supplies and dressings you may need for at home care.

THE FIRST WEEK AFTER SURGERY

AVOID PHYSICAL ACTIVITY AND EXERTION. Excessive physical activity raises the blood pressure and can cause nasal bleeding.

OBTAIN ADDITIONAL REST. Even though your operation is relatively short, you may be tired and fatigued.

NASAL CARE. Do not blow the nose for the first seven days. If there is blood or mucus in the nose, gently sniff it back into the throat.

At the start of your recovery, you will have increased nasal drainage, often with some bright red bleeding. Do not be alarmed. A small amount of bleeding is not unusual and may continue through the first week. If you find it necessary to change your nasal dressing more than every 10 minutes, call Dr. Levine. Old blood which accumulates in the nose during surgery is reddish brown in color, drains from the nose for a week or more and is of no worry.

A moderate amount of thick and discolored drainage may continue from four to six weeks after surgery. The small mustache-dressing under your nose is for your convenience and may need to be changed frequently. When the drainage slows, you will not need to wear it. Gently wipe or dab your nose with a soft facial tissue.

You will have a stuffy, congested nose for several weeks.

Do not insert anything into the nose. If some dried blood has accumulated within your nostrils, gently remove it with a cotton tipped applicator moistened in hydrogen peroxide.

SNEEZING. If you must sneeze, do so with your mouth open so there will be less pressure within your nose.

DRY NOSE. You must use a salt-water nasal spray (e.g. Ocean®, AYR®, Afrin Saline®) 4 to 5 times per day to keep the nose moist. When the air is dry, a cool mist vaporizer will also help keep the nose moist. DRY LIPS. Dry lips caused by breathing through your mouth can be moistened with Vaseline® or baby oil.

AIR TRAVEL. Airplanes are dry and you must be sure to keep your nose moist by using a salt-water (saline) nasal spray frequently during your flight. If you experience facial pressure during air travel, a decongestant pill (e.g. Sudafed®) or using a nasal spray (e.g. Afrin®, Neo-Synephrine®) may provide comfort.

DISCOMFORT AFTER SURGERY. You will have some discomfort after surgery which will be more of an ache and pressure, rather than sharp pain. As the week passes, discomfort may increase due to increased swelling and accumulation of secretions in the sinuses. Keeping your head elevated and sleeping with an extra pillow helps decrease swelling, provides for better nasal drainage and gives you added comfort.

THE FIRST OFFICE VISIT AFTER SURGERY

It is important to keep your follow-up appointment. If you do not have one, please call the office. During your first office visit after surgery, you will have a nasal endoscopic examination. Some patients are anxious about this visit and you may be too. However, there is little or no discomfort involved with the nasal examination because your nose will be anesthetized. Unless other nasal procedures were done, there are no stitches to remove.

THE FIRST MONTHS AFTER SURGERY

PHYSICAL ACTIVITY. Aerobic activity may be resumed after one week. However, DO NOT SWIM for two weeks since water in your nose may cause a nasal infection. If bright red bleeding occurs, decrease these activities for a few days.

THE RECOVERY PROCESS. Your nasal breathing will not be its best until about six weeks after surgery. Some days, the breathing will be good. Other days, it will not. During this time, it is common for your nasal breathing to alternate from one side of the nose to the other.

Remember, your recovery is a process, not an event.

Date of Surgery: _____

Surgery Center: _____

Surgery Center Phone Number: _____

First Appointment after Surgery: _____

HOWARD L. LEVINE, M.D., F.A.C.S.
CLEVELAND NASAL-SINUS & SLEEP CENTER
5555 TRANSPORTATION BOULEVARD
CLEVELAND, OHIO 44125
216-518-3298 OR 800-24-SINUS

FIGURE 26–1 *(Continued)*

Patients undergoing local anesthesia do not require any preoperative testing. Healthy pediatric patients age 16 years or younger require no screening laboratory testing. African Americans who have not previously been screened for sickle cell disease must have a sickle cell prep performed. If a pediatric patient has a medical problem, appropriate tests may be done to clarify the extent or severity of that particular problem.

Adult patients are grouped into two categories. Those <35 years of age require complete blood count, glucose, potassium, BUN, and serum glutamic-oxaloacetic transaminase (SGOT); electrocardiogram (ECG) is obtained as indicated by the patient's medical history. In those patients >35 years of age, the same blood work is performed, and ECG is mandatory. A screening chest x-ray is required only if indicated by a patient's medical condition. Because many patients undergoing endoscopic sinus surgery have chronic obstructive pulmonary disease, chronic bronchitis, or a recent pulmonary infection, a chest x-ray may be obtained in these individuals.

Adult patients are required by the Joint Commission on Accreditation of Hospitals to have a completed history and physical examination in the chart prior to a surgical or endoscopic procedure. This is accomplished through the preadmission testing office, where a nurse practitioner is responsible for completion of this history and physical.

Children who do not undergo laboratory testing are examined by the nurse practitioner on the day of surgery, unless special arrangements have been made in advance with the patient's pediatrician or specialist. Pediatric patients and their families often visit with a child life specialist to introduce them to the surgical procedures and facility.

As with any surgical procedure, it is of the utmost importance to maintain an open dialogue with the anesthesia staff who are responsible for the patients at each individual facility to resolve potential conflicts before they have a negative impact on the surgery schedule.

As a final step before surgery, the patient's office chart is completed and reviewed by the operating surgeon and/or nurse. Those who are responsible for interacting with third-party payors quickly realize the utility of such information in the documentation of care. It becomes a permanent component of the patient's medical records.

Of course, there are exceptions to these guidelines, which must be based on the patient's medical condition and the problem that is being treated. Patient care is of paramount importance, and by following these guidelines, perioperative morbidity will be minimized in the outpatient surgical setting.

■ Perioperative Care

A transition from the preoperative area to the operating room and finally to the postanesthesia room and postoperative recovery area must be arranged in a fashion that will allow the patient to feel as comfortable as possible on the day of surgery. Minimal emphasis is placed on the actual preparation of the patient for surgery. Most of these issues have been addressed prior to the day of surgery. Instead, the patient is supported by the nursing staff, attending anesthesiologist and certified registered nurse anesthetist, attending surgeon, nurse clinician, and child life worker.

Preoperative sedation is generally not needed, but for the anxious patient intravenous midazolam (Versed) may be given. Oxymetazoline or an appropriate topical decongestant may be placed in the nose during this time to begin nasal decongestion. All eye makeup should be removed prior to entering the surgical suite so that the globe may be easily observed during surgery.

The anesthesia team may choose to use medications such as metoclopramide (Reglan) or ordansetron (Zofran) for the patient who has had a previous experience with nausea or vomiting following surgery. This allows for more rapid anesthesia recovery and avoids the occasional hospital transfer for nausea, vomiting, or fluid management.

The actual surgical procedure takes place much in the same way as it would in a standard inpatient facility. The technique generally utilizes propofol (Diprivan) for induction because of its short half-life. The patient experiences a shorter time in the postanesthesia recovery area and is able to return home in an expedient manner. Moreover, this maintains the tempo of the ambulatory surgery facility that is usually more rapid than that of its inpatient counterpart.

During surgery, the blood pressure is maintained using inhalation gases and other pharmacological modalities when necessary at the lowest possible level that is safe for each particular patient. This greatly facilitates the dissection, improves surgical visualization, and keeps blood loss to a minimum.

The instrumentation that is available may vary among institutions and surgeons. Arrangements must be made in advance if special equipment is required, such as image-guided triplanar navigation, surgical lasers, irrigation devices, microshavers, and drills. The attending surgeon must be familiar with the instrumentation that is available in each ambulatory surgery center. Ideally, video equipment should be stored together in single rolling cabinet to minimize setup time and to reduce maintenance.

A special surgical nursing team designated to and specifically trained to assist with endoscopic sinus surgery can greatly enhance the efficiency of performing multiple procedures on a given day. These personnel should be specifically trained to handle the video equipment, light sources, printers, and endoscopes. Departments such as biomedical engineering, which are normally found in larger inpatient settings, are usually not available in smaller freestanding ambulatory settings.

During surgery, the use of video imaging maintains the appropriate level of interest by others in the operating room, such as the anesthesiologist, circulating nurse, and scrub technician. This may aid the anesthesiologist in lowering the blood pressure if excessive bleeding is seen and in predicting the conclusion of the procedure, which promotes operating room efficiency by not delaying the wake-up time of the patient. Video imaging assists the skilled scrub technician in anticipating the surgeon's instrumentation needs.

The use of the video equipment also provides documentation for the patient's chart through the use of photographs or videotape. This helps during postoperative office visits in recalling specifics of the operation and unique intraoperative findings.

■ Postoperative Period

Following surgery, the patient is transferred to the postanesthesia recovery room. Preprinted written orders are provided to the postanesthesia nursing staff that are concerned with both general and specific aspects of the care of the patient who has undergone ESS. These order sheets have "fill in the blank" categories to customize the recovery orders for the specific patient needs (Fig. 26–2). These include vital signs, intravenous fluids, diet, analgesia, antibiotics (when applicable), antinausea medications, dressing changes, oxygen, and humidity. Special considerations are given to the surgical patient with pulmonary problems for the use of appropriate aerosol treatments. Freestanding ambulatory surgical centers may limit the physician's access to both the patient and the medical resources. The operating physician may have left the facility while the patient is still recovering and must have some method of communicating with the

GENERIC DRUG EQUIVALENT AUTHORIZED UNLESS OTHERWISE INDICATED

DRUG SENSITIVITY -

PRESS HARD WITH BALL POINT PEN ONLY

DATE	HOUR	ORDERS
		POSTOP
		1. Vital Signs per ASC Routine
		2. IV Therapy: DC PRN
		3. Diet: CLEAR LIQUIDS, THEN ADVANCE
		4. Activity: OOB WITH ASSIST, THEN AD LIB
		5. PRN Medications in ASC:
		A. Pain:
		1. Tylenol #3, 1-2 po Q4H PRN for pain
		2. Tylenol (2) po Q4H PRN for pain
		B. Nausea/Vomiting:
		Tigan, 200 mg IM/Supp Q6H
		6. Ice to Operative Area: Yes___ No___
		7. Dressing: Non-Sterile 2X2, 1/2" Micropore tape
		8. Void Before Discharge: Yes X No___
		9. Follow-Up Appointment:
		10. Discharge Instructions: SALINE NASAL SPRAY 5XDAILY
		SEND HOME WITH POST-OP BAG
		11. Discharge from ASC:
		12. Other:
		***ONLY THOSE ORDERS DATED, CHECKED, AND SIGNED BY M.D.
		WILL BE CARRIED OUT BY THE NURSING STAFF***

PHYSICIANS SIGNATURE/DATE _____

FIGURE 26–2 The postoperative order sheet, using a "fill in the blank" format tailored to the individual patient.

ambulatory unit. The nursing staff are often the ones to provide immediate assessment and attention to problems to ensure early intervention and the prevention of permanent postoperative morbidity. Therefore, the postoperative nursing team must become knowledgeable about nasal and, most importantly, sinus surgery. An understanding of what occurs intraoperatively and how this can effect the postoperative period is extremely helpful. This can best be accomplished through in-service training and observation of actual surgical procedures. In this way, the anatomy of the region and the potential complications are better understood.

The postoperative nursing team should become familiar with how much nasal bleeding to expect following surgery. This is usually best assessed by the frequency of dressing changes. Supplies and equipment to manage nasal hemorrhage must be available if needed by the nursing staff, nurse clinician, or operating surgeon. The nasal dressings that are removed by the nursing staff or nurse clinician and any unusual drainage are noted and reported to the surgeon.

The presence of ophthalmologic problems requires careful assessment by the postoperative nurses and often

immediate management. If a patient exhibits proptosis, orbital ecchymosis, or subconjunctival hemorrhage associated visual impairment, the attending physician or nurse clinician should be notified immediately. An ophthalmologic consultation may be needed to assess the patient. Because an ophthalmologist may not always be available in the ambulatory surgical facility one should be contacted and notified of the impending problems. In the interim, the operating surgeon and nursing staff must be able to initiate care to avert further problems.

Most patients achieve adequate pain control through the use of acetaminophen with codeine or an equivalent narcotic analgesic. Occasionally, patients require the use of parenteral pain medication, such as MSO 4 or meperidine. Orders for these medications are included in the standard nasal and sinus physicians' postoperative sheet. The nurse or surgeon is notified for any pain that is not adequately controlled with these medications. The findings of postural headaches or severe ocular pain need to be evaluated by the nurse or surgeon prior to the patient's discharge from the center.

Family members of patients < age 16 are permitted in the postanesthesia recovery area. They provide a familiar face for the patient recovering from anesthesia and generally make the postoperative nurse's task easier.

At the time of discharge, the nurse reviews with the patient and a responsible adult the postoperative home-going instruction booklet that had been given to the patient at the time of the initial preoperative counseling. It includes avoidance of excessive exertion, bending, or lifting, refraining from sneezing and expectoration through the nose, and strict avoidance of the use of aspirin and nonsteroidal anti-inflammatory drugs. If excessive headache, bleeding, or other unusual symptoms occur, patients are instructed to call the surgeon immediately.

Patients are given a home-going care supply bag (Fig. 26–3), which contains nasal cotton tip applicators to clean away any accumulated blood in the vestibule of the nose, 2 × 2 inch gauze dressings, ½ inch nonallergic paper tape to catch any nasal drainage, and a starter bottle of saline nasal spray to be used several times a day. The

supply bag also includes the office telephone number for contact staff if there is any problem. A written prescription for acetaminophen and codeine tablets or another appropriate analgesic is also included in this package. Antibiotics and steroids are used selectively depending on the specific patient problem.

■ Outpatient Care

Patients are instructed to consider taking a dose of their home-going pain medication 30 minutes before each of the several office visits following their surgery. During the first visit, if nasal splints or middle meatus dressing was used, it is removed following topical application of an aerosol anesthetic and decongestant. During this and subsequent visits, crusts, clots, secretions, and absorbable dressing materials are removed endoscopically using specially designed postoperative suctions and forceps. Intraoperative culture results are reviewed, and any necessary changes in the antibiotic regimen are undertaken at this time. Patients are counseled to expect continued expectoration and drainage of secretions and clot material and to have nasal congestion intermittently for several weeks following surgery.

■ Conclusion

Endoscopic sinus surgery represents a significant advance in the treatment of paranasal sinus disease and has allowed major sinus surgical procedures to be done in the ambulatory surgical setting. ESS can be done with great efficacy and safety. Perhaps no other procedure in the specialty of otolaryngology–head and neck surgery has evolved so closely with the transition of much of the surgical practice to outpatient-based facilities. Treatment of paranasal sinus diseases is ideally suited for either the freestanding surgical center or an outpatient facility that exists as part of a larger inpatient center. Regardless of the facility that is available, ESS requires considerable preoperative preparation, instrumentation, and personnel who are familiar with surgical techniques and perioperative care. Careful attention to coordination between office staff and personnel at the outpatient surgical facility will ensure a smooth and efficient flow that facilitates safe and successful surgery.

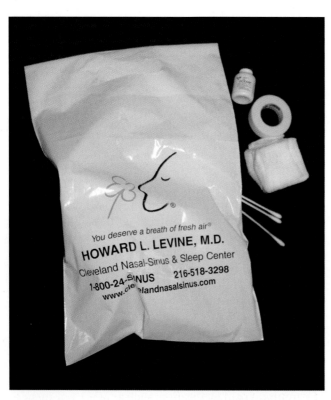

FIGURE 26–3   Postoperative home-going supplies.

Index

Abscess, pediatric rhinosinusitis complications, 127

Acanthamoeba infection, immunosuppressed patients, 116

Acoustic rhinometry, combined microscopic and endoscopic surgery, 170

Acquired immunodeficiency syndrome (AIDS) patients, rhinosinusitis, 114

   allergic *vs.* infective, 115–116

Acute sinusitis

   combined microscopic and endoscopic surgery, 166, *167*

   imaging studies, 72, *72*

   pediatric rhinosinusitis, surgical management, 125

Adenoidectomy, pediatric rhinosinusitis, 125

α-Adrenergic agonists, allergic rhinitis management, 101–102

Agger nasi

   combined microscopic and endoscopic surgery, frontal sinusotomy, 189–192, *191–193*

   endoscopic view, *53*, 54–55

   ethmoid sinus anatomy, 39, 41–42

   frontal recess anatomy, 21

   headache diagnosis, 136, *136*

   macroscopic anatomy, 21

   minimally invasive endoscopic sinus surgery, 213, *215*

Allergic bronchopulmonary aspergillosis (ABPA)

   allergic fungal sinusitis, differential diagnosis, 290, 294

   steroid therapy, 144–145

Allergic fungal sinusitis (AFS)

   combined microscopic and endoscopic surgery, 168

   diagnosis, *105–106*, 105–107

     allergic rhinitis, 296, *296*

     asthma, 296

     clinical presentation, 295–296

     criteria for, 298

     eosinophilic mucin sinusitis, differential diagnosis, 292

     fungal cultures, 293–294e

     fungal serology, 294

     fungal source geography and exposure, 297

     histopathology, 291–292

     imaging studies, *297*, 297–298

     immunologic evaluation, 294

     intracranial findings, 296

     lower airway association, 294–295

     Mayo Clinic case study, 292–293

     mechanical characteristics, 295

     ocular findings, 296

     paranasal manifestations, 290, *291*

     pathophysiology, 294–295

     saprophytic fungal colonization, EMRS non-AFS patients, 293

     staging system, 296–297, *297*

   etiology/pathogenesis, 105

   imaging studies, *76*, 77

   management, 107

     antifungal therapy, 145

     immunotherapy, 145–146

     overview, 141–142, *142–143*

     steroid therapy, 144–145

     surgical management, 144

Allergic rhinitis

   allergic fungal sinusitis, differential diagnosis, 296

   clinical findings/diagnosis, 101

   etiology/pathogenesis, 100–101

   management, *101*, 101–102

Allergy, sinus disease and, 103–105

Allergy testing, rhinosinusitis diagnosis, 95–99

Amoxicillin-clavulanate, pediatric rhinosinusitis, 124

Amphotericin B, allergic fungal sinusitis therapy, 145

Anamnesis, rhinosinusitis, immunosuppressed patients, 116–117

Anesthesia
    avoidance of ophthalmological complications, 286
    combined microscopic and endoscopic surgery, 163
        protocols for, 177–179, *178–179*
    minimally invasive endoscopic sinus surgery, 209–210
    sinus surgery
        coexisting clinical conditions, 320
        management protocols, *317–319*, 317–320
        preoperative evaluation, 316–317

Anterior arch (turbinates), revision endoscopic sinus surgery assessment, 262

Anterior cerebral artery, surgical bleeding from, 275

Anterior ethmoid air cell, computed tomographic imaging, 69

Anterior ethmoid sinus
    combined microscopic and endoscopic surgery, 162
    minimally invasive endoscopic sinus surgery, 214

Anterior nasal polyposis, Nd:YAG laser surgery, 249–250, *251*

Antibiotics
    pediatric rhinosinusitis, 124
    rhinosinusitis therapy, 98–99
    sinus disease and allergy and, 104–105

Antifungal therapy, allergic fungal sinusitis, 145

Antigen immunotherapy
    allergic fungal sinusitis, 107
    allergic rhinitis management, 102
    sinus disease and allergy and, 104–105

Antigen-presenting cells (AP cells), paranasal sinus physiology, immune defense, 61

Antigen testing, allergic fungal sinusitis diagnosis, *296*

Antihistamines, allergic rhinitis management, *101*, 101–102

Antimicrobials, pediatric rhinosinusitis, 124

Antral choanal polyps, laser surgery, 244

Archiving information, Medtronic Xomed LandmarX system, 224

Asthma
    allergic fungal sinusitis diagnosis, 296
    rhinosinusitis, 91–99
        pediatric rhinosinusitis, 123
    sinusitis and
        eosinophil mechanisms, 108
        epidemiology, 107–108
        inflammatory mediators, 108–109
        medical therapy, 109, *109*
        neural reflexes, 108
        surgical therapy, 109–110

Atopy, allergic fungal sinusitis and, 106–107

Autonomic innervation, nasal cavity, 23–25, *28–29*

Backbiter forceps, minimally invasive endoscopic sinus surgery, 213, *214*

Bacterial infection, rhinosinusitis, 98–99
    HIV patients, 115–116

Barosinusitis, headache and, *139*, 139–140

Basal lamellae
    computed tomographic imaging, 69, *69*
    ethmoid sinus anatomy, 37–39, *39–40*, 41
    meatal system anatomy, 39, 41–42

Bifrontal craniotomy, cerebrospinal fluid leak management, 303–304

Binocular Zeiss operating microscope, combined microscopic and endoscopic surgery, 162

Biophysics, Nd:YAG laser, 245–246

Blakesley forceps, endoscopic orbital decompression, 308, *308*

Bleeding
    ophthalmologic complications involving, 287
    as surgical complication, 275

Bone pathology, imaging studies, 83–84, *83–84*

Bony anatomy
    ethmoid sinus, 33, *34*, 35, 37–43, *38–42*
    frontal sinus, *43–46*, 43–47
    maxillary sinus, 27, 29–33, *29–33*
    nasal cavity, 13, *14*
    paranasal sinus, 27, *29*
    sphenoid sinus, 45, 47, *48–50*, 49–50

Bony structures, maxillary sinus, 27, 29, 31–33, *31–34*, 35

Boyer's cell, ethmoid sinus anatomy, 39–42

BrainLab's VectorVision, stereotactic surgery, 224–227, *225–227*

Bronchial hyperresponsiveness (BHR), asthma and sinusitis, 109, *109*

Bullar system, anatomy, 39–43, *41*

Burs, Micro-Debrider tool, 209

Caldwell-Luc procedure, endoscopic orbital decompression, 306

Calibration protocols, BrainLab's VectorVision, 226

Carbon dioxide (CO_2) laser
    nasal and sinus surgery, 241
    vs. Nd:YAG laser, 245–246
    turbinate dysfunction, 242–243

Carbon dioxide pressure (pCO_2), paranasal sinus physiology, 60

Carotid artery
    bleeding as surgical complication, 275
    sphenoid sinus anatomy, 49, *49*

Cartilage, medial nasal cavity wall, 13, *14*

Cavernous sinus thrombosis
    imaging studies, 79–80
    pediatric rhinosinusitis complications, 127

Cellulitis, pediatric rhinosinusitis complications, 127

Cerebrospinal fluid leak, endoscopic sinus surgery, 300–305, *301–304*

Cerebrospinal fluid rhinorrhea, combined microscopic and endoscopic surgery, 168

Change-coupled device (CCD) video camera, combined microscopic and endoscopic surgery, 172

Charcot-Leyden crystals, allergic fungal sinusitis, histopathology, *291*, 291–292

Choanal atresia
    developmental anatomy, 4–5
    Nd:YAG laser surgery
        indications, 251–252
        results, 254

Chronic fungal sinusitis, defined, 141

Chronic obstructive pulmonary disease, anesthesia for sinus surgery and, 320

Chronic rhinosinusitis (CRS), allergic fungal sinusitis, differential diagnosis, 292–293
Chronic sinusitis
  asthma and
    eosinophils and, 108
    epidemiology, 107–108
    inflammatory mediators, 108–109
    medical therapy, 109, *109*
    neural reflexes, 108
    surgical therapy, 109–110
  combined microscopic and endoscopic surgery, 164–166
  headache pain and, 137–140
  imaging studies, 72–75, *73–75*
  odontogenic pathology, imaging studies, 84, *84*
  pediatric rhinosinusitis, surgical management, 125–126
  revision endoscopic sinus surgery assessment, 261–262
Ciliary dysfunction, pediatric rhinosinusitis, 123
Classification issues, combined microscopic and endoscopic surgery, 199–200
Clear ESS system, endoscopic surgery, 151–152, *152*
Clindamycin, pediatric rhinosinusitis, 124
Clivus, sphenoid sinus anatomy, 47, 49
Cluster headaches, epidemiology, 138
Cocaine
  endoscopic orbital decompression, 307
  minimally invasive endoscopic sinus surgery, 209
Combined microscopic and endoscopic technique (COMET)
  anesthesia considerations, 177–179, *178–179*
  classification, standardization and results documentation, 199–200
  complications, 203, *203*
  ergonomic performances, 175–176, *175–176*
  ethmoidectomy, *185*, 185–189, *187–190*
  frontal sinusotomy, 189–190, *191*, 192, *192–193*
  historical evolution, 162–163
  indications for, 166, *167*, 168
  inferior turbinate, 195–197, *196–197*
  instrumentation, *171*, 171–172
  major/minor nasal unit concept, 198–199
  maxillary antrostomy, 181–185, *186*
  middle turbinate management, 180, *181*
  optical performances, 173–175, *173–175*
  optical principles, 172–173
  patient positioning, 176–177, *176–177*
  planning protocols, 170–171
  postoperative care, *197*, 197–198
  preoperative evaluation, *169*, 169–170
  results evaluation, 198–203, *200–202*
  septoplasty and/or rhinoplasty, 179–180
  sphenoidotomy, 192–195, *193–195*
  strategic approach, 179, *179*
  surgical principles, *163*, 163–166, *165–166*
  uncinectomy, 181, *182–184*
Complement system, paranasal sinus physiology, immune defense, 61
Complications
  anesthesia for sinus surgery, 319–320
  avoidance strategies, 276–282
    anteroposterior ethmoid dissection, 279–280, *280*
    frontal sinusitis surgical approach, 281, *282*
    imaging techniques, 277
    instrumentation selection, 277–278, *278*
    lateral nasal wall anatomy knowledge, *276*, 276–277
    posteroanterior upper ethmoid level dissection, 281–282
    sphenoid sinus anterior wall dissection, 280–281, *280–281*
    surgical techniques, 278–282, *279–282*
  bleeding, 275
  classification, 269–276
  combined microscopic and endoscopic surgery, 203, *203*
  dacryocystorhinostomy, 314–315
  endoscopic orbital decompression, 310–311
  ethmoid roof/cribrifrom plate injuries, 272–275, *273–274*
  frontal sinusitis, post-paranasal surgery, 275–276
  internal carotid artery bleeding, 275
  intraconal orbital injuries, 270–271
  lacrimal duct/sac injujry, 270, *270*
  lid hematoma, 270
  myospherulosis, 275
  Nd:YAG laser surgery, 252–253
  ophthalmologic complications, research overview, 285–289, *286–288*
  research overview, 269
  retrobulbar postseptal hematoma, 271–272, *272*
Computed tomography (CT)
  allergic fungal sinusitis
    diagnosis, *297*, 297–298
    surgical assessment, 144
  BrainLab's VectorVision, 226, *226*
  combined microscopic and endoscopic surgery, 163
    preoperative evaluation, 170
  endonasal endoscopy, 148–150
  functional endoscopic surgery, 64, *64–67*, 66–67
  intraoperative computer-assisted guidance, 88
  Medtronic Xomed LandmarX system, 222–223
  ophthalmological surgical complications, *288*, 288–289
  paranasal sinus
    anatomical variations, 70
    basic principles, 64–67, *64–67*
    dental implants, 84–85, *85*
    ethmoid variants, 71, *71*
    inflammatory/infectious disease, 72–77
      acute sinusitis, 72
      chronic sinusitis, 72–75, *73–75*
      fungal sinusitis, 75, *76*, 77
      granulomatous sinusitis, *76*, 77
    inflammatory polyps, 78, *78*
    intraoperative computer-assisted guidance, 88
    magnetic resonance imaging, 67–68
    middle turbinate variants, 70, *70–71*
    mucocele, 77, *78*
    mucous retention cyst, 77, *77*
    nasal masses, 85–86, *85–86*
    normal anatomy, *68–69*, 68–70
    nuclear medicine, 68
    odontogenic/bone pathology, 83–84, *84–85*
    orbital complications, 79–80
    osteomyelitis, 80, *81–82*, 83
    postoperative assessment, 86–87
    septal variants, 70, *70*

Computed tomography (CT), paranasal sinus *(Continued)*
  sphenoid variants, 71, *72*
    surgical complications, 87, *87–88*
    uncinate variants, 70–71, *71*
  pediatric rhinosinusitis, 123
  revision endoscopic sinus surgery assessment, *261*, 261–262
  rhinosinusitis
    diagnosis, *95–98*, 95–99
    immunosuppressed patients, 119
    surgical management, staging systems, 256–257
  VTI InstaTrak, 221–222
Computer requirements
  Medtronic Xomed LandmarX system, 222
  Stryker Navigation System, 228, *229*
  VTI InstaTrak, 220
Concha bulla
  chronic sinusitis, imaging studies, 73–74
  ethmoid sinus anatomy, 37–38
Concha bullosa, endoscopic sinus surgery, *158*, 158–159
Corticosteroids. *See* Steroids
Cranial fossa, frontal sinus anatomy, 43, *44*
Cribriform plate
  ethmoid sinus anatomy, 35, *36*, 37
  surgical injury to, 272–274, *273–274*
Crista galli, ethmoid sinus anatomy, 35, *36*
Cromolyn, allergic rhinitis management, 102
Cutter instrumentation
  Micro-Debrider tool, 208–209
  minimally invasive endoscopic sinus surgery, characteristics and positioning, 207–208
Cystic fibrosis
  chronic sinusitis, imaging studies, 74
  pediatric rhinosinusitis, 123
  rhinosinusitis and, 91
Cytokines
  asthma, eosinophil activity and, 108
  sinus disease and allergy and, 104
Cytomegalovirus (CMV), rhinosinusitis, HIV patients, 115–116

Dacryocystorhinostomy
  endoscopic anatomy, 312, *313*
  postoperative care, 314
  results evaluation, 314–315
  surgical technique, 313–314, *314*
Decompression techniques, ophthalmological surgical complications, 289
Dematiaceous fungi, allergic fungal sinusitis diagnosis, 293–294
Dental implants, imaging studies, 84–85, *85*
Depth of field, combined microscopic and endoscopic surgery, 173
Developmental anatomy
  paranasal sinus, 1–12
    ethmoid sinus, 7–9, *8–10*
    frontal sinus, 10–11, *11*
    maxillary sinus, 7, *7*
    nose development, 1–6, *2–5*
    sinus development, *6*, 6–7
    sphenoid sinus, 11–12, *11–12*
  pediatric rhinosinusitis, 122
Diplopia, as surgical complication, 287, *287*

Documentation, combined microscopic and endoscopic surgery, 199–200
Doppler laser velocimetry, mucociliary clearance assessment, 60
Drillout technique, endoscopic surgery, frontal sinus, 238
Drug rebound headache, 138
Dysthyroid orbitopathy, endoscopic orbital decompression, 306–310, *307*

Electromagnetic transmitter/receiver, VTI InstaTrak, 221
Endonasal endoscopic surgery
  anterior ethmoid sinus, 153, *154*
  dressing and packing, 160–161
  frontal sinus, 155
  general principles, 151–152, *152*
  historical evolution, 148
  image-guided triplanar localization, 159, *160*
  marsupialization technique, 156
  maxillary sinus, 155, *156*
  minimally invasive techniques, 156, *157*
  nasal septal surgery, 151
  nasal turbinates, 156–159
    inferior turbinate, *157*, 157–158
    middle turbinate, *158*, 158–159
    superior turbinate, 159
  operating room protocols, 149–151, *149–151*
  patient preparation, 148–149
  posterior ethmoid sinus, 153–154, *154*
  posterior Wigand approach, 155–156
  sphenoid sinus, 154–155, *155*
  traditional approach, 152
  uncinate process, 152–153, *153*
Endoscopic anatomy
  dacryocystorhinostomy, 312, *313*
  paranasal sinus, *50–54*, 50–55
Endoscopic equipment
  combined microscopic and endoscopic surgery, 172
  Nd:YAG laser surgery, 247–248
Endoscopic orbital decompression
  classification, *307*
  research overview, 306
  results evaluation, 310–311
  surgical technique, 307–310, *307–310*
Endoscopic sinus surgery (ESS)
  allergic fungal sinusitis management, 141–142, *142–143*, 144
  complications
    avoidance strategies, 276–282
    classification, 269–276
  meningoencephaloceles and cerebrospinal fluid leak, 300–305, *301–304*
  minimally invasive techniques, powered instrumentation
    agger nasi to frontal sinus, 213, *216*
    anesthesia, 209
    anterior ethmoid sinus, 214
    cocaine administration, 209
    cutter characteristics and positioning, 207–208
    ethmoid bulla, 213–214, *216*
    frontal sinus locations, 213, *216*
    hiatus semilunaris posterior, 214, 216, *217*
    historical background, 207–208

injection techniques, 209–210
micro-debrider tool development, 208–209
middle turbinate, 211–212, *211–212*
oxymetazoline administration, 209
posterior ethmoid sinus, 216
postoperative care, 218–219
sphenoid sinus, 217–218
techniques, *210,* 210–211
uncinate/maxillary ostium, 212–213, *214–215*
ophthalmological complications, 285–289, *286–288*
outpatient nursing care, 325–330
outpatient care, 330
perioperative care, 328
postoperative period, 328–330
preoperative evaluation, 325
preoperative teaching, 325–328, *326–327*
pediatric rhinosinusitis, 125–126
postoperative care, 322–324, *323*
revision ESS
ethmoid revision, 264, *264*
frontal sinus, 266–267, *266–267*
maxillary sinus, 263–264, *264*
medical and surgical failures, 262–263
research overview, 260–262, *261*
sphenoid sinus, *265,* 265–266
traditional approach, 152
Endoscopic techniques, paranasal sinus physiology, 60
Energy dosage, endonasal laser surgery, 242
Environmental factors, rhinosinusitis, 90–91
Eosinophilic mucin sinusitis, allergic fungal sinusitis,
    differential diagnosis, 292
Eosinophils
asthma mechanisms and, 108
nasal polyposis, laser surgery, 243–244, *244*
Epistaxis
laser surgery, 243
Nd:YAG laser surgery
indications, 250, *251*
results, 254
Equipment, Nd:YAG laser surgery, 247–248
Ergonomics, combined microscopic and endoscopic surgery,
    175–176, *175–176*
Ethmoid bulla
anatomy, 39–43, *41*
combined microscopic and endoscopic surgery,
    ethmoidectomy, 186–188, *188–190*
computed tomographic imaging, 69, *69*
macroscopic anatomy, 21
minimally invasive endoscopic sinus surgery, 213–214,
    216
surgical strategies involving, 278–282, *279*
anteroposterior dissection, 279–280, *280*
Ethmoidectomy
combined microscopic and endoscopic surgery, 185–186,
    188–189, *188–190*
endoscopic orbital decompression, 308
Ethmoid foramina, ethmoid sinus anatomy, 35, 37, *38*
Ethmoid infundibulum, macroscopic anatomy, 19–20
Ethmoid labyrinth, anatomy, 35, 37–40, *39–40*
Ethmoid roof injury, etiology and management, 272–274,
    273–274

Ethmoid sinus. *See also* Anterior ethmoid sinus
bony anatomy, vasculature, and innervation, 35, *36,* 37–43,
    38–42, 50–51
computed tomographic imaging, variants, 71, *71*
developmental anatomy, 7–9, *8–10*
endoscopic surgery
anterior, 153, *154*
posterior, 153–154, *154*
headache and, 132–133, *133*
minimally invasive endoscopic sinus surgery, posterior view,
    216, *217*
revision endoscopic surgery, 264, *264*
surgical strategies for
anteroposterior dissection, 279–280, *280*
posteroanterior dissection, 281–282
Ethmoturbinals, developmental anatomy, 8–10
Eustachian tube pathology, Nd:YAG laser surgery, 252
Evolutionary theory, paranasal sinus physiology, 57
Exophthalmos, combined microscopic and endoscopic
    surgery, 168
Extraocular motion (EOM) impairment, pediatric
    rhinosinusitis complications, 127
Extropia, as surgical complication, 288, *288*

Facial components, developmental anatomy, 3–6, *3–6*
Facial pressure, headache pain and, 137
Failed surgery and medicine, revision surgery assessment,
    262–263
Fiber properties, Nd:YAG laser surgery, 247
Fiducial markers, BrainLab's VectorVision, 225
Fine control techniques, minimally invasive endoscopic sinus
    surgery, 211
Focal distance, combined microscopic and endoscopic
    surgery, 173
Forced expiratory volume (FEV_1), asthma mechanisms,
    109
Frontal recess
endoscopic surgery, frontal sinus, 231, *232*
macroscopic anatomy, 20–21
Frontal recess (FR), normal anatomy, 68–70, *69–70*
Frontal sinus
developmental anatomy, 10–11, *11*
endoscopic surgery, 155–156
anatomy, 231–233, *231–235*
drillout techniques, 238
embryology, 231
indications/contraindications, 238
irrigation problems, *237,* 237–238
landmarks for, 238–239, *239*
objective abnormalities, 236–237, *237*
pathophysiology, 233, 235, *235*
theoretical background, 235–236, *236*
minimally invasive endoscopic sinus surgery, 213, *216*
mucociliary transport, 60
operative complications, imaging studies, 87, *87*
pediatric rhinosinusitis complications, 128
revision endoscopic surgery, 266–267, *266–267*
surgical anatomy, *43–46,* 43–47
surgical strategies for, 282, *282*
vasculature and innervation, 50
Frontal sinusitis, as surgical complication, 275–276

Frontal sinusotomy, combined microscopic and endoscopic surgery, 189–192, *191–193*
Frontonasal communication, macroscopic anatomy, 19, *20*
Frontonasal process, developmental anatomy, 1–2, *2*
Functional endoscopic surgery (FESS)
  asthma and chronic sinusitis, 109–110
  defined, 148
  frontal sinus, theoretical background, 235–236, *236*
  imaging studies
    anatomical variations, 70
    computed tomography, 64–67, *64–67*
    dental implants, 84–85, *85*
    ethmoid variants, 71, *71*
    inflammatory/infectious disease, 72–77
      acute sinusitis, 72
      chronic sinusitis, 72–75, *73–75*
      fungal sinusitis, 75, *76*, 77
      granulomatous sinusitis, *76*, 77
    inflammatory polyps, 78, *78*
    intraoperative computer-assisted guidance, 88
    magnetic resonance imaging, 67–68
    middle turbinate variants, 70, *70–71*
    mucocele, 77, *78*
    mucous retention cyst, 77, *77*
    nasal masses, 85–86, *85–86*
    normal anatomy, *68–69*, 68–70
    nuclear medicine, 68
    odontogenic/bone pathology, 83–84, *84–85*
    orbital complications, 79–80
    osteomyelitis, 80, *81–82*, 83
    postoperative assessment, 86–87
    septal variants, 70, *70*
    sphenoid variants, 71, *72*
    surgical complications, 87, *87–88*
    ultrasound, 68
    uncinate variants, 70–71, *71*
  revision, assessment and indications, 260–262, *261*
Functional theory, paranasal sinus physiology, 58
Fungal cultures
  allergic fungal sinusitis diagnosis, *293*, 293–294
  source geography and exposure, 297
Fungal serology, allergic fungal sinusitis diagnosis, 294
Fungal sinusitis
  HIV patients, 116, *116*
  imaging studies, 75, *75–76*, 77
  management, 141–142, *142–143*
  paranasal manifestations, 290, *291*

Gaseous exchange, paranasal sinus physiology, 59
Gliklich and Metson staging system, rhinosinusitis surgical management, 257–258
Granulocyte macrophage colony-stimulating factor (GM-CSF), sinus disease and allergy and, 104
Granulomatous sinusitis
  imaging studies, *76*, 77
  invasive sinusitis, defined, 141
Graves' disease, endoscopic orbital decompression, 306–310

Haller's cells
  ethmoid sinus anatomy, 39, 41–42
  ethmoid sinus development, 10, *10*

Hand positioning, minimally invasive endoscopic sinus surgery, 211
Headache, rhinosinusitis and, 132–140, *132–140*
Headset, VTI InstaTrak, 220–221, *221*
Hereditary hemorrhagic telangiectasia
  laser surgery, 243
  Nd:YAG laser surgery, 250, *251*
Hiatus semilunaris
  macroscopic anatomy, 19
  minimally invasive endoscopic sinus surgery, posterior view, 214, 216, *218*
High-energy particulate air (HEPA) filter, allergic rhinitis management, 101–102
Histamines
  allergic rhinitis etiology/pathogenesis, 100–101
  asthma mechanisms, 108–109
Histocompatibility system (HLA-DR), paranasal sinus physiology, immune defense, 61
Hounsfield unit (HU), computed tomographic imaging, 66, *66*
Ho:YAG laser, nasal and sinus surgery, 241
Human immunodeficiency virus (HIV) infection, rhinosinusitis
  clinical signs and symptoms, 115–119, *116–118*
  epidemiology, *114*, 114–115
  treatment, 119
Hypertrophic rhinitis, Nd:YAG laser surgery
  indications, 249, *250*
  results, 253

Image-guided sinus surgery
  revision assessment, 262
  triplanar localization
    basic techniques, 159–160, *159–160*
    Micro-Debrider tool, 209
Imaging studies
  allergic fungal sinusitis
    clinical signs, *76*, 77
    diagnosis, *297*, 297–298
  avoidance of surgical complications with, 277
  cerebrospinal fluid leak management, 302–304, *303*
  Nd:YAG laser surgery, 248
Immune defense
  paranasal sinus physiology, 60–62
  pediatric rhinosinusitis, developmental anatomy, 123
Immunoglobulin E (IgE)
  allergic fungal sinusitis, 105–107
  allergic rhinitis etiology/pathogenesis, 100–101
  EMRS non-AFS patients, 293
  sinus disease and allergy and, 103
Immunoglobulin G (IgG)
  allergic fungal sinusitis, 105–107
  immunocompromised hosts, rhinosinusitis epidemiology, 113, *114*
Immunoglobulins, paranasal sinus physiology, immune defense, 61
Immunologic evaluation, allergic fungal sinusitis diagnosis, 294
Immunosuppressed patients
  computed tomographic imaging, 66–67
  rhinosinusitis, 91, Human immunodeficiency virus general epidemiology, 113, *114*

Immunotherapy
    allergic fungal sinusitis, 107, 145–146
    allergic rhinitis management, 102
    sinus disease and allergy and, 104–105
Incisor lesions, imaging studies, 83–84, *83–84*
Inferior turbinate
    combined microscopic and endoscopic surgery, *195–196,*
        195–197
    endoscopic view, 51, *51*
    macroscopic anatomy, 21–22, *22*
Inflammatory/infectious disease
    orbital complications, imaging studies, *79,* 79–80
    paranasal sinus imaging studies, 72–77
        acute sinusitis, 72
        chronic sinusitis, 72–75, *73–75*
        fungal sinusitis, 75, *76,* 77
        granulomatous sinusitis, *76,* 77
    rhinosinusitis, 91–99
Inflammatory mediators, asthma and, 108–109
Inflammatory polyps, imaging studies, 78, *78*
Inflammatory response, rhinosinusitis, HIV infection, 115
Infraorbital foramen, maxillary sinus anatomy, 32
Infratemporal fossa, maxillary sinus anatomy, 32–33, *33*
Injection techniques, anesthesia, minimally invasive
        endoscopic sinus surgery, 209–210
Instrumentation
    avoidance of surgical complications with, 277, *278*
    BrainLab's VectorVision, 227, *227*
    cerebrospinal fluid leak management, *302,* 302–303
    combined microscopic and endoscopic surgery, 171–172,
        178
    laser surgery, 242
    Medtronic Xomed LandmarX system, 224
    Stryker Navigation System, 228, *229*
    VTI InstaTrak, 222
Insufflating xenon, mucociliary clearance assessment, 60
Interferons, paranasal sinus physiology, immune defense, 61
Interleukins
    allergic rhinitis etiology/pathogenesis, 100–101
    sinus disease and allergy and, 104
Internal frontal ostium, endoscopic surgery, frontal sinus,
    231
Internal maxillary artery, nasal cavity vascular anatomy, 22–23,
    24
Intracerebral bleeding, as surgical complication, 275
Intraconal injury, etiology and management, 270–271
Intracranial complications
    allergic fungal sinusitis diagnosis, 296
    pediatric rhinosinusitis complications, 127–128
Intranasal/intrasinus scar formation, laser surgery, 244
Intraoperative computer-assisted guidance, imaging
        techniques, 88
Intraorbital retrobulbar hematoma, 287
Intrasinus/local complications, pediatric rhinosinusitis,
    126–127
Intravenous contrast, computed tomographic imaging, 66
In vitro testing, allergic rhinitis diagnosis, 101
Ipratropium, allergic rhinitis management, 102
Irrigation techniques
    frontal sinus, endoscopic surgery, *237,* 237–238
    Micro-Debrider tool, 208

Itraconazole, allergic fungal sinusitis therapy, 145

Kaposi's lesions, rhinosinusitis, 114
Kartagener's syndrome, chronic sinusitis, imaging studies, 75,
    75
Kiesselbach's plexus, nasal cavity vasculature, 23, *25*
Kolibri ENT system, stereotactic surgery, 227–228, *228*
KTP/532 laser, nasal and sinus surgery
    antral choanal polyps, 244
    energy dosage, 242
    historical background, 241–242
    instrumentation, 242, *242*
    intranasal/intrasinus scar formation, 244
    laser comparisons, *242*
    nasal polyposis/eosinophilia, 243–244, *244*
    postoperative management, 244
    safety issues, 242
    turbinate dysfunction, 242–243
    vascular disorders, 243

Lacrimal duct/sac, surgical injury to, 270, *270*
Lamellae
    developmental anatomy, 8, *8*
    ethmoid sinus anatomy, 35, *36,* 37–43
    macroscopic anatomy, 15, *16,* 17
    surgical injury to, 272–274, *273–274*
Lamina papyracea
    endoscopic orbital decompression, 308, *308*
    endoscopic sinus surgery, uncinate process, 153, *153*
    revision endoscopic sinus surgery assessment, 262
Laryngeal mask airway (LMA)
    endonasal endoscopy, 150–151, *150–151*
    sinus surgery, *317–318,* 317–320
Laser surgery
    nasal and sinus surgery
        antral choanal polyps, 244
        energy dosage, 242
        historical background, 241–242
        instrumentation, 242, *242*
        intranasal/intrasinus scar formation, 244
        laser comparisons, *242*
        nasal polyposis/eosinophilia, 243–244, *244*
        postoperative management, 244
        safety issues, 242
        turbinate dysfunction, 242–243
        vascular disorders, 243
    overview, 241
Lateral sinus, macroscopic anatomy, 21
Leukotriene receptor antagonist, allergic rhinitis
        management, 102
Leukotrienes, asthma mechanisms, 108–109
Lid hematoma, etiology and management, 270
Light source, Nd:YAG laser surgery, 248
Limen nasi, macroscopic anatomy, 12
Long-term care, endoscopic sinus surgery, 323–324
Lothrop procedure, frontal sinus, 267, *267*
Lower airway association, allergic fungal sinusitis diagnosis,
    294–295
Lower respiratory tract (LRT), pediatric rhinosinusitis and, 128
Luminance, combined microscopic and endoscopic surgery,
    175

Lund and McKay staging system, rhinosinusitis surgical
    management, 258–259
Lymphatic drainage
    naval cavity, 27
    paranasal sinuses, 49–50
Lysozyme, paranasal sinus physiology, immune defense, 61

Macrophages, paranasal sinus physiology, immune defense, 61
Magnetic resonance imaging (MRI)
    acute sinusitis, 72
    chronic sinusitis, 72–75, *74–75*
    functional endoscopic surgery, 67–68
    fungal sinusitis, 75, *75–76*, 77
    inflammatory polyps, 78, *78*
    intraoperative computer-assisted guidance, 88
    mucous retention cyst, 77, *77*
    nasal masses, 85–86, *85–86*
    orbital complications, 79–80
    pediatric rhinosinusitis, 123
    rhinosinusitis, immunosuppressed patients, 119
Major/minor nasal unit concept, combined microscopic and
    endoscopic surgery, 198–199
Malignant tumors, combined microscopic and endoscopic
    surgery, 168
Marsupialization endoscopic sinus surgery (MESS),
    applications, 156
Mast cells
    allergic rhinitis etiology/pathogenesis, 100–101
    paranasal sinus physiology, immune defense, 61
Maxillary antrostomy
    combined microscopic and endoscopic surgery, 181–185,
        185–187
    revision endoscopic sinus surgery assessment, 262
Maxillary nerve, nasal cavity anatomy, 23, *26–27*
Maxillary ostium, minimally invasive endoscopic sinus surgery,
    212–213, *214–215*
Maxillary process, developmental anatomy, 2–5, *4*
Maxillary sinus
    developmental anatomy, 7, *7*
    endoscopic orbital decompression, *307*, 307–308
    endoscopic surgery, 155, *156*
    headache and, 132, *132–133*
    mucociliary transport, 60
    revision endoscopic surgery, 263–264, *264*
    surgical anatomy, 27, 29, 31–33, *31–34*, 35
    surgical strategies involving, 278–279, *279*
    vasculature and innervation, 27, *28*, 29, 31–33, *31–34*, 35,
        50–51
Mayo Clinic case study, allergic fungal sinusitis, differential
    diagnosis, 292–293
Mayo stand, endonasal endoscopy, 149–151, *149–151*
Meatal system
    anatomy, 39–43, *41*
    endoscopic view, 51, *52–53*, 54
Medical therapy
    asthma and sinusitis, 109, *109*
    headaches, 138–139
    pediatric rhinosinusitis, 123–124
Medtronic Xomed LandmarX system, stereotactic surgery,
    222–224, *223–224*
Meningitis, pediatric rhinosinusitis and, 128

Meningoencephaloceles, endoscopic sinus surgery and,
    300–305, *301–304*
Microbiology, pediatric rhinosinusitis, 123
Micro-Debrider
    allergic fungal sinusitis, 144
    development of, 208–209
    minimally invasive endoscopic sinus surgery, techniques,
        210–212, *210–212*
Microsporidia, rhinosinusitis, immunosuppressed patients,
    116
Middle turbinate flap, cerebrospinal fluid leak management,
    303–304, *304*
Middle turbinates
    combined microscopic and endoscopic surgery, 180–181,
        180–181
    computed tomographic imaging, variants, 70, *70–71*
    endoscopic orbital decompression, 308
    minimally invasive endoscopic sinus surgery, 211–212,
        211–213
Midinspiratory flow (MIF_{50}), asthma mechanisms, 109
Migraine headaches, epidemiology, 137–138
Minimally invasive endoscopic sinus surgery
    basic techniques, 156, *157*
    powered instrumentation
        agger nasi to frontal sinus, 213, *216*
        anesthesia, 209
        anterior ethmoid sinus, 214
        cocaine administration, 209
        cutter characteristics and positioning, 207–208
        ethmoid bulla, 213–214, *216*
        frontal sinus locations, 213, *216*
        hiatus semilunaris posterior, 214, 216, *217*
        historical background, 207–208
        injection techniques, 209–210
        micro-debrider tool development, 208–209
        middle turbinate, 211–212, *211–212*
        oxymetazoline administration, 209
        posterior ethmoid sinus, 216
        postoperative care, 218–219
        sphenoid sinus, 217–218
        techniques, *210*, 210–211
        uncinate/maxillary ostium, 212–213, *214–215*
Monitored anesthesia care (MAC), sinus surgery, 317
Montelukast, allergic rhinitis management, 102
Muciprocin ointment, for surgical dressing, 275
Mucocele
    combined microscopic and endoscopic surgery, 168
    imaging studies, 77, *78*
Mucociliary transport (MCT), paranasal sinus physiology,
    59–60
Mucociliary transport time (MCTt)
    paranasal sinus physiology, 60
    rhinosinusitis, HIV infection, 115
Mucormycosis
    immunosuppressed patients, 116, *117–118*
    management, 141–142, *142–143*
Mucosa
    combined microscopic and endoscopic surgery
        frontal sinusotomy, 192, *193*
        scarring effects, 164–166, *165*
    nasal cavity innervation, 25, *29*

Mucosal inflammation, sinus disease and allergy and, 103–104
Mucosal vasoconstriction, combined microscopic and
     endoscopic surgery, 179, *179*
Mucous retention cyst, imaging studies, 77, *77*
Mycetoma, imaging studies, *76*, 77
Mycotic rhinosinusitis, immunosuppressed patients, 116
Myospherulosis, as surgical complication, 275

Nasal associated local immune tissue (NALT), paranasal sinus
     physiology, immune defense, 61
Nasal capsule, developmental anatomy, *5*, 5–6
Nasal cavity
    developmental anatomy, 5
    endoscopic view, 51, *51*
    macroscopic anatomy, 12–21
        ethmoid bulla, 21
        floor, 14
        frontal recess, 20–21
        hiatus semilunaris, 19
        lateral wall, 15, *15*, 17
        medial wall, 13, *14*
        roof, *12*, 12–13
        uncinate process, 17, 19, *20*
        vasculature, innervation, and lymphatic drainage, 23–27,
             23–27
Nasal endoscopy
    equipment, 50–51
    rhinosinusitis diagnosis, 92–99, *93–98*
    sinonasal anatomical variations, 50, *50*
    surgical technique, 50–55, *52*
Nasal masses, imaging studies, 85–86, *85–86*
Nasal pits, developmental anatomy, 3
Nasal polyps
    headache and, 138–139
    laser surgery, 243–244, *244*
    Nd:YAG laser surgery
        indications, 249–250
        results, *253*, 253–254
Nasal septum
    bony and cartilaginous segment, 13, *15*
    endoscopic surgery, 151
    endoscopic view, 51–52, *52*
    headache and, 139–140, *140*
    sensory innervation, 23–27, *27*
    vasculature, 22–24, *25*
Nasal valve, macroscopic anatomy, 12, *12*
Nasal wall
    developmental anatomy, 6–7, *6–7*
    endonasal surgery preconditions, complication avoidance,
         276, 276–277
    maxillary sinus anatomy, 31–33, *32–34*, 35
    nasal cavity
        lateral wall, 15, *15*, 17
        medial wall, 14, *14*
Nasofrontal duct, endoscopic surgery, frontal sinus, 231
Nasolacrimal duct. *See also* Lacrimal duct/sac
    combined microscopic and endoscopic surgery, 168
    maxillary sinus anatomy, 31
Nasopalatine nerve, nasal cavity innervation, 23, *27–28*
Nasopharynx
    endoscopic view, rhinosinusitis diagnosis, 92–99, *93–98*

pathology, Nd:YAG laser surgery, 254–255
Navigational instrumentation
    allergic fungal sinusitis surgery, 144
    Stryker Navigation System, 230
Neodymium:yttrium-aluminum-garnet (Nd:YAG) laser
    nasal and sinus surgery
        anterior nasal polyposis, 249–250, *251*, 253–254
        biophysics, 245–246
        carbon dioxide laser comparisons, 246
        choanal atresia, 251–252, 254
        clinical considerations, 248–249
        complications, 252–253
        endoscope specifications, 247–248
        equipment, 247
        eustachian tube pathology, 252
        fiber characteristics, 247
        historical background, 241
        hypertrophic rhinitis, 249, 253
        imaging techniques, 248
        light source, 248
        limitations and contraindications, 248
        nasopharyngeal pathology, 254–255
        pathological applications, 245
        posterior nasopharyngeal wall, 252
        preoperative preparation, 246–247
        recurrent epistaxis, 250–251, *251*, 254
        results evaluation, 253–255
        synechiae, 251, *251*, 254
        techniques, 248–249
        therapeutic indications, 247
        tissue interaction, 246
    vascular disorders, 243
Nervous system anatomy
    maxillary sinus, 27, *28*, 29, 31–33, *31–34*, 35
    naval cavity, 23–25, 27, *27–29*
    paranasal sinus, 27, *29*, 50–51
    sphenoid sinus, 50
Neural reflexes, asthma and, 108
Neutropenia, immunosuppressed patients, 116
Neutrophils, paranasal sinus physiology, immune defense, 61
Nose, developmental anatomy, 1–6, *2–5*
Nuclear medicine, functional endoscopic surgery, 68
Numerical aperture, combined microscopic and endoscopic
     surgery, 173

Objective abnormalities, frontal sinus, endoscopic surgery,
     236–237, *237*
Ocular characteristics, allergic fungal sinusitis diagnosis,
     296
Odontogenic pathology, imaging studies, 83–84, *83–84*
Olfactometry, combined microscopic and endoscopic surgery,
     preoperative assessment, 170
Olfactory bulb, nasal cavity innervation, 25, *27*
Olfactory cleft, macroscopic anatomy, 12
One-stage integrated nose/paranasal sinus treatment,
     combined microscopic and endoscopic surgery, *163*,
     163–166
Onodi cell
    ethmoid sinus anatomy, 38–39, 42–43
    sphenoid sinus anatomy, 46–47, *48*
        endoscopic surgery, 154–155, *155*

Operating room requirements
  BrainLab's VectorVision, 226–227
  Medtronic Xomed LandmarX system, 223
  Nd:YAG laser surgery, 248
  VTI InstaTrak, 222
Operative complications, imaging studies, 87, *87–88*
Ophthalmic artery, nasal cavity vascular anatomy, 23–24, *24*
Ophthalmic nerve, nasal cavity anatomy, 23, *26*
Ophthalmological complications, endoscopic sinus surgery, 285–289, *286–288*
Optical digitizers, Kolibri ENT system, 227–228
Optical performance requirements, combined microscopic and endoscopic surgery, 173–175, *173–175*
Optical principles, combined microscopic and endoscopic surgery, 172–173
Optic nerve, sphenoid sinus anatomy, 50
Oral decongestants, allergic rhinitis management, 101–102
Orbital air cell, ethmoid variants, computed tomographic imaging, 71, *71*
Orbital bones
  maxillary sinus anatomy, 32–33, *33*, 35
  paranasal sinus anatomy, 27, 29, *30*
Orbital complications
  endoscopic orbital decompression
    classification, *307*
    research overview, 306
    surgical technique, 307–310, *307–310*
  imaging studies, 79–80
  immunosuppressed patients, rhinosinusitis, 118–119
  intraconal injuries, 270–271
  pediatric rhinosinusitis, 127
Ostiomeatal complex
  combined microscopic and endoscopic surgery, 165–166
  computed tomographic imaging, 64, *64–66*, 66
    septal variants, 70, *70*
  endoscopic view, rhinosinusitis diagnosis, 92–99, *93–98*
  headache diagnosis, *135*, 135–136, *139*, 139–140
  macroscopic anatomy, 17, *18*
  normal anatomy, 68–70, *69–70*
Osteomyelitis
  imaging studies, 80, *80–82*, 83
  pediatric rhinosinusitis, 127
Osteoplastic flap surgery, frontal sinus, 266–267, *266–267*
Ostial obstruction
  pediatric rhinosinusitis, abnormalities, 123
  sinus disease and allergy and, 103–104
Ostium
  combined microscopic and endoscopic surgery, maxillary antrostomy, 182–185, *185–187*
  paranasal sinus physiology, ventilatory function, *58*, 58–59
Outpatient nursing care, endoscopic sinus surgery, 325–330
  outpatient care, 330
  perioperative care, 328
  postoperative period, 328–330
  preoperative evaluation, 325
  preoperative teaching, 325–328, *326–327*
Oxycel cotton, endoscopic sinus surgery, 160–161
Oxygen absorption, paranasal sinus physiology, 59–60

Oxymetazoline
  endonasal endoscopy, *150*, 150–151
  minimally invasive endoscopic sinus surgery, 209

Pain localization, headache, 133, *134*
Palatal shelves, developmental anatomy, *4*, 5
Papilloma virus, Nd:YAG laser surgery, 252–253
Paranasal sinus
  bony anatomy, *9*
  combined microscopic and endoscopic surgery
    general principles, 163–166
    indications for, *166*, 166–168
  developmental anatomy, 1–12
    ethmoid sinus, 7–9, *8–10*
    frontal sinus, 10–11, *11*
    maxillary sinus, 7, *7*
    nose development, 1–6, *2–5*
    sinus development, *6*, 6–7
    sphenoid sinus, 11–12, *11–12*
  endoscopic anatomy, *50–54*, 50–55
    nasal endoscopy, 50–55, *51–54*
  fungal manifestations in, 290, *291*
  imaging studies
    anatomical variations, 70
    computed tomography, 64–67, *64–67*
    dental implants, 84–85, *85*
    ethmoid variants, 71, *71*
    inflammatory/infectious disease, 72–77
      acute sinusitis, 72
      chronic sinusitis, 72–75, *73–75*
      fungal sinusitis, 75, *76*, 77
      granulomatous sinusitis, *76*, 77
    inflammatory polyps, 78, *78*
    intraoperative computer-assisted guidance, 88
    magnetic resonance imaging, 67–68
    middle turbinate variants, 70, *70–71*
    mucocele, 77, *78*
    mucous retention cyst, 77, *77*
    nasal masses, 85–86, *85–86*
    normal anatomy, *68–69*, 68–70
    nuclear medicine, 68
    odontogenic/bone pathology, 83–84, *84–85*
    orbital complications, 79–80
    osteomyelitis, 80, *81–82*, 83
    postoperative assessment, 86–87
    septal variants, 70, *70*
    sphenoid variants, 71, *72*
    surgical complications, 87, *87–88*
    ultrasound, 68
    uncinate variants, 70–71, *71*
  macroscopic anatomy
    agger nasi, 21
    bony structures, 27, 29–33, *29–33*, 35
    inferior turbinate, 21–22, *22*
    lateral sinus, 21
    nasal cavity, 12–21
      ethmoid bulla, 21
      floor, 13
      frontal recess, 21
      hiatus semilunaris, 19

lateral wall, 15, *15*, 17
medial wall, 13, *14*
roof, 12–13
uncinate process, 17, 19, *20*
vasculature, innervation, and lymphatic drainage,
23–27, *23–27*
physiology
evolutionary theory, 57–58
functional theory, 58
immune defense, 60–62, *62*
mucociliary clearance, 59–60
structural theory, 57–58
ventilatory function, *58*, 58–59
surgical complications, frontal sinusitis, 275–276
vasculature, innervation, and lymphatic drainage, 49–50
Patient characteristics, allergic fungal sinusitis, *295*, 295–296
Patient education, outpatient endoscopic sinus surgery,
325–328, *326–327*
Patient positioning, combined microscopic and endoscopic
surgery, 176–177, *176–177*
Pediatric patients
allergic fungal sinusitis, steroid therapy, 144–145
combined microscopic and endoscopic surgery, 164–166
Nd:YAG laser surgery contraindications, 248
rhinosinusitis
antimicrobial therapy, 125
complications, 127–129
intracranial, 128–129
intrasinus/local, 127–128
lower respiratory tract, 129
periorbital, 128
definition and clinical presentation, 121–122
developmental anatomy, 122
differential diagnosis, 122
imaging studies, 124
medical therapy, 124–125
microbiology, 124
pathogenesis and predisposing factors, 122–123
patient history, 123
physical examination, 123–124
steroids, 125
surgical management
acute rhinosinusitis, 126
chronic rhinosinusitis, 126–127
Perioperative care, outpatient endoscopic sinus surgery, 328
Periorbital complications, pediatric rhinosinusitis, 127
Periorbital incisions, endoscopic orbital decompression, *309*,
309–310
Peroxidase, paranasal sinus physiology, immune defense, 61
Pharyngeal mucosa, asthma and sinusitis and, 109
Plasma cells, paranasal sinus physiology, immune defense, 61
Platform requirements, Stryker Navigation System, 228, *229*
Plethysmography, mucociliary clearance assessment, 60
Pneumatization
frontal sinus development, 10–11
paranasal sinus development, 8
sphenoid sinus anatomy, 50
variants, 71, *72*
sphenoid sinus development, 12
Postanesthesia recovery unit (PACU), sinus surgery, 320

Posterior nasopharyngeal wall, Nd:YAG laser surgery, 252, *252*
Posterior Wigand approach, endoscopic sinus surgery,
155–156
Posterosuperior fontanelle, maxillary sinus anatomy, 31
Postoperative care
anesthesia management and, 319–320
combined microscopic and endoscopic surgery, 166
basic guidelines, 197–198, *198*
dacryocystorhinostomy, 314
endoscopic sinus surgery, 322–324, *323*
imaging, basic principles, *86*, 86–87
laser surgery, 244
minimally invasive endoscopic sinus surgery, 217–218
outpatient endoscopic sinus surgery, 328–330, *329–330*
pediatric rhinosinusitis, 126
revision endoscopic sinus surgery assessment, 260–262,
261
Powered instrumentation, minimally invasive endoscopic
sinus surgery
agger nasi to frontal sinus, 213, *216*
anesthesia, 209
anterior ethmoid sinus, 214
cocaine administration, 209
cutter characteristics and positioning, 207–208
ethmoid bulla, 213–214, *216*
frontal sinus locations, 213, *216*
hiatus semilunaris posterior, 214, 216, *217*
historical background, 207–208
injection techniques, 209–210
micro-debrider tool development, 208–209
middle turbinate, 211–212, *211–212*
oxymetazoline administration, 209
posterior ethmoid sinus, 216
postoperative care, 218–219
sphenoid sinus, 217–218
techniques, *210*, 210–211
uncinate/maxillary ostium, 212–213, *214–215*
Preoperative assessment
allergic fungal sinusitis, 144
combined microscopic and endoscopic surgery, 169–170,
170
frontal sinus, endoscopic surgery, 236
Nd:YAG laser surgery, 246–247
outpatient endoscopic sinus surgery, 325–328, *326–327*
Pressure system, Micro-Debrider tool, 208
Proetz displacement method, Nd:YAG laser surgery, 250
Prostaglandin D_2 (PGD_2), asthma mechanisms, 108–109
Pterygoid plates, sphenoid sinus anatomy, 47, 49
Pterygopalatine fossa, maxillary sinus anatomy, 32–33, *32–34*
Pulmonary disease, anesthesia for sinus surgery and, 320

Quartz fiber, Nd:YAG laser surgery, 247

Radiofrequency (RF) turbinate reduction, inferior turbinate,
157–158, *157–158*
Radiology requirements
BrainLab's VectorVision, *226*, 226
Medtronic Xomed LandmarX system, 222–223
Stryker Navigation System, 228
VTI InstaTrak, 221–222

Recirculation problems, revision endoscopic surgery, maxillary sinus, 263–264, *264*

Registration process
Medtronic Xomed LandmarX system, 223
Stryker Navigation System, 229, *230*

Renal dysfunction, computed tomographic imaging, contraindications for contrast procedures, 66

Rendu-Osler-Weber syndrome
laser surgery, 243
Nd:YAG laser surgery, 250, *251*

Resolution, combined microscopic and endoscopic surgery, 175

Results evaluation
combined microscopic and endoscopic surgery, *200–202,* 200–203
dacryocystorhinostomy, 314–315
endoscopic orbital decompression, 310–311
frontal sinus, endoscopic surgery, 239, *239*
rhinosinusitis surgical management, 259

Retrobulbar postseptal hematoma, etiology and management, 271–272, *272*

Revision endoscopic sinus surgery
ethmoid revision, 264, *264*
frontal sinus, 266–267, *266–267*
maxillary sinus, 263–264, *264*
medical and surgical failures, 262–263
research overview, 260–262, *261*
sphenoid sinus, 265, *265–266*

Rhinomanometry
combined microscopic and endoscopic surgery, preoperative evaluation, 170
rhinosinusitis diagnosis, 95

Rhinopathic headache, combined microscopic and endoscopic surgery, 168

Rhinoplasty, combined microscopic and endoscopic surgery, *179,* 179–180

Rhinosinusitis
allergy and asthma (*See* Allergic rhinitis; Asthma)
diagnosis and management, *91–98,* 91–99
epidemiology, 90–91
etiology, 98, *98*
headache and, 132–140, *132–140*
HIV infection
clinical signs and symptoms, 115–119, *116–118*
epidemiology, *114,* 114–115
treatment, 119
immunocompromised hosts, general epidemiology, 113, *114*
pediatric patients
antimicrobial therapy, 125
complications, 127–129
intracranial, 128–129
intrasinus/local, 127–128
lower respiratory tract, 129
periorbital, 128
definition and clinical presentation, 121–122
developmental anatomy, 122
differential diagnosis, 122
imaging studies, 124
medical therapy, 124–125
microbiology, 124
pathogenesis and predisposing factors, 122–123
patient history, 123
physical examination, 123–124
steroids, 125
surgical management
acute rhinosinusitis, 126
chronic rhinosinusitis, 126–127
surgical management
Gliklich and Metson system, 257–258
Lund and McKay system, 258–259
results evaluation, 259
staging systems, 256–257

Rosenmüller's fossa, endoscopic view, 51–52, *52*

Safety issues, laser surgery, 242

Saprophytic fungal growth
allergic fungal sinusitis, 142
EMRS non-AFS patients, 293

Sarcoidosis, fungal sinusitis, imaging studies, *76, 77*

Scar formation
combined microscopic and endoscopic surgery, 164–166, *166*
laser surgery, 244

Self-irrigation system, Micro-Debrider tool, 208

Septal mucoperichondrial flaps, cerebrospinal fluid leak management, 303–304

Septal variants, computed tomographic imaging, 70, *70*

Septoplasty, combined microscopic and endoscopic surgery, *179,* 179–180

Single photon emission computed tomography (SPECT), osteomyelitis, 80, *81–82,* 83

Sinonasal gaseous exchange, paranasal sinus physiology, *58,* 58–59

Sinonasal polyposis, combined microscopic and endoscopic surgery, 168

Sinus disease, allergy and, 103–105

Sinusitis. *See* Asthma; specific sinusitis, e.g. Acute sinusitis

Skin testing
allergic fungal sinusitis, 106–107
allergic rhinitis diagnosis, 101

Somnoplasty reduction, inferior turbinate, 157–158, *158*

Sphenoethmoid cell
ethmoid sinus anatomy, 39, 41–43
sphenoid sinus anatomy, 46–47, *48*

Sphenoethmoid recess (SER)
headache diagnosis, 135
normal anatomy, 68–70, *69–70*

Sphenoid bone
frontal sinus anatomy, 45–46, *46*
maxillary sinus anatomy, 32
sphenoid sinus anatomy, 46–47, *48–50,* 49–50

Sphenoidotomy, combined microscopic and endoscopic surgery, 192–195, *193–195*

Sphenoid sinus
computed tomographic imaging, 70
variants, 71, *72*
developmental anatomy, *11,* 11–12
endoscopic surgery, 154–155, *155*
headache and, 132–133, *134*

minimally invasive endoscopic sinus surgery, 216–217
operative complications, imaging studies, 87, *88*
revision endoscopic surgery
    assessment, 262
    techniques, *265*, 265–266
surgical anatomy, 46–47, *48*, 49–50, *49–50*
surgical strategies involving, 280–281, *280–281*
vasculature and innervation, 49–50
Sphenopalatine artery, nasal cavity vascular anatomy, 22–23, *24*
Staging systems
allergic fungal sinusitis diagnosis, 296–297, *296–297*
rhinosinusitis surgical management, 256–257
    Gliklich and Metson system, 257–258
    Lund and McKay system, 258–259
    results evaluation, 259
Standardization, combined microscopic and endoscopic
        surgery, 199–200
Stereotactic surgery
BrainLAB's VectorVision and Kolibri ENT, 224–228, *225–228*
historical background, 219
Medtronic Xomed LandmarX
    basic components, 222–224, *223–224*
    triplanar screen image, 219, *220*
Stryker Navigation System, 228–230, *229–230*
VTI InstaTrak, 219–222
Steroids
allergic fungal sinusitis
    histopathology, 292
    management with, 144–145
nasal sprays
    allergic fungal sinusitis, 107
    allergic rhinitis management, 102, *102*
    sinus disease and allergy and, 104–105
pediatric rhinosinusitis, 124
Stopcock system, Micro-Debrider tool, 208
Structural theory, paranasal sinus physiology, 57
Stryker Navigation System, stereotactic surgery, 228–230
Subperiosteal abscess, pediatric rhinosinusitis complications,
        127
Substance abuse, rhinosinusitis and, 91–92
Substance P, headache pain and, 136, *136*
Suction apparatus, Micro-Debrider tool, 208
Superior ophththalmic vein (SOV), orbital complications
        involving, imaging studies, *79*, 79–80
SurfaceMerge algorithm, Medtronic Xomed LandmarX
        system, 223
Surgical management
allergic fungal sinusitis, 107, 144
asthma and sinusitis, 109–110
avoidance of complications and, 278–282
dacryocystorhinostomy, 313–314, *313–314*
Medtronic Xomed LandmarX system, 223–224, *224*
pediatric rhinosinusitis, 125–126
Swimming, rhinosinusitis, 91
Synechiae, Nd:YAG laser surgery
indications, 251, *251*
results, 254

Technetium imaging, osteomyelitis, 80
Tension headaches, epidemiology, 138

Tissue interactions, Nd:YAG laser, 245–246
Tissue trap, Micro-Debrider tool, 208
T lymphocytes
allergic rhinitis etiology/pathogenesis, 100–101
paranasal sinus physiology, immune defense, 61
rhinosinusitis, HIV infection, 115
sinus disease and allergy and, 104
"True" sinus, frontal sinus development, 11
Turbinates. *See also* Inferior turbinates; Middle turbinates
computed tomographic imaging, 69–70
    middle turbinate variants, 70, *70–71*
developmental anatomy, 6–7
endonasal laser surgery, 242–243
endoscopic sinus surgery, 157–159
    inferior, 157–158, *157–158*
    middle turbinate, *158*, 158–159
    superior turbinates, 159
endoscopic view, 51–52, *52–54*, 54–55
    rhinosinusitis diagnosis, 92–99, *93–98*
headache diagnosis, *135–136*, 135–140
macroscopic anatomy, 15, *15–19*, 17
    inferior turbinate, 21–22, *22*
minimally invasive endoscopic sinus surgery, Micro-
        Debrider techniques, 210–212, *210–212*

Ulcerations, headache and, 133, 135, *135*
Ultrasound imaging, functional endoscopic surgery, 68
Uncinate process
combined microscopic and endoscopic surgery, 166, 168
computed tomographic imaging, variants, 70–71, *71*
developmental anatomy, 8–10
endoscopic orbital decompression, 307, *307*
endoscopic sinus surgery, 152–153, *153*
endoscopic surgery, frontal sinus, 232, *233i*
ethmoid sinus anatomy, 37–38
headache diagnosis, 135, *136*
macroscopic anatomy, 17, 19, *19*
minimally invasive endoscopic sinus surgery, 212–213,
        214–215
surgical strategies involving, 278–282, *279*
Uncinate system, anatomy, 39–43, *41*
Uncinectomy, combined microscopic and endoscopic surgery,
        181, *182–184*
Upper respiratory tract infection (URI), pediatric patients
antimicrobial therapy, 125
complications, 127–129
    intracranial, 128–129
    intrasinus/local, 127–128
    lower respiratory tract, 129
    periorbital, 128
definition and clinical presentation, 121–122
developmental anatomy, 122
differential diagnosis, 122
imaging studies, 124
medical therapy, 124–125
microbiology, 124
pathogenesis and predisposing factors, 122–123
patient history, 123
physical examination, 123–124
steroids, 125

Upper respiratory tract infection (URI), pediatric patients
  (Continued)
  surgical management
    acute rhinosinusitis, 126
    chronic rhinosinusitis, 126–127

Vascular disorders, laser surgery, 243
Vasculature
  naval cavity, 22–27, *23–25*
  paranasal sinus, 25, 29, *30,* 50–51
  sphenoid sinus anatomy, 50
Vasoconstriction, nasal cavity innervation, 25, *28–29*
Venous drainage, nasal cavity vasculature, 22–23
Ventilatory function, paranasal sinus physiology, *58,* 58–59
Video system positioning, minimally invasive endoscopic sinus
    surgery, 211
Viral disease, rhinosinusitis, 91–99
  HIV patients, 115–116

VTI InstaTrak, stereotactic surgery, 219–222
VTI intraoperative imaging equipement, endoscopic sinus
    surgery, 159–160, *159–160*

Walsh-Ogura procedure, endoscopic orbital decompression,
    306
Wegener's granulomatosis, imaging studies, *76,* 77
Wigand approach, endoscopic sinus surgery, 155–156
Wrist/arm positioning, minimally invasive endoscopic sinus
    surgery, 211

Xomed XPS microshaver, endoscopic surgery, 151–152, *152*

Zeiss operating microscope, combined microscopic and
    endoscopic surgery, *171,* 171–172
Z-touch laser registration, BrainLab's VectorVision, *225,*
    225–226
Zygomatic bone, maxillary sinus anatomy, 32